I0065793

Recent Progress in Osteoarthritis

Recent Progress in Osteoarthritis

Edited by Willard Leopold

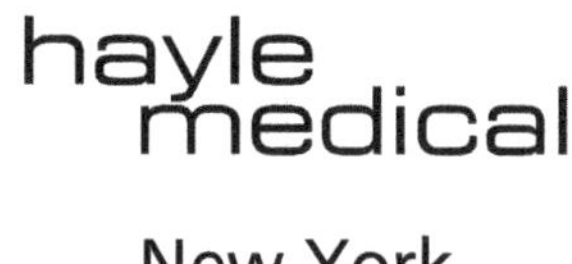

New York

Hayle Medical,
750 Third Avenue, 9th Floor,
New York, NY 10017, USA

Visit us on the World Wide Web at:
www.haylemedical.com

ISBN: 978-1-63241-721-3

Cataloging-in-Publication Data

Recent progress in osteoarthritis / edited by Willard Leopold.
p. cm.
Includes bibliographical references and index.
ISBN 978-1-63241-721-3
1. Osteoarthritis. 2. Osteoarthritis--Diagnosis. 3. Osteoarthritis--Treatment.
I. Leopold, Willard.
RC931.O67 R43 2019
616.722 3--dc23

Table of Contents

Preface

This book was inspired by the evolution of our times; to answer the curiosity of inquisitive minds. Many developments have occurred across the globe in the recent past which has transformed the progress in the field.

Osteoarthritis is a joint disease, which is caused by a breakdown of the joint cartilage and underlying bone. It mainly affects the joints of the lower back, hips, neck, base of the thumbs, and the ones which are near the ends of the fingers. In osteoarthritis, the joints on one side of the body are usually more affected than the ones on the other side. Its symptoms include joint pain, swelling and stiffness. It is generally caused due to mechanical stress on the joints and low grade inflammatory processes. Medications, including, naproxen and ibuprofen are quite effective in reducing the pain caused due to osteoarthritis. Other treatment methods include physical therapy, joint injections and joint replacement therapy. This book includes some of the vital pieces of work being conducted across the world, on various topics related to osteoarthritis. It consists of contributions made by international experts. This book, with its detailed analyses and data, will prove immensely beneficial to practicing doctors and medical students.

This book was developed from a mere concept to drafts to chapters and finally compiled together as a complete text to benefit the readers across all nations. To ensure the quality of the content we instilled two significant steps in our procedure. The first was to appoint an editorial team that would verify the data and statistics provided in the book and also select the most appropriate and valuable contributions from the plentiful contributions we received from authors worldwide. The next step was to appoint an expert of the topic as the Editor-in-Chief, who would head the project and finally make the necessary amendments and modifications to make the text reader-friendly. I was then commissioned to examine all the material to present the topics in the most comprehensible and productive format.

I would like to take this opportunity to thank all the contributing authors who were supportive enough to contribute their time and knowledge to this project. I also wish to convey my regards to my family who have been extremely supportive during the entire project.

Editor

Evoked Temporal Summation in Cats to Highlight Central Sensitization Related to Osteoarthritis-Associated Chronic Pain

Martin Guillot[1,2], Polly M. Taylor[3], Pascale Rialland[1,2], Mary P. Klinck[1,2], Johanne Martel-Pelletier[2], Jean-Pierre Pelletier[2], Eric Troncy[1,2*]

1 Groupe de Recherche en Pharmacologie Animale du Québec (GREPAQ), Department of Biomedical Sciences, Faculty of Veterinary Medicine – Université de Montréal, Saint-Hyacinthe, Quebec, Canada, **2** Osteoarthritis Research Unit, Université de Montréal Hospital Centre, Notre-Dame Hospital, Montreal, Quebec, Canada, **3** Topcat Metrology, Gravel Head Farm, Downham Common, Little Downham, Nr Ely, Cambridgeshire, United Kingdom

Abstract

In cats, osteoarthritis causes significant chronic pain. Chronicity of pain is associated with changes in the central nervous system related to central sensitization, which have to be quantified. Our objectives were 1) to develop a quantitative sensory testing device in cats for applying repetitive mechanical stimuli that would evoke temporal summation; 2) to determine the sensitivity of this test to osteoarthritis-associated pain, and 3) to examine the possible correlation between the quantitative sensory testing and assessment using other pain evaluation methods. We hypothesized that mechanical sub-threshold repetitive stimuli would evoke temporal summation, and that cats with osteoarthritis would show a faster response. A blinded longitudinal study was performed in 4 non-osteoarthritis cats and 10 cats with naturally occurring osteoarthritis. Quantification of chronic osteoarthritis pain-related disability was performed over a two week period using peak vertical force kinetic measurement, motor activity intensity assessment and von Frey anesthesiometer-induced paw withdrawal threshold testing. The cats afflicted with osteoarthritis demonstrated characteristic findings consistent with osteoarthritis-associated chronic pain. After a 14-day acclimation period, repetitive mechanical sub-threshold stimuli were applied using a purpose-developed device. Four stimulation profiles of predetermined intensity, duration and time interval were applied randomly four times during a four-day period. The stimulation profiles were different ($P<0.001$): the higher the intensity of the stimulus, the sooner it produced a consistent painful response. The cats afflicted with osteoarthritis responded more rapidly than cats osteoarthritis free ($P=0.019$). There was a positive correlation between the von Frey anesthesiometer-induced paw withdrawal threshold and the response to stimulation profiles #2 (2N/0.4 Hz) and #4 (2N/0.4 Hz): $Rho_s=0.64$ ($P=0.01$) and 0.63 ($P=0.02$) respectively. This study is the first report of mechanical temporal summation in awake cats. Our results suggest that central sensitization develops in cats with naturally occurring osteoarthritis, providing an opportunity to improve translational research in osteoarthritis-associated chronic pain.

Editor: Sam Eldabe, The James Cook University Hospital, United Kingdom

Funding: This study was supported in part by a Pilot Study grant from the Quebec Bio-Imaging Network (#5886) of the Fonds de recherche du Québec – Santé (Pr. Eric Troncy), by a Discovery grant (#327158-2008, #441651-2013, supporting salaries) and a Collaborative Research and Development grant (#RDCPJ 418399-11, supporting operations and salaries) in partnership with ArthroLab, Inc. from the Natural Sciences and Engineering Research Council (NSERC) of Canada (Pr. Eric Troncy), as well as an ongoing New Opportunities Fund grant (#9483) and a Leader Opportunity Fund grant (#24601), supporting pain/function equipment from the Canada Foundation for Innovation (Pr. Eric Troncy). The funding sources were not involved in the study design, collection, analysis and interpretation of data, writing of the manuscript, nor in the decision to submit the manuscript for publication. Dr. Martin Guillot was the recipient of an Alexander Graham Bell NSERC Canada Graduate Scholarship for doctorate research, and a Doctoral Scholarship from the Canadian Institutes of Health Research – MENTOR Strategic Training Initiative in Health Research Program. Dr. Pascale Rialland received a doctoral Industrial Innovation Scholarship from a partnership including NSERC of Canada (#406726), Fonds de recherche du Québec – Nature et Technologies (#144812) and ArthroLab, Inc. Dr. Mary Klinck was the recipient of a Zoetis – Morris Animal Foundation (#D10-901) doctoral scholarship. The funders had no role in study design, data collection and analysis, decision to publish, or preparation of the manuscript.

Competing Interests: The authors have the following interests. This study was partly supported by a Collaborative Research and Development grant (#RDCPJ 418399-11, supporting operations and salaries) in partnership with ArthroLab Inc from the Natural Sciences and Engineering Research Council (NSERC) of Canada. Dr. Pascale Rialland received a doctoral Industrial Innovation Scholarship from a partnership including NSERC of Canada, Fonds de recherche du Québec – Nature et Technologies and ArthroLab, Inc. Polly M. Taylor is a director of Topcat Metrology, Ltd. There are no patents, products in development or marketed products to declare. This does not alter the authors' adherence to all the PLOS ONE policies on sharing data and materials, as detailed online in the guide for authors.

* E-mail: eric.troncy@umontreal.ca

Introduction

Feline osteoarthritis (OA) develops with ageing in diarthrodial joints, predominantly the elbow, coxofemoral and stifle joints, and causes chronic pain [1–4]. Assessment of chronic pain in animals with OA takes into account the impact of pain on both physical ability and quality of life. Owners of cats with OA observe a number of altered behaviour patterns such as decreased daily activity and a reluctance to jump or to walk up stairs [5–8]. Objective functional methods have also been developed to evaluate OA-associated disability in cats. The peak vertical ground reaction force (PVF) quantifies limb impairment that may be related to decreased use because of pain [9–11]. In addition, accelerometer-based motor activity (MA) assessment enables objective quantification of the impairment of normal function related to OA-associated chronic pain [10,12,13].

Central sensitization is expressed as pain hypersensitivity, particularly dynamic tactile allodynia, secondary punctate hyperalgesia, aftersensations, and enhanced temporal summation (TS) [14] and is present in OA [15,16]. Quantitative sensory testing (QST) is used to characterize these abnormal sensations [17]. Until recently, little attention had been paid to detailed assessment of sensory abnormalities in animals. Neurology texts describe the gross assessment of sensory function (*e.g.*, the response to pinching skin in various dermatomes) [18] and pain management texts refer to the theory of altered sensory processing (peripheral and central sensitization) associated with acute injury or chronic disease [18]. Most information on QST is based on rodent models and the human literature; in particular regarding the (mechanical) pressure pain threshold in painful OA [19,20]. Several studies in humans suggest that QST to detect mechanical allodynia and hyperalgesia should be an integral part of the assessment of OA-associated chronic pain [15,19–23]. Quantitative ST using von Frey anesthesiometer-induced paw withdrawal threshold (vFWT) in dogs [22] and cats [10] with natural OA represents one of the first attempts to evaluate the changes in central processing in companion animals suffering chronic pain.

Low frequency repetition of a fixed-intensity stimulus increases the action potential discharge of dorsal horn neurons followed by after discharges; this activity-dependent facilitation is called spinal windup [24]. The early phase of windup is denoted as TS, and has been widely used to investigate spinal cord excitability [14,25]. Windup is considered to be an intrinsic part of the early plastic changes in the central nervous system leading to chronicity, hence TS is an ideal target for studying chronic pain [14].

Our objectives were 1) to develop a QST device in cats for applying repetitive mechanical stimuli that would evoke TS; 2) to determine the sensitivity to OA pain (discriminatory ability) of a number of stimulation profiles, and 3) to examine the correlation between the repetitive stimuli QST responses and assessment using other objective chronic pain evaluation methods (PVF, MA monitoring, and vFWT).

We hypothesized that mechanical sub-threshold repetitive stimuli QST with a controlled profile would evoke TS, and that cats with OA would show an enhanced response.

This study aimed to provide insight about central sensitization in cats with naturally occurring OA. Using an innovative QST technique, this study results suggest that central sensitization is a feature of feline OA-associated chronic pain.

Methods

Ethics statement

The Institutional Animal Care and Use Committee (*Comité d'Éthique et d'utilisation des Animaux* (CÉUA) of *Université de Montréal*) approved the study protocol (# Rech-1482), and the Canadian Council on Animal Care guidelines were followed for all cat care and procedures undertaken. Furthermore, this study adhered to the guidelines of the Committee for Research Ethical Issues of the IASP [26], and the ARRIVE guidelines for reporting animal research [27].

Animals and experimental design

This study used 4 normal healthy, non-OA cats (one neutered female, and three neutered males), and 10 cats with naturally occurring OA (5 neutered females, and 5 neutered males) belonging to the colony of a contract research organization (ArthroLab, Inc., Montreal, QC, Canada) accredited by the Canadian Council on Animal Care. The cats were housed together in a dedicated room (floor area approximately 8×12 m). The room's environment and the cats' health were monitored and recorded daily. The cats were fed a standard certified commercial cat food (Hill's Prescription Diet w/d Feline, Hill's Pet Nutrition, Inc., Mississauga, ON, Canada) once daily in the afternoon according to the food manufacturer's recommendations. Water was supplied *ad libitum*. The cats were loose-housed, with free access to toys, raised platforms, and a large window. Beds in a quiet area were also freely accessible.

No abnormalities were detected upon neurologic evaluation, complete blood count, blood biochemical profile (including T4), and urine analysis; nor were there any limb deformities or signs of acute musculoskeletal disease. All cats were free from both feline immunodeficiency and leukemia viruses. The extent of radiographic OA was graded by a veterinary radiologist as previously described [9–11,28], using computed radiographs of the stifle, coxofemoral, carpal and tarsal joints (mediolateral and caudocranial projections), and of the shoulders and elbows joints (mediolateral projections). These radiographs were performed under sedation using medetomidine (0.02 mg/kg; Domitor 1 mg/mL, Zoetis Canada, Kirkland, QC, Canada) and morphine (0.1–0.2 mg/kg; Morphine Sulfate Injection 10 mg/mL, Sandoz, Boucherville, QC, Canada), administered intramuscularly.

On the first day of this longitudinal study, a certified veterinary behaviourist, blinded to the radiographic grade and age of the cats, performed a behavioural examination. This examination aimed to detect changes in gait, posture, and the presence of subjective joint pain. Cats designated "non-OA" had no abnormalities detected during this examination, and selected "OA cats" were considered subjectively to be in pain (refer to Table 1).

The cats were acclimated and trained for one week only immediately prior to the study, as they already had six months experience with all the procedures except repetitive stimuli QST. Chronic OA pain-related disability was quantified over a two-week period using functional methods that consisted of PVF measurement and MA intensity assessment. During the same period, objective chronic pain evaluation was undertaken using mechanical QST with vFWT testing to assess secondary punctate tactile allodynia [10]. Finally, several repeated mechanical stimuli QST protocols were tested after a further 14-day acclimation period. This comprised positive reinforcement for progressive habituation to the evaluation environment: being in the evaluation cage, wearing the stimulation device, and being stimulated by the device.

Measurement of PVF

The cats' PVF were recorded twice, a week apart. Measurements were performed within 60 sec of approximately 3 minutes of stair exercise. This consisted of running up and down, and again up a 10 m long staircase; this acquisition protocol decreases data variability and optimizes effect sizes [11]. Post-exercise PVF were acquired using a floor mat-based plantar force measurement system (Walkway System WE4, Tekscan Inc., Boston, MA) while the cats trotted across the walkway at a comfortable speed (0.8–1.4 m/sec). Speed was computed by the software, using length and duration of a given stride. Equilibration and calibration of the system were performed prior to each acquisition session, as previously described [9–11]. A maximum of 3 valid trials (with the cat moving across the entire mattress undisturbed, consistently, in a straight line, and at the correct speed) were obtained for each

Table 1. Age, body weight, radiographic and clinical features of the selected cats.

Features		Non-OA cats	OA cats
Mean age (range; year)		**3.4 (1.5–4.5)**	**9.3 (7.0–12.0)**
Mean body weight (range; kg)		5.1 (3.5–7.1)	4.8 (3.1–6.2)
Median radiographic scores (range)	Forelimbs	0 (0–0)	2 (0–4)
	Hind limbs	0 (0–0)	2 (0–9)
Median radiographic OA-affected joint number (range)	Forelimbs	0 (0–0)	1 (0–2) [a]
	Hind limbs	0 (0–0)	2 (0–4) [b]
Presence of gait alteration		**0/4**	**5/10**
Presence of posture alteration	Forelimbs	0/4	1/10
	Hind limbs	**0/4**	**4/10**
Presence of subjective pain	Forelimbs	0/4	2/10
	Hind limbs	**0/4**	**10/10**

[a]Affected joints were shoulder (6/10), elbow (5/10), and carpal (1/10) joints.
[b]Affected joints were coxofemoral (9/10), stifle (5/10), and tarsal (5/10) joints.

cat, with an *a priori* maximum of 16 consecutive trials allowed. The number of trials needed to obtain the 3 valid trials was recorded [10].

The analysis focused on the hind limbs, as the subjective pain evaluation indicated that these were the only painful limbs. The PVF data management used the most affected hind limb, determined as the hind limb that generated the lower PVF value [expressed in % body weight (BW)] most frequently (maximum of 2×3 = 6 trials) [11]. If an equal number of lower values was detected for each hind limb, the hind limb with the lower average PVF was chosen.

Motor activity assessment

The MA intensity was assessed using a collar-mounted accelerometer-based activity sensor (ActiWatch, Minimitter/Respironics, distributed by Bio-Lynx Scientific Equipment Inc., Montreal, QC, Canada) maintained in place for two weeks. The device was set for local time and configured to create 1 count per 2 minutes. The amplitude of each count was subsequently translated into a numeric value (from 0 to infinite) describing the MA intensity. In common with previous studies [9,10], and to avoid the effects of human interference, analysis of the cats' activity was restricted to 3 days per week (Friday, Saturday and Sunday), between 5:00 pm and 7:00 am. Data were expressed as the average total intensity count. The final MA intensity was calculated for each cat by taking the median of the three days recorded.

Secondary punctate tactile allodynia quantification

Secondary punctate allodynia was quantified twice, at a week's interval, using a mechanical von Frey polypropylene probe (Rigid Tip, surface area 0.7 mm^2, IITC Life Science, Woodland Hills, CA) fitted onto the hand-held force transducer of a paw withdrawal threshold monitoring anesthesiometer. With the cat standing in a meshed cage (Model 55035, Hunter Brand, Inc., Montreal, QC, Canada; dimensions 33" ×22" ×37"), the probe tip was placed perpendicular to the plantar surface of the foot (Fig. 1), and an increasing force was applied without manipulating the limb. The four limbs were tested in a predefined order with a 60-s interval between stimuli. The same evaluator performed all evaluations, and was blinded to the cat's OA status. The stimulus was stopped as soon as the paw was withdrawn, and the peak force recorded. Duplicate measurements were obtained from each paw. Data under 2 g were discarded, and a maximum cut off value of 200 g was applied. For both evaluations (one week apart), the vFWT was expressed as the average of the available threshold values (maximum of 2×4 = 8 values).

Mechanical repetitive stimuli quantitative sensory testing

Repeated mechanical stimuli of sub-threshold intensity (that is, for which a single stimulus would not elicit pain behaviour) were applied using a purpose-made device (Topcat Metrology Ltd; Cambs, UK). Available protocols of TS in humans and animals were used to devise the stimulation set profiles used in this study [29–32], and the profiles were refined during a pilot study in three cats (2 with OA; data not shown). The device supplied repeated mechanical stimuli at a predetermined intensity, duration and time interval. The mechanical stimulus was produced by hemispherical-ended metallic pin (2.5 mm diameter, 10 mm length) mounted on a rolling diaphragm actuator, adapted from a validated mechanical threshold testing system [33]. The actuator was mounted on the anterolateral aspect of the right or left mid metacarpus, held by

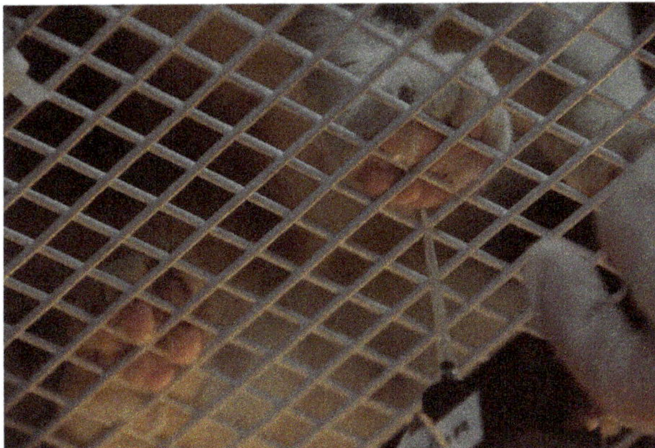

Figure 1. Photograph of the placement of the von Frey probe. During evaluation, the cats stood in a meshed cage, the probe tip was placed perpendicular to the plantar surface of the foot, and an increasing force was applied without manipulating the limb.

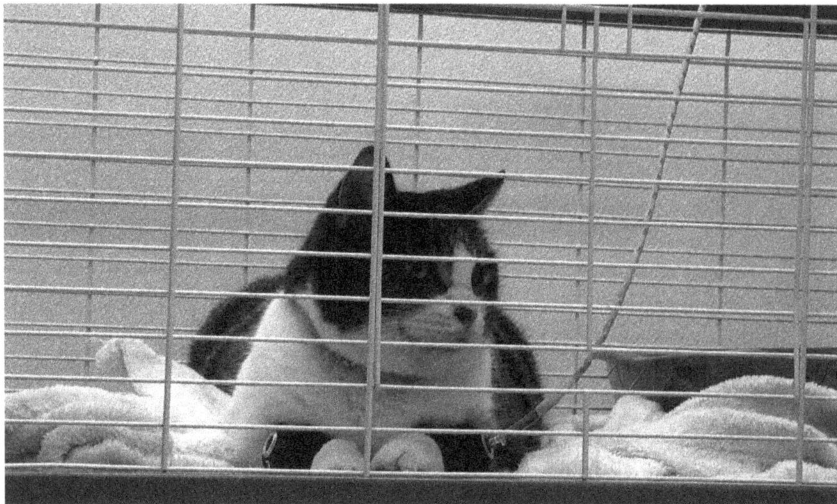

Figure 2. Photograph of the mechanical repetitive stimuli quantitative sensory testing experimental setting. Cats were placed in a meshed cage. The mechanical stimulator, which was embedded in a small band, was placed around the distal aspect of the cat's foreleg (left in this photograph) and connected to the stimulator device, while a dummy band was installed on the contralateral leg (right in this photograph).

a narrow band around the leg; a dummy was installed on the contralateral leg. During testing, the cats were free to move about in the same meshed cage (Fig. 2).

Each cat underwent four separate testing sessions (two sessions on the right leg, and two on the left), each separated by one day. Two of these sessions were conducted in the morning, and two during the afternoon. Before each testing session, the evaluator spent 5 minutes watching the normal behaviour of the cat once it had been placed in the cage, wearing the stimulator device. During each testing session one series of each of four sets of stimulation profiles was completed in a randomized order, with a 5-minute interval between each set of stimuli. Each stimulation set comprised up to 30 stimuli with one the four profiles of intensity and/or frequency; the power of the stimulation set increased from profile #1 to 4 (Table 2). The evaluator was blinded to the cat's OA status and the stimulation profile. During each set of stimuli, testing was either stopped by the evaluator as soon as clear pain behaviour was seen (*e.g.* vocalization, agitation, biting at the limb band, vigorously shaking the leg or jumping away from it) or stimulation was stopped automatically when the maximum number of stimuli (30) was reached. The number of stimuli (NS) reached was noted for each test. The response to each stimulation profile was defined as the NS for each cat by taking the median of the four NS recorded for each stimulation profile.

Statistical methods

All analyses were two-sided with an α threshold of 0.05 using a statistical software program (SAS system, version 9.3, SAS Institute Inc., Cary, NC, USA). Continuous data distribution was assessed using the Shapiro-Wilk test (normal distribution) and kernel density estimation. The NS data sets comprised count data that were assumed to be Poisson distributed by nature.

Mixed model analyses for repeated measures were conducted to compare the PVF and vFWT between non-OA and OA cats [34,35]. Generalized linear mixed model analyses for repeated measures were conducted using conditional models to compare the MA intensity (Weibull distributed data) between non-OA and OA cats, and to compare the responses of the mechanical repeated NS (Poisson distributed data) between stimulation profiles and between non-OA and OA cats [36,37]. Whole model details are shown in Table 3. These models provided fixed effect estimates by restricted likelihood modelling. Homogeneity of variance was assessed using the absolute values of the residuals of the mixed model, and the best structure of the covariance model was assessed using a graphical method (plots of covariance *versus* lag in time between pairs of observations compared to different covariance models in mixed models), as well as using information criteria that measure the relative fit of competing covariance models (mixed models, and generalized linear mixed models). Also, residuals of the models were thoroughly studied to assess the model's validity. A Bonferroni adjustment provided adjusted p-values (adj-*P*), and adjusted 95% confidence interval (95% CI) for multiple comparisons when appropriate.

Exploratory correlations between PVF expressed as %BW, MA intensity, vFWT (the mean value of the two evaluations were used in this analysis for the three above outcomes), and the NS from the

Table 2. Characterization of the mechanical stimuli provided by each stimulation profile.

Stimulation profile	Intensity (N)	Duration (s)	Frequency (Hz)	Interval (s)	Maximal number
#1	2	1.5	0.4	2.5	30
#2	4	1.5	0.4	2.5	30
#3	6	1.5	0.125	8	30
#4	6	1.5	0.4	2.5	30

Table 3. Details of the mixed model analyses.

Data	Data distribution	Data transformation*	Fixed effects	Random effects	Covariance structures	Tested covariates
PVF	Normal	Log-transformed	Cat group, evaluation day, and cat group × evaluation day	Cat	Compound symmetry	Age, BW, Velocity and Maximum number of trials
MA	Weibulll	None		Cat, and evaluation day	Compound symmetry	Age, and BW
vFWT	Normal	Log-transformed		Cat	Type 1 autoregressive	
NS	Poisson	None	Cat group, stimulation profile, cat group × stimulation profile	Stimulation profile, and cat × stimulation profile	Compound symmetry	

*Outcome transformations were recommended following residual analysis results to correct for data heteroscedasticity; PVF: ; MA: motor activity; vFWT: von Frey anesthesiometer-induced paw withdrawal threshold; NS: number of stimuli, BW: body weight.

four stimulation profiles were carried out using Spearman's rank correlations.

Results

PVF after exercise in the most affected hindlimb tended to be lower in the OA cats compared with the non-OA cats (Fig. 3A; cat group effect $P=0.070$): least squares means estimate difference (LSD; 95% CI) = −0.059 kg (−0.124, 0.005). PVF analyses also identified some significant covariates: BW ($P<0.0001$) and the inverse of the maximum number of trials ($P<0.001$). However, the evaluation day effect was not significant ($P=0.79$), nor was there a significant interaction between cat group and evaluation day ($P=0.41$).

MA intensity was not significantly lower in OA cats than in non-OA cats (Fig. 3B; cat group effect $P=0.12$): LSD (95% CI) = −95 (−216, 27). The analyses neither showed a significant evaluation day effect ($P=0.72$) nor an interaction of cat group with evaluation day ($P=0.78$).

vFWT was significantly lower in OA cats than in non-OA cats (Fig. 3C; cat group effect $P=0.007$): LSD (95% CI) = −53 g (−88, −18). There was no significant evaluation day effect ($P=0.76$) nor any interaction between cat group and evaluation day ($P=0.79$).

Sustained pain behaviours persisting for several seconds after the end of the stimulation set were observed with all stimulation profiles. Analysis of the mechanical repetitive stimuli QST data identified significant differences between the profiles (stimulation set effect $P<0.001$): the higher the intensity of the stimulus, the sooner (lower NS) it produced a consistent painful response (Fig. 4A). Planned comparisons showed that stimulation profiles #4 and #3 enhanced the response (lower NS) compared with both profile #2 (LSD [adjusted 95% CI] = −0.62 [−1.03, −0.21], and LSD [adjusted 95% CI] = −0.82 [−1.25, −0.39] respectively; adj-$P<0.001$ for both) and #1 (LSD [adjusted 95% CI] = −1.00 [−1.40, −0.61], and LSD [adjusted 95% CI] = −1.20 [−1.62, −0.79] respectively; adj-$P<0.001$ for both). In addition, profile #2 led to a lower NS than profile #1 (LSD [adjusted 95% CI] = −0.38 [−0.73, −0.03]; adj-$P=0.031$).

The response in OA cats was enhanced (lower NS) compared to the non-OA cats (cat group effect $P=0.019$): LSD [95% CI] = −0.52 [−0.94, −0.10]. In addition, interaction of the stimulation set with the cat group was not significant ($P=0.18$). This indicated a similar effect across stimulation profiles for each group (equality of the slopes). However, when it (profile of stimulation × group of cat) was tested for the presence of slopes not equal to zero (same model but without the profile effect term), the interaction was significant ($P<0.001$) permitting the following interpretation of planned OA *versus.* non-OA cat comparisons for the different stimulation profiles (Fig. 4B; each stimulation profile was considered independent, implying that no adjustment for multiple comparisons was needed): the response to stimulation profiles #1 and #3 was similar in both OA and non OA cats (LSD [95% CI] = −0.20 [−0.69, 0.28], and LSD [95% CI] = −0.53 [−1.14, 0.08] respectively; $P=0.39$, and 0.089 respectively), but NS was lower in OA cats than non-OA cats with stimulation profiles #2 and #4 (LSD [95% CI] = −0.76 [−1.26, −0.25], and LSD [95% CI] = −0.60 [−1.17, −0.02] respectively; $P=0.005$, and 0.043 respectively).

There was no significant association between chronic pain measurements and age in any of the above models (PVF, MA intensity, vFWT or stimulation NS) ($P>0.15$). There was a highly significant positive correlation between the vFWT and NS profiles #2 and #4 ($Rho_s=0.64$, and 0.63, respectively; $P=0.01$, and 0.02, respectively), but not between PVF or MA intensity and any of the profile responses (all $P>0.10$).

Discussion

The objective methods PVF, MA intensity and vFWT used in this study to evaluate OA-associated chronic pain enabled non-OA, non painful cats, and painful OA cats to be distinguished. These three evaluation methods were used in a previous study using a larger sample, where both PVF and vFWT discriminated between OA and non-OA cats [10]. Although MA intensity was not sensitive to the presence of OA [10], it was still included in the present study as an objective measure of the effect of OA pain on physical activity and function; MA was significantly affected by both administration of the analgesic non-steroidal anti-inflammatory drug (NSAID) meloxicam [10,13] and also by feeding an analgesic therapeutic diet [12]. The sample of OA cats used in our study therefore truly characterized cats with OA-related chronic pain. Although the study was slightly underpowered with regards to PVF evaluation, testing the discriminatory ability of PVF in OA cats was not a primary objective.

In the previous study, a four-week NSAID treatment did not eliminate the difference in vFWT between the OA and non-OA cats (OA cats were lower) [10]. Approximately 25% of the OA cats (n = 39) were classified as allodynic based on a repeated duplicate vFWT measurement recorded below a cut-off of 40 g for the front

A

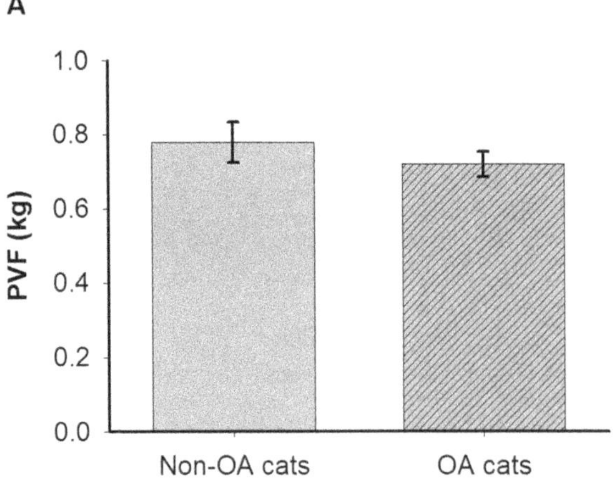

B

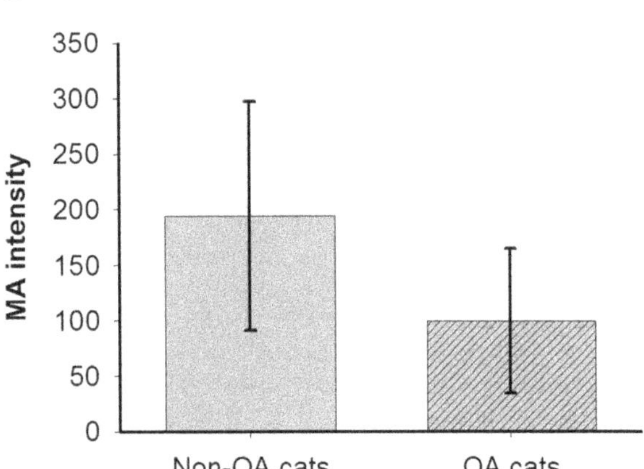

C

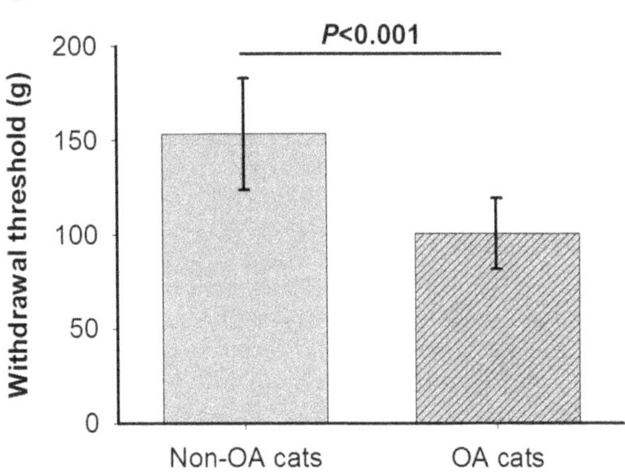

Figure 3. Characterization of osteoarthritis (OA) using chronic pain evaluation methods: A- Least squares means and 95% confidence interval of the log-transformed most affected limb peak vertical ground reaction force (PVF) after-exercise by OA status. B- Least squares means and 95% confidence interval of the motor activity (MA) intensity by OA status. C- Least squares means and 95% confidence interval of the log-transformed von Frey anesthesiometer-induced paw withdrawal threshold by OA status.

paws and 50 g for the hind paws (first quartile values of the sample of OA cats under placebo) [10]. Most of the OA cats responded favourably to meloxicam, but in those classified as allodynic the response was poor or negligible [10]. This is not surprising in view of the recognized low efficacy of NSAIDs against centralized neuropathic pain [14,15] and supports the supposition that central sensitization occurs in feline OA-associated chronic pain, similar to humans [15,20,21,23]. While the vFWT was also reliable in OA cats [10], this is primarily only a reflexive evaluation of hypersensitivity [38,39]. In contrast, evaluation of TS provides the opportunity to evaluate central sensitization with conscious perception since it is based on pain behaviour, implying cortical integration.

We were able to evoke TS in conscious cats, which has not been previously reported in this species. Repetition of sub-threshold mechanical stimuli summated and facilitated pain as detected through observation of pain behaviour, and also detected different responses between OA and non-OA cats. Temporal summation involves conduction of impulses *via* Aδ and C-fibers in wide dynamic range neurons of the dorsal horn, and primarily results from progressive and prolonged dorsal horn C-fibre neuron discharge (windup) [25,30]. Wind-up and central sensitization are not identical phenomena, but depend on similar pathways, where wind-up initiates and maintains central sensitization [14,25]. Evoked TS of pain was enhanced (faster) in OA compared to non-OA cats, thereby suggesting that central sensitization plays a role in feline OA-associated chronic pain.

Increasing the stimulus intensity enhanced the cats' response. This is consistent with the supposed mechanism of induced TS, and is in accordance with previous studies [29,31]. With repeated brief stimuli, the transient first pain response tends to decrease, while second pain increases in intensity and duration, corresponding to prolonged C-fibre discharge [30]. The intensity-dependent response observed in this group of cats suggests that higher intensity stimulation enhanced C-fiber recruitment. The observation of sustained pain behaviours after the end of the stimulation set supports the likelihood that C-fibers were activated. These behaviours persisted for several seconds, consistent with the 15 s aftersensations induced by TS in normal humans [40] and a return to baseline after 30 s in rats [29]. In human patients afflicted with fibromyalgia, aftersensations lasted for up to 120 s after TS of pain was established [40]. This led to the choice of the 5-min delay we imposed between two stimulation sets, preventing persistence of pain into the start of a new stimulation set. Randomization also protected against a potential carry over effect.

Augmentation of stimulation frequency between stimulation profiles #3 and #4 did not affect the time to appearance of pain behaviour, as might be expected [29,31]. A possible explanation is that the 6N intensity was already close to a single-stimulus pain threshold, so the cats very rapidly experienced pain.

Temporal summation was enhanced in OA cats, particularly with stimulation profiles #2 and #4. This suggests that OA cats with chronic pain have developed central sensitization and the associated pain facilitation. It is noteworthy that the response to both these stimulation profiles correlated positively with the vFWT, supporting the suggestion that profiles #2 and #4 are the best for characterizing central sensitization. The lack of correlation between NS after any stimulation profiles and the other objective evaluation methods of OA-associated disability (PVF and MA intensity) suggests that they can be regarded as complementary assessment methods. This was expected, because TS is specific to central sensitization, which is not correlated with the severity of structural or functional impairment related to chronic pain. The effect of NSAID treatment on MA intensity [10,13] leads to a similar conclusion, suggesting that MA intensity may be more closely related to the inflammatory component of feline OA pain.

We acknowledge that the cat groups were small and the reported enhancement of mechanical TS in OA cats requires

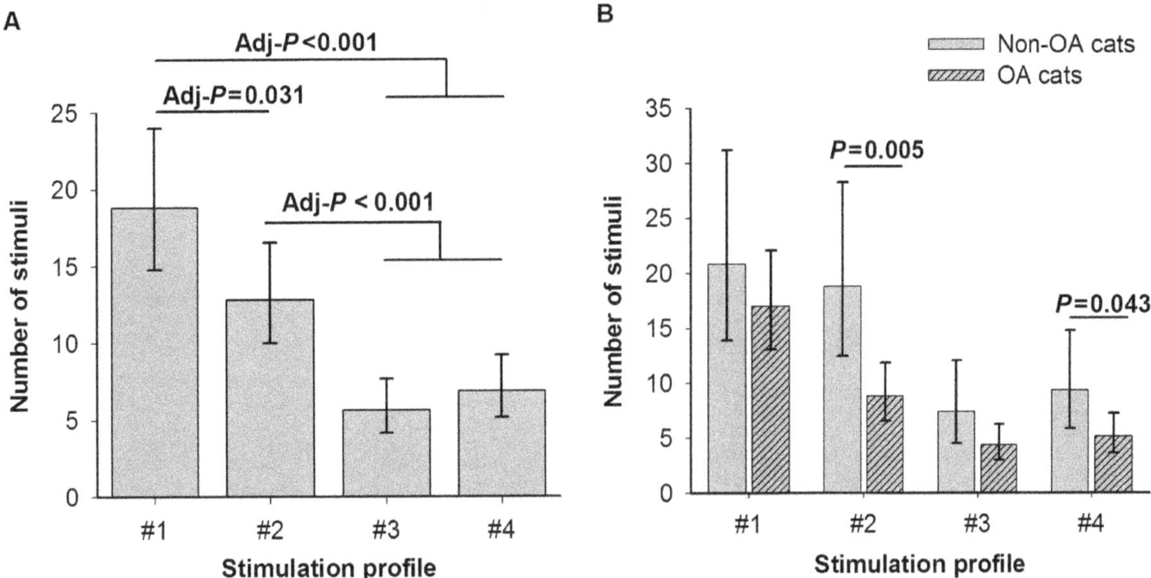

Figure 4. Number of stimuli reached and 95% confidence interval (inverse link of the least squares means estimates and 95% confidence interval obtained using the Poisson generalized linear modelling) following repetitive mechanical stimuli: A- by stimulation profiles (#1 to 4); B- by stimulation profiles and osteoarthritis (OA) status. Adj-*P*= adjusted p-value.

confirmation in a larger study. However, this is the first report of mechanical TS in conscious cats, which was challenging from both a technical and subject acclimation standpoint. Moreover, the use of naturally occurring OA improves the translational potential of these results. This study highlights similarities between cat and human OA-associated chronic pain, which may share similar nociceptive mechanisms. Temporal summation appears to be *N*-methyl-D-aspartate (*N*MDA) receptor-dependent in both animals [41] and humans [42]. Temporal summation QST is a well-recognized mechanism-based evaluation technique for musculoskeletal pain in humans [14,20,21,23]. Hence, evoked TS has considerable potential for effective translational research [43]. A further advantage of investigation into central sensitization is that this phenomenon is potentially reversible. The inefficiency of numerous treatments of human OA-induced chronic pain highlights the need for development of drugs targeting central sensitization (*e.g.*, ionic channel or *N*MDA-receptor blockers, serotonin/noradrenaline reuptake inhibitors) [14–17]. The positive results obtained recently in humans using duloxetine, a dual-reuptake inhibitor of serotonin and noradrenaline encourage this approach [44].

In conclusion, our results suggest that central sensitization is a feature of feline OA-associated chronic pain. Use of evoked TS in cats with naturally occurring OA provides a unique opportunity to improve translational research in OA-associated chronic pain, and supports the concept of using naturally occurring disease in animals as an ethical and highly relevant alternative to the use of induced models of pain [45].

Acknowledgments

The authors wish to acknowledge the wonderful technical support provided by the personnel of both ArthroLab, Inc. and the GREPAQ, namely Mrs Carolle Sylvestre, Pascale St-Onge, Audrey Raymond, Dafné LeCorre-Laliberté, Dominique Gauvin, and Mélissa d'Auteuil.

Author Contributions

Conceived and designed the experiments: MG PMT PR JMP JPP ET. Performed the experiments: MG PMT PR MPK ET. Analyzed the data: MG PMT ET. Contributed reagents/materials/analysis tools: PMT. Wrote the paper: MG PMT PR MPK JMP JPP ET.

References

1. Bennett D, Zainal Ariffin SM, Johnston P (2012) Osteoarthritis in the cat: 1. how common is it and how easy to recognise? J Feline Med Surg 14: 65–75.
2. Hardie EM, Roe SC, Martin FR (2002) Radiographic evidence of degenerative joint disease in geriatric cats: 100 cases (1994–1997). J Am Vet Med Assoc 220: 628–632.
3. Lascelles BD (2010) Feline degenerative joint disease. Vet Surg 39: 2–13.
4. Beale BS (2005) Orthopedic problems in geriatric dogs and cats. Vet Clin North Am Small Anim Pract 35: 655–674.
5. Bennett D, Morton C (2009) A study of owner observed behavioural and lifestyle changes in cats with musculoskeletal disease before and after analgesic therapy. J Feline Med Surg 11: 997–1004.
6. Klinck MP, Frank D, Guillot M, Troncy E (2012) Owner-perceived signs and veterinary diagnosis in 50 cases of feline osteoarthritis. Can Vet J 53: 1181–1186.
7. Slingerland LI, Hazewinkel HA, Meij BP, Picavet P, Voorhout G (2011) Cross-sectional study of the prevalence and clinical features of osteoarthritis in 100 cats. Vet J 187: 304–309.
8. Zamprogno H, Hansen BD, Bondell HD, Sumrell AT, Simpson W, et al. (2010) Item generation and design testing of a questionnaire to assess degenerative joint disease-associated pain in cats. Am J Vet Res 71: 1417–1424.
9. Guillot M, Moreau M, d'Anjou MA, Martel-Pelletier J, Pelletier JP, et al. (2012) Evaluation of osteoarthritis in cats: novel information from a pilot study. Vet Surg 41: 328–335.
10. Guillot M, Moreau M, Heit M, Martel-Pelletier J, Pelletier JP, et al. (2013) Characterization of osteoarthritis in cats and meloxicam efficacy using objective chronic pain evaluation tools. Vet J 196: 360–367.
11. Moreau M, Guillot M, Pelletier JP, Martel-Pelletier J, Troncy E (2013) Kinetic peak vertical force measurement in cats afflicted by coxarthritis: data management and acquisition protocols. Res Vet Sci 95: 219–224.
12. Lascelles BD, DePuy V, Thomson A, Hansen B, Marcellin-Little DJ, et al. (2010) Evaluation of a therapeutic diet for feline degenerative joint disease. J Vet Intern Med 24: 487–495.
13. Lascelles BD, Hansen BD, Roe S, DePuy V, Thomson A, et al. (2007) Evaluation of client-specific outcome measures and activity monitoring to measure pain relief in cats with osteoarthritis. J Vet Intern Med 21: 410–416.

14. Woolf CJ (2011) Central sensitization: implications for the diagnosis and treatment of pain. Pain 152: S2–15.
15. Mease PJ, Hanna S, Frakes EP, Altman RD (2011) Pain mechanisms in osteoarthritis: understanding the role of central pain and current approaches to its treatment. J Rheumatol 38: 1546–1551.
16. Staud R (2011) Evidence for shared pain mechanisms in osteoarthritis, low back pain, and fibromyalgia. Curr Rheumatol Rep 13: 513–520.
17. Arendt-Nielsen L, Graven-Nielsen T (2011) Translational musculoskeletal pain research. Best Pract Res Clin Rheumatol 25: 209–226.
18. Lascelles BD (2013) Getting a sense of sensations. Vet J 197: 115–117.
19. Hendiani JA, Westlund KN, Lawand N, Goel N, Lisse J, et al. (2003) Mechanical sensation and pain thresholds in patients with chronic arthropathies. J Pain 4: 203–211.
20. Suokas AK, Walsh DA, McWilliams DF, Condon L, Moreton B, et al. (2012) Quantitative sensory testing in painful osteoarthritis: a systematic review and meta-analysis. Osteoarthritis Cartilage 20: 1075–1085.
21. Arendt-Nielsen L, Nie H, Laursen MB, Laursen BS, Madeleine P, et al. (2010) Sensitization in patients with painful knee osteoarthritis. Pain 149: 573–581.
22. Brydges NM, Argyle DJ, Mosley JR, Duncan JC, Fleetwood-Walker S, et al. (2012) Clinical assessments of increased sensory sensitivity in dogs with cranial cruciate ligament rupture. Vet J 193: 545–550.
23. Imamura M, Imamura ST, Kaziyama HH, Targino RA, Hsing WT, et al. (2008) Impact of nervous system hyperalgesia on pain, disability, and quality of life in patients with knee osteoarthritis: a controlled analysis. Arthritis Rheum 59: 1424–1431.
24. Mendell LM, Wall PD (1965) Responses of Single Dorsal Cord Cells to Peripheral Cutaneous Unmyelinated Fibres. Nature 206: 97–99.
25. Herrero JF, Laird JM, Lopez-Garcia JA (2000) Wind-up of spinal cord neurones and pain sensation: much ado about something? Prog Neurobiol 61: 169–203.
26. Zimmermann M (1983) Ethical guidelines for investigations of experimental pain in conscious animals. Pain 16: 109–110.
27. Kilkenny C, Browne WJ, Cuthill IC, Emerson M, Altman DG (2010) Improving bioscience research reporting: the ARRIVE guidelines for reporting animal research. PLoS Biol 8: e1000412.
28. D'Anjou MA, Moreau M, Troncy E, Martel-Pelletier J, Abram F, et al. (2008) Osteophytosis, subchondral bone sclerosis, joint effusion and soft tissue thickening in canine experimental stifle osteoarthritis: comparison between 1.5 T magnetic resonance imaging and computed radiography. Vet Surg 37: 166–177.
29. Lomas LM, Picker MJ (2005) Behavioral assessment of temporal summation in the rat: sensitivity to sex, opioids and modulation by NMDA receptor antagonists. Psychopharmacology (Berl) 180: 84–94.
30. Price DD, Hu JW, Dubner R, Gracely RH (1977) Peripheral suppression of first pain and central summation of second pain evoked by noxious heat pulses. Pain 3: 57–68.
31. Vierck CJ Jr., Cannon RL, Fry G, Maixner W, Whitsel BL (1997) Characteristics of temporal summation of second pain sensations elicited by brief contact of glabrous skin by a preheated thermode. J Neurophysiol 78: 992–1002.
32. Yeomans DC, Cooper BY, Vierck CJ Jr. (1995) Comparisons of dose-dependent effects of systemic morphine on flexion reflex components and operant avoidance responses of awake non-human primates. Brain Res 670: 297–302.
33. Dixon MJ, Taylor PM, Slingsby L, Hoffmann MV, Kastner SB, et al. (2010) A small, silent, low friction, linear actuator for mechanical nociceptive testing in veterinary research. Lab Anim 44: 247–253.
34. Brown H, Prescott R (2006) Repeated Measures Data. In: Brown H, Prescott R, editors. Applied mixed models in medicine. Chichester, England: John Wiley & Sons Ltd. 215–270.
35. Littell RC, Milliken GA, Stroup WW, Wolfinger RD, Schabenberger O (2006) Analysis of repeated measure data, in SAS for mixed models. In: Littell RC, Milliken GA, Stroup WW, Wolfinger RD, Schabenberger O, editors. SAS for mixed models, second edition. Second ed. Cary, NC: SAS institute Inc. 159–204.
36. Brown H, Prescott R (2006) Generalised linear mixed models. In: Brown H, Prescott R, editors. Applied mixed models in medicine. Chichester, England: John Wiley & Sons Ltd. 107–152.
37. Stroup WW (2013) Correlated errors, Part I: Repeated Measures. In: Stroup WW, editor. Generalized linear mixed models: Modern concepts, methods and applications. Boca Raton, FL: CRC Press, Taylor and Francis Group. 413–442.
38. Boyce-Rustay JM, Zhong C, Kohnken R, Baker SJ, Simler GH, et al. (2010) Comparison of mechanical allodynia and the affective component of inflammatory pain in rats. Neuropharmacology 58: 537–543.
39. Navratilova E, Xie JY, King T, Porreca F (2013) Evaluation of reward from pain relief. Ann N Y Acad Sci 1282: 1–11.
40. Staud R, Vierck CJ, Cannon RL, Mauderli AP, Price DD (2001) Abnormal sensitization and temporal summation of second pain (wind-up) in patients with fibromyalgia syndrome. Pain 91: 165–175.
41. Dickenson AH, Sullivan AF (1987) Evidence for a role of the NMDA receptor in the frequency dependent potentiation of deep rat dorsal horn nociceptive neurones following C fibre stimulation. Neuropharmacology 26: 1235–1238.
42. Price DD, Mao J, Frenk H, Mayer DJ (1994) The N-methyl-D-aspartate receptor antagonist dextromethorphan selectively reduces temporal summation of second pain in man. Pain 59: 165–174.
43. Arendt-Nielsen L, Mansikka H, Staahl C, Rees H, Tan K, et al. (2011) A translational study of the effects of ketamine and pregabalin on temporal summation of experimental pain. Reg Anesth Pain Med 36: 585–591.
44. Frakes EP, Risser RC, Ball TD, Hochberg MC, Wohlreich MM (2011) Duloxetine added to oral nonsteroidal anti-inflammatory drugs for treatment of knee pain due to osteoarthritis: results of a randomized, double-blind, placebo-controlled trial. Curr Med Res Opin 27: 2361–2372.
45. Dolgin E (2010) Animalgesic effects. Nat Med 16: 1237–1240.

2

Pathogenic Role of Basic Calcium Phosphate Crystals in Destructive Arthropathies

Hang-Korng Ea[1,2], Véronique Chobaz[3], Christelle Nguyen[1], Sonia Nasi[3], Peter van Lent[4], Michel Daudon[5], Arnaud Dessombz[6], Dominique Bazin[6], Geraldine McCarthy[7], Brigitte Jolles-Haeberli[8], Annette Ives[3], Daniel Van Linthoudt[3], Alexander So[3], Frédéric Lioté[1,2], Nathalie Busso[3]*

1 INSERM, UMR-S 606, Hospital Lariboisière,Paris, France, **2** University Paris Diderot (UFR de Médecine), Sorbonne Paris Cité, Paris, France, **3** Department of Musculoskeletal Medicine, Service of Rheumatology, CHUV and University of Lausanne, Lausanne, Switzerland, **4** Department of Rheumatology, Rheumatology Research and Advanced Therapeutics, Radboud University Nijmegen Medical Centre, Nijmegen, The Netherlands, **5** Service des Explorations Fonctionnelles, Hôpital Tenon, AP-HP, Paris, France, **6** Laboratoire de Physique des Solides, Université Paris Sud, Orsay, France, **7** Mater Misericordiae University Hospital, Dublin, Ireland, **8** Service de chirurgie orthopédique et traumatologique de l'appareil moteur, Department of Musculoskeletal Medicine, CHUV and University of Lausanne, Lausanne, Switzerland

Abstract

Background: basic calcium phosphate (BCP) crystals are commonly found in osteoarthritis (OA) and are associated with cartilage destruction. BCP crystals induce in vitro catabolic responses with the production of metalloproteases and inflammatory cytokines such as interleukin-1 (IL-1). In vivo, IL-1 production induced by BCP crystals is both dependant and independent of NLRP3 inflammasome. We aimed to clarify 1/ the role of BCP crystals in cartilage destruction and 2/ the role of IL-1 and NLRP3 inflammasome in cartilage degradation related to BCP crystals.

Methodology/ Principal Findings: synovial membranes isolated from OA knees were analysed by alizarin Red and FTIR. Pyrogen free BCP crystals were injected into right knees of WT, NLRP3 -/-, ASC -/-, IL-1α -/- and IL-1β-/- mice and PBS was injected into left knees. To assess the role of IL-1, WT mice were treated by intra-peritoneal injections of anakinra, the IL-1Ra recombinant protein, or PBS. Articular destruction was studied at d4, d17 and d30 assessing synovial inflammation, proteoglycan loss and chondrocyte apoptosis. BCP crystals were frequently found in OA synovial membranes including low grade OA. BCP crystals injected into murine knee joints provoked synovial inflammation characterized by synovial macrophage infiltration that persisted at day 30, cartilage degradation as evidenced by loss of proteoglycan staining by Safranin-O and concomitant expression of VDIPEN epitopes, and increased chondrocyte apoptosis. BCP crystal-induced synovitis was totally independent of IL-1α and IL-1β signalling and no alterations of inflammation were observed in mice deficient for components of the NLRP3-inflammasome, IL-1α or IL 1β. Similarly, treatment with anakinra did not prevent BCP crystal effects. In vitro, BCP crystals elicited enhanced transcription of matrix degrading and pro-Inflammatory genes in macrophages.

Conclusions/ Significance: intra-articular BCP crystals can elicit synovial inflammation and cartilage degradation suggesting that BCP crystals have a direct pathogenic role in OA. The effects are independent of IL-1 and NLRP3 inflammasome.

Editor: Dimitrios Zeugolis, National University of Ireland Galway, Ireland

Funding: This work was supported by the Fonds national suisse de la recherche scientifique (grant 310030-130085/1), from the Fondation Jean and Linette Warnery, from the Fondation pour la Recherche Médicale (FRM DV020081013483, call for bids Vieillissement, 2008-2011), INSERM, University Paris Diderot, Faculty of Medicine (Institut Claude Bernard), the Société Française de Rhumatologie, the Association pour la Recherche en Pathologie Synoviale (ARPS), Prévention et Traitement des Décalcifications - Cristaux et Cartilage, and Rhumatisme et Travail. The funders had no role in study design, data collection and analysis, decision to publish, or preparation of the manuscript.

Competing Interests: The authors have declared that no competing interests exist.

* E-mail: Nathalie.Busso@chuv.ch

Introduction

Basic calcium phosphate (BCP) crystals including carbonated-apatite (CA), hydroxyapatite (HA), octacalcium phosphate (OCP), tricalcium phosphate and whitlockite crystals are associated with osteoarthritis (OA), calcific tendinitis, acute arthritis and atherosclerosis (reviewed in [1]). They are identified in the synovial fluid of rapidly destructive OA, as illustrated by the Milwaukee shoulder syndrome [2], and are also highly prevalent in cartilage obtained from affected OA joints at the time of knee joint replacement surgery [3].

Some investigators still consider articular BCP crystals as "innocent bystanders" and/or markers of end-stage OA. Indeed, many cartilage injuries allow subchondral bone mineral to be released into the joint that subsequently deposit onto the cartilage or synovium. However, numerous clinical and experimental reports suggest that cartilage calcification is, in fact, an active process, and can occur in mild OA lesions, and in normal and young cartilage [3,4,5]. Furthermore, Sun *et al* have shown that OA meniscal cells upregulate genes involved in the calcification process, that can facilitate crystal formation [6]. Similarly, Fuerst *et al* demonstrated that chondrocytes isolated from OA cartilage generate BCP crystals in conjunction with chondrocyte hypertrophy [3]. This data suggests that both hyaline and fibrous cartilage calcification may be an early and active phenomenon that affects the whole joint and occurs before evidence of cartilage breakdown. Indeed, the guinea pig and STR/Ort murine models of spontaneous OA support this theory, as time-course studies using these animal models demonstrated that, indeed, calcification of the cartilage or menisci as well as the ligaments occur prior to any cartilage breakdown (reviewed in [1]). Finally, in Sprague-Dawley rat, articular cartilage calcification is common and alters cartilage biomechanical properties favouring cartilage destruction [7].

Currently, the mechanisms by which BCP crystals contribute to OA pathogenesis still require further investigation, but it is clear that BCP crystals have multiple effects on articular cells. They are able to induce cellular proliferation, proto-oncogene stimulation, and inflammation related events such as the production and/or activation of cytokines (IL-1 and TNF-β), metalloproteases (MMP), cyclo-oxygenases -1 and -2 and prostaglandin E2 [8,9], the production of nitric oxide, and the induction of apoptosis in synovial fibroblasts, and articular chondrocytes [10,11]. They initiate both IL-1β -mediated inflammatory processes through NLRP3 (NACHT-, LRR- and PYD-containing Protein 3)-inflammasome as well as inflammasome-independent pathways [12,13]. However, despite experimental evidence that suggests the importance of IL-1β in OA pathogenesis [14], clinical studies using IL-1 inhibition in OA treatment have not yielded convincing results [15,16].

In order to demonstrate the pathogenic role of BCP crystals in the process of destructive arthropathies, we injected HA and OCP crystals, the latter being the most phlogistic one amongst BCP crystals, into murine knee joints. We also explored the mechanisms underlying intra-articular OCP crystals' effects *in vivo*, taking advantage of mice deficient for different components of the inflammasome, for IL-1α and IL-β, and for Toll-like receptors (TLRs).

Materials and Methods

Mice

Female C57BL/6J mice were purchased from Harlan (Horst, The Netherlands). IL-1α-/- and IL-1β-/- mice were a gift from Dr YoichiroIwakura (University of Tokyo, Japan) [17]. Toll-like receptors (TLR) 1, 2, 4, 6 and MyD88 (Myeloid differentiation factor 88) deficient mice were kindly provided by Dr Thierry Roger (Department of infectious diseases, CHUV, Lausanne, Switzerland). ASC-/- (apoptosis-associated speck-like protein containing a CARD) [18] and NLRP3-/- [19] mice were obtained from the late J. Tschopp's laboratory (Biochemistry Institute, University of Lausanne, Switzerland). All mice were backcrossed onto the C57BL/6 background for at least 9 generations and were compared to WT littermates. Mice were breed under conventional, non-SPF conditions. Mice between 8–12 weeks of age were used for experiments. Animal experiments were performed in strict accordance to the Swiss Federal Regulations. The protocol was approved by the "Service de la consommation et des affaires vétérinaires du Canton de Vaud", Switzerland (Permit Number: 1908.2). All efforts were made to minimize suffering and minimize the number of mice needed to assess statistical significance and experimental reproducibility.

Crystal-induced arthritis

Sterile, pyrogen-free HA and OCP crystals were synthesized as previously described [20]. The nature of BCP crystals were checked before and after sterilisation by X-ray diffraction and infrared spectroscopy. X-ray diffraction patterns were recorded with Co-Kalpha (λ = 1.78892Å) using Inel CPS 120 diffractometer operating at 45 kV and 28 mA. Infrared spectra were obtained over the 4000-400 cm^{-1} range, using Nicolet FT-IR 5700 spectrometer with KBr pellet. HA and OCP crystal sizes and Ca/(P+CO3) ratios were determined as previously and were for HA 1.1 ± 0.3 µm and 1.56 and for OCP crystals 1.5 ± 0.5 and 1.33, respectively [20]. Crystals were suspended in sterile PBS and dispersed by brief sonication. All crystals were determined to be endotoxin free (<0.01 EU/10 mg) by Limulus amebocyte cell lysate assay. Crystals (OCP used at 20 or 200 µg in 20 µl endotoxin-free PBS, HA used at 20 µg in 20 µl endotoxin-free PBS) were injected into the right knee joint (i.a.) of mice anaesthetised with 2.5% isoflurane, the left knee joint injected with 20 µl of PBS as a control.

Anakinra treatment

Anakinra, the recombinant form of IL-1Ra, was injected i.p. twice daily at a dose of 200 µg/mouse for 4 days, the first injection being 30 min prior to intra-articular BCP crystal injection into the knee.

Isotopic quantification of joint inflammation

Joint inflammation was measured by ^{99m}Technetium (Tc) uptake in the knee joint, as previously described [21]. The ratio of Tc uptake in the inflamed arthritic knee versus Tc uptake in the ipsilateral control knee was calculated. A ratio higher than 1:1 indicated joint inflammation.

Histological examination of knee joints

Mice were sacrificed, the knees dissected, and fixed in 10% buffered formalin for 4 days. Fixed tissues were decalcified in 5% formic acid, dehydrated, and embedded in paraffin. Sagittal sections (6 µm) of the whole knee joint were stained with Safranin-O and counterstained with fast green/iron hematoxylin. Histological sections were graded by two independent observers (VC and NB) unaware of animal genotype or handling. Two different parameters, synovial inflammation and cartilage PG loss were scored on a scale of 0 to 6 in proportion to severity. Von Kossa staining was performed on knees embedded in methyl-methacrylate as described [22].

Immunohistochemistry

Macrophage and neutrophil (PMN) infiltrates and endothelial cells in knee synovium were detected using anti- Mac-2, anti-MPO or anti-ICAM primary antibodies (all from Sigma-Aldrich, Buchs Switzerland), and visualized using the avidin-biotin-horseradish peroxidase (HRP) complex (Vectastain Elite ABC kit; Vector Laboratories, Burlingame, CA, USA). The color was developed by 3,3′-diaminobenzidine (Sigma-Aldrich, Buchs, Switzerland) containing 0.01% H2O2. Slides were counterstained with Papanicolaou (Merck AG, Dietikon, Switzerland). Apoptotic cells were detected with apopTag Kit (S7100) according to manufacturer's instructions (Chemicon, Temecula, California, USA). Briefly, DNA fragments labelled in situ by terminal deoxynucleotidyl transferase (TdT) and digoxigenin-nucleotide were detected by anti-digoxigenin antibody conjugated to peroxydase. Negative control sections were performed without TdT. Apoptotic chondrocytes were counted per field (180×140 µm, 3 different fields/mouse) by an observer (VC) who was blinded with regard to mice groups.

MMP-induced neoepitope VDIPEN staining was performed with affinity-purified anti-VDIPEN IgG overnight at 4°C as previously described [23]. Scoring was performed by two independent observers (VC and NB) on an arbitrary scale from 0 to 3 according to the immunostained areas.

Macrophage stimulation experiments and real-time PCR

C57BL/6 mice were sacrificed and bone marrow cells recovered from tibial and femoral bones. The cells were cultured for 7 days in L929 conditioned media to allow differentiation into macrophages, as described previously [13]. Bone marrow derived macrophages (BMDM) were then stimulated with 500 μg/ml of OCP crystals for 4 hours in RPMI with 1% penicillin/streptomycin (Invitrogen™). RNA was extracted (RNA Clean & Concentrator5-Zymoresearch), reverse transcribed (Superscript II- Invitrogen™), and quantitative Real Time PCR (qRT-PCR) with gene specific primers using the LightCycler480®system (Roche Applied Science) was performed (Table 1). Data was normalized against Tbp and Gapdh references genes, with fold induction of transcripts calculated against the unstimulated control cells.

OA synovial membrane analysis

OA synovial membranes from 31 patients with different radiographic OA Kellgren-Lawrence scores were collected during knee arthroscopy (scores 0 to 3) or total knee joint replacement (score 4), fixed in 10% buffered formalin for 4 days, dehydrated, and embedded in paraffin. All the patients signed informed consent for obtaining synovial specimens of the operative tissue. The study was approved by the ethics committee of the University Hospital of Lausanne. Sections (6 μm) were stained with alizarin-red. For some OA synovial membranes, consecutive sections were analysed by immunohistochemistry. Macrophages, PMNs and endothelial cells in the synovium were detected using anti-CD68, anti-MPO or CD31 (all from Sigma-Aldrich, Buchs Switzerland) primary antibodies, respectively, and visualized as described in the immunohistochemistry section above. Synovial membrane tissues were also examined by Fourier-transform infrared spectroscopy (FTIR). Mineral phase was evaluated by FT-IR Bruker Vector 22 (BruckerSpectrospin, Wissembourg), according to analytical procedure using the KBr pellet method, as previously described [24,25].

Statistical analysis

All values are expressed as the mean ± SEM. Variation between data sets was evaluated using the Student's t test or one-way ANOVA test, where appropriate, with a 95% confidence interval. Differences were considered statistically significant for a value of $p < 0.05$. Data was analysed with GraphPad Prism software (GraphPad software).

Results

1. Intra-articular injection of BCP crystals induces synovial inflammation in mice

To assess the role of BCP crystals in cartilage degradation, we performed intra-articular injections of OCP crystals into mouse right knees and an equivalent volume of PBS into the contralateral knee. Joints were evaluated up to 30 days, using immuno/histology methods. We observed a persistent, significant increase in the degree of inflammation (up to day 30) as compared to PBS controls (which showed almost no inflammation at all time points examined), with peak inflammation observed at day 4 (Figure 1A and 1B). OCP crystals were still present in the joints 30 days post-injection, and were predominantly found within the synovial membrane as evidenced by Von Kossa staining (Figure 1C). At 6h, neutrophils predominated the inflammatory infiltrate (results not shown). At later times (d4 onwards), neutrophils were no longer abundant but the membranes showed prominent macrophage

Table 1 Gene specific primers for Real time PCR analysis.

Gene	Forward Primer (5′ 3′)	Reverse Primer (5′ 3′)
Ccl3	CCA AGT CTT CTC AGC GCC AT	TCC GGC TGT AGG AGA AGC AG
Tbp	CTT GAA ATC ATC CCT GCG AG	CGC TTT CAT TAA ATT CTT GAT GGT C
Sdc4	TCT TTG AGA GAA CTG AGG TCT TG	GTC GTA ACT GCC TTC GTC
Sdc1	GTG GCT GTA AAT GTT CCT CC	ACA GAA GGG AAG GAG TAC AT
S100a8	CCA TGC CCT CTA CAA GAA TGA	ATC ACC ATC GCA AGG AAC TC
S100a9	TTA CTT CCC ACA GCC TTT GC	AGG ACC TGG ACA CAA ACC AG
Rage Gapdh	ACA TGT GTG TCT GAG GGA AGC CTC ATG ACC ACA GTC CAT GC	AGC TCT GAC CGC AGT GTA AAG CAC ATT GGG GGT AGG AAC AC
Mmp3	ATA CGA GGG CAC GAG GAG	AGA AGT AGA GAA ACC CAA ATG CT
Mmp13	GCA GTT CCA AAG GCT ACA AC	GCT GGG TCA CAC TTC TCT G
Mmp9	AAT AAA GAC GAC ATA GAC GGC A	AAG AGC CCG CAG TAG GG
Mmp14 Il1a	CAG TAT GGC TAC CTA CCT CC AAA CAC TAT CTC AGC ACC ACT TG	TTG ATC TCA GTC CCA AAC TTA TCC GGT CGG TCT CAC TAC CTG TG
Il1b	CCA CCA ACA AGT GAT ATT CTC CAT G	GTG CCG TCT TTC ATT ACA CAG
Il6	CTG GAC CTC TGC CCT CTG G	TCC ATG GCC ACA ACA ACT GA
Tnfa	CAT CTT CTC AAA ATT CGA GTG ACA A	TGG GAG TAG ACA AGG TAC AAC CC
Adamst4	GCC CGA GTC CCA TTT CCC GC	GCC ATA ACC GTC AGC AGG TAG CG
Adamts5	GAC AGA CCTA CGA TGC CAC CCA GC	ATG AGC GAG AAC ACT GAC CCC AGG
Nos2	ACT ACT ACC AGA TCG AGC C	ACC ACT TTC ACC AAG ACT CTA
Ccl5	TCT CCC TAG AGC TGC CT	TCC TTG AAC CAA CTT CTT CTC TG
Cxcl1	GCC TAT CGC CAA TGA G	CTATGACTTCGGTTTGGG
Cxcl2	ATC CAG AGC TTG AGT GTG ACG C	AAG GCA AAC TTT TTG ACC GC

infiltration and the presence of occasional multinucleated giant cells with internalized crystals (Figure 1D). Almost no neovascularisation was found, as evidenced by ICAM staining (Figure 1D). We also assessed inflammation by ^{99m}Technetium (Tc) scintigraphy. OCP crystal injection induced a small but significant increase in Tc uptake in the knee joints that occurred as an early transient event that peaked at 24 hours, and returned to normal by 72 hours (Figure 1E). Similar histological features of inflammation were also observed with lower doses of OCP and HA crystals (20 μg) into the mouse knee (Figure 1F).

2. Intra-articular calcium crystals induced cartilage degradation

We evaluated the effects of crystal injection on cartilage integrity at different times following intra-articular injection. PBS injection into the contralateral knee served as a control. OCP crystals induced cartilage proteoglycan loss (PG) as evidenced by loss of Safranin-O staining (Figure 2A, and D) that was already present at day 4 and persisted through to d30. Signs of MMP-mediated aggrecan degradation were also observed by positive VDIPEN staining, that was prominent on d4 and d17, returning to near normal levels at d30 (Figure 2B and E). This was accompanied by chondrocyte apoptosis (Fig 2 C and F), which was maximal at d4. Therefore the sustained PG loss induced by BCP crystals (up to day 30) seemed to be accounted for by both early chondropoptosis (at day 4) and increased MMP activity (at day 4 and 17). However, no typical features of OA such as fissurations or fibrillations of cartilage were found. Taken together, these results indicate that calcium crystals are potent inducers of cartilage degradation as well as synovial inflammation.

3. Articular effects of BCP crystals are independent of IL-1 secretion or signalling

Previous data suggested that IL-1 might play a crucial role in the pathogenesis of OA, and that inflammasome activation leading to IL-1β secretion may be important. We investigated the contributions of IL-1 signalling to synovial inflammation and cartilage degradation in this model, using mice deficient for components of the inflammasome, IL-1α and IL-1β. We also tested if IL-1 inhibition using IL-1ra (anakinra) modified the joint pathology.

Knee joints of NLRP3 and ASC deficient mice injected with BCP crystals had similar inflammation, PG loss and VDIPEN-staining scores compared to WT mice (Figure 3A, B, C, D). These results suggest that the NLRP3-inflammasome pathway of IL-1β production is not necessary in crystal-mediated cartilage destruction. To test if either IL-1α or-β were directly involved, we then injected crystals into knee joints of IL-1β or IL-1α deficient mice or WT mice. We observed no significant reduction of inflammation or cartilage damage in the deficient mice (Figure 3E). Finally, we investigated the effects of IL-1Ra, which blocks the binding of both IL-1α and -β to the IL-1 receptor (IL-1R). Mice were injected

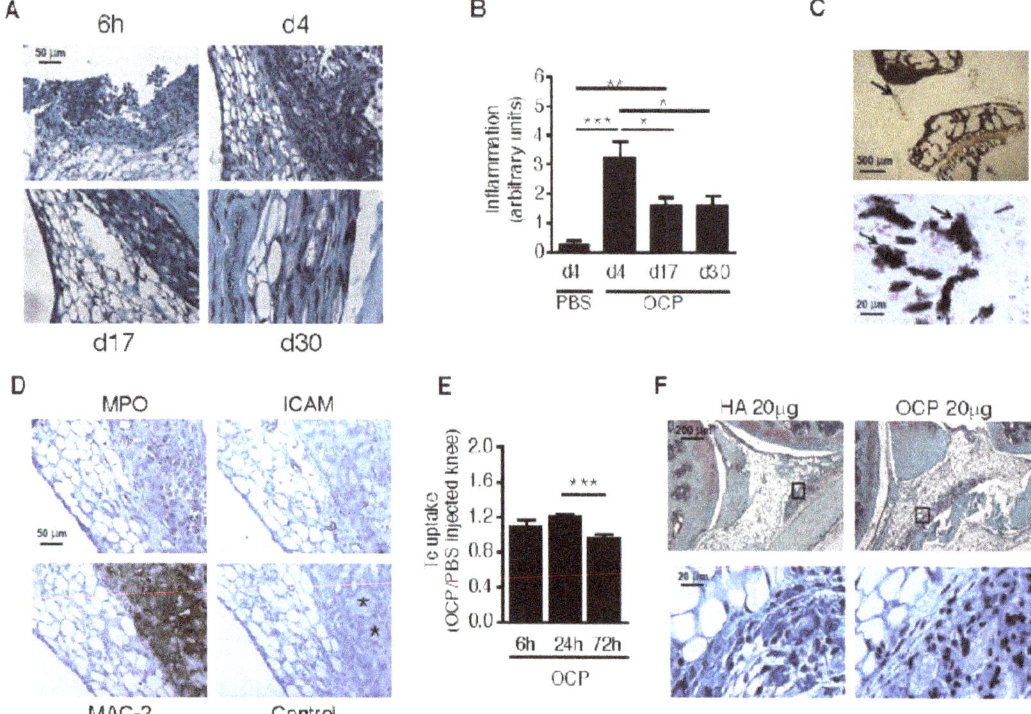

Figure 1. Intra-articular BCP crystals induce synovial inflammation and cartilage proteoglycan loss in mice. OCP crystals (200 μg/20 μl) were injected into right knees of C57BL/6 mice whereas 20 μl PBS was injected into the left knees (A–E). Knees were harvested at different times (day 4, 17 and 30 n = 8 mice per group). Sections were stained with fast green/iron hematoxylin (A) and the degree of inflammation was assessed at the different time points (B). Since the inflammation was very low and similar at all time points in the PBS-injected control knees, only data from PBS-injected knees at day 4 was shown in B. OCP crystal deposition in the synovial membrane was evidenced at day 30 after OCP crystals injection by Von Kossa staining (see arrows) (C). Macrophage, endothelial and PMN cells were detected using antibodies for MAC-2, ICAM, and MPO, respectively, at day 4 after OCP injection (D). Isotype controls allowed the identification of giant cells that had engulfed tissue crystal deposits (*) (D). Ratio of Tc uptake between OCP-injected (n = 8) versus PBS controls was calculated (E). Fast green/iron hematoxylin staining of knees injected with 20 μg/20 μl of HA or OCP crystal at day 4 (F). Results are expressed as mean ± S.E.M with significance being at * $p<0.05$, ** $p<0.01$, *** $p<0.001$.

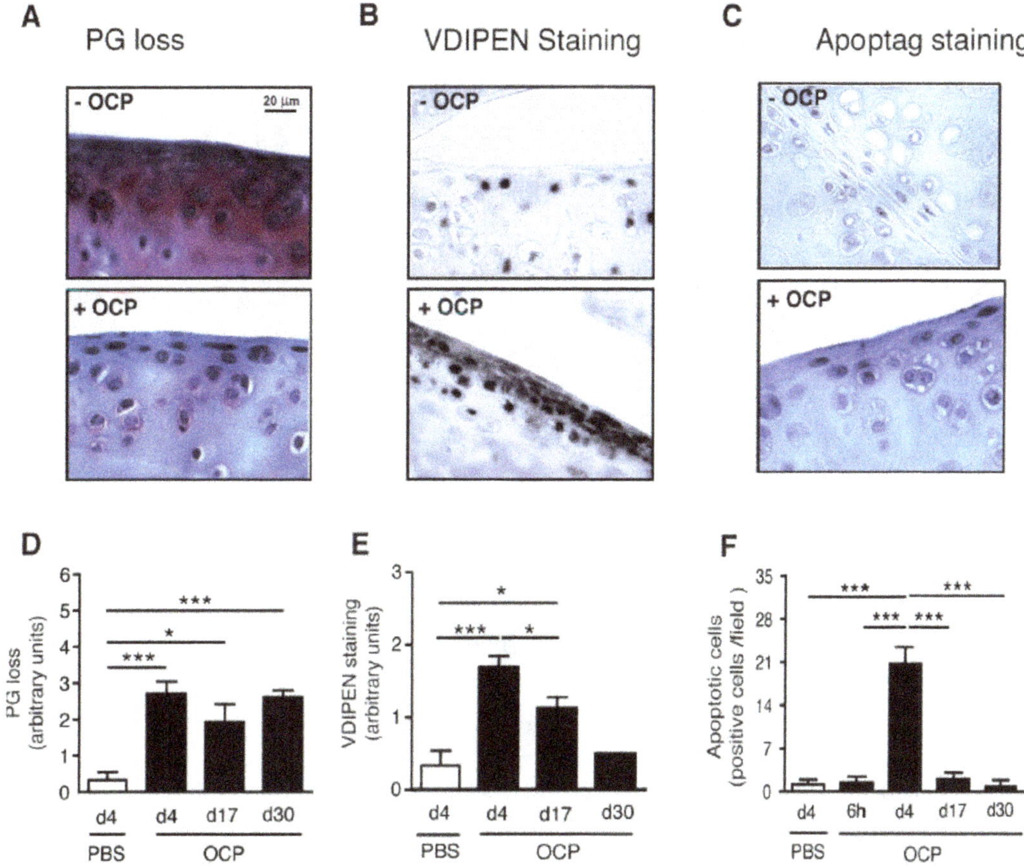

Figure 2. OCP crystals induce cartilage degradation. C57BL/6 mice were injected with OCP crystals (OCP+) or PBS (OCP-). Knees harvested at different times (day 4, 17 and 30 n=8 mice per group) were assessed for cartilage PGs with Safranin-O (A), aggrecan degradation via VDIPEN immunohistochemistry (B) and apoptosis (C). Since at all time points, data from PBS-injected control knees were similar, only data from PBS-injected knees at day 4 were shown in D, E, and F. Scoring of PG loss and VDIPEN staining was performed on sections, using a scale of 0 to 6 and 0 to 3, respectively (D and E). Apoptotic chondrocytes were counted per field of view (F). Results are expressed as mean ± S.E.M with significance being at * $p<0.05$, ** $p<0.01$, *** $p<0.001$

twice daily i.p. with recombinant anakinra at 200 µg per mouse for 4 days prior to sacrifice, at day 5. The treatment had no effect on crystal-induced synovial inflammation, PG depletion, or VDIPEN staining (Figure 3F).

4. OCP crystals induce the expression of matrix degrading genes by macrophages

In view of the predominant macrophage infiltrate within the synovium of OCP injected mice, we hypothesized that crystals induce the expression of macrophage genes that lead to cartilage damage. We stimulated bone marrow derived macrophages from mice with OCP crystals, and analysed by qRT-PCR the expression of inflammatory cytokine and matrix modifying genes (Figure 4).We found dramatically increased expression (>10x compared to control) of *ADAMTS4*, syndecan 1 (*SDC1*), *MMP3* and *9*, *CXCL1* and *CXCL2*, as well as the cytokines *ILA, IL1B, IL6 and TNFA*. The alarmins *S100A8* and *A9* were also upregulated significantly (Figure 4).

5. BCP crystals and synovial inflammation in OA patients

In parallel to the murine joints evaluation, we analyzed synovial membranes from six OA patients obtained at time of knee joint replacement. All synovial tissues stained positively by alizarin red. In addition, we observed that calcium crystal deposits were surrounded by inflammatory cells, mainly macrophages, as shown by CD68 immunohistochemistry, while neutrophil and endothelial staining was much less abundant (Figure 5A). Analysis with Fourier-transformed infrared spectroscopy (FTIR) clearly showed the presence of BCP crystals, specifically CA (Figure 5B) (17, 18). Thus, the histological findings in human OA synovium were very similar to those observed in the mouse knee joint injected with BCP crystals. Finally, we explored the presence of calcium crystals in a series of synovial membranes harvested during arthroscopy performed in patients with different OA severity stages (Kellgren-Lawrence grades from 0 to 4). Calcium crystals were detected at all stages (except grade 3, were only 2 synovial membranes were analysed). Very interestingly, a significant proportion of synovial membranes from patients not yet diagnosed for OA, were alizarin-red positive (Figure 5C).

Discussion

The role of calcium phosphate crystals in the pathogenesis of OA is still under debate. Although BCP crystals are highly prevalent in the cartilage of patients presenting for knee and hip surgery in advanced OA [3,26], there has only been one report of BCP crystals in the synovium [27]. In this study, we showed that calcium-containing microcrystals are found in the 6 synovial membranes in OA at time of joint replacement. We also detected

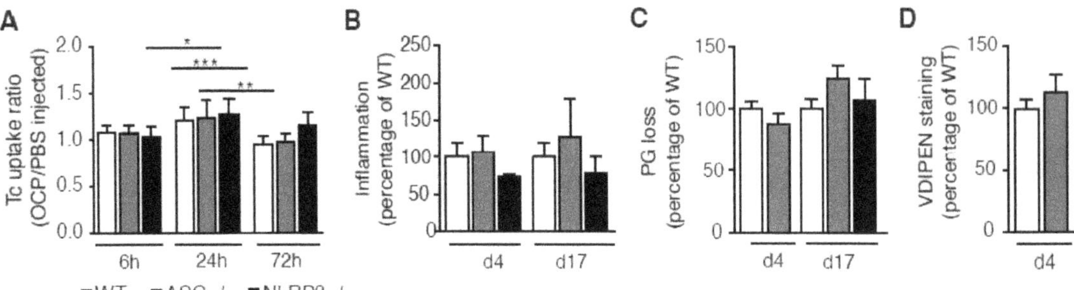

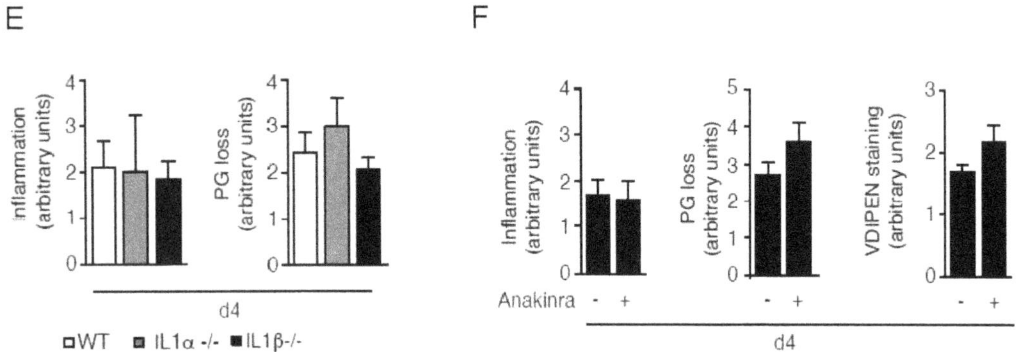

Figure 3. OCP crystal-induced inflammation and cartilage degradation is NLRP3 inflammasome- and IL-1 independent. WT (n = 6), ASC-/- (n = 4), NLRP3-/- (n = 6), IL-1α-/- (n = 5) and IL-1β-/- (n = 6) mice were injected i.a. with OCP crystals (200 µg in 20 µl) or PBS. In a second set of experiment, anakinra, the recombinant form of IL-1Ra, or PBS were injected for 4 days (7 mice per group), the first injection being 30 min prior to OCP injection into the knee of WT (F). Ratio of isotope uptake into OCP injected knee versus PBS-injected ones was calculated at different time points (A). Synovial inflammation (B, E, F), cartilage PG loss (C, E, F) and VDIPEN immunohistochemistries (D, F) were assessed. Results are expressed as % of scores against WT (B,C,D) or in arbitrary units (E, F), and represent mean ± S.E.M. of at least n = 4 mice per group. For p values, * = $p<0.05$, ** = $p<0.01$, *** = $p<0.001$.

crystals in synovial membrane from low-grade OA (Kellgren-Lawrence score 1–2) and from non affected OA knees (Kellgren-Lawrence score 0). In some cases, we confirmed their composition as BCP using FTIR spectroscopy. The presence of BCP crystals in

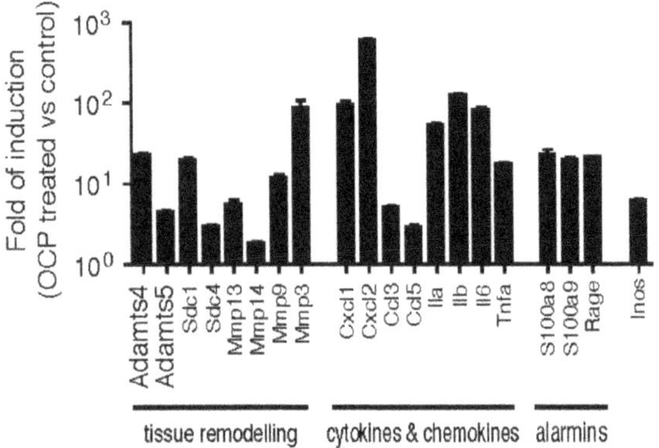

Figure 4. OCP crystals induce macrophage expression of genes involved in inflammation and cartilage degradation. Bone marrow derived macrophages were stimulated *in vitro* with 500 µg/ml of OCP crystals for 4 hours. RNA was extracted, reverse transcribed and qRT-PCR performed using gene specific primers with Tbp, and Gapdh as reference genes. Results are expressed as the fold induction of OCP treated over unstimulated macrophages, using the mean ± S.E.M of triplicate samples.

the synovium suggests that they may be a cause of low-grade inflammation as well as a stimulus for cartilage breakdown. To investigate these effects in more detail, we decided to develop an animal model whereby BCP crystals were injected into the knee joint in vivo. Our findings suggest that BCP crystals do exert a biological effect that is relevant to the pathogenesis of OA.

Following injection of BCP crystals, we observed an early, transient increase in neutrophil recruitment in the synovium at 6 hours post -injection, which was then replaced by a macrophage and multinucleated giant cell rich infiltrate that persisted till day 30. This was observed using different concentrations of OCP crystals as well as a low dose of HA. We also found that the injected crystals persisted within the joint, and were still detectable at up to 30 days when the synovium was stained using von Kossa or alizarin. In the human OA samples, BCP crystal deposits in the synovium co-localized frequently with macrophage infiltration. Similar histological changes have been reported in patients with BCP-associated arthropathy, such as the Milwaukee shoulder syndrome [28] and in canine knee joints that had been injected with calcium pyrophosphate crystals [29]. Additionally, calcium pyrophosphate crystals injected into rabbit knees worsened cartilage OA lesions induced by meniscectomy along with same pattern of synovial inflammation including macrophage infiltration and formation of multinucleated giant cells [30]. Altogether, these results suggest that synovial deposition of calcium-containing crystals leads to synovial inflammation and may enhance joint damage.

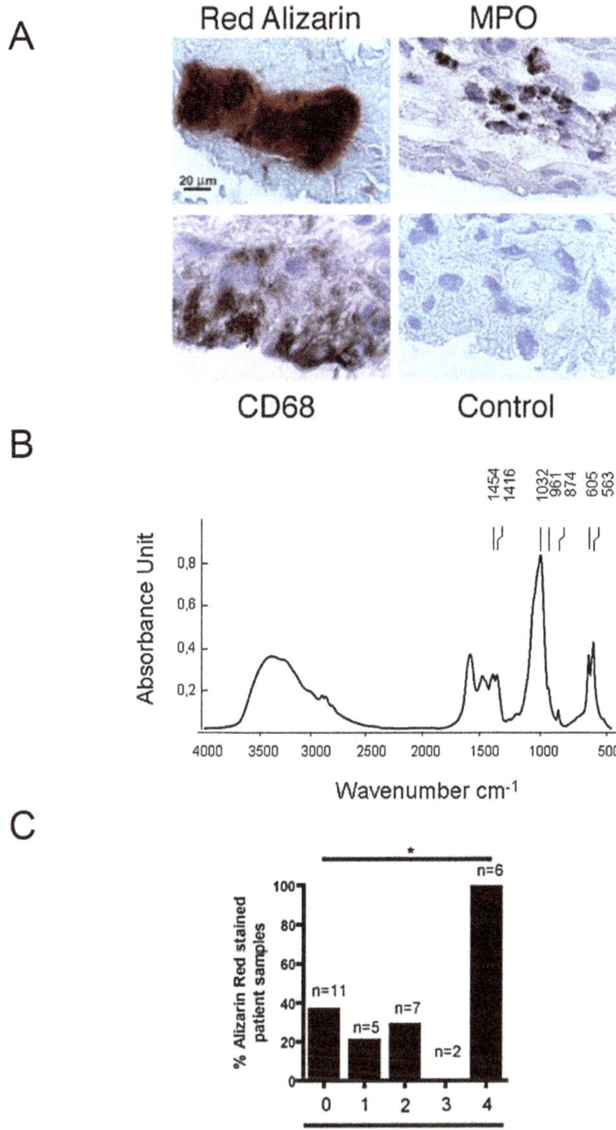

Figure 5. OA synovial membranes contained BCP crystals. Consecutive paraffin sections of OA synoviums were analyzed with alizarin-red staining or by immunohistochemistry using anti-CD68 and anti-MPO primary antibodies (A). Biochemical composition of calcium-containing crystals in OA synovial membranes was assessed by FTIR spectroscopy, displaying a characteristic spectrum of Carbonated apatite (CA), with an absorption band peak at approximately 1035 cm-1 (B). Synovial membranes of different OA grades as assessed by Kellgren Lawrence score were harvested during arthroscopy. FTIR analysis showed the frequent presence of CA crystals in synovium membranes (C).

Crystal-induced synovitis was accompanied by loss of Safranin-O staining and the appearance of the VDIPEN epitope in cartilage. This epitope, generated by MMPs' degradation of aggrecan, provides evidence that matrix degradation enzymes are activated within the joint. The cellular sources of these enzymes are multiple. Synovial fibroblasts, synovial macrophages, PMNs and chondrocytes can all produce MMPs, but macrophages are likely to be a major source. We confirmed that transcription of a range of molecules implicated in tissue remodelling was upregulated in BMDM following contact with BCP crystals. The genes include MMPs and ADAMTs. Increased MMP activities have been detected in the synovial fluid of patients with BCP-associated arthropathy [28] and are produced by several cell types.

Other molecules that have been demonstrated to participate in cartilage metabolism or to play a role in the development of experimental OA include the syndecans, the alarmins S100A8 and A9 as well as the inflammatory cytokines IL-1α and -β, TNF-α and IL-6. Their transcription was strongly upregulated by BCP crystals.

As there is a body of evidence that suggests that IL1 plays an important role in OA, and BCP crystals can stimulate IL-1β release by activation of the NLRP3-inflammasome, we expected that mice deficient for components of these pathways would demonstrate an attenuated phenotype following intra-articular injection. Surprisingly, all the deficient strains tested did not demonstrate a reduction in signs of synovial inflammation nor cartilage degradation. We have also tested mice that are deficient in MyD88, TLR-1, -2, -4 and -6 and found no difference in the histological findings (supplement results Fig S1). These results could be explained either by the involvement of cytokines other than IL-1, such as IL-6 and TNF-α, that have been shown to have catabolic effects on cartilage [14] or by pathways of chondrocyte activation that are independent of cytokines. Thus, it was recently shown that mechanical-induced MMP production and cartilage destruction was independent of NLRP3 inflammasome and IL-1 [31]. Monosodium urate (MSU) crystals have been shown to activate Syk kinase following interaction with phospholipids of cell membrane in a receptor independent manner [32], and aluminium crystals as well as MSU activate Syk kinase, PIP3 kinase and prostaglandin synthesis in an inflammasome-independent manner [33]. Very recently, Cunningham et al. showed that BCP crystals induced the production of inflammatory cytokines (IL-1β, IL-1α and TNF-α) by macrophages via Syk and PIP 3 kinase pathways [34]. However, Ng et al. have suggested that Syk was not involved by BCP crystals in dentritic cells [32,35]. These differences may be secondary to cell types and the characteristics of BCP crystals. Furthers investigations are warranted to clarify this important finding.

In summary, we provide evidence that intra-articular BCP crystals in mouse knees induce synovial inflammation, cartilage degradation and chondrocyte apoptosis and these processes could play a part in the pathogenesis of OA. The findings closely resemble the histological picture seen in patients with moderate and severe OA and suggest that they are of pathologic relevance. The effects observed were independent of the inflammasome-IL-1 pathway that had been described for microcrystal-induced inflammation. We suggest this model may be useful in furthering our understanding of how microcrystals participate in the development or progression of OA.

Supporting Information

Figure S1 OCP crystal-induced effects are not mediated by TLRs and MyD88. Wild-type (WT, n = 10) or knock-out (KO) mice for TLR-1 (n = 8), -2 (n = 12), -4 (n = 10), and -6 (n = 9) and Myd88 (n = 8) mice were injected i.a with 200 µg of OCP crystals into the right knee, the left knee being injected with PBS. Mice were sacrificed at day 4 and histology was performed on the knee joints for inflammation using fast green/iron hematoxylin (A), or PG loss using Safranin O (B). Results are expressed as the mean ± S.E.M with significance being at * $p<0.05$, ** $p<0.01$, *** $p<0.001$.
(TIF)

Acknowledgments

We thank Dr Thierry Roger (Department of infectious diseases, CHUV, Lausanne, Switzerland) for his continuous support, Dr. Catherine Ronet (Department of Biochemistry, University of Lausanne- Switzerland) for her expertise in real time PCR. All the authors (except PVL and BJH) are members of the European Crystal Research Network formed after the 1st European Crystal Workshop in Paris on 11 & 12 March, 2010 (convenors: Prof. Frédéric Lioté, Paris; and Prof. Alexander So, Lausanne).

Author Contributions

Obtained permission for human synovial study: AS BJH DVL NB. Permission for animal studies: HKE FL AS NB. Funding: HKE FL AS NB. Conceived and designed the experiments: HKE VC CN GM BJH DVL AS FL NB. Performed the experiments: HKE VC CN SN PVL MD AD DB BJH AI DVL. Analyzed the data: HKE VC SN PVL MD AD DB GM BJH AI DVL AS FL NB . Contributed reagents/materials/analysis tools: VC SN PVL MD AD DB BJH DVL AI. Wrote the paper: HKE PVL MD DB GM BJH DVL AI AS FL NB.

References

1. Ea HK, Nguyen C, Bazin D, Bianchi A, Guicheux J, et al. (2011) Articular cartilage calcification in osteoarthritis: insights into crystal-induced stress. Arthritis Rheum 63: 10–18.
2. Halverson PB, Cheung HS, McCarty DJ, Garancis J, Mandel N (1981) "Milwaukee shoulder"--association of microspheroids containing hydroxyapatite crystals, active collagenase, and neutral protease with rotator cuff defects. II. Synovial fluid studies. Arthritis Rheum 24: 474–483.
3. Fuerst M, Bertrand J, Lammers L, Dreier R, Echtermeyer F, et al. (2009) Calcification of articular cartilage in human osteoarthritis. Arthritis Rheum 60: 2694–2703.
4. Mitsuyama H, Healey RM, Terkeltaub RA, Coutts RD, Amiel D (2007) Calcification of human articular knee cartilage is primarily an effect of aging rather than osteoarthritis. Osteoarthritis Cartilage 15: 559–565.
5. Scotchford CA, Greenwald S, Ali SY (1992) Calcium phosphate crystal distribution in the superficial zone of human femoral head articular cartilage. J Anat 181 (Pt 2): 293–300.
6. Sun Y, Mauerhan DR, Honeycutt PR, Kneisl JS, Norton HJ, et al. (2010) Calcium deposition in osteoarthritic meniscus and meniscal cell culture. Arthritis Res Ther 12: R56.
7. Roemhildt ML, Beynnon BD, Gardner-Morse M (2012) Mineralization of articular cartilage in the Sprague-Dawley rat: characterization and mechanical analysis. Osteoarthritis Cartilage 20: 796–800.
8. Ea HK, Liote F (2009) Advances in understanding calcium-containing crystal disease. Curr Opin Rheumatol 21: 150–157.
9. Molloy ES, Morgan MP, Doherty GA, McDonnell B, O'Byrne J, et al. (2009) Microsomal prostaglandin E2 synthase 1 expression in basic calcium phosphate crystal-stimulated fibroblasts: role of prostaglandin E2 and the EP4 receptor. Osteoarthritis Cartilage 17: 686–692.
10. Ea HK, Monceau V, Camors E, Cohen-Solal M, Charlemagne D, et al. (2008) Annexin 5 overexpression increased articular chondrocyte apoptosis induced by basic calcium phosphate crystals. Ann Rheum Dis 67: 1617–1625.
11. Ea HK, Uzan B, Rey C, Liote F (2005) Octacalcium phosphate crystals directly stimulate expression of inducible nitric oxide synthase through p38 and JNK mitogen-activated protein kinases in articular chondrocytes. Arthritis Res Ther 7: R915–926.
12. Narayan S, Pazar B, Ea HK, Kolly L, Bagnoud N, et al. (2011) Octacalcium phosphate crystals induce inflammation in vivo through interleukin-1 but independent of the NLRP3 inflammasome in mice. Arthritis Rheum 63: 422–433.
13. Pazar B, Ea HK, Narayan S, Kolly L, Bagnoud N, et al. (2011) Basic calcium phosphate crystals induce monocyte/macrophage IL-1beta secretion through the NLRP3 inflammasome in vitro. J Immunol 186: 2495–2502.
14. Kapoor M, Martel-Pelletier J, Lajeunesse D, Pelletier JP, Fahmi H (2011) Role of proinflammatory cytokines in the pathophysiology of osteoarthritis. Nat Rev Rheumatol 7: 33–42.
15. Bacconnier L, Jorgensen C, Fabre S (2009) Erosive osteoarthritis of the hand: clinical experience with anakinra. Ann Rheum Dis 68: 1078–1079.
16. Chevalier X, Goupille P, Beaulieu AD, Burch FX, Bensen WG, et al. (2009) Intraarticular injection of anakinra in osteoarthritis of the knee: a multicenter, randomized, double-blind, placebo-controlled study. Arthritis Rheum 61: 344–352.
17. Horai R, Asano M, Sudo K, Kanuka H, Suzuki M, et al. (1998) Production of mice deficient in genes for interleukin (IL)-1alpha, IL-1beta, IL-1alpha/beta, and IL-1 receptor antagonist shows that IL-1beta is crucial in turpentine-induced fever development and glucocorticoid secretion. J Exp Med 187: 1463–1475.
18. Mariathasan S, Newton K, Monack DM, Vucic D, French DM, et al. (2004) Differential activation of the inflammasome by caspase-1 adaptors ASC and Ipaf. Nature 430: 213–218.
19. Martinon F, Petrilli V, Mayor A, Tardivel A, Tschopp J (2006) Gout-associated uric acid crystals activate the NALP3 inflammasome. Nature 440: 237–241.
20. Prudhommeaux F, Schiltz C, Liote F, Hina A, Champy R, et al. (1996) Variation in the inflammatory properties of basic calcium phosphate crystals according to crystal type. Arthritis Rheum 39: 1319–1326.
21. Busso N, Peclat V, Van Ness K, Kolodziesczyk E, Degen J, et al. (1998) Exacerbation of antigen-induced arthritis in urokinase-deficient mice. J Clin Invest 102: 41–50.
22. Horn DA, Garrett IR (2004) A novel method for embedding neonatal murine calvaria in methyl methacrylate suitable for visualizing mineralization, cellular and structural detail. Biotech Histochem 79: 151–158.
23. van Lent P, Blom A, Schelbergen R, Sloetjes A, Lafeber F, et al. (2011) Active involvement of "alarmins" S100A8 and S100A9 in regulation of synovial activation and joint destruction during mouse and human osteoarthritis. Arthritis Rheum.
24. Estepa-Maurice L, Hennequin C, Marfisi C, Bader C, Lacour B, et al. (1996) Fourier transform infrared microscopy identification of crystal deposits in tissues: clinical importance in various pathologies. Am J Clin Pathol 105: 576–582.
25. Nguyen C, Ea HK, Thiaudiere D, Reguer S, Hannouche D, et al. (2011) Calcifications in human osteoarthritic articular cartilage: ex vivo assessment of calcium compounds using XANES spectroscopy. J Synchrotron Radiat 18: 475–480.
26. Fuerst M, Niggemeyer O, Lammers L, Schafer F, Lohmann C, et al. (2009) Articular cartilage mineralization in osteoarthritis of the hip. BMC Musculoskelet Disord 10: 166.
27. Van Linthoudt D, Beutler A, Clayburne G, Sieck M, Fernandes L, et al. (1997) Morphometric studies on synovium in advanced osteoarthritis: is there an association between apatite-like material and collagen deposits? Clin Exp Rheumatol 15: 493–497.
28. Halverson PB, Garancis JC, McCarty DJ (1984) Histopathological and ultrastructural studies of synovium in Milwaukee shoulder syndrome--a basic calcium phosphate crystal arthropathy. Ann Rheum Dis 43: 734–741.
29. McCarty DJ, Jr., Phelps P, Pyenson J (1966) Crystal-induced inflammation in canine joints. I. An experimental model with quantification of the host response. J Exp Med 124: 99–114.
30. Fam AG, Morava-Protzner I, Purcell C, Young BD, Bunting PS, Lewis AJ (1995) Acceleration of experimental lapine osteoarthritis by calcium pyrophosphate microcrystalline synovitis. Arthritis Rheum 38: 201–210.
31. Bougault C, Gosset M, Houard X, Salvat C, Godmann L, et al. (2012) Stress-induced cartilage degradation does not depend on NLRP3 inflammasome in osteoarthritis. Arthritis Rheum.
32. Ng G, Sharma K, Ward SM, Desrosiers MD, Stephens LA, et al. (2008) Receptor-independent, direct membrane binding leads to cell-surface lipid sorting and Syk kinase activation in dendritic cells. Immunity 29: 807–818.
33. Kool M, Willart MA, van Nimwegen M, Bergen I, Pouliot P, et al. (2011) An unexpected role for uric acid as an inducer of T helper 2 cell immunity to inhaled antigens and inflammatory mediator of allergic asthma. Immunity 34: 527–540.
34. Cunningham CC, Mills E, Mielke LA, O'Farrell LK, Lavelle E et al. (2012) Osteoarthritis-associated basic calcium phosphate crystals induce pro-inflammatory cytokines and damage-associated molecules via activation of Syk and PI3 kinase. Clin Immunol 144: 228–236.
35. Shi Y, Evans JE, Rock KL (2003) Molecular identification of a danger signal that alerts the immune system to dying cells. Nature 425: 516–521.

3

Synovial Fluid Progenitors Expressing CD90+ from Normal but Not Osteoarthritic Joints Undergo Chondrogenic Differentiation without Micro-Mass Culture

Roman J. Krawetz[1,2*], Yiru Elizabeth Wu[1], Liam Martin[3], Jerome B. Rattner[2], John R. Matyas[4], David A. Hart[1]

1 Department of Surgery, University of Calgary, Calgary, Alberta, Canada, 2 Department of Cell Biology and Anatomy, University of Calgary, Calgary, Alberta, Canada, 3 Department of Medicine, University of Calgary, Calgary, Alberta, Canada, 4 Department of Comparative Biology and Experimental Medicine, Faculty of Veterinary Medicine, University of Calgary, Calgary, Alberta, Canada

Abstract

Objective: Mesenchymal progenitor cells (MPCs) can differentiate into osteoblasts, adipocytes, and chondrocytes, and are in part responsible for maintaining tissue integrity. Recently, a progenitor cell population has been found within the synovial fluid that shares many similarities with bone marrow MPCs. These synovial fluid MPCs (sfMPCs) share the ability to differentiate into bone and fat, with a bias for cartilage differentiation. In this study, sfMPCs were isolated from human and canine synovial fluid collected from normal individuals and those with osteoarthritis (human: clinician-diagnosed, canine: experimental) to compare the differentiation potential of CD90+ vs. CD90− sfMPCs, and to determine if CD90 (Thy-1) is a predictive marker of synovial fluid progenitors with chondrogenic capacity *in vitro*.

Methods: sfMPCs were derived from synovial fluid from normal and OA knee joints. These cells were induced to differentiate into chondrocytes and analyzed using quantitative PCR, immunofluorescence, and electron microscopy.

Results: The CD90+ subpopulation of sfMPCs had increased chondrogenic potential compared to the CD90− population. Furthermore, sfMPCs derived from healthy joints did not require a micro-mass step for efficient chondrogenesis. Whereas sfMPCs from OA synovial fluid retain the ability to undergo chondrogenic differentiation, they require micro-mass culture conditions.

Conclusions: Overall, this study has demonstrated an increased chondrogenic potential within the CD90+ fraction of human and canine sfMPCs and that this population of cells derived from healthy normal joints do not require a micro-mass step for efficient chondrogenesis, while sfMPCs obtained from OA knee joints do not differentiate efficiently into chondrocytes without the micro-mass procedure. These results reveal a fundamental shift in the chondrogenic ability of cells isolated from arthritic joint fluids, and we speculate that the mechanism behind this change of cell behavior is exposure to the altered milieu of the OA joint fluid, which will be examined in further studies.

Editor: Irina Kerkis, Instituto Butantan, Brazil

Funding: This study was supported by research grants from Pfizer, Alberta Innovates-Health Solutions team grant in osteoarthritis, and Canadian Institutes for Health Research (MOP 79384). The funders had no role in study design, data collection and analysis, decision to publish, or preparation of the manuscript.

Competing Interests: The authors have the following interest: This study was partly funded by Pfizer Inc. There are no patents, products in development or marketed products to declare. This does not alter the authors' adherence to all the PLOS ONE policies on sharing data and materials, as detailed online in the guide for authors.

* E-mail: rkrawetz@ucalgary.ca

Introduction

Within the last decade, the synovium and synovial fluid have been identified as a source of mesenchymal progenitor/stem cells (sMPCs) that are functionally distinct from bone marrow MPCs [1–7]. Furthermore, these synovial membrane (smMPCs) and sfMPCs can assist in cartilage repair both *in vivo* and *in vitro* [8–11]. There is compelling evidence that these cells can be used effectively to promote cartilage repair [1–11]. sfMPCs reportedly have increased chondrogenic potential [12,13] compared to bone marrow-derived mesenchymal stem cells (bmMPCs), including increased expression of the hyaluronan receptor CD44 [13,14] and uridine diphosphoglucose dehydrogenase (UDPGD), an enzyme required for hyaluronan synthesis. Notably, bmMPCs and other MPC populations do not express UDPGD [13,14]. Evidence from *in vivo* studies have demonstrated that when partial-thickness defects in the articular cartilage of rabbits are formed, a continuous cell layer extending from the synovial membrane is observed to contribute to the repair of the cartilage either with or without chondrogenic inducers present [9,10]. In addition, pig and human sfMPCs have been transformed *in vitro* into scaffolds termed Tissue Engineering Constructs (TECs) that can be used to repair cartilaginous defects (in pigs) *in vivo* [6,7]. Additionally, another group has recently demonstrated that smMPCs have the ability to bind directly to cartilage *ex vivo* in minutes, and are able to contribute to cartilage repair in a defect model [11]. Human sfMPCs are typically characterized using cluster of differentiation (CD) antigens [15]: CD105 (Endoglin), CD90 (Thy-1), CD73 (Ecto-5′-nucleotidase) and CD44 are present on the surface of MPCs/MSCs, while CD45 (Protein tyrosine phosphatase, receptor type, C) and CD11b (Integrin alpha M) are not expressed by this cell population [15]. The present study focuses on CD90 (Thy-1), which has been shown to interact with Integrins, tyrosine kinases, growth factors, and cytokines thereby promoting downstream cellular events including: adhesion, apoptosis, proliferation, and migration [16]. CD90 is commonly used as a marker of MPCs/MSCs, though it is also expressed by many other cell types including neurons, endothelial cells, T-cells, and other immune/non-immune cell types [16]. More recently, CD90 has been utilized as a selection marker of multi-potent progenitors from bone marrow, synovial tissues, fat, amnion and other tissues [17]. However, the exact role of CD90 on the surface of this class of cells remains unknown.

A number of recent studies have begun to explore the role of sfMPCs in diseases, including arthritis. Initial reports suggested that there was no difference in the chondrogenic potential of sfMPCs derived from healthy joints and joints with osteoarthritis (OA) or rheumatoid arthritis (RA) [2], notwithstanding the increase in number of sfMPCs in the OA knees [2]. A more recent study by the same group reported that the inflammatory intra-articular environment in RA joints is responsible for the reduced chondrogenic potential of sfMPCs [18]. As OA is generally viewed primarily as a degenerative rather than an inflammatory joint disease, it seems that the milieu of RA and OA joints has a fundamentally different influence on the capacity of sfMPCs to proliferate and differentiate. If, as has been speculated, sfMPCs participate in processes of joint maintenance or repair after injury [9,10], a fuller understanding of sfMPCs is warranted as they are potential therapeutic targets for these common and debilitating joint diseases.

In a recent study where synovial membrane stem cells were obtained from OA patients and differentiated using a micro-mass tissue culture, a significant positive correlation was observed between CD90 expression and chondrogenic differentiation [19]. Therefore, the aim of the present study is a comparison of the chondrogenic potential of sfMPCs (human and canine) isolated from normal and osteoarthritic synovial fluid.

Results

Differentiation potential of normal and OA derived sfMPCs

To evaluate the chondrogenic potential of human sfMPCs (CD105+, CD73+, CD44+, CD45−. CD11b−) and canine sfMPCs (CD45−, CD34−) derived from normal and OA synovial fluid, the cells were differentiated into chondrocytes with media supplements over a 14 day period with a prior micro-mass aggregation step. At days 0, 3, 5, 8 and 14, mRNA was collected and probed using qRT-PCR for Sox9, Collagen 2, and Aggrecan (Figure 1 A,E,H,L). By day 14, Sox9, Collagen 2 and Aggrecan were significantly elevated compared to day 0 controls in normal (Figure 1 A,E) and OA (Figure 1 H,L) sfMPCs derived from human and canine synovial fluid. Immunofluorescence confirmed the qRT-PCR data using a Collagen 2 antibody on day 14. sfMPC-derived chondrogenic masses from normal (Figure 1 B,F) and OA (Figure 1 I,M) fluid expressed Collagen 2 protein on day 14. Secondary antibody alone controls demonstrated minimal non-specific staining in human (Figure 1 C) and canine (Figure 1 J) sfMPCs. Furthermore, the micro-masses generated from all conditions stained with Alcian blue (Figure 1 D,G,K,N).

Enhanced Chondrogenic Differentiation of CD90+ sfMPCs

Since the human and canine sfMPCs contained CD90 positive and negative cells, the chondrogenic potential of the CD90-positive and CD90-negative fractions within the sfMPC population were studied. Previously isolated sfMPCs (Figure 2) were further enriched for CD90 using immuno-magnetic separation, with the resultant CD90-positive and CD90-negative fractions induced to differentiate into chondrocytes utilizing a micro-mass step (Figure 2). CD90+ sfMPCs from normal individuals (human and canine) behaved in a similar fashion to the total sfMPC population, displaying significantly increased levels of Sox9, type II Collagen, and Aggrecan mRNA (Figure 2 A,K) and demonstrated positive staining for Alcian blue (Figure 2 B,L) and Collagen 2 (Figure 2 C,M) by day 14. The CD90-negative fraction displayed reduced levels of Sox9, Collagen 2 and Aggrecan mRNA (although significantly increased compared to day 0)(Figure 2 A,K), as well as less intense alcian blue (Figure 2 D,N) and Collagen 2 (Figure 2 E, O) staining at day 14 of differentiation compared to the CD90+ population. Similarly, human and canine CD90+ sfMPCs from OA fluid demonstrated increased Sox9, Collagen 2 and Aggrecan mRNA expression (Figure 2 F,P), as well as staining with alcian blue (Figure 2 G,Q) and Collagen 2 (Figure 2 H,R) compared to the CD90− sfMPCs. Specifically, the mRNA level (Figure 2 F,P) and staining with alcian blue (Figure 2 I,S) and Collagen 2 (Figure 2 J,T) were decreased in the CD90− sfMPCs compared to the CD90+ sfMPCs.

To examine if there were any differences in the osteogenic or adipogenic capacity of CD90+/− human sfMPCs (normal & OA), the cells were placed in adipogenic or osteogenic conditions and allowed to differentiate for 20 days (Figure 3). After 20 days of differentiation, the cells were stained for Alkaline phosphatase (Figure 3 A) or Oil Red-O (Figure 3 B), and assayed using qPCR for Adiponectin, PPAR-gamma, Osteonectin and Osterix (Sp7) (Figure 3 C–F). Using these outcome measures, no differences in osteogenic or adipogenic differentiation capacity were observed between normal and OA sfMPCs, or CD90+/− sub-populations of either group.

Chondrogenesis of normal CD90-positive sfMPCs without a prior micro-mass step

Based on the foregoing results, the chondrogenic potential of normal and OA sfMPSc were studied without micro-mass culture. Without a prior micro-mass step, normal sfMPCs from human (Figure 4 A) and canine (Figure 4 D) up-regulated Sox 9, Collagen 2 and Aggrecan mRNA during differentiation. In contrast, the Sox 9, Collagen 2 and Aggrecan mNRA levels in OA sfMPCs were significantly lower (Figure 4 A,D). Normal (human and canine) sfMPCs aggregated into small tissue-like structures during differentiation (Figure 4 B,G); OA-derived sfMPCs (human and canine) did not aggregate (Figure 4 C,F).

CD90-positive Cells Form a Tissue-like Structure

The tissue-like structures formed by normal CD90+ sfMPCs stained positively with antibodies against Aggrecan (Figure 5 A) and Collagen 2 (Figure 5 C). When visualized with TEM, these

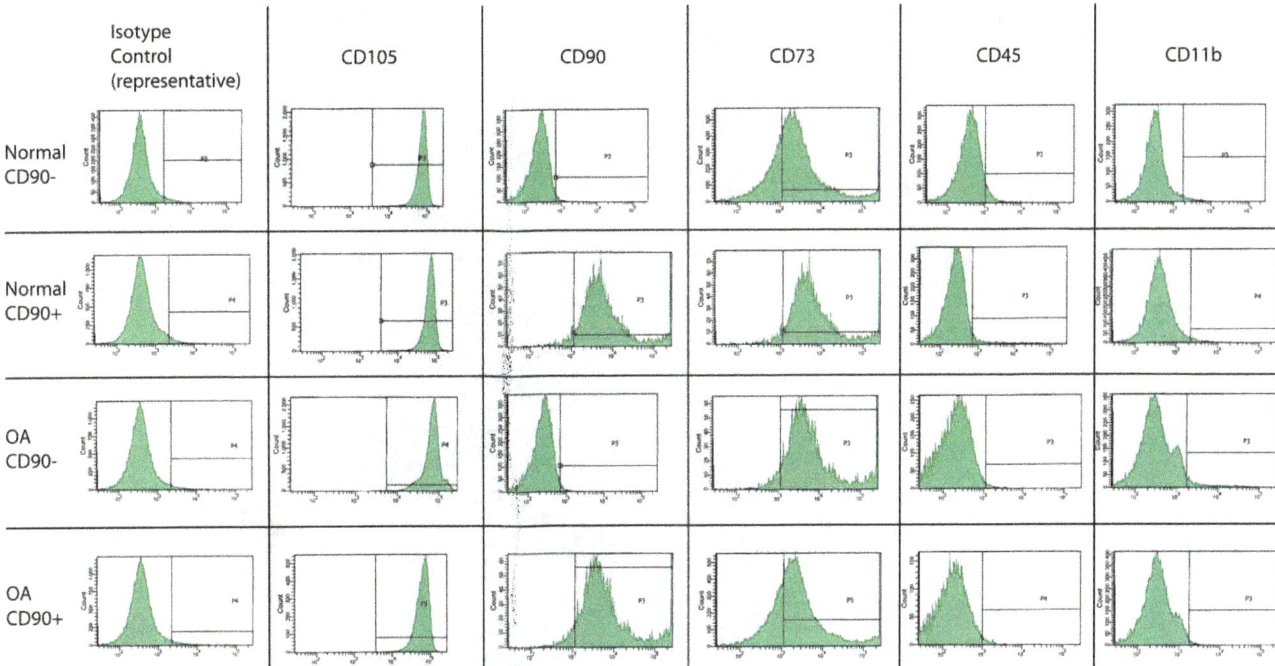

Figure 1. Micro-mass differentiation of sfMPCs. Normal (human N = 5 A–D & canine N = 2 H–K) and OA (human N = 5 E–G & canine N = 2 L–N) derived sfMPCs where aggregated using the micro-mass technique and induced to differentiate over a 14 day period with media supplements. qRT-PCR results demonstrated that Sox9, Collagen 2 and Aggrecan are significantly elevated at days 3, 5, 8 and 14 of differentiation (A,E,H,L), furthermore, at day 14 Collagen 2 protein is expressed in the cell cultures (B,F,I,M). Secondary controls (C,J) demonstrate minimal non-specific staining. Scale bars represent 50 μM. * = p>0.05.

tissue-like structures were highly cellular (Figure 5 E). TEM analysis demonstrated that the cells were in close association with each other (Figure 5 F), and were also in proximity to collagen fibres (Figure 5 G). The cells in these self-assembled structures were attached to the surrounding collagen fibre network of the extracellular matrix (Figure 5 E and F).

Discussion

OA is a degenerative disorder of synovial joints characterized by articular cartilage degradation and meager evidence of repair or regeneration. Although evidence of cartilage stem/progenitor cells has been difficult to obtain, which may explain this response, recent animal studies have raised the possibility that MPCs present in the synovial membrane or joint fluid may play a role in repair cartilage *in vivo* [9,10].

MPCs are of particular interest to regenerative medicine as they have the ability to generate bone, cartilage, and muscle under certain conditions. Indeed, properly harnessed, these MPCs could be utilized *in-vivo* to promote the repair or replacement of tissue damaged by trauma or disease. MPCs for skeletal regeneration are most commonly sourced from the bone marrow or fat, and it is increasing recognized that many adult tissues have resident stem cell populations. Although seemingly the ideal source of MPCs for cartilage regeneration, it has been claimed that adult articular cartilage uniquely lacks 'true' MPCs [21]. Interestingly, MPC populations have been isolated from the synovial membrane and synovial fluid bathing the joint [14]. Moreover, when compared to MPC populations isolated from bone marrow or fat [12], sfMPCs demonstrate an increased chondrogenic capacity compared to MPC populations isolated from bone marrow or fat [12].

This current study demonstrates that normal and OA (human and canine) derived sfMPCs undergo effective chondrogenesis when a micro-mass step is included in the differentiation protocol, which corroborates previously published findings [2]. Furthermore, when sfMPCs (normal/OA) are enriched for the CD90-positive fraction, enhanced chondrogenesis is observed compared to the CD90-depleted fraction. This is of particular interest as a recent study by Nagase et al. reports that the chondrogenic potential of adult stem cells decrease with the subsequent loss of CD90 [19], while another study seems to contradict this observation [22]. The results of the present study supports those of Nagase et al. suggesting that CD90 is a cell surface marker that correlates positively with chondrogenic potential [19]. It is also noteworthy that patients with even advanced OA have sfMPCs, and in some cases with numbers far exceeding normal individuals [2], which could be interpreted as a cellular repair response.

A particularly noteworthy finding in the present study is that CD90-positive sfMPCs (normal/OA) can differentiate into chondrocytes without a micro-mass step. However, whereas whole populations of sfMPCs from normal individuals aggregate and express high levels of chondrogenic markers, whole populations of sfMPCs from OA joints do not aggregate spontaneously, grow only as a monolayer, and express low levels of chondrogenic markers during differentiation. The exact functional significance of micromass aggregation is unclear, yet micro-mass-induced aggregation clearly increases the efficiency of chondrogenesis [23,24], possibly by mimicking embryonic tissue condensation. Although the promotion of cell differentiation by aggregation is not limited to sfMPCs and chondrogenesis, (having been demonstrated with pancreatic, hepatic, fibroblastic, bone marrow, and cord blood MPCs [25–30]), it seems curious that all normal and OA sfMPCs behave differently in non-aggregating culture even though they

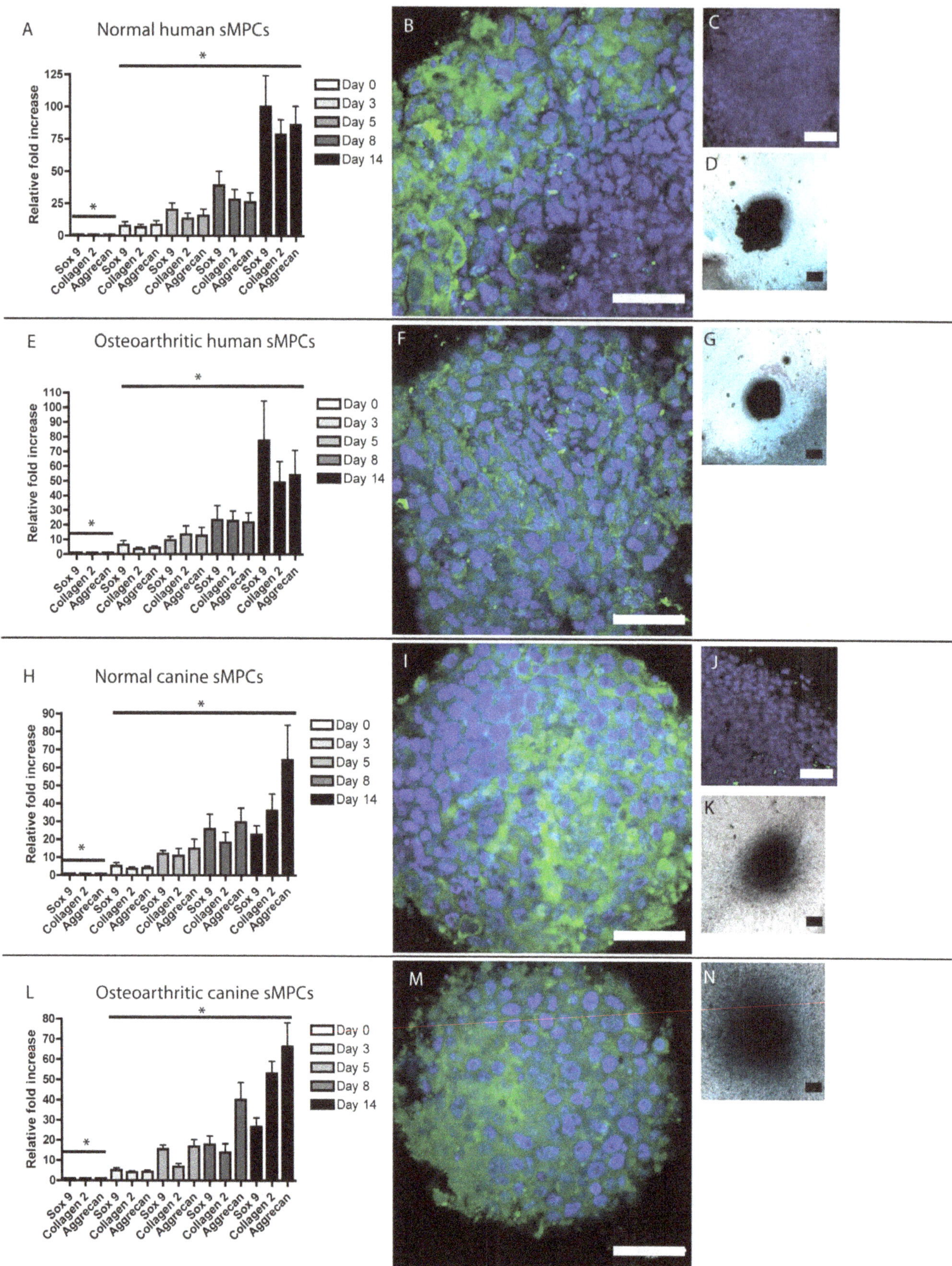

Figure 2. Chondrogenic Differentiation of CD90+/− sfMPCs. sfMPCs derived from normal synovial fluid were enriched/depleted for CD90 and induced to differentiate into chondrocytes. The CD90+ fraction expressed (A,F,K,P) similar levels of Sox9, Collagen 2 and Aggrecan mRNA on day 14 to the total sMPC population (Figure 2), whereas the CD90− fraction demonstrated reduced levels of Sox9, Collagen 2 and Aggrecan (A,F,K,P). Alcian

blue (D,I,N,S) and Collagen 2 (E,J,O,T) staining intensity was also decreased in the CD90− negative fraction compared to the CD90+ fraction (Alcian blue: B,G,L,Q, Collagen 2:C,H,M,R) on day 14. Scale bars represent 250 μM.

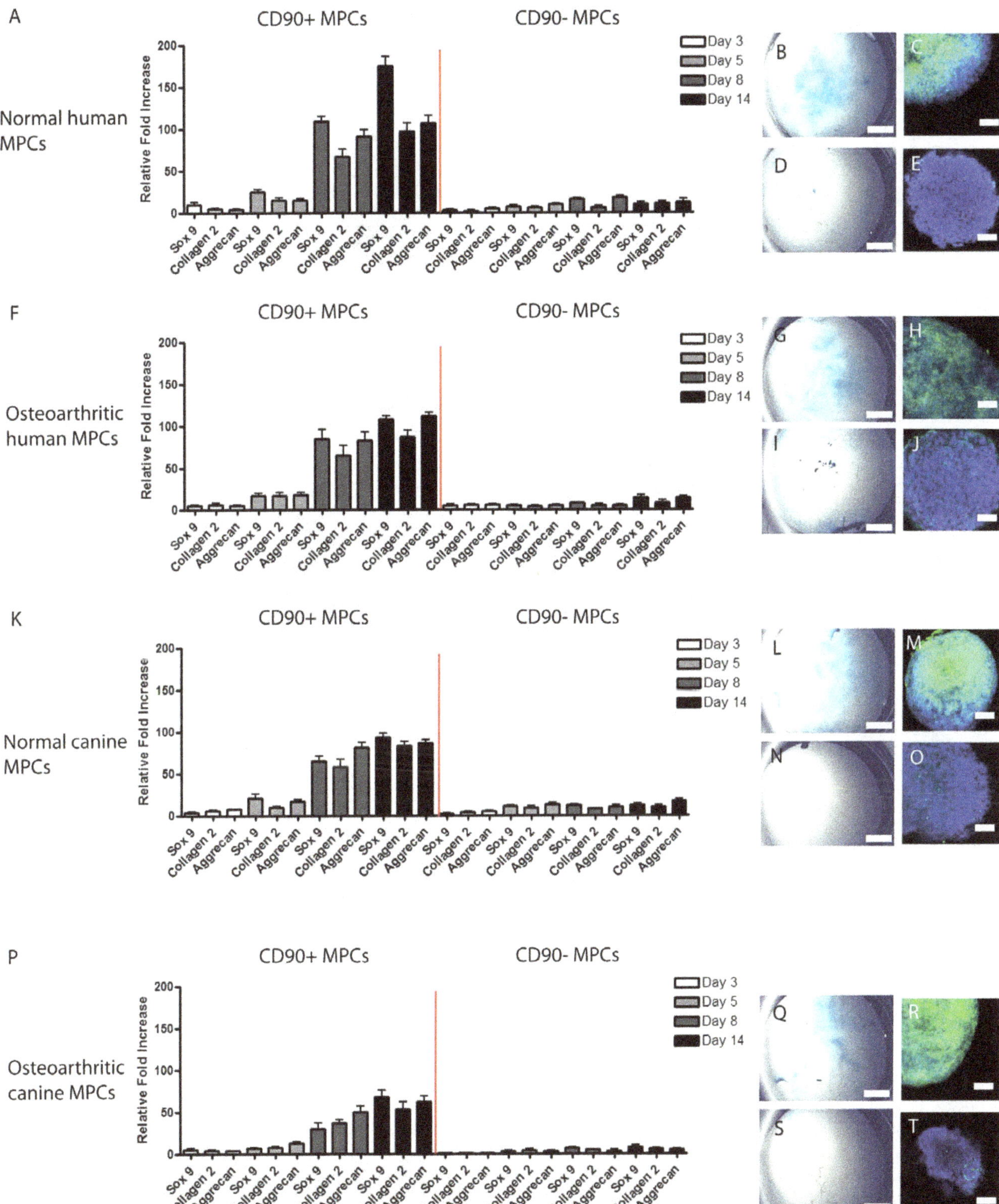

Figure 3. Multi-potent differentiation of CD90+/− sfMPCs. Normal and OA CD90+ or CD90− sfMPCs were induced to differentiate into osteoblasts or adipocytes and stained with Akaline phosphatase (A) to indentify osteoblasts, or Oil Red-O (B) to identify lipid-containing cells (adipocytes). qRT-PCR was used to determine the relative level of adipocyte specific genes (Adiponectin, PPAR-gamma, [C]) and osteoblastic specific genes (Osteonectin, Sp7/Osterix [D]). * = p>0.05.

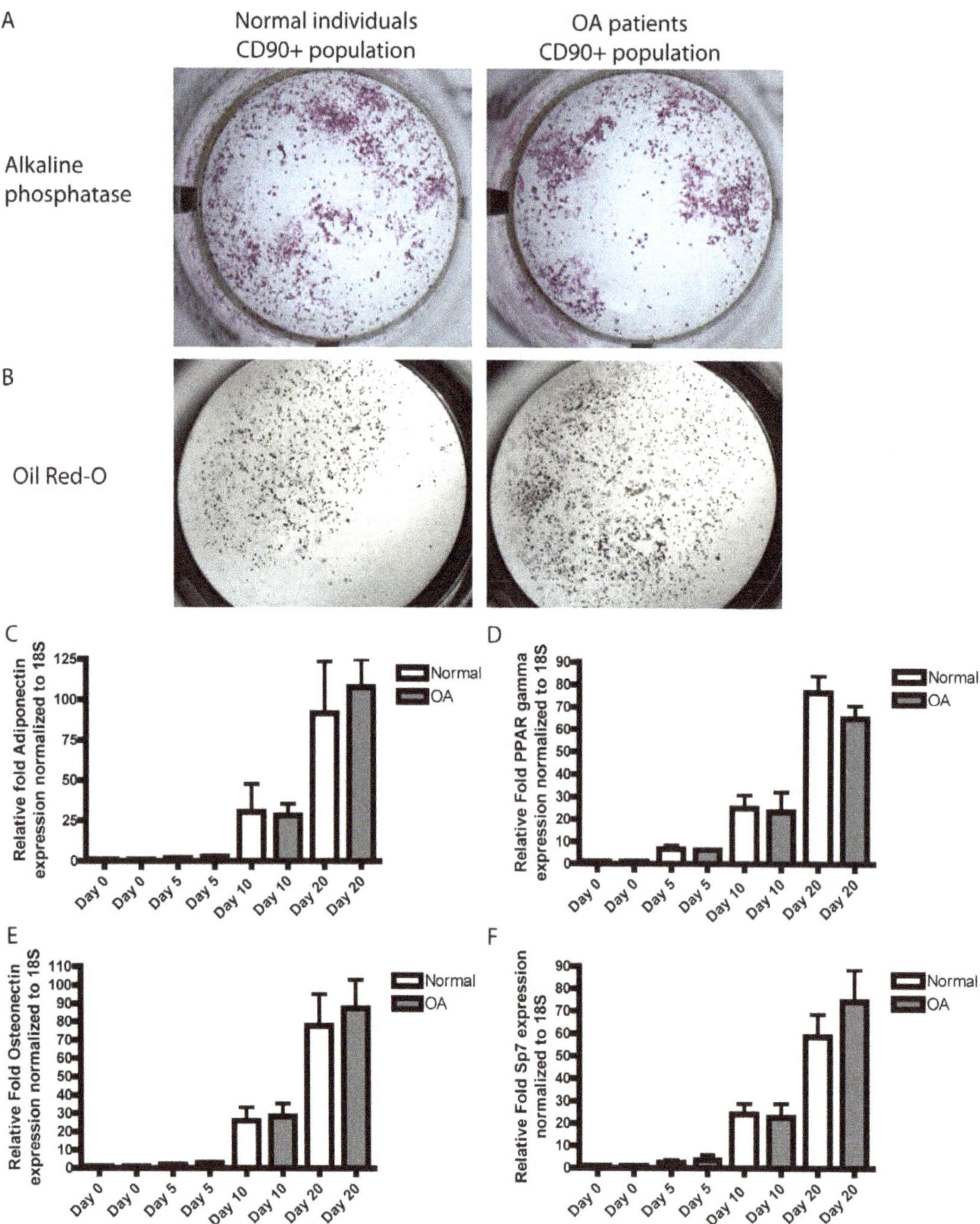

Figure 4. Aggregation and Chondrogenesis of sfMPCs. Normal and OA CD90+ sfMPCs were induced to differentiate without prior micro-mass aggregation. By day 14 normal sfMPCs expressed Sox9, Collagen2 and Aggrecan mRNA (A,D) while OA sfMPCs expressed severely reduced levels (A,D). Furthermore, normal sfMPCs generated a tissue-like structure that stained positive for Alcian Blue (B,G), whereas OA sfMPCs did not (C,F) and remained as a monolayer. Scale bars represent 200 μM.

were otherwise derived and cultured under identical conditions. Moreover, it would appear that this aggregation behaviour (which was consistent across the 5 human and 2 canine normal individuals tested) is lost within the OA phenotype (again consistent across the 5 OA patients and 2 canines tested). We speculate that MPCs in the OA joint might be missing, or have masked, a cell surface receptor necessary for spontaneous aggregation. In continuing studies, we will examine if OA sfMPCs demonstrate any changes in gene expression compared to normal sfMPCs, specifically in genes related to pre-condensation (CCN-1, CNN-2) and/or within condensation (N-CAM, Tenascin C) [31]. To complement this line of investigation, micro-array studies comparing the global gene expression patterns of normal vs. OA sfMPCs have been completed and the data analysis is underway. Previously, studies have demonstrated that chondrocyte aggregation is mediated by β1-Integrin [32], while Cadherins seem to play a dominant role in the aggregation of MSCs during chondrogenesis [33]. Therefore, the mechanism behind the failure of OA sfMPCs aggregation should be studied further to determine if genes expressed during the normal chondrogenic developmental process are aberrantly expressed.

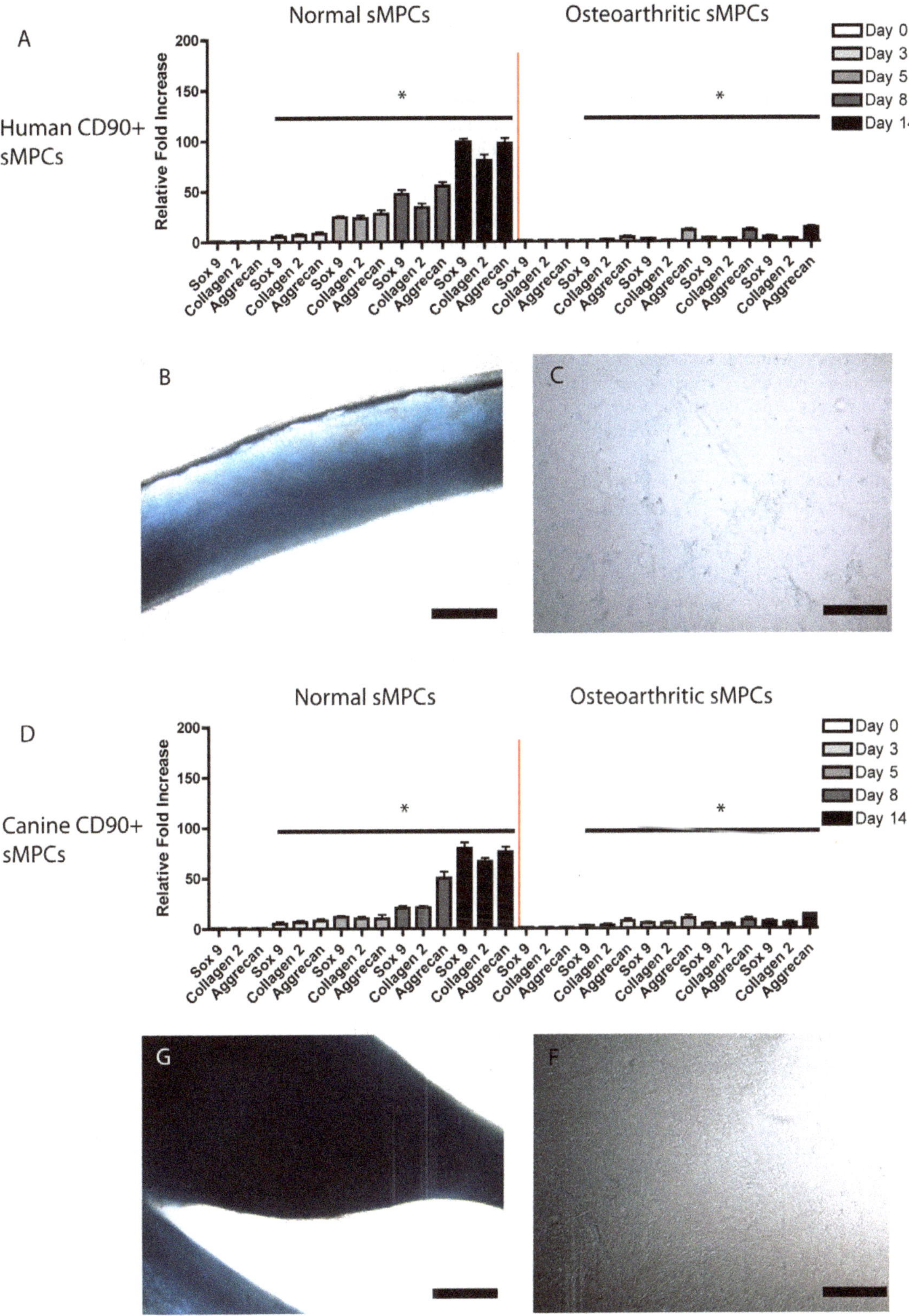

Figure 5. Staining and TEM of Derived Tissue from Normal sfMPCs. The resultant tissue-like masses were stained with antibodies to Collagen 2 (A) and Aggrecan (C), nuclei were stained with TOTO3 (B, D). Cells were found in closer association to each other (E), with higher magnification showing production of collagen fibres (F). Cells were also found in proximity with the produced collagen ECM (E, F). Scale bars represent 200 μM.

Since OA leads to a progressive loss of cartilage and synovial progenitors cells have the potential to contribute to articular cartilage repair *in vivo* [34], the inability of OA sfMPCs to spontaneously differentiate into chondrocytes suggests that cell-to-cell aggregation and/or communication may be impaired in OA and somehow dampen the normal mechanism of chondrocyte replenishment from the synovium or synovial fluid. Should the cells of the synovium or synovial fluid be a reservoir of stem cells for normal articular cartilage maintenance and repair, these endogenous sources of chondro-biased cells would be a fundamental and new strategy for treating OA and cartilage injury if this loss of aggregation & differentiation phenotype can be overcome.

Methods

Ethics Statements

Human: Informed consent to participate was obtained by written agreement. The study protocol was approved by the University of Calgary Research Ethics Board (Application number: 21987).

Canine: All procedures received approval by the institutional ethics board (University of Calgary, Animal Care Committee) and were carried out under the supervision of a veterinarian according to the guidelines of the Canadian Council on Animal Care.

Human Subjects

Patients with clinical and radiographic OA [20] with no other co-morbidities consented to arthrocentesis and had synovial fluid aspirated from their knees (mean volume 63.4 ml+/−12.6 ml) during a visit to the University of Calgary Foothills Medical Clinic (N = 5, 3 males age: 47, 50, 52; 2 females age 52, 54; Ethics ID #21987). Synovial fluid from macroscopically normal knees was aspirated (mean volume 5.6 ml+/−2.2 ml) from cadavers less than 4 hrs after death (N = 5, 2 males age: 47, 54; 3 female age 46, 51, 52 Ethics ID #21987). Tissue donors were received by the Southern Alberta Organ and Tissue Donation Program (SAOTDP), which obtains the medical history of every donor, including current medication, previous history of joint diseases, and other co-morbidities (e.g., cancer, diabetes, inflammatory diseases). All donor knees received x-ray and macroscopic examination of the joint surfaces. Any abnormalities (cracking, blistering, darkening, abnormal wear) prompted exclusion from the study. In total seven cadaveric joints were examined and two were excluded from the study.

Animals

Animals were adult, outbred, skeletally mature canines ranging in age from 18–54 months. Briefly, unilateral cruciate ligament transection was performed through a lateral peripatellar athrotomy (N = 2, 1 male, 1 female). Eight weeks after surgery, animals were euthanized, and sterile samples of joint fluid were withdrawn with a syringe. The volume of joint fluid from un-operated control knee joints ranged from 150–300 micro-liters; the volume of joint fluid from knees with cruciate transection ranged from 5–8 ml. Joint fluid was kept at 4°C and transported to the laboratory within 2 hours of necropsy. All knee and hip joints were inspected for morphological abnormalities, which were not observed in any of the ipsilateral or contralateral hips, nor in any of the ipsilateral (control) knee joints.

sMPC derivation and purification

Human: Fresh synovial fluid was plated in untreated culture dishes and after 1–2 hrs at 37°C/5%CO_2 culture media was added. sMPC culture media consisted of DMEM (Invitrogen # 11965), 10% FBS, 1% Pen/Strep, 1% Non-essential amino acids (NEAA), 0.2% Beta-mercaptoethanol (BME) (all Invitrogen, Carlsbad, CA). Once cells had adhered to the plastic and reached 30–40% confluence, the media was changed and the cells were allowed to reach 60–70% confluence. At this point the cells were dissociated and resuspended in Dulbecco's PBS (DPBS) at 1 million cells/ml. Primary labeled FACS antibodies (Table 1) to CD105, CD73, CD44, CD45, CD11b (All Becton, Dickinson and Company (BD), Franklin Lakes, NJ) were added to the suspension and the cells were sterilely sorted (University of Calgary, Flow Cytometry Core Facility). This CD105+, CD73+, CD44+, CD45−, CD11b− population accounted for 47.4%(+/−5.4%) of the total cells isolated from normal joints, and 67.2%(+/−3.1%) from joints with OA. Both normal and OA CD105+, CD73+, CD44+, CD45−, CD11b− cell populations were over 80% positive for CD90 before magnetic purification. The CD105+, CD73+, CD44+, CD45−, CD11b− cell population was returned to culture for 1 passage and then prepared for magnetic enrichment (an aliquot of this population was tested for multi-potency, with differentiation into fat, bone and cartilage assayed with oil red, alizarin red and Alcian blue respectively). Purified sfMPCs were dissociated and treated with anti-CD90 (BD) and then a magnetically labeled secondary (BD), and subsequently exposed to a magnetic field for enrichment following the manufacturer's instructions. CD90-positive and CD90-negative fractions were cultured for one additional passage and then induced to differentiate. An aliquot of the cells at this passage were

Table 1. Primary antibodies used for analyses.

Marker	Source	Identifies	Species	Cell target
CD105	Becton Dickinson	Endoglin	Human	MPC
CD73	Becton Dickinson	5′-nucleotidase	Human	MPC
CD44	Becton Dickinson	CD44	Human	MPC
CD45	Becton Dickinson	Protein tyrosine phosphatase, receptor type, C	Human	hematopoietic cells
CD11b	Becton Dickinson	Integrin alpha M	Human	hematopoietic cells
CD90	Becton Dickinson	Thy-1	Human/Canine	MPC
CD34	Becton Dickinson	CD34	Canine	hematopoietic cells
CD45	Aviva Systems Biology	Protein tyrosine phosphatase, receptor type, C	Canine	hematopoietic cells
Collagen 2	Hybridoma Bank, Iowa	Collagen 2	Human/Canine	Chondrocytes
Aggrecan	Santa Cruz	Aggrecan	Human/Canine	Chondrocytes

analyzed using FACS to confirm the presence or absence of CD105, CD90, CD73, CD44, CD45, CD11b (Figure 6).

Canine: Fresh synovial fluid was plated in untreated culture dishes and after 1–2 hrs at 37°C/5%CO_2 culture media was added. sMPC media (as above) was used. Once cells had adhered to the plastic and reached 30–40% confluence, the media was changed and the cells were allowed to reach 60–70% confluence. At this point the cells were dissociated and resuspended in Dulbecco's PBS (DPBS) at 1 million cells/ml. The total cell population was negatively purified using biotin-labeled antibodies to canine CD45 (Aviva Systems Biology, San Diego, CA) and CD34 (BD) following the manufacturer's instructions. This cell population was then selected for the CD90+ (BD) fraction using magnetic separation. CD90-positive and CD90-negative fractions were cultured for one additional passage and then induced to differentiate.

Adipogenic Differentiation

sfMPCs were plated in triplicate (100,000 cells/well/24 well dish) and exposed to adipogenic differentiation media for 20 days. Differentiation media consisted of sMPC culture media with 0.5 mM isobutylmethylxanthine, 1 µM dexamethasone, 10 µM insulin, 200 µM indomethacin (all Sigma). Media was changed every three days during the 20 day differentiation period.

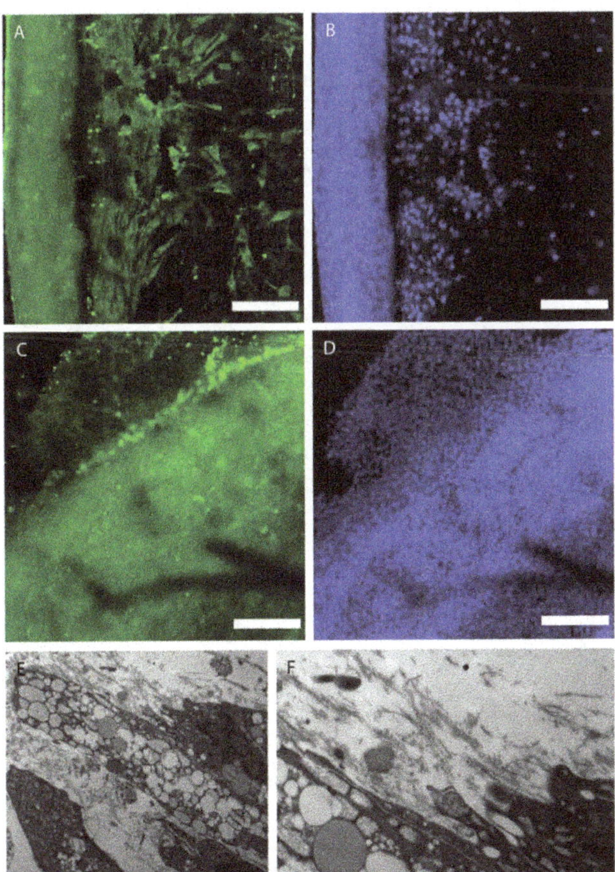

Figure 6. FACS characterization of human sfMPCs. Normal and OA CD90+ and CD90− subpopulations were assayed for expression of CD105, CD90, CD73, CD45 and CD11b prior to chondrogenic differentiation.

Osteogenic Differentiation

sfMPCs were plated in triplicate (100,000 cells/well/24 well dish) and exposed to osteogenic differentiation media for 20 days. Differentiation media consisted of sMPC culture media with 0.1 µM dexamethasone and 50 µM ascorbate-2-phosphate. Media was changed every three days during the 20 day differentiation period.

Chondrogenic Differentiation

sfMPCs were plated in triplicate (100,000 cells/well/24 well dish) and exposed to chondrogenic media for 14 days with or without micro-mass aggregation. Aggregation was achieved by placing 100,000 cells in a 1.5 ml sterile tube at 37°C overnight. Differentiation media consisted of sMPC culture media with 500 ng/mL BMP-2 (Peprotech, Rocky Hill, NJ), 10 ng/mL TGF-β3 (Peprotech), 10^{-8} M dexamethasone (Sigma, St. Louis, MO), 50 µg/mL ascorbic acid (Sigma), 40 µg/mL proline (Invitrogen), 100 µg/mL pyruvate (Sigma) and supplemented with insulin, transferrin, and selenium (Sigma). Media was changed every three days during the 14-day differentiation period.

Analysis of Differentiation

Differentiation was assessed using quantitative RT-PCR (qRT-PCR) and immunofluorescence (IF).

qRT-PCR: RNA was collected using Trizol (Invitrogen) and converted to cDNA using a High Capacity cDNA kit (Applied Biosystems (ABS), Carlsbad, CA). The cDNA was probed using pre-validated Taqman^{TM} primer-sets for human Sox9, Collagen 2, Aggrecan, Osterix (SP7), Osteocalcin, PPAR-gamma, Adiponectin, and canine Sox9, Collagen 2 and Aggrecan (Table 2) on an ABI 7900HT using 18S as the internal control and the ddCT method included within the ABI software to analyze results.

IF: Aggregates/tissues generated from sfMPCs were washed in PBS and fixed in 4% para-formaldehyde (PFA) in PBS at 4°C overnight. Aggregates were then permeabilized in 0.5% saponin (Sigma) in PBS at 4°C overnight, rinsed once in PBS, then blocked in 3% BSA at 4°C overnight. Primary antibodies (Collagen 2: Developmental Studies Hybridoma Bank, Iowa. Aggrecan: Santa Cruz, Santa Cruz, CA) (Table 1) were diluted 1:50 in 3% BSA, added to the cell samples and incubated overnight at 4°C. The aggregates were then washed 3 times with PBS and blocked again overnight at 4°C. Following the block, the aggregates were incubated with an appropriate Alexa-fluor 488 secondary antibody (Molecular Probes, Carlsbad, CA) and Toto-3^{TM} (Molecular Probes) overnight at 4°C. After incubation, the aggregates were washed thrice with PBS and mounted on slides with mountant (9:1 glycerol:PBS). Slides were analyzed using a Zeiss 510 confocal

Table 2. qRT-PCR probes used for analysis.

Marker	Source	Cell Target
Sox 9	ABI (human and canine probes)	Chondrocytes
Collagen 2	ABI (human and canine probes)	Chondrocytes
Aggrecan	ABI (human and canine probes)	Chondrocytes
Osterix (SP7)	ABI (human)	Osteoblasts
Osteocalcin	ABI (human)	Osteoblasts
PPAR-gamma	ABI (human)	Adipocytes
Adiponectin	ABI (human)	Adipocytes

Microscope with 488, 568 and 633 nm filters. Images were prepared using Zeiss LSM image browsing software.

Transmission Electron Microscopy

For transmission electron microscopy (TEM), pre-cartilaginous tissue-like aggregates were collected after differentiation, and then washed in PBS before fixation with 4% glutaraldehyde in Millonig's phosphate buffer for 1 hour at room temperature. Post-fixation was carried out in 2% OsO_4 for 20 minutes. The tissues were then dehydrated in ethanol, and subsequently infiltrated with Polybed 812 resin (Polysciences). Polymerization was performed at 37°C for 24 hours. Silver-gray sections were cut with an ultramicrotome equipped with a diamond knife, and sections were stained with uranyl acetate and lead citrate, then examined in an H-7000 Hitachi electron microscope.

Statistical Analysis

Each treatment (cell differentiation) and assay (IF, qRT-PCR) was performed in triplicate. Statistical analysis (ANOVA) was performed on qRT-PCR data using GraphPad Prism4 (GraphPad Software) and significance was set at $p<0.05$.

Acknowledgments

We would like to thank Scott Ewald, Gary Rockl and the SAOTDP for assisting with the collection of cadaveric tissues.

Author Contributions

Conceived and designed the experiments: RJK JBR JRM DAH. Performed the experiments: RJK YEW JBR JRM. Analyzed the data: RJK. Contributed reagents/materials/analysis tools: LM JRM. Wrote the paper: RJK YEW.

References

1. McGonagle D, Jones E (2008) A potential role for synovial fluid mesenchymal stem cells in ligament regeneration. Rheumatology (Oxford) 47:1114–6.
2. Jones EA, Crawford A, English A, Henshaw K, Mundy J, et al. (2008) Synovial fluid mesenchymal stem cells in health and early osteoarthritis: detection and functional evaluation at the single-cell level. Arthritis Rheum 58:1731–40.
3. Horie M, Sekiya I, Muneta T, Ichinose S, Matsumoto K, et al. (2009) Intra-articular Injected synovial stem cells differentiate into meniscal cells directly and promote meniscal regeneration without mobilization to distant organs in rat massive meniscal defect. Stem Cells 27:878–87.
4. Morito T, Muneta T, Hara K, Ju YJ, Mochizuki T, et al. (2008) Synovial fluid-derived mesenchymal stem cells increase after intra-articular ligament injury in humans. Rheumatology (Oxford) 47:1137–43.
5. Koga H, Muneta T, Ju YJ, Nagase T, Nimura A, et al. (2007) Synovial stem cells are regionally specified according to local microenvironments after implantation for cartilage regeneration. Stem Cells 25:689–96.
6. Ando W, Tateishi K, Hart DA, Katakai D, Tanaka Y, et al. (2007) Cartilage repair using an in vitro generated scaffold-free tissue-engineered construct derived from porcine synovial mesenchymal stem cells. Biomaterials 28:5462–70.
7. Ando W, Tateishi K, Katakai D, Hart DA, Higuchi C, et al. (2008) In vitro generation of a scaffold-free tissue-engineered construct (TEC) derived from human synovial mesenchymal stem cells: biological and mechanical properties and further chondrogenic potential. Tissue Eng Part A 14:2041–9.
8. Kanamoto T, Nakamura N, Nakata K, Yoshikawa H (2008) Articular cartilage regeneration using stem cells Clin Calcium 18:1744–9.
9. Hunziker EB, Rosenberg LC (1996) Repair of partial-thickness defects in articular cartilage: cell recruitment from the synovial membrane. J Bone Joint Surg Am 78:721–33.
10. Hunziker EB (2001) Growth-factor-induced healing of partial-thickness defects in adult rticular cartilage. Osteoarthritis Cartilage 9:22–32.
11. Koga H, Shimaya M, Muneta T, Nimura A, Morito T, et al. (2008) Local adherent technique for transplanting mesenchymal stem cells as a potential treatment of cartilage defect. Arthritis Res Ther 10:R84.
12. Koga H, Muneta T, Nagase T, Nimura A, Ju YJ, et al. (2008) Comparison of mesenchymal tissues-derived stem cells for in vivo chondrogenesis: suitable conditions for cell therapy of cartilage defects in rabbit. Cell Tissue Res 333:207–15.
13. Archer CW, Dowthwaite GP, Francis-West P (2003) Development of synovial joints. Birth Defects Res C Embryo Today 69:144–55.
14. Fan J, Varshney RR, Ren L, Cai D, Wang DA (2009) Synovium-derived mesenchymal stem cells: a new cell source for musculoskeletal regeneration. Tissue Eng Part B Rev 15:75–86.
15. Dominici M, Le BK, Mueller I, Slaper-Cortenbach I, Marini F, et al. (2006) Minimal criteria for defining multipotent mesenchymal stromal cells. The International Society for Cellular Therapy position statement. Cytotherapy 8:315–317.
16. Barker TH, Hagood JS (2009) Getting a grip on Thy-1 signaling. Biochim Biophys Acta 1793:921–3.
17. Mafi P, Hindocha S, Mafi R, Griffin M, Khan W (2011) Adult mesenchymal stem cells and cell surface characterization - a systematic review of the literature. Open Orthop J (Suppl 2):253–60.
18. Jones E, Churchman SM, English A, Buch MH, Horner EA, et al. (2010) Mesenchymal stem cells in rheumatoid synovium: enumeration and functional assessment in relation to synovial inflammation level. Ann Rheum Dis 69:450–7.
19. Nagase T, Muneta T, Ju YJ, Hara K, Morito T, et al. (2008) Analysis of the chondrogenic potential of human synovial stem cells according to harvest site and culture parameters in knees with medial compartment osteoarthritis. Arthritis Rheum 58:1389–98.
20. Altman R, Alarcón G, Appelrouth D, Bloch D, Borenstein D, et al. (1986) The American College of Rheumatology criteria for the classification and reporting of osteoarthritis of the knee. Arthritis Rheum 29:1039–49.
21. Koelling S, Miosge N (2009) Stem cell therapy for cartilage regeneration in osteoarthritis. Expert Opin Biol Ther 9:1399–405.
22. Han HS, Lee S, Kim JH, Seong SC, Lee MC (2010) Changes in chondrogenic phenotype and gene expression profiles associated with the in vitro expansion of human synovium-derived cells. J Orthop Res 28:1283–91.
23. Mackay AM, Beck SC, Murphy JM, Barry FP, Chichester CO, et al. (1998) Chondrogenic differentiation of cultured human mesenchymal stem cells from marrow. Tissue Eng 4:415–28.
24. Pittenger MF, Mackay AM, Beck SC, Jaiswal RK, Douglas R, et al. (1999) Multilineage potential of adult human mesenchymal stem cells. Science 284:143–7.
25. Luo W, Shitaye H, Friedman M, Bennett CN, Miller J, et al. (2008) Disruption of cell-matrix interactions by heparin enhances mesenchymal progenitor adipocyte differentiation. Exp Cell Res 314:3382–91.
26. Lim JJ, Scott L Jr, Temenoff JS (2011) Aggregation of bovine anterior cruciate ligament fibroblasts or marrow stromal cells promotes aggrecan production. Biotechnol Bioeng 108:151–62.
27. Okura H, Komoda H, Saga A, Kakuta-Yamamoto A, Hamada Y, et al. (2010) Properties of hepatocyte-like cell clusters from human adipose tissue-derived mesenchymal stem cells. Tissue Eng Part C Methods 16:761–70.
28. Wei C, Geras-Raaka E, Marcus-Samuels B, Oron Y, Gershengorn MC (2006) Trypsin and thrombin accelerate aggregation of human endocrine pancreas precursor cells. J Cell Physiol 206:322–8.
29. Gao F, Wu DQ, Hu YH, Jin GX, Li GD, et al. (2008) In vitro cultivation of islet-like cell clusters from human umbilical cord blood-derived mesenchymal stem cells. Transl Res 151:293–302.
30. Heng BC, Cowan CM, Basu S (2008) Temperature and calcium ions affect aggregation of mesenchymal stem cells in phosphate buffered saline. Cytotechnology 58:69–75.
31. Lorda-Diez CI, Montero JA, Diaz-Mendoza MJ, Garcia-Porrero JA, Hurle JM (2011) Defining the earliest transcriptional steps of chondrogenic progenitor specification during the formation of the digits in the embryonic limb. PLoS One 6:e24546.
32. Gigout A, Jolicoeur M, Nelea M, Raynal N, Farndale R, et al. (2008) Chondrocyte aggregation in suspension culture is GFOGER-GPP- and beta1 integrin-dependent. J Biol Chem 283:31522–30.
33. Bradley EW, Drissi MH (2011) Wnt5b regulates mesenchymal cell aggregation and chondrocyte differentiation through the planar cell polarity pathway. J Cell Physiol 226:1683–93.
34. Kurth TB, Dell'accio F, Crouch V, Augello A, Sharpe PT, et al. (2011) Functional mesenchymal stem cell niches in adult mouse knee joint synovium in vivo. Arthritis Rheum 63:1289–300.

Adiponectin and Leptin Induce VCAM-1 Expression in Human and Murine Chondrocytes

Javier Conde[1], Morena Scotece[1], Verónica López[1], Rodolfo Gómez[2], Francisca Lago[3], Jesús Pino[4], Juan Jesús Gómez-Reino[1], Oreste Gualillo[1]*

1 NEIRID Lab (NeuroEndocrine Interaction in Rheumatology and Inflammatory Diseases), SERGAS, Santiago University Clinical Hospital, Institute of Medical Research (IDIS), Santiago de Compostela, Spain, 2 Division of Rheumatology, Fundación Jiménez Diaz, Madrid, Spain, 3 Research Laboratory 7 (Molecular and Cellular Cardiology), SERGAS, Santiago University Clinical Hospital, Institute of Medical Research (IDIS), Santiago de Compostela, Spain, 4 Division of Orthopaedics Surgery and Traumatology, SERGAS, Santiago University Clinical Hospital, Santiago de Compostela, Spain

Abstract

Background: Osteoarthritis (OA) and rheumatoid arthritis (RA), the most common rheumatic diseases, are characterized by irreversible degeneration of the joint tissues. There are several factors involved in the pathogenesis of these diseases including pro-inflammatory cytokines, adipokines and adhesion molecules.

Objective: Up to now, the relationship between adipokines and adhesion molecules at cartilage level was not explored. Thus, the aim of this article was to study the effect of leptin and adiponectin on the expression of VCAM-1 in human and murine chondrocytes. For completeness, intracellular signal transduction pathway was also explored.

Methods: VCAM-1 expression was assessed by quantitative RT-PCR and western blot analysis upon treatment with leptin, adiponectin and other pertinent reagents in cultured human primary chondrocytes. Signal transduction pathways have been explored by using specific pharmacological inhibitors in the adipokine-stimulated human primary chondrocytes and ATDC5 murine chondrocyte cell line.

Results: Herein, we demonstrate, for the first time, that leptin and adiponectin increase VCAM-1 expression in human and murine chondrocytes. In addition, both adipokines have additive effect with IL-1β. Finally, we demonstrate that several kinases, including JAK2, PI3K and AMPK are at a play in the intracellular signalling of VCAM-1 induction.

Conclusions: Taken together, our results suggest that leptin and adiponectin could perpetuate cartilage-degrading processes by inducing also factors responsible of leukocyte and monocyte infiltration at inflamed joints.

Editor: Nuno M. Neves, University of Minho, Portugal

Funding: The work of O.G. and F.L. is funded by the Instituto de Salud Carlos III and the Xunta de Galicia (SERGAS) through a research-staff stabilization contract. O.G. is supported by Instituto de Salud Carlos III and Xunta de Galicia. This work was also partially supported by RETICS Program, RD08/0075 (RIER) from Instituto de Salud Carlos III (ISCIII), within the VI NP of R+D+I 2008–2011. The funders had no role in study design, data collection and analysis, decision to publish, or preparation of the manuscript.

Competing Interests: The authors have declared that no competing interests exist.

* E-mail: oreste.gualillo@sergas.es

Introduction

Osteoarthritis (OA), one of the most common rheumatic diseases, is a pathology characterized by irreversible joint cartilage destruction. Biochemical, genetic and mechanical factors [1] affect the onset and progression of OA. The role of obesity in OA is known from time. Actually, the dysfunction of adipose tissue associated with altered adipokine secretion pattern is emerging as relevant factor that affect joint structures [2,3,4].

Chondrocytes are the unique cell type of adult human articular cartilage capable to maintain extracellular matrix components integrity and turnover [5]. In osteoarthritis, due to abnormal environmental insults, chondrocytes produce a wide range of inflammatory mediators leading cartilage loss [6] including adipokines and vascular cell adhesion molecules (VCAM) [7,8].

VCAM-1 is an inducible surface glycoprotein that belongs to immunoglobulin gene superfamily (IgSF) [9]. VCAM-1 serves as surface ligand for VLA-4 ($\alpha_4\beta_1$) integrin [10] and this adhesion molecule plays a main role in the adhesion of lymphocytes to endothelium in the site of inflammation [11].

VCAM-1 expression is increased in RA and OA synovial tissue [12,13]. Synovial fibroblast and chondrocytes express VCAM-1 [7,14] and pro-inflammatory cytokines such as IL-1β and TNF-α are able to up-regulate VCAM-1 expression in primary cultures of human articular chondrocytes [7]. VCAM-1 might contribute to adhesion of T-lymphocytes to chondrocytes, and thus participate in host defense mechanisms during inflammatory joint conditions such as rheumatoid arthritis or osteoarthritis and/or after cartilage transplantation [7,15]. Recently, it has been described that VCAM-1 is a strong and independent predictor of the risk of knee and hip joint replacement due to severe OA

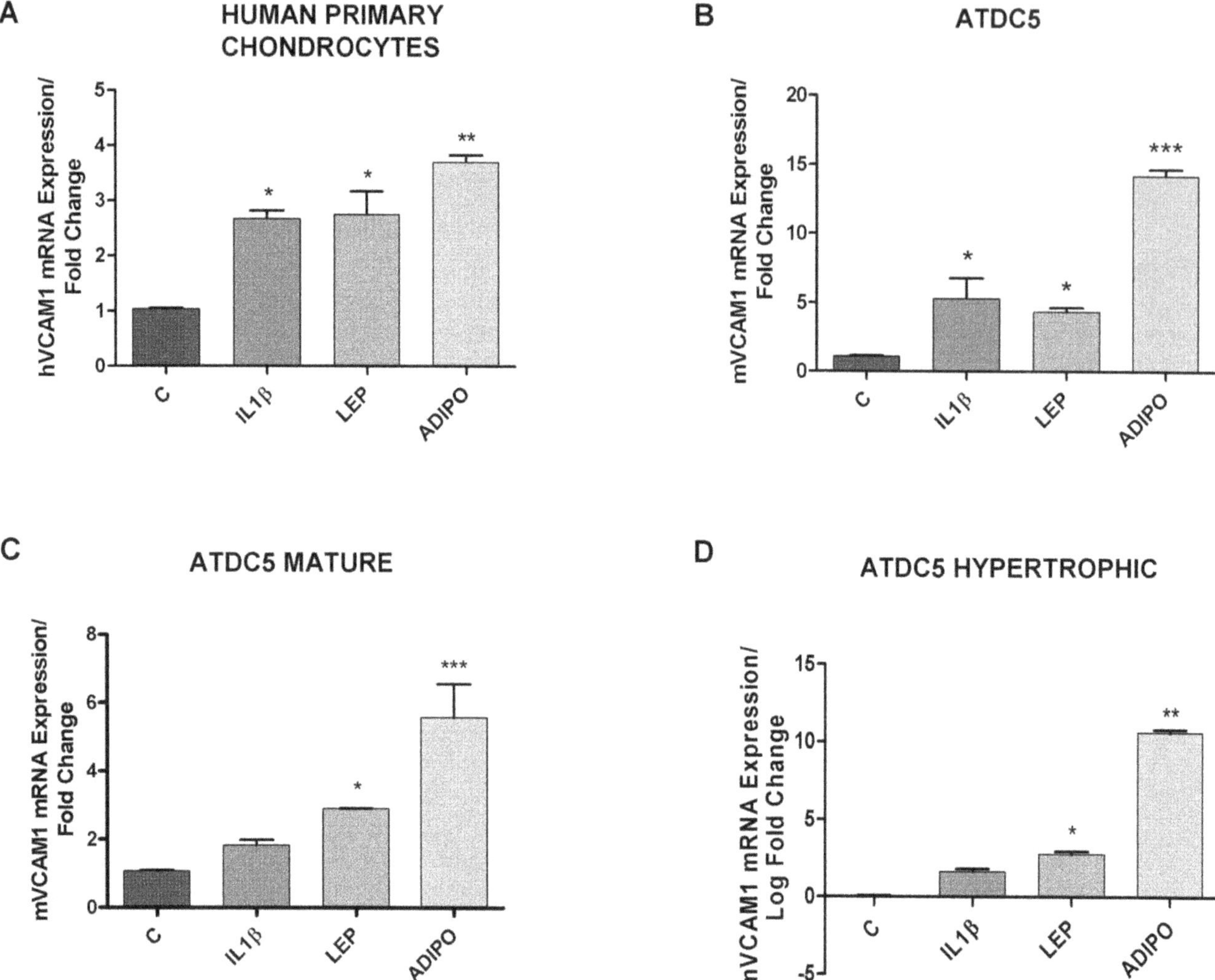

Figure 1. Determination of hVCAM-1 and mVCAM-1 mRNA expression by quantitative real-time PCR. A. hVCAM-1 expression after IL-1β (10 ng/ml), leptin (800 nM) and adiponectin (10 μg/ml) treatment in human primary chondrocytes, during 24 hours. **B,C,D.** mVCAM-1 expression after IL-1β (10 ng/ml), leptin (800 nM) and adiponectin (10 μg/ml) treatment in undifferentiated ATDC-5 cells (B), mature ATDC-5 cells (C) and hypertrophic ATDC-5 cells, during 24 hours.

[16]. In addition, serum level of soluble VCAM-1 was associated with hand OA [17].

In earlier studies we demonstrated that adipokines are novel and potent factors able to modulate chondrocytes physiology. Thus, the aim of this study was to describe the effect of different adipokines (adiponectin leptin and visfatin) on the expression of VCAM-1 in chondrocytes and to elucidate the potential intracellular mechanism involved in the signalling pathway triggered by adipokines.

Materials and Methods

Reagents

All culture reagents were from Sigma (MO, USA), and Lonza, (Switzerland). For RT-PCR, a First Strand Kit, Master mix, primers for VCAM-1 and GAPDH were purchased from SABiosciences (MD, USA). Nucleospin kits for RNA and protein isolation were from Macherey-Nagel (Germany). Mouse and human recombinant leptin, mouse and human recombinant IL-1β, tyrphostin AG490, LY294002, PD098059 and compound C were from Sigma (MO, USA), and recombinant mouse and human adiponectin and visfatin from BioVendor (Germany).

Cell Culture and Treatments

Human primary chondrocytes and the murine ATDC-5 cell line culture were developed as previously described [18,19,20]. Briefly, normal human articular cartilage samples were obtained from the knee joints of 10 patients undergoing knee amputations for peripheral vascular disease or total knee replacement surgery (with permission from the local ethics committee). Cartilage samples were obtained from the joint area of minimal load with normal morphologic examination (i.e., no change in color and no fibrillation). Human chondrocytes were cultured in DMEM/Ham's F12 medium supplemented with 10% of fetal bovine serum, L-glutamine, and antibiotics (50 units/ml penicillin and 50 μg/ml streptomycin). Cells were seeded in monolayer up to the high density and used freshly in order to avoid dedifferentiation.

Murine chondrogenic cell line ATDC-5, passage 30–50 (purchased from RIKEN Cell Bank, Tsukuba, Japan), were cultured in DMEM–Ham's F-12 medium supplemented with 5%

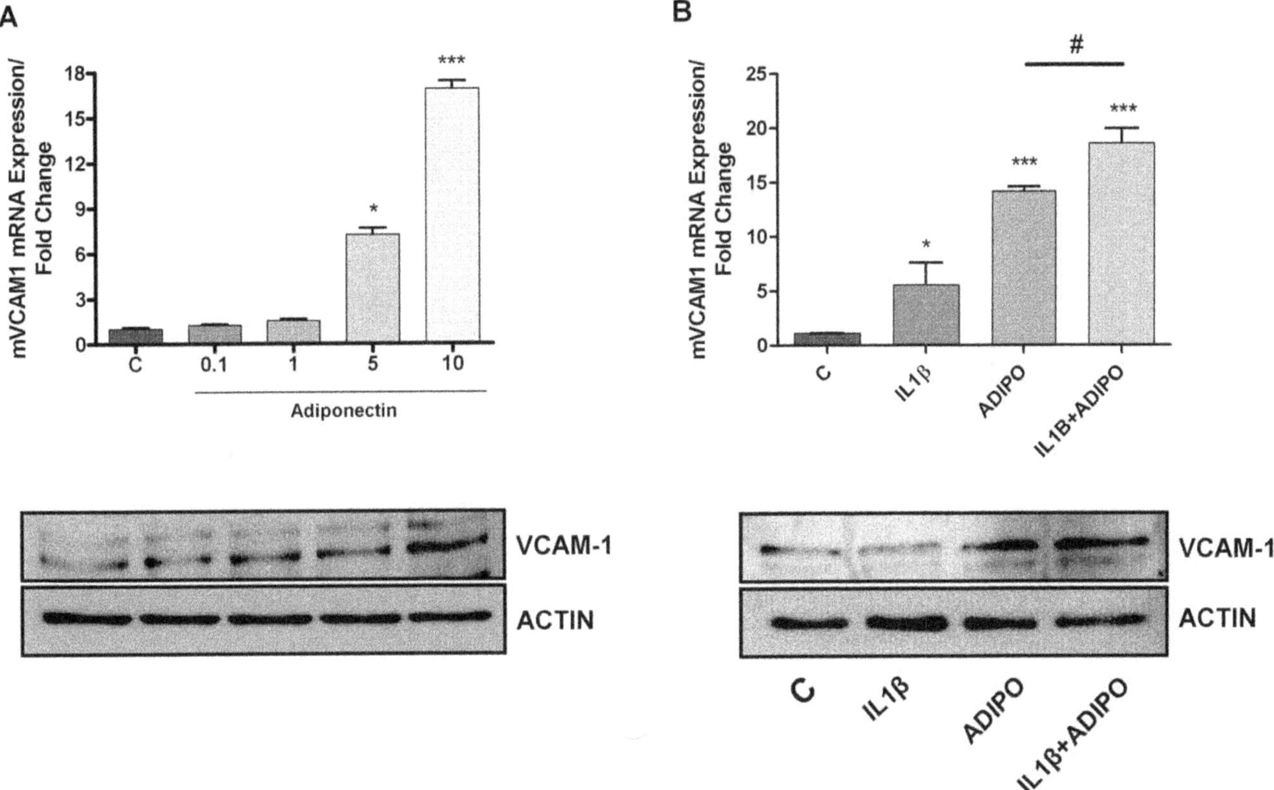

Figure 2. Determination of mVCAM-1 mRNA and protein expression by quantitative real-time PCR and western blot. A. mVCAM-1 expression after adiponectin (0.1, 1, 5, 10 µg/ml) treatment in ATDC-5 cell line, during 24 hours. **B**. mVCAM-1 expression after IL-1β (10 ng/ml), adiponectin (10 µg/ml) and the combination of IL-1β (10 ng/ml) plus adiponectin (10 µg/ml) challenge in ATDC-5 cell line, during 24 hours.

fetal bovine serum, 10 µg/ml human transferrin, 3×10^{-8} M sodium selenite, and antibiotics (50 units/ml penicillin and 50 µg/ml streptomycin). ATDC-5 cells were differentiated into mature chondrocytes and hypertrophic chondrocytes. Briefly, cells were seeded at a density of 6×10^3/cm^2 in 6-well plates with the ATDC-5 standard media supplemented with insulin (10 µg/mL). The differentiation media was replaced every two days for 14 days. On day 15, the culture medium was switched to α-MEM up to day 21 in order to obtain hypertrophic cells. Differentiation was qualitatively characterized by increased formation of cell nodules and enhanced staining with Alcian blue, which are indicative of proteoglycan accumulation. In other experiments (data not shown), differentiation was further analyzed by sequential increase in the levels of type II collagen, aggrecan and type X collagen mRNA, as previously published [18,19].

For RT-PCR and western blot, cells were seeded in P6 multiwell plates until complete adhesion and then incubated overnight in serum-free conditions. Cells were treated with mouse or human IL-1β (10 ng/ml), mouse or human leptin (400 or 800 nM), mouse or human adiponectin (0.1, 1, 5 and 10 µg/ml), mouse or human visfatin (500 ng/ml). Specific pharmacological inhibitors were added 1 h before stimulation: tyrphostin AG490 (10 µM) for JAK2 inhibition, PD098059 (30 µM) for mitogen-activated protein kinase kinase (MEK1) inhibition, LY294002 (10 µM) for phosphatidylinositol 3-kinase (PI3K) inhibition and compound C (10 µM) for AMPK inhibition.

RNA Isolation and Real-time Reverse Transcription–polymerase Chain Reaction (RT-PCR)

Human and murine VCAM-1 mRNA levels were determined using SYBR Green–based quantitative PCR. RNA was extracted using a NucleoSpin kit, according to the manufacturer's instructions. For cDNA synthesis, we performed a RT reaction with a SABiosciences First Strand Kit, using 1 µg of RNA. Next, real-time PCR was performed using specific primers (for human VCAM-1, 141 bp, PPH00623E, reference position 2879, GenBank accession no. NM_001078.2; for mouse VCAM-1, 146 bp, PPM03208B, reference position 2870, GenBank accession no. NM_011693.3; for mouse GAPDH, 140 bp, PPM02946E, reference position 309–328, GenBank accession no. NM_008084.2; for human GAPDH, 175 bp, PPH00150E, reference position 1287–1310, GenBank accession no. NM_002046.3) and Master mix (SABiosciences, MD, USA). All reagents used for RT-PCR were added at the concentrations provided by the manufacturer: 12.5 µL of Master mix, 10.5 µL of water and 1 µL of primers were used by each sample. Results of comparative real-time PCRs were analyzed using MxPro software (Stratagene, CA, USA).

Western Blot Analysis

Proteins were extracted using a NucleoSpin kit, according to the manufacturer's instructions; electrophoresis and blotting procedures have been described previously (4). Immunoblots were incubated with the appropriate antibody (anti-VCAM-1 diluted 1:500, Santa Cruz, CA,USA; anti-phospho-JAK2 diluted 1:1000, Cell Signalling, MA, USA; anti-JAK2 diluted 1:1000, Cell Signalling, MA, USA; anti-phospho-PI3K diluted 1:1000, Cell

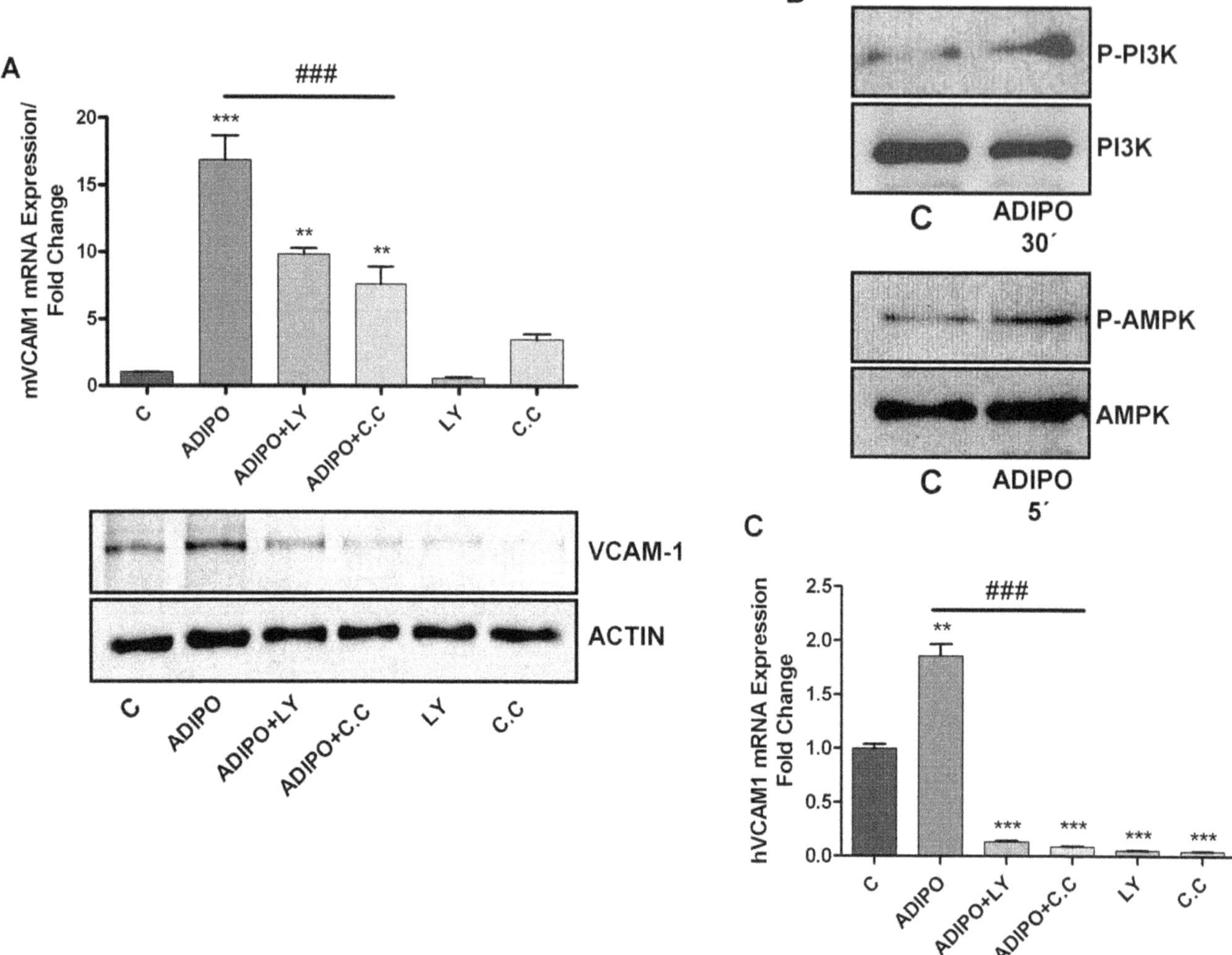

Figure 3. Determination of VCAM-1 mRNA and protein expression by quantitative real-time PCR and western blot. A. mVCAM-1 expression after 1 hour pre-treatment with LY294002 (10 μM) and compound C (10 μM), followed by a 24 hours of adiponectin (10 μg/ml) challenge in ATDC-5 cells. **B**. Determination of the phosphorylation of PI3K and AMPK by western blot. **C**. hVCAM-1 expression after 1 hour pre-treatment with LY294002 (10 μM) and compound C (10 μM), followed by a 24 hours of adiponectin (10 μg/ml) challenge in human primary chondrocytes.

Signalling, MA, USA; anti-PI3K diluted 1:1000, Cell Signalling, MA, USA; anti-phospho-AMPK diluted 1:1000, Cell Signalling, MA, USA; anti-AMPK diluted 1:1000, Cell Signalling, MA, USA) and visualized using an Immobilon Western kit (Millipore, MA, USA) and anti-goat (Santa Cruz, CA, USA) or anti-rabbit (GE Healthcare, UK) horseradish-peroxidise-labelled secondary antibody diluted 1:2000. To confirm equal loading for each sample, after stripping in glycine buffer at pH3, membranes were reblotted with anti-actin antibody diluted 1:5000 (Sigma, MO, USA). Autoradiographs were analyzed with an EC3 imaging system (UVP, CA, USA).

Statistical Analysis

Data are reported as the mean ± SEM of at least 3 independent experiments. The comparison method for RT-PCR was performed as previously (18). Statistical analyses were performed by analysis of variance, followed by post-hoc comparison testing (using the unpaired *t*-test and Student-Newman-Keuls test) using the GraphPad Prism 4 computerized package (GraphPad Software). P values less than 0.05 were considered significant.

Results

VCAM-1 Induction by Cytokines and Adipokines in Human Primary Chondrocytes and ATDC-5 Chondrocytes

As shown in figure 1, IL-1β (10 ng/ml), leptin (800 nM) and adiponectin (10 μM) are able to significantly induce the VCAM-1 mRNA expression in human primary chondrocytes (A) and in ATDC-5 chondrocytes at different stages of differentiation (B–C–D) after 24 hours treatment. To note, adiponectin was the most potent adipokine in inducing VCAM-1.

VCAM-1 Induction by Adiponectin in ATDC5 Cell Line

As shown in figure 2A, adiponectin was able to induce VCAM-1 expression in a dose- dependent manner.

When cells have been stimulated with a combination of IL-1β and adiponectin, the expression of VCAM-1 was significantly higher than in the cells stimulated with IL-1β or adiponectin alone (figure 2B).

These results were confirmed also in terms of protein expression (figure 2A–B low panels).

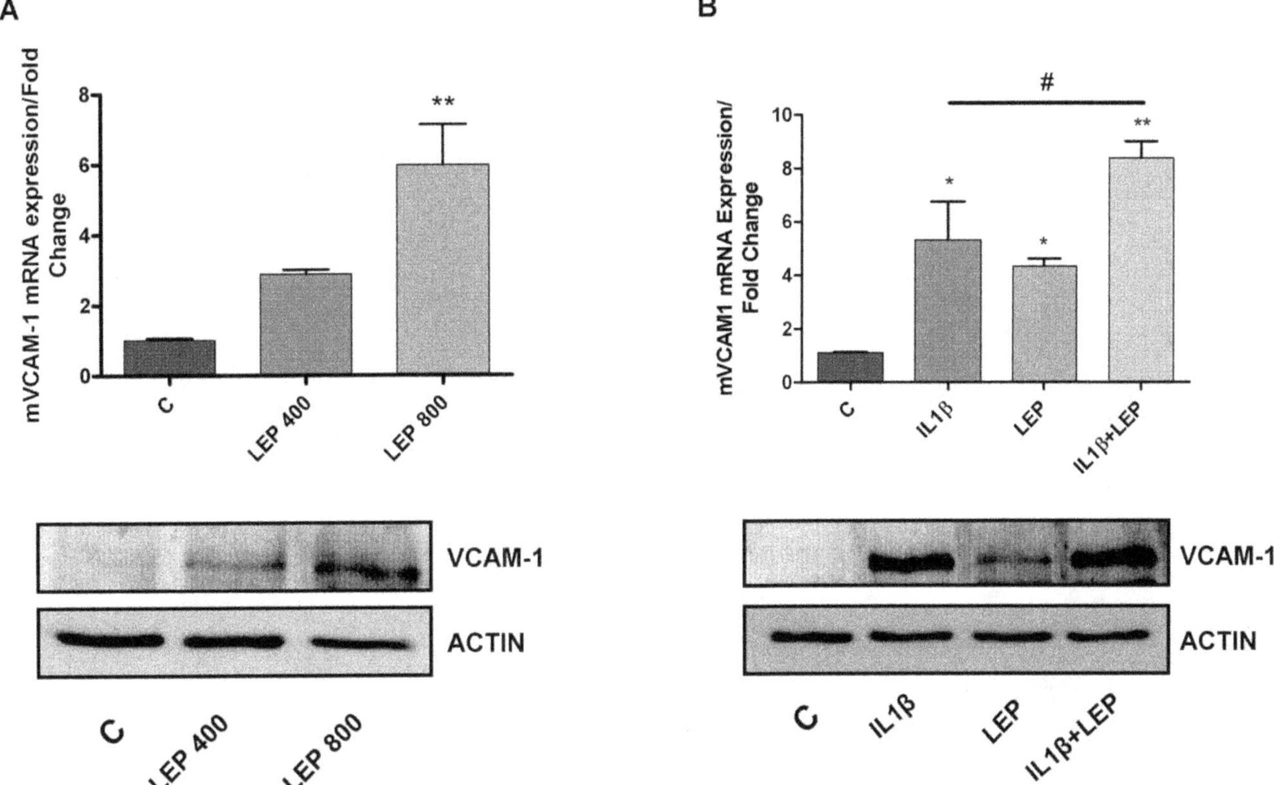

Figure 4. Determination of mVCAM-1 mRNA and protein expression by quantitative real-time PCR and western blot. A. mVCAM-1 expression after leptin (400 and 800 nM) treatment in ATDC-5 cell line, during 24 hours. B. mVCAM-1 mRNA expression after IL-1β (10 ng/ml), leptin (800 nM) and the combination of IL-1β (10 ng/ml) plus leptin (800 nM) challenge in ATDC-5 cell line, during 24 hours.

Effect of the Specific Signalling Pathway Inhibitors on Adiponectin-induced VCAM-1 Expression

To gain further insights into the intracellular mechanism(s) responsible for VCAM-1 induction by adiponectin, we evaluated the effect of specific pharmacological inhibitors of relevant kinases such as MEK1, PI3K and AMPK.

As shown in figure 3A, addition of LY294002 and compound C (inhibitors of PI3K and AMPK respectively), one hour before adiponectin treatment, resulted in a significant decrease in mVCAM-1 expression in the ATDC-5 cell line (figure 3A).

The phosphorylation of PI3K and AMPK by adiponectin was confirmed by also western blot (figure 3B).

Inhibition of PI3K and AMPK by LY294002 and compound C respectively, also decreased adiponectin-induced hVCAM-1 in human primary chondrocytes (figure 3C).

VCAM-1 Induction by Leptin in ATDC5 Cell Line

As shown in figure 4A, leptin was able to induce VCAM-1 expression in a dose- dependent manner.

When cells have been stimulated with a combination of IL-1β and leptin, the expression of VCAM-1 was significantly higher than the cells stimulated with IL-1β or leptin alone (figure 4B).

These results were also confirmed in terms of protein expression (figure 4A–B low panels).

Effect of the Specific Signalling Pathway Inhibitors on Leptin-induced VCAM-1 Expression

To gain further insights into the intracellular mechanism(s) responsible for VCAM-1 induction by leptin, we evaluated the effect of specific pharmacological inhibitors of relevant kinases such as JAK2 and PI3K.

As shown in figure 5A, cell stimulation with leptin in presence of tyrphostin AG490 and LY294002 (inhibitors of JAK2 and PI3K respectively), one hour before adipokine challenge, significantly decrease mVCAM-1 expression in the ATDC-5 cell line. The phosphorylation of JAK2 and PI3K by leptin was confirmed by western blot (figure 5B).

Inhibition of JAK2 and PI3K by tyrphostin AG490 and LY294002 respectively, also decreased leptin-induced hVCAM-1 in human primary chondrocytes (figure 5C).

Discussion

Recently chondrocytes have been recognized to synthesize also adipokines such as adiponectin and leptin [21,22]. This novel superfamily of metabolic factors mediates prevalently inflammatory processes at joint cartilage level. For instance, it has been reported that adiponectin induces NOS2, MMP-3, MMP-9 and IL-6 in chondrocytes [4]. Moreover adiponectin plasma levels are associated with markers of cartilage degradation and these levels are higher in patients with most severe OA [22] and adiponectin levels are increased in RA patients as well [23]. Similarly, leptin and IL-1 induce synergistically nitric oxide in chondrocytes [24]. The inflammatory environment that exists in the joint, produced

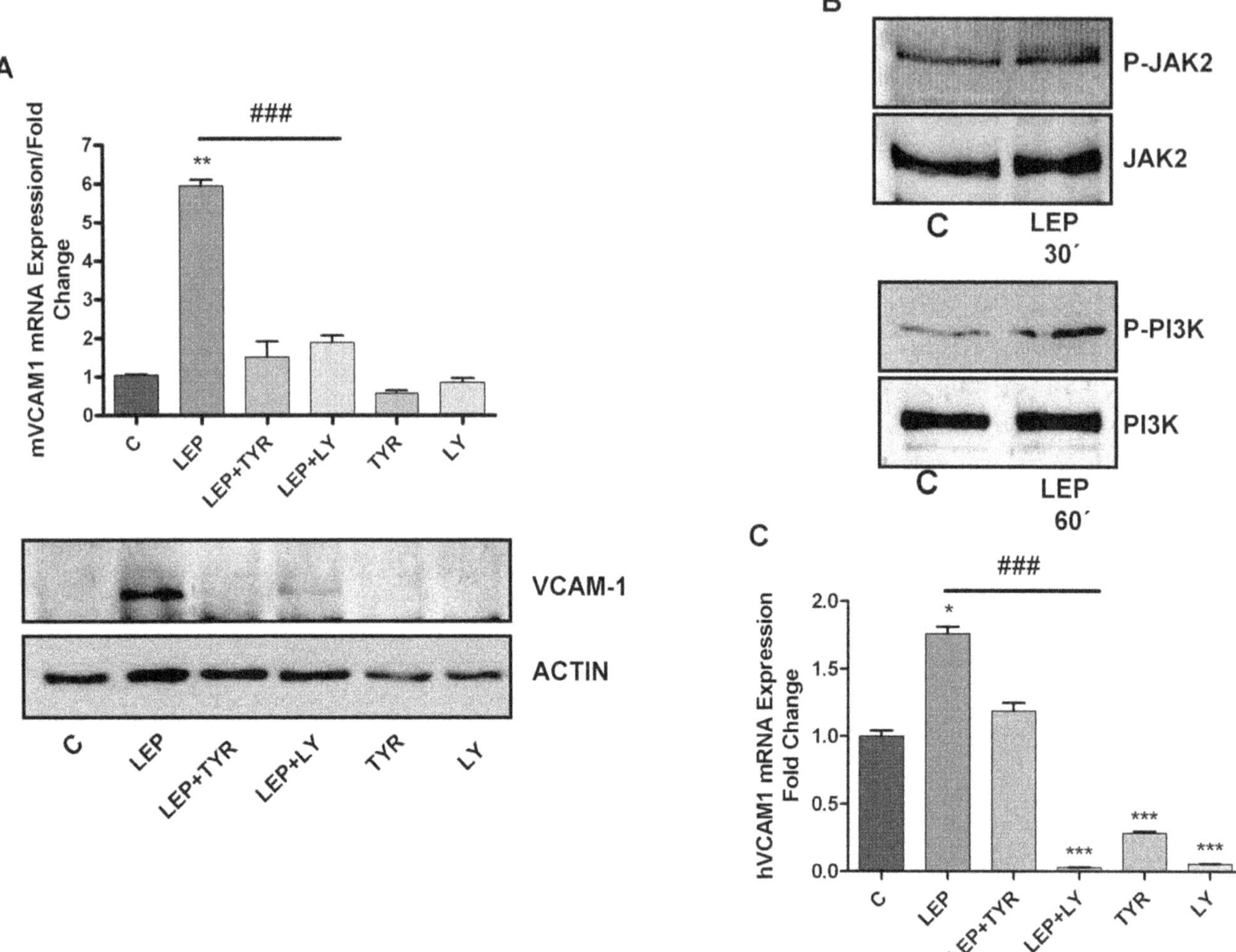

Figure 5. Determination of VCAM-1 mRNA and protein expression by quantitative real-time PCR and western blot. A. mVCAM-1 expression after 1 hour pre-treatment with tyrphostin AG490 (10 μM) and LY294002 (10 μM), followed by a 24 hours of leptin (800 nM) challenge in ATDC-5 cells. **B.** Determination of the phosphorylation of JAK2 and PI3K by western blot. **C.** hVCAM-1 expression after 1 hour pre-treatment with tyrphostin AG490 (10 μM) and LY294002 (10 μM), followed by a 24 hours of leptin (10 μg/ml) challenge in human primary chondrocytes.

in part by adipokines, generates changes in the synovium, including synovial hypertrophy and inflammatory cells infiltration [25].

Therefore extravasation of leukocytes from circulating blood to inflamed tissue is crucial in inflammatory processes and this complex event is regulated by adhesion molecules such as VCAM-1 [26]. The expression of this adhesion molecule affects the binding and recruitment of leucocytes into inflamed joints. For instance, antibody blockade of VCAM-1 decreased significantly the binding of lymphocytes to joint vessels [27]. Similarly, other author demonstrated that incubating synovial fluid with anti-VCAM-1 resulted in a significant inhibition of monocyte chemotaxis [28].

Due to the relevance of adipokines and VCAM-1 respectively in the joint inflammatory processes, we investigated, for the first time, the relationship between these factors. An earlier article reported the induction of VCAM-1 by IL-1β in chondrocytes [7]; thus, we have used the stimulation with this cytokine as our positive control of VCAM-1 induction. Our current study shows, for the first time, a clear VCAM-1 mRNA induction by leptin and adiponectin in human primary chondrocytes. Similar results were obtained in ATDC5 cell line, being adiponectin the most potent inductor, even more than IL-1β. The intracellular pathway/s involved in the adiponectin-induced VCAM-1 expression was, up to now, unknown. Thus we have explored, by using specific pharmacological inhibitors the potential involvement of several intracellular kinases. Our results clearly show that AMPK and PI3K are at play in the VCAM-1 induction by adiponectin. In the same way, JAK2 and PI3K are involved in VCAM-1 induction by leptin.

Moreover, in this study we observed that treatment with adiponectin or leptin in combination with IL-1β, resulted in an additive induction of VCAM-1. Noteworthy, our group demonstrated that leptin is able to synergize with IL-1β in the production of nitric oxide [24]. We also tested the effect of visfatin on VCAM-1 expression, and any modulation was observed neither in human primary chondrocytes nor in ATDC-5 cells (data not shown).

Several lines of evidence suggest that adipokines are clearly involved in degenerative joint disease such as RA and OA. This study extends our current knowledge of adipokine functions by specifically demonstrating that both leptin and adiponectin are able to induce VCAM-1 directly in cultured human and murine chondrocytes, thus contributing to a better understanding of disease etiology. So, it is reasonable to depict a scenario in which adipokines may perpetuate cartilage degrading processes by inducing also factors responsible of leukocyte and monocyte infiltration at inflamed joints.

Author Contributions

Conceived and designed the experiments: FL OG. Performed the experiments: JC MS VL JP. Analyzed the data: JC FL JJGR OG. Contributed reagents/materials/analysis tools: RG JP. Wrote the paper: JC RG FL OG. Acquisition of data, analysis and interpretation of data and critical revision of the manuscript: JC. Acquisition of data, drafting of the manuscript and statistical analysis: MS VL JP. Participated in drafting the manuscript: JJGR Scientific supervision of experiments: OG FL.

References

1. Martel-Pelletier J (2004) Pathophysiology of osteoarthritis. Osteoarthritis Cartilage 12 Suppl A: S31–33.
2. Felson DT (2005) Relation of obesity and of vocational and avocational risk factors to osteoarthritis. J Rheumatol 32: 1133–1135.
3. Lago F, Dieguez C, Gomez-Reino J, Gualillo O (2007) Adipokines as emerging mediators of immune response and inflammation. Nat Clin Pract Rheumatol 3: 716–724.
4. Lago R, Gomez R, Otero M, Lago F, Gallego R, et al. (2008) A new player in cartilage homeostasis: adiponectin induces nitric oxide synthase type II and pro-inflammatory cytokines in chondrocytes. Osteoarthritis Cartilage 16: 1101–1109.
5. Martin JA, Buckwalter JA (2002) Aging, articular cartilage chondrocyte senescence and osteoarthritis. Biogerontology 3: 257–264.
6. Heinegard D, Saxne T (2011) The role of the cartilage matrix in osteoarthritis. Nat Rev Rheumatol 7: 50–56.
7. Kienzle G, von Kempis J (1998) Vascular cell adhesion molecule 1 (CD106) on primary human articular chondrocytes: functional regulation of expression by cytokines and comparison with intercellular adhesion molecule 1 (CD54) and very late activation antigen 2. Arthritis Rheum 41: 1296–1305.
8. Francin PJ, Guillaume C, Humbert AC, Pottie P, Netter P, et al. (2011) Association between the chondrocyte phenotype and the expression of adipokines and their receptors: evidence for a role of leptin but not adiponectin in the expression of cartilage-specific markers. J Cell Physiol 226: 2790–2797.
9. Golias C, Tsoutsi E, Matziridis A, Makridis P, Batistatou A, et al. (2007) Review. Leukocyte and endothelial cell adhesion molecules in inflammation focusing on inflammatory heart disease. In Vivo 21: 757–769.
10. Elices MJ, Osborn L, Takada Y, Crouse C, Luhowskyj S, et al. (1990) VCAM-1 on activated endothelium interacts with the leukocyte integrin VLA-4 at a site distinct from the VLA-4/fibronectin binding site. Cell 60: 577–584.
11. Albelda SM (1991) Endothelial and epithelial cell adhesion molecules. Am J Respir Cell Mol Biol 4: 195–203.
12. Tak PP, Thurkow EW, Daha MR, Kluin PM, Smeets TJ, et al. (1995) Expression of adhesion molecules in early rheumatoid synovial tissue. Clin Immunol Immunopathol 77: 236–242.
13. Morales-Ducret J, Wayner E, Elices MJ, Alvaro-Gracia JM, Zvaifler NJ, et al. (1992) Alpha 4/beta 1 integrin (VLA-4) ligands in arthritis. Vascular cell adhesion molecule-1 expression in synovium and on fibroblast-like synoviocytes. J Immunol 149: 1424–1431.
14. Kriegsmann J, Keyszer GM, Geiler T, Brauer R, Gay RE, et al. (1995) Expression of vascular cell adhesion molecule-1 mRNA and protein in rheumatoid synovium demonstrated by in situ hybridization and immunohistochemistry. Lab Invest 72: 209–214.
15. Sommaggio R, Manez R, Costa C (2009) TNF, pig CD86, and VCAM-1 identified as potential targets for intervention in xenotransplantation of pig chondrocytes. Cell Transplant 18: 1381–1393.
16. Schett G, Kiechl S, Bonora E, Zwerina J, Mayr A, et al. (2009) Vascular cell adhesion molecule 1 as a predictor of severe osteoarthritis of the hip and knee joints. Arthritis Rheum 60: 2381–2389.
17. Kalichman L, Pantsulaia I, Kobyliansky E (2011) Association between vascular cell adhesion molecule 1 and radiographic hand osteoarthritis. Clin Exp Rheumatol 29: 544–546.
18. Gomez R, Lago F, Gomez-Reino JJ, Dieguez C, Gualillo O (2009) Expression and modulation of ghrelin O-acyltransferase in cultured chondrocytes. Arthritis Rheum 60: 1704–1709.
19. Thomas DP, Sunters A, Gentry A, Grigoriadis AE (2000) Inhibition of chondrocyte differentiation in vitro by constitutive and inducible overexpression of the c-fos proto-oncogene. J Cell Sci 113 (Pt 3): 439–450.
20. Conde J, Gomez R, Bianco G, Scotece M, Lear P, et al. (2011) Expanding the adipokine network in cartilage: identification and regulation of novel factors in human and murine chondrocytes. Ann Rheum Dis 70: 551–559.
21. Iliopoulos D, Malizos KN, Tsezou A (2007) Epigenetic regulation of leptin affects MMP-13 expression in osteoarthritic chondrocytes: possible molecular target for osteoarthritis therapeutic intervention. Ann Rheum Dis 66: 1616–1621.
22. Koskinen A, Juslin S, Nieminen R, Moilanen T, Vuolteenaho K, et al. (2011) Adiponectin associates with markers of cartilage degradation in osteoarthritis and induces production of proinflammatory and catabolic factors through mitogen-activated protein kinase pathways. Arthritis Res Ther 13: R184.
23. Otero M, Lago R, Gomez R, Lago F, Dieguez C, et al. (2006) Changes in plasma levels of fat-derived hormones adiponectin, leptin, resistin and visfatin in patients with rheumatoid arthritis. Ann Rheum Dis 65: 1198–1201.
24. Otero M, Lago R, Lago F, Reino JJ, Gualillo O (2005) Signalling pathway involved in nitric oxide synthase type II activation in chondrocytes: synergistic effect of leptin with interleukin-1. Arthritis Res Ther 7: R581–591.
25. Smith MD, Triantafillou S, Parker A, Youssef PP, Coleman M (1997) Synovial membrane inflammation and cytokine production in patients with early osteoarthritis. J Rheumatol 24: 365–371.
26. Kluger MS (2004) Vascular endothelial cell adhesion and signaling during leukocyte recruitment. Adv Dermatol 20: 163–201.
27. Salmi M, Jalkanen S (2001) Human leukocyte subpopulations from inflamed gut bind to joint vasculature using distinct sets of adhesion molecules. J Immunol 166: 4650–4657.
28. Tokuhira M, Hosaka S, Volin MV, Haines GK, 3rd, Katschke KJ Jr, et al. (2000) Soluble vascular cell adhesion molecule 1 mediation of monocyte chemotaxis in rheumatoid arthritis. Arthritis Rheum 43: 1122–1133.

Development and Validation of a Questionnaire Assessing Fears and Beliefs of Patients with Knee Osteoarthritis: The Knee Osteoarthritis Fears and Beliefs Questionnaire (KOFBeQ)

Mathilde Benhamou[1], Gabriel Baron[2], Marie Dalichampt[2], Isabelle Boutron[2], Sophie Alami[3], François Rannou[1,4], Philippe Ravaud[2], Serge Poiraudeau[1,4]*

1 Service de Rééducation et Réadaptation de l'Appareil Locomoteur et des Pathologies du Rachis, Assistance Publique-Hôpitaux de Paris; Université Paris Descartes; INSERM IFR 25 Handicap, Paris, France, **2** Centre d'Epidémiologie Clinique, Assistance Publique-Hôpitaux de Paris; Université Paris Descartes, Paris, France, **3** Department of Sociology, Université Paris Descartes, Interlis, Paris, France, **4** Section Arthrose de la Société Française de Rhumatologie, Paris, France

Abstract

Objective: We aimed to develop a questionnaire assessing fears and beliefs of patients with knee OA.

Design: We sent a detailed document reporting on a qualitative analysis of interviews of patients with knee OA to experts, and a Delphi procedure was adopted for item generation. Then, 80 physicians recruited 566 patients with knee OA to test the provisional questionnaire. Items were reduced according to their metric properties and exploratory factor analysis. Reliability was tested by the Cronbach α coefficient. Construct validity was tested by divergent validity and confirmatory factor analysis. Test–retest reliability was assessed by the intra-class correlation coefficient (ICC) and the Bland and Altman technique.

Results: 137 items were extracted from analysis of the interview data. Three Delphi rounds were needed to obtain consensus on a 25-item provisional questionnaire. The item-reduction process resulted in an 11-item questionnaire. Selected items represented fears and beliefs about daily living activities (3 items), fears and beliefs about physicians (4 items), fears and beliefs about the disease (2 items), and fears and beliefs about sports and leisure activities (2 items). The Cronbach α coefficient of global score was 0.85. We observed expected divergent validity. Confirmation factor analyses confirmed higher intra-factor than inter-factor correlations. Test–retest reliability was good, with an ICC of 0.81, and Bland and Altman analysis did not reveal a systematic trend.

Conclusions: We propose an 11-item questionnaire assessing patients' fears and beliefs concerning knee OA with good content and construct validity.

Editor: Steve Milanese, University of South Australia, Australia

Funding: This study was funded by an unlimited grant from Pfizer. The funders had no role in study design, data collection and analysis, decision to publish, or preparation of the manuscript.

Competing Interests: This study was funded by an unlimited grant from Pfizer. Co-authors François Rannou and Isabelle Boutron are PLOS ONE Editorial Board members. There are no patents, products in development or marketed products to declare. This does not alter the authors' adherence to all the PLOS ONE policies on sharing data and materials.

* E-mail: serge.poiraudeau@cch.aphp.fr

Introduction

Fear is an emotional response generated during dangerous or painful experiences and can include potentially useful survival mechanisms such as escape and avoidance behaviours [1,2]. After fearful experiences, anticipated or actual exposure to similar situations can re-elicit a fear response, even when these exposures are not dangerous or painful], a situation called classical conditioning. Fear can also be learned through vicarious exposure, including observing others (modelling) [3], and through information or instruction [4,5]. Although emotion-based fear may be a relevant factor in some people, reason-based beliefs are important to all people. Beliefs are defined as convictions of the truth of propositions without their verification and therefore are subjective, mental interpretations derived from perceptions, reasoning or communications. All adults have measurable beliefs about diseases or their management that involve thoughts about the pathology or process responsible for the disease [6]. Beliefs are derived by processing information from multiple sources, including personal experiences, family, acquaintances, societal attitudes, media, literature, internet research, and encounters with the health care system [7]. Because human behaviours are shaped by beliefs, beliefs directly influence decisions to follow or not management strategies, including treatments. Of greatest importance, beliefs encompass ongoing reasoning and are therefore amenable to change in response to new information and new experiences [8].

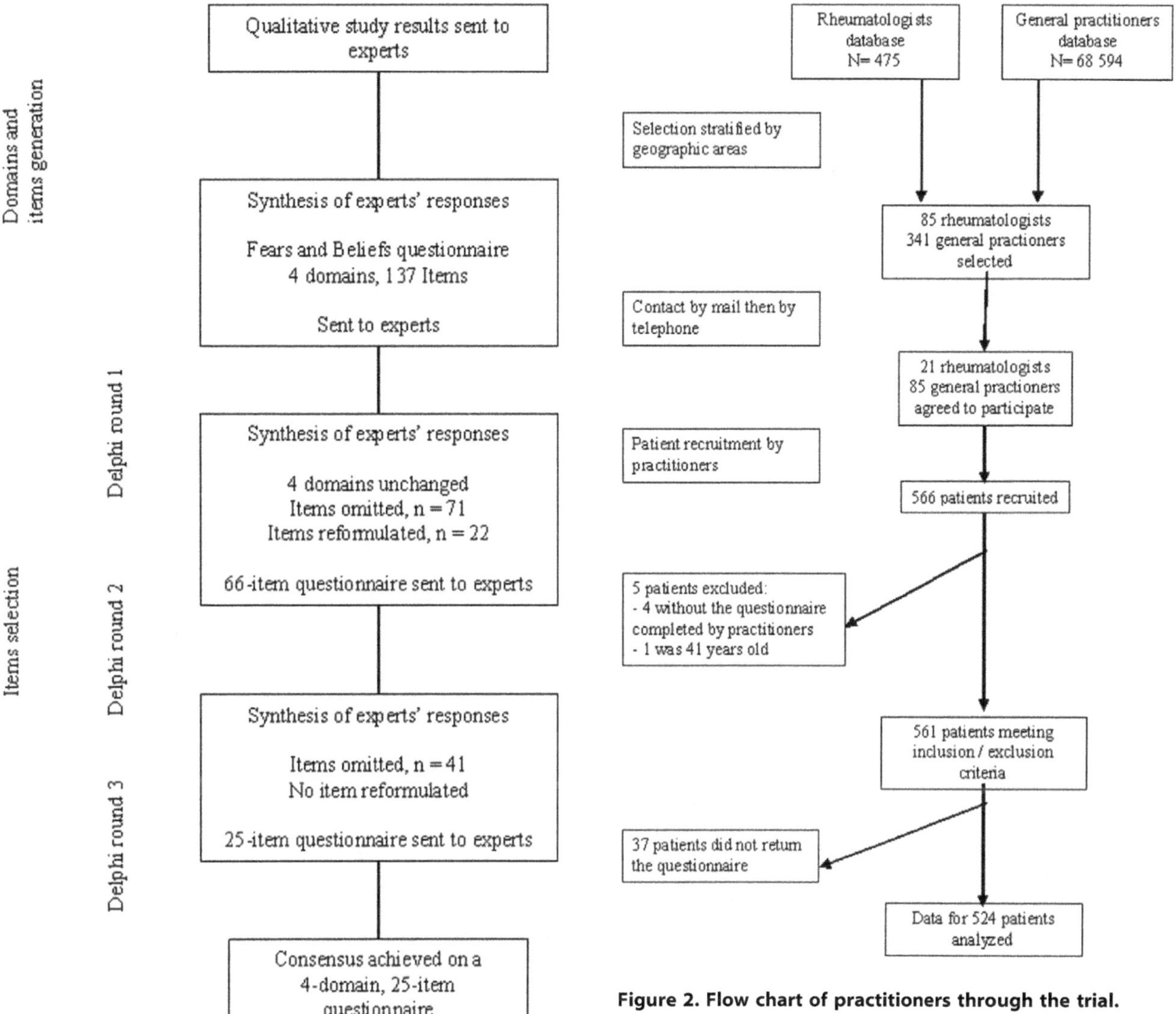

Figure 1. Development of the Knee Osteoarthritis Fears and Beliefs Questionnaire.

Figure 2. Flow chart of practitioners through the trial.

Fears and beliefs have been mostly studied in patients with low back pain and have been shown to be important prognostic factors and to influence treatment adherence [9–13].

Arthritis (mainly osteoarthritis [OA]) is the most common cause of reported disability [14,15] in developed societies and similar to chronic low back pain, is a chronic musculoskeletal painful situation. A recent survey suggested that the burden of knee OA in primary care is substantial [16], and a substantial decrease in health-related quality of life was also reported in a family practice setting [17]. Fears and beliefs of patients concerning knee OA management have been seldom studied. The Tampa scale of kinesiophobia (TSK) has been used in one cohort study and its score shown to be associated with psychological disability and walking at fast speed [18], and the metric properties of a brief fear of movement scale derived from the TSK have been recently published [19]. Although a modified version for knee OA of the fear-avoidance beliefs questionnaire has been used in one study [20], to our knowledge, no validated questionnaire has been specifically designed to assess fears and beliefs in OA patients.

We aimed to develop a questionnaire assessing fears and beliefs of patients with knee OA: the Knee Osteoarthritis Fears and Beliefs Questionnaire (KOFBeQ).

Methods

The general methodology used to develop this questionnaire have been previously published [21].

1) Development of the provisional questionnaire

We adopted a Delphi procedure to select items for the provisional questionnaire. We used previously described general methods for instrument development [22]. The process consists of 3 main steps: definition of the aim of the questionnaire, generating items, and selecting items.

Aim of the questionnaire

The general purpose of this questionnaire is to facilitate the patient–physician relationship and patient education by recording patient fears and beliefs in routine practice and clinical research. The specific purposes are to better define patients' unrealistic fears and beliefs to try to modulate barriers to treatment adherence and help plan disease management.

Table 1. Characteristics of patients with knee osteoarthritis (OA) surveyed in developing the Knee Osteoarthritis Fears and Beliefs Questionnaire.

Sociodemographic characteristics	N	
Age, years, mean (SD)	524	68.2 (10.1)
Female sex	524	327 (62.5)
Married	524	294 (56.4)
Level of education	524	
- primary		272 (52.4)
- secondary		171 (32.9)
- post-graduate		76 (14.6)
Employment status	524	
- job activity		96 (18.4)
- retired		374 (71.8)
- no job activity		29 (5.6)
- unemployed		4 (0.8)
- invalidity		18 (3.5)
Living area	524	
- rural		210 (41.4)
- urban		297 (58.6)
Level of physical activity	524	
- professional sports activity		12 (2.3)
- intensive sports activity		13 (2.5)
- regular sport activity		69 (13.2)
- occasional sport activity		88 (16.8)
- no sport activity		342 (65.3)
Medical characteristics		
Body mass index, kg/m^2, mean (SD)	520	28.3 (4.9)
Duration of disease, years, mean (SD)	520	6.6 (5.3)
Co-morbidities	524	
- cardiovascular abnormality		293 (55.9)
- metabolic and endocrinal disorders		166 (31.7)
- joint and bone disorders (except knee OA)		48 (9.2)
- gastrointestinal disorders		72 (13.7)
- respiratory function		35 (6.7)
Medial femoro-tibial knee OA	524	219 (52.9)
Lateral femoro-tibial knee OA	524	73 (39.5)
Femoro-patellar knee OA	524	145 (53.1)
Physician scale of severity of knee OA (0–10), mean (SD)	523	5.9 (1.8)
Pain intensity (0–10), mean (SD)	405	5.6 (2.1)
Medical drugs for OA		
- analgesics	496	459 (92.5)
- nonsteroidal anti-inflammatory drugs	475	234 (49.2)
- slow-acting drugs for OA	484	312 (64.5)
Physical treatments for OA		
- exercise	455	126 (27.7)
- physiotherapy	466	153 (32.8)
- alternative medicine	458	46 (10.0)
Functional status		
WOMAC score, mean (SD), range	476	31.8 (12.9), 1–62
SF-12, mean (SD)	461	
-physical score (range 0–100)		35.4 (8.0)
-mental score (range 0–100)		44.4 (10.3)

Data are number (%) unless indicated.

Generating items

The Delphi consensus method was used to generate and select items [22], with the initial development in French. For extracting items related to fears and beliefs, a detailed document reporting on the qualitative analysis of interviews with patients was sent to 10 experts (1 general practitioner, 5 rheumatologists, 1 sociologist, 1 orthopaedic surgeon, 1 physical therapist, and 1 physical and rehabilitation medicine physician) [23]. Experts were asked to read the documents and extract the most relevant items concerning patient fears and beliefs. To help experts, several domains were proposed: the disease, its causes and outcomes (triggering and worsening factors); impact of knee OA on daily living, sports, leisure and professional activities; treatments; and physicians. Experts were invited to add domains if they wished.

Selecting items

For each generated item, experts were asked to rate on two 11-point Likert scales (0, disagree, to 10, agree) whether they believed the item should be selected in the final tool and the degree of agreement with the formulation of the item. Experts who disagreed with the formulation of the item were asked to propose a new formulation. Experts were also invited to add items to domains. Items with median relevance score ≤7 were excluded, as were redundant items.

For the second Delphi round, experts were asked to re-rank their agreement with each item; they could change their score in

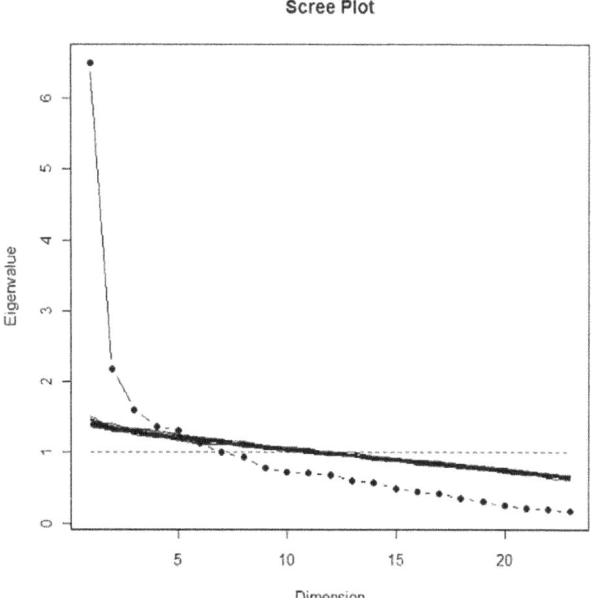

Figure 3. Exploratory factor analysis of the Knee Osteoarthritis Fears and Beliefs Questionnaire.

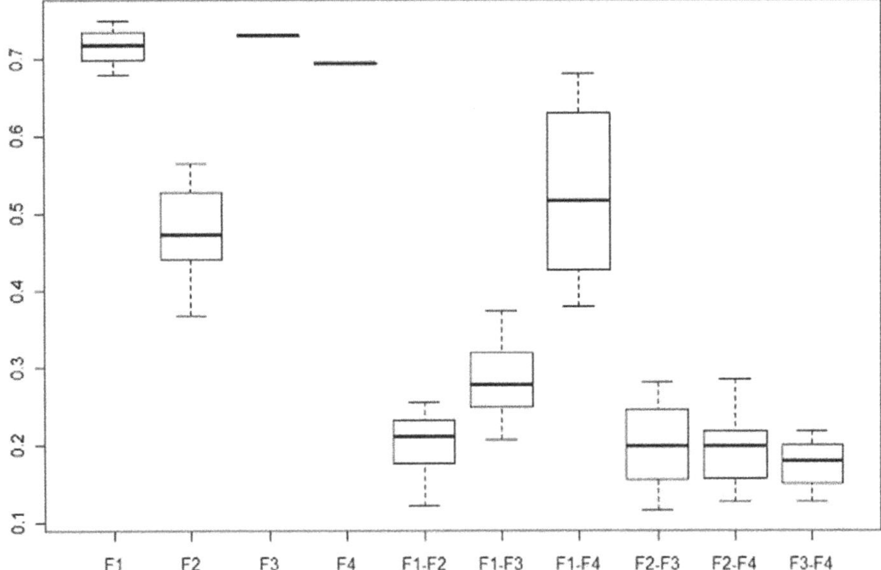

Figure 4. Confirmatory factor analysis of the Knee Osteoarthritis Fears and Beliefs Questionnaire.

view of the group's response to the previous round but could not conform to the group's median response. A rewording of some items was proposed. Further, an explanation for the questionnaire and the modalities of answers were developed. Items with median relevance score ≤8 were excluded. A rewording of some items was proposed.

During the third and last round, experts commented on the final checklist and modalities of answers. Agreement was obtained with the third Delphi round.

Analysis of items

The responses for each Delphi round were reported as the percentage of experts choosing each value of the 11-point Likert scale. Experts' comments on each item were recorded. After each round, the steering group (IB, SA, SP) discussed experts' qualitative and quantitative answers. From these answers, redundant items were combined, categories of items with insufficient consensus rates were excluded, items proposed by experts were added, and items were modified or expanded.

English translation of the provisional questionnaire

To provide a version of the questionnaire for English-speaking patients, the French version was translated by the forward and backward translation procedure [24,25]. Two independent bilingual translators, whose native language was English, translated the French version of the questionnaire into English. As recommended, the translators were encouraged to strive for idiomatic rather than word-for-word translation. Two bilingual investigators (SP, FR) compared the 2 translated versions, with consensus. Two other independent translators who had not participated in the first stage and whose native language was French then back-translated the English version of the questionnaire into French. The investigators (SP, FR) then compared the translated version, with consensus.

2) Reduction of items in the provisional questionnaire and validation of the final questionnaire

The aim was to select items with the best metric qualities from the provisional questionnaire and to assess the reliability and construct validity of the final questionnaire. Therefore, we conducted a national multicenter cross-sectional survey of patients in a primary care setting.

Recruitment of physicians and patients

Physicians. Rheumatologists and general practitioners (GPs) were randomly selected from 2 national databases of 475 and 68 594 practitioners, respectively, who had not previously refused to participate in studies or surveys. The assigned physicians were

Table 2. Divergent validity: correlation of the global score of the Knee Osteoarthritis Fears and Beliefs Questionnaire with other outcome measures.

	Spearman correlation coefficients
Knee OA severity (0–10) assessed by physicians	0.30
Knee pain (0–10)	0.38
Function WOMAC score	0.52
SF-12 physical score	−0.36
SF-12 mental score	−0.38

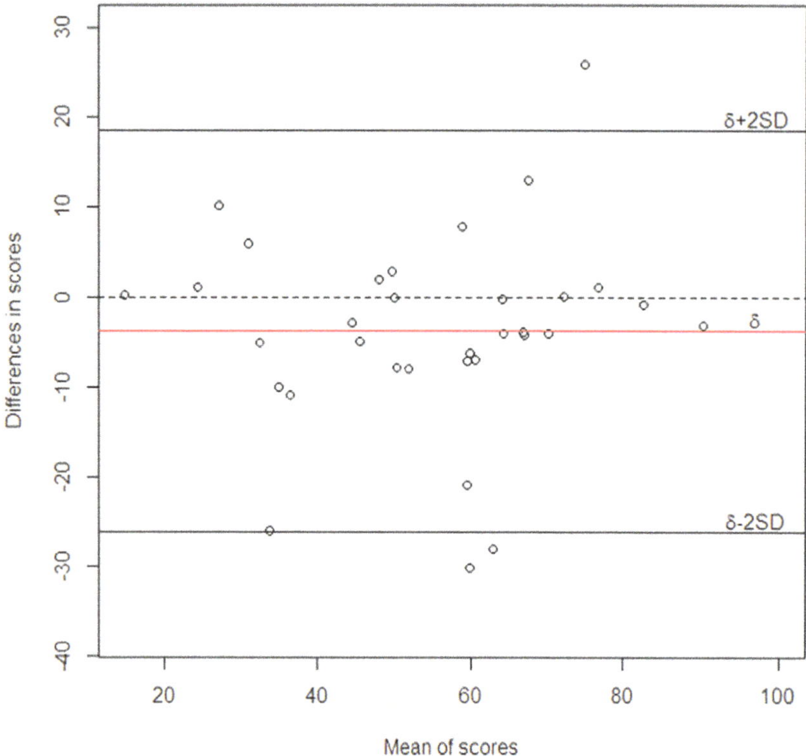

Figure 5. Bland and Altman analysis of test-retest reliability.

contacted by mail, then telephone calls if they did not respond. The randomisation was stratified by geographic area. Each physician was asked to include 5 consecutive patients.

Patients. Each patient consulting one of the participating physicians for knee OA during the period of inclusion and meeting the inclusion criteria was asked to participate in the study.

The inclusion criteria were age 45 years and older, knee OA defined by the American College of Rheumatology criteria [26], whatever knee OA activity status or treatment used, and written consent to participate in the study. The exclusion criteria were absence of knee radiographs and inability to complete a questionnaire.

Patients were included from September 2009 to March 2010.

Data collection

Data recorded were patient characteristics: socio-demographic (age, sex, marital status, level of education, employment status, living area), medical (body mass index, duration of disease, co-morbidities, type of knee OA [medial femoro-tibial, lateral femoro-tibial, femoro-patellar]), level of physical activity, pharmacological and physical treatments for OA, and OA activity and function (pain intensity on an 11-point numeric scale [0–10], physician opinion of severity on an 11-point numeric scale [0–10], WOMAC functional scale, and SF-12 physical and mental scales). The questionnaires were completed on paper or electronically according to patient preference.

Sample size calculation

We expected a Cronbach α coefficient of 0.7 to 0.9 for the KOFBeQ. We needed to include 400 patients for a coefficient of 0.7 with 0.05 accuracy and one of 0.9 with 0.015 accuracy. This number of 400 patients was also sufficient for excellent accuracy of the coefficients on factorial analysis.

We assumed that each physician would include 5 patients. Therefore, we planned to enrol 80 physicians (80% [64] GPs, and 20% [16] rheumatologists). We hypothesized that 25% of the physicians contacted would agree to participate and that 75% of these would include patients.

Statistical analysis

We used descriptive statistics to examine the response distribution to each item. The scoring system was 10-points Likert scale

Table 3. Test-retest reliability for the global score.

	N	Mean baseline (SD)	Mean 2 weeks (SD)	Δ mean (SD)	Limits of agreement	ICC (95%CI)	SEM	SDC
Global score	33	52.4 (19.0)	56.2 (18.2)	−3.79 (1.95)	−26.2 to 18.6	0.81 (0.64–0.90)	8.2	22.8

SD = Standard Deviation, ICC = intraclass correlation coefficient for agreement, CI = Confidence Interval, SEM = Standard Error of Measurement, SDC = Smallest Detectable Change.

(0–9). Items with the following characteristics were removed: low response rate (≤95%); floor or ceiling effect, defined by more than 50% of the respondents choosing an extreme positive or negative response category, respectively; and high inter-item correlation (>0.70) assessed by Spearman correlation coefficient.

We used explanatory factor analyses with principal component analysis (PCA) to examine the construct validity of the KOFBeQ. Oblique promax rotation was selected because the factors were not expected to be completely independent of each other [27]. Factors generated by PCA were extracted if eigenvalues were greater than the randomly generated factors from Horn's parallel analysis [28]. Items were included in the factors if they revealed loadings greater than 0.5. In the case of multiple loading of an item on several factors, the item was included in the factor with a better conceptual relationship.

We assessed the internal consistency of the KOFBeQ by the Cronbach α coefficient to examine the degree to which the items in a scale measured the same concept [29]; a Cronbach α >0.70 was considered acceptable, 0.71 to 0.80 respectable, and >0.8 very good. The 95% confidence interval (95% CI) of the Cronbach α was assessed by the bootstrap technique with 1000 replications.

For confirmatory factor analysis, the multi-trait method was used to test the significantly higher correlation of each item with items of its hypothesized factor than with items of the other factors [27] in a different sample of 40 patients. Distributions of intra- and inter-factor correlations were compared by a boxplot graphic.

Divergent validity was assessed by Spearman correlation of the global score of the KOFBeQ and other outcome measures (knee OA severity assessed by physicians, knee pain, function WOMAC score and SF-12 physical and mental scores).

For test-retest reliability, patients from the cross-sectional survey could not participate because a visit to the physician might modify expectations. Therefore, we selected a sample of 40 patients from the files of the physical and rehabilitation medicine department and mailed them a questionnaire to complete at 2-week intervals. Test–retest reliability was assessed by the intra-class correlation coefficient (ICC) by a two-way random-effects model (an ICC ≥0.75 is considered excellent reproducibility) [30] and the Bland and Altman method, by calculating the mean difference (δ) between 2 measurements and the standard deviation (SD) of the difference [31]. The 95% limits of agreement were defined as the mean difference between the measurements ±1.96 SD of the differences. By definition, if differences are normally distributed, 95% of individual differences are within 2 SD of the mean difference (i.e., within the limits of agreement). The Bland-Altman plot is useful to search for any systematic bias, assess random error and reveal whether the difference between scores depends on the level of scores. We computed the standard error of measurement (SEM: essentially, the average SD among observations from the same subject) [31]. The SEM was estimated by calculating the square root of the within-subject variance ($SEM = \sqrt{\sigma_{between\ measurement} + \sigma_{residual}}$). From the same set of data, the smallest detectable change (SDC) was calculated by the formula $SDC = 1.96 * \sqrt{2} * SEM$. SDC allows to be 95% confident that the observed change is a real change.

Data analysis involved use of R 2.10.1 and SAS 9.1.

Ethical considerations

All patients gave their written informed consent to participate in the study. The study protocol was approved by the ethics committee of Cochin Hospital, Paris. Investigations were conducted according to the principles of the Declaration of Helsinki.

Results

1) Development of the questionnaire assessing fears and beliefs of patients with knee OA (Figure 1)

The experts did not generate new domains for the questionnaire. Synthesis of experts' responses to the analysis of the qualitative study led to the extraction of 137 items concerning fears and beliefs.

Selection of items. For the first Delphi round, the 137-item questionnaire was mailed to experts. Experts' responses were synthesized, items with median relevance ≤7 were eliminated, and redundant items were combined, for a 66-item questionnaire. We reformulated 22 items. Domains were combined into 4 categories: causes and evolution of the disease, impact on daily activities, treatments, and physicians.

For the second Delphi round, the 66-item questionnaire was sent back to experts, along with the median scores for relevance and quality of the formulation of each item obtained during the first round, with minimum and maximum scores. Experts were asked again to rate the relevance and quality of the formulation of each item on two 11-point scales. After synthesis of experts' responses, a 25-item questionnaire assessing patient fears and beliefs for knee OA management (Appendix S1) was sent to experts for the third Delphi round. Consensus was achieved at this stage.

We identified few discrepancies between each translation by the forward and backward translation procedure, and consensus was easily reached. Therefore, the translated versions and the original versions explored the same dimensions.

2) Reduction of items and validation of the questionnaire

Patients. Physicians recruited 566 patients to test the questionnaire (Figure 2). Five patients were excluded (4 because the physician questionnaire could not be retrieved for verification of inclusion and exclusion criteria and 1 because he was 41 years old), 37 patients did not return their questionnaire; finally, data for 524 patients were analysed.

The mean (SD) age of patients was 68.2 (10.1) years, disease duration 6.6 (5.3) years, pain intensity 5.6 (2.1; 0–10 scale), and WOMAC score 31.8 (12.9, range 1–62) (Table 1).

The 38 patients not included in the validation of the questionnaire were somewhat younger (5 years younger, on average), had less disease duration (28.9% vs. 45.5% had OA for more than 5 years), and were taking more nonsteroidal anti-inflammatory drugs (66.7% vs. 49.2%) than patients whose data were analyzed (data not shown).

Item reduction

In total, data for 524 patients were analyzed at this step. Concerning the 25-item provisional questionnaire, no missing values occurred for 455 cases (86.8%).

Fourteen items were omitted after the item reduction process, for an 11-item questionnaire (score range 0–99, Appendix S2). We omitted 1 item with a non-response rate >5% (item 16 of the provisional questionnaire, Appendix S1). We omitted 1 item with a ceiling effect (item 3 of the provisional questionnaire, Appendix S1); no item had a floor effect. Two pairs of items were highly correlated (Spearman correlation coefficients 0.7–0.8) and 2 items were omitted (items 4 and 11 of the provisional questionnaire, Appendix S1).

Exploratory factor analysis extracted 4 main factors with eigenvalues of 6.51, 2.19, 1.60, and 1.37 explaining 41% of the variance (Figure 3). Each factor was easily characterized, factor 1 (3 items) representing fears and beliefs about daily living activities, factor 2 (4 items) fears and beliefs about physicians, factor 3 (2 items) fears and beliefs about the disease, and factor 4 (2 items) fears and beliefs about sports and leisure activities. Another 10 items (items 1, 2, 7–9, 17–20, and 22 of the provisional questionnaire, Appendix S1) were eliminated because of weak correlation (<0.5) for each factor.

Validity of the questionnaire

Overall reliability was excellent, with a Cronbach α coefficient of 0.85 (95% CI 0.83–0.87). Reliability of each factor was good, with Cronbach α coefficients of 0.89 (0.80–0.89) for factor 1, 0.78 (0.74–0.82) for factor 2, 0.85 (0.80–0.89) for factor 3, and 0.84 (0.80–0.87) for factor 4. Confirmatory multi-trait analyses confirmed higher intra- than inter-factor correlations (Figure 4).

Expected divergent validity was observed with knee pain score (r = 0.38), WOMAC function score (r = 0.52), and physical and mental component scores of the SF-12 (r = 0.36 and r = 0.38, respectively) (table 2).

Test-retest validity

Test–retest reliability was good (table 3), with an ICC of 0.81 (95% CI 0.64–0.90), and Bland and Altman analysis revealed a slight bias in mean differences (−3.79 [1.95]) without a systematic trend (Figure 5). The variability was random and uniform throughout the range of values (Figure 5). With the limits of agreement, 95% of the differences between the 2 measurements could be expected to lie between −26.2 and 18.6 points (2 SD of the mean difference). From the value of the SEM, the SDC for the global score was 22.8 points, which in a maximum of 99 points equates to a 23.0% score change.

Scoring of the KOFBeQ

The principal component analysis showed a first eigenvalue substantially higher than the others explaining 28.3% of the variance. According to the latter result and those of reliability analyses, an overall score can be used (0–99). The global score is obtained by adding scores of each of the 11 items. The metric properties of the global score should be tested in another sample of patients with knee OA.

Discussion

To our knowledge, this is the first questionnaire assessing patients' fears and beliefs concerning knee OA. For musculoskeletal conditions, fears and beliefs have been mainly studied in low back pain and shown to be important predictors of severity and outcome [13]. Therefore, measuring fears and beliefs in patients with knee OA may help in developing treatment approaches such as education and behavioral therapy and better define prognosis at the individual level.

The main strength of this study is probably the design adopted to generate items. The in-depth interviews about views of patients with knee OA and its management provide a relevant qualitative database to select items that really matter to the patient when building a patient-reported questionnaire. This approach is strongly recommended by the US Food and Drug Administration [32] because it increases the content validity of the instrument. Most patient-reported outcomes widely used with OA were developed in the 1980s and 1990s mainly by selecting items from expert viewpoints and/or pre-existing questionnaires [33–37]. Because patient and physician views differ on what is important or what matters [38–40], the content validity of these questionnaires is questionable. Another strength is that the sample is likely to be representative of patients with knee OA in primary care. Physicians were asked to include 5 consecutive patients and demographic and clinical characteristics of the patients are similar of those previously published in a primary care French context [16].

The Delphi design adopted to select items from the qualitative study is a classical recommended method [22] that allows experts to give an opinions blinded to the opinions of other experts in a first step and achieve consensus anonymously in a second step. The method prevents a "leading expert" effect. Items generated in the provisional questionnaire we developed seemed understandable and acceptable in view of the very low rate of missing answers to the provisional scale.

We translated the provisional questionnaire in English rather than the final one to let researchers from other English-speaking countries test the item reduction step in their own country if they feel it could be relevant in a different background.

The Delphi procedure preserved the 4-domain structure that the steering group proposed to help experts select items: the disease, its causes and outcomes (triggering and worsening factors); impact of knee OA on daily living, sports, leisure and professional activities; treatments; and physicians. Therefore the final questionnaire explores important domains of fears and beliefs that may have an impact on the burden of the disease and its management.

The metric performances of the questionnaire are promising. It has excellent internal validity (reliability) and test–retest reproducibility. It is likely to have satisfactory construct validity because we observed the expected divergent validity, and the factorial structure seems robust, with 4 factors identified and easily characterized after exploratory factor analysis and confirmed by confirmatory factor analysis. Patient fears and beliefs are organized around 4 axes: daily living activities; physicians; the disease; and sports and leisure activities.

This study has limitations. The main limitation is that we did not include patients in the group of experts for the Delphi procedure. Although knee OA is a frequent clinical situation, a patient association is lacking in France, and the identification and selection of patients implicated in the disease and its management is far from obvious. Furthermore, we did not test face validity of the final 11-item questionnaire with a different sample of patients. Another limitation is that this questionnaire has been developed in a strict French context and its content validity should be verified in other groups of patients with different cultural backgrounds. However, the French society is a highly multicultural one, and this limitation applies to every patient-reported outcome because none of them has been developed simultaneously in different countries with different languages and cultures. For assessment of the validity of the questionnaire, we assessed divergent validity but not convergent validity. However, no other instrument exists to assess fears and beliefs or a concept close to fears and beliefs in this context.

Finally, use of this questionnaire may be helpful for two different approaches: a qualitative individualized analysis of responses in routine practice may help increase the quality of patient education by providing relevant information to physicians to adapt attitudes, educational messages, and treatment strategies according to patient fears and beliefs, and a quantitative analysis may provide useful information in clinical research into the effect of high or low level of fears and beliefs or their modification on compliance with treatment, outcomes of treatments, and disease evolution. In this perspective, sensitivity to change of the instrument should be first demonstrated.

In conclusion, we propose a new 11-item patient self-reported questionnaire assessing patient fears and beliefs about knee OA. This questionnaire has robust metric properties, particularly content and construct validity. Its usefulness in the clinic and in clinical research remains to be demonstrated.

Supporting Information

Appendix S1 The provisional questionnaire assessing fears and beliefs of patients with knee osteoarthritis for disease management.

Appendix S2 The Knee Osteoarthritis Fears and Beliefs Questionnaire (KOFBeQ).

Acknowledgments

The authors acknowledge Philippe Anract, Francis Berenbaum, Xavier Chevalier, Thierry Conrozier, Dominique Desjeux, Romain Forestier, Yves Henrotin, Alain Lorenzo, Rémy Nizard and Pascal Richette for their participation in the Delphi process.

Author Contributions

Critical review of the manuscript: MB GB MD IB SA FR PR SP. Conceived and designed the experiments: IB SA FR PR SP. Performed the experiments: GB MD IB. Analyzed the data: GB MD IB SP. Wrote the paper: MB GB SP.

References

1. Davis M (2006) Neural systems involved in fear and anxiety measured with fear-potentiated startle. Am Psychol 61: 741–56.
2. Vlaeyen JW, Kole-Snijders AM, Boeren RG (1995) Fear of movement/(re)injury in chronic low back pain and its relation to behavioral performance. Pain 62: 363–72.
3. Askew C, Field AP (2007) Vicarious learning and the development of fears in childhood. Behav Res Ther 45: 2616–27.
4. Rachman S (1977) The conditioning theory of fear-acquisition: a critical examination. Behav Res Ther 15: 375–87.
5. Field AP, Lawson J (2003) Fear information and the development of fears during childhood: effects on implicit fear responses and behavioural avoidance. Behav Res Ther 41: 1277–93.
6. Waddell G, Newton M, Henderson I (1993) A Fear-Avoidance Beliefs Questionnaire (FABQ) and the role of fear-avoidance beliefs in chronic low back pain and disability. Pain 52: 157–68.
7. Buchbinder R, Jolley D (2004) Population based intervention to change back pain beliefs: three year follow up population survey. BMJ 328: 321.
8. Turner JA, Franklin G, Fulton-Kehoe D (2006) Worker recovery expectations and fear-avoidance predict work disability in a population-based workers' compensation back pain sample. Spine 31: 682–9.
9. Boersma K, Linton SJ (2006) Psychological processes underlying the development of a chronic pain problem: a prospective study of the relationship between profiles of psychological variables in the fear-avoidance model and disability. Clin J Pain 22: 160–6.
10. Woby SR, Watson PJ, Roach NK (2004) Adjustment to chronic low back pain–the relative influence of fear-avoidance beliefs, catastrophizing, and appraisals of control. Behav Res Ther 42: 761–74.
11. Elfving B, Andersson T, Grooten WJ (2007) Low levels of physical activity in back pain patients are associated with high levels of fear-avoidance beliefs and pain catastrophizing. Physiother Res Int 12: 14–24.
12. Gheldof EL, Vinck J, Vlaeyen JW (2005) The differential role of pain, work characteristics and pain-related fear in explaining back pain and sick leave in occupational settings. Pain 113: 71–81.
13. Rainville J, Smeets RJ, Bendix T (2011) Fear-avoidance beliefs and pain avoidance in low back pain–translating research into clinical practice. Spine J 11: 895–903.
14. LaPlante MP (1991) The demographics of disability. Milbank Q 69: 55–77.
15. Badley EM, Rasooly I, Webster GK (1994) Relative importance of musculoskeletal disorders as a cause of chronic health problems, disability, and health care utilization: findings from the 1990 Ontario Health Survey. J Rheumatol 21: 505–14.
16. Boutron I, Rannou F, Jardinaud-Lopez M (2008) Disability and quality of life of patients with knee or hip osteoarthritis in the primary care setting and factors associated with general practitioners' indication for prosthetic replacement within 1 year. Osteoarthritis Cartilage 16: 1024–31.
17. van der Waal JM, Terwee CB, van der Windt DA (2005) Health-related and overall quality of life of patients with chronic hip and knee complaints in general practice. Qual Life Res 14: 795–803.
18. Somers TJ, Keefe FJ, Pells JJ, Dixon KE, Waters SJ, et al. (2009) Pain catastrophizing and pain-related fear in osteoarthritis patients: relationships to pain and disability. J Pain Symptom Manage 37: 863–72.
19. Shelby RA, Somers TJ, Keefe FJ, DeVellis BM, Patterson C, et al (2012) Brief Fear of Movement Scale for osteoarthritis. Arthritis Care Res 64: 862–71.
20. Scopaz KA, Piva SR, Wisniewski S, Fitzgerald GK (2009) Relationships of fear, anxiety, and depression with physical function in patients with knee osteoarthritis. Arch Phys Med Rehabil 90: 1866–73.21.
21. Benhamou M, Boutron I, Dalichampt M (2012) Elaboration and validation of a questionnaire assessing patient expectations about management of knee osteoarthritis by their physicians: the Knee Osteoarthritis Expectations Questionnaire. Ann Rheum Dis. [Epub ahead of print].
22. Stewart J, O'Halloran C, Harrigan P (1999) Identifying appropriate tasks for the preregistration year: modified Delphi technique. BMJ 319: 224–9.
23. Alami S, Boutron I, Desjeux D (2011) Patients' and practitioners' views of knee osteoarthritis and its management: a qualitative interview study. PLoS One 6: e19634.
24. Guillemin F, Bombardier C, Beaton D (1993) Cross-cultural adaptation of health-related quality of life measures: literature review and proposed guidelines. J Clin Epidemiol 46: 1417–32.
25. Beaton DE, Bombardier C, Guillemin F (2000) Guidelines for the process of cross-cultural adaptation of self-report measures. Spine 25: 3186–91.
26. Altman R, Asch E, Bloch D (1986) Development of criteria for the classification and reporting of osteoarthritis. Classification of osteoarthritis of the knee. Diagnostic and Therapeutic Criteria Committee of the American Rheumatism Association. Arthritis Rheum 29: 1039–49.
27. Costello A, Osborne J (2005) Best practices in exploratory factor analysis: four recommendations for getting the most from your analysis. Practical Assessment Research & Evaluation 10: 1–9.
28. Dinno A (2009) Exploring the Sensitivity of Horn's Parallel Analysis to the Distributional Form of Random Data. Multivariate Behav Res 44: 362–88.
29. Bland JM, Altman DG(1997) Cronbach's alpha. BMJ 314: 572.
30. Ware JE, Jr., Gandek B (1998) Methods for testing data quality, scaling assumptions, and reliability: the IQOLA Project approach. International Quality of Life Assessment. J Clin Epidemiol 51: 945–52.
31. Bland JM, Altman DG (1986) Statistical methods for assessing agreement between two methods of clinical measurement. Lancet 1: 307–10.
32. FDA (2009) Patient-Reported Outcome Measures: Use in Medical Product Development to Support Labeling Claims. Clinical/Medical 74: (65) 132–133.
33. Bellamy N, Buchanan WW, Goldsmith CH (1988) Validation study of WOMAC: a health status instrument for measuring clinically important patient relevant outcomes to antirheumatic drug therapy in patients with osteoarthritis of the hip or knee. J Rheumatol 15: 1833–40.
34. Lequesne MG, Mery C, Samson M (1987) Indexes of severity for osteoarthritis of the hip and knee. Validation–value in comparison with other assessment tests. Scand J Rheumatol 65: 85–9.
35. Bellamy N, Campbell J, Haraoui B (2002) Dimensionality and clinical importance of pain and disability in hand osteoarthritis: Development of the Australian/Canadian (AUSCAN) Osteoarthritis Hand Index. Osteoarthritis Cartilage 10: 855–62.
36. Duruoz MT, Poiraudeau S, Fermanian J (1996) Development and validation of a rheumatoid hand functional disability scale that assesses functional handicap. J Rheumatol 23: 1167–72.
37. Dreiser RL, Maheu E, Guillou GB (1995) Validation of an algofunctional index for osteoarthritis of the hand. Rev Rhum 62: 43S–53S.
38. Wylde V, Hewlett S, Learmonth ID (2006) Personal impact of disability in osteoarthritis: patient, professional and public values. Musculoskeletal Care 4: 152–66.
39. Hewlett S, Smith AP, Kirwan JR (2001) Values for function in rheumatoid arthritis: patients, professionals, and public. Ann Rheum Dis 60: 928–33.
40. Tugwell P, Bombardier C, Buchanan WW (1990) Methotrexate in rheumatoid arthritis. Impact on quality of life assessed by traditional standard-item and individualized patient preference health status questionnaires. Arch Intern Med 150: 59–62.

6

SMAD3 Is Associated with the Total Burden of Radiographic Osteoarthritis: The Chingford Study

Erfan Aref-Eshghi[1], Yuhua Zhang[1], Deborah Hart[2], Ana M. Valdes[2], Andrew Furey[1], Glynn Martin[1], Guang Sun[1], Proton Rahman[1], Nigel Arden[3], Tim D. Spector[2], Guangju Zhai[1,2]*

1 Faculty of Medicine, Memorial University of Newfoundland, St. John's, Newfoundland, Canada, **2** Department of Twin Research & Genetic Epidemiology, King's College London, London, United Kingdom, **3** Musculoskeletal Epidemiology and Biobank, University of Oxford, Oxford, United Kingdom

Abstract

Background: A newly-described syndrome called Aneurysm-Osteoarthritis Syndrome (AOS) was recently reported. AOS presents with early onset osteoarthritis (OA) in multiple joints, together with aneurysms in major arteries, and is caused by rare mutations in *SMAD3*. Because of the similarity of AOS to idiopathic generalized OA (GOA), we hypothesized that *SMAD3* is also associated with GOA and tested the hypothesis in a population-based cohort.

Methods: Study participants were derived from the Chingford study. Kellgren-Lawrence (KL) grades and the individual features of osteophytes and joint space narrowing (JSN) were scored from radiographs of hands, knees, hips, and lumbar spines. The total KL score, osteophyte score, and JSN score were calculated and used as indicators of the total burden of radiographic OA. Forty-one common SNPs within *SMAD3* were genotyped using the Illumina HumanHap610Q array. Linear regression modelling was used to test the association between the total KL score, osteophyte score, and JSN score and each of the 41 SNPs, with adjustment for patient age and BMI. Permutation testing was used to control the false positive rate.

Results: A total of 609 individuals were included in the analysis. All were Caucasian females with a mean age of 60.9 ± 5.8. We found that rs3825977, with a minor allele (T) frequency of 20%, in the last intron of *SMAD3*, was significantly associated with total KL score ($\beta = 0.14$, $P_{permutation} = 0.002$). This association was stronger for the total JSN score ($\beta = 0.19$, $P_{permutation} = 0.002$) than for total osteophyte score ($\beta = 0.11$, $P_{permutation} = 0.02$). The T allele is associated with a 1.47-fold increased odds for people with 5 or more joints to be affected by radiographic OA ($P_{permutation} = 0.046$).

Conclusion: We found that *SMAD3* is significantly associated with the total burden of radiographic OA. Further studies are required to reveal the mechanism of the association.

Editor: Masaru Katoh, National Cancer Center, Japan

Funding: The study was supported financially by Newfoundland and Labrador RDC Ignite program, and Memorial University of Newfoundland. EAE was supported by The Dean's Fellowship of Faculty of Medicine, Memorial University of Newfoundland. The Chingford Study was supported by Welcome Trust and Arthritis Research UK. The funders had no role in study design, data collection and analysis, decision to publish, or preparation of the manuscript.

Competing Interests: The authors have declared that no competing interests exist.

* E-mail: guangju.zhai@med.mun.ca

Introduction

Osteoarthritis (OA) is the most common form of arthritis in the elderly, characterized pathologically by focal areas of damage to the articular cartilage centered on load-bearing areas. It is associated with new bone formation at the joint margins (osteophytosis), changes in the subchondral bone, variable degrees of mild synovitis, and thickening of the joint capsule [1] which lead to the presentation of pain, stiffness and disability. Its prevalence—already high—is increasing due to population aging and the increase in obesity. Eighty percent of individuals over 75 years of age have radiographic OA changes in at least one of their joints [2]. According to a report from the Arthritis Community Research & Evaluation Unit in April 2010, the prevalence of self-reported and physician-diagnosed OA in individuals over age 45 ranged from 2.3%–11% in the third world to 8%–16% in the USA [3]. In the same year it affected 27 million people in the USA, imposing a burden of over 11 million dollars on outpatient visits and over 13 billion dollars on OA-related job absence [4]. Half of all adults will develop symptomatic OA of the knee at some points in their lives [5].

OA is a multifactorial disease whose etiology is incompletely understood. It is believed that a number of different environmental and genetic factors interact in its initiation and progression [6]. Evidence suggests that genetic factors play a major role in OA, although they may be site- and sex-specific. From twin studies, this genetic influence has been estimated to be between 40% and 65% on hand and knee OA [7]. First-degree relatives of individuals with spine, hand, hip, or polyarticular OA have a two- to three-fold increased risk of the disease [8,9]. The nature of the genetic influence in OA is still unclear but it is likely to involve a combination of effects on structure (i.e. collagen), alterations in cartilage, bone metabolism and inflammation [10]. Although the genetic influence on OA was recognized more than 130 years ago [11], genetic variants identified so far account only for a small fraction of its heritability [12]. This may reflect several factors including the heterogeneous nature of the disease, the tendency to use less severe phenotypes in genetic searches and the reliance on underpowered studies [13]. Generalized OA—a subtype of primary OA—is characterized by the involvement of multiple joints, and is believed to have a stronger genetic component than individual joint OA [14]. However, genetic data on generalized OA are limited.

Recently, a new syndrome called Aneurysm-Osteoarthritis Syndrome (AOS) was reported [15]. Patients with AOS present with early-onset OA affecting multiple joints including feet/ankle, hand/wrist, knee, hip, facet joints, uncovertebral joints and also exhibit degeneration of the intervertebral discs [15,16]. Eight rare mutations in the *SMAD3* gene (Similar to Mothers Against Decapentaplegic type 3) were identified as responsible for AOS in eight unrelated families.[15, 16] Subsequent studies reported additional *SMAD3* mutations [17,18] and also a CNV (copy number variant) [19] linked to AOS. The *SMAD3* gene encodes a protein that belongs to the SMAD protein family, that are downstream mediators of the transforming growth factor beta (*TGF-β*) signaling pathway [20], which inhibits terminal hypertrophic differentiation of chondrocytes and is essential for maintaining the integrity of articular cartilage [20,21]. This regulatory pathway also stimulates osteogenesis and bone formation [22]. *SMAD3* knock-out mice develop degenerative joint disease similar to human OA [23]. Although a few studies on *SMAD3* and single-joint OA have been reported, no data are available regarding the role *SMAD3* plays in generalized OA. Because of the similarity with AOS, in which multiple joints are also affected, we hypothesized that the *SMAD3* gene plays a role in idiopathic generalized OA. We tested our hypothesis in a large population-based cohort of individuals who had radiographic assessment of multiple joints.

Methods and Subjects

Subjects

The study subjects were women aged 43-67 years at baseline (1988–1989) who were participating in the Chingford Study, a prospective population-based study of OA and osteoporosis. The Chingford Study cohort comprises 1003 women derived from the register of a large general practice in North London, who are similar to the UK population for most demographic variables [24].

Height, weight and details of concomitant diseases, operations and medications were recorded for all subjects. DNA was extracted from blood by standard phenol or salting-out methods. At both baseline and 10 years later, all subjects completed a standardized medical history questionnaire.

Ethics

The Guys & St Thomas' Trust and the Waltham Forest Trust ethics committees approved the study protocol. Written consent was obtained from all participants.

Radiography

Plain films of all joints were obtained from a standard postero-anterior view at baseline and again 9–11 years later. The distal interphalangeal (DIP), proximal interphalangeal (PIP) and first carpometacarpal (CMC) joints of the thumbs, the knee- and hip-joints, as well as four lumbar spinal joints (L1–L5) were assessed for radiographic OA according to the Kellgren & Lawrence (KL) score using a 0–4 scale [25]. Joint Space Narrowing (JSN) and osteophyte characteristics were each scored on a 0–3 scale using a standard atlas [26]. All radiographs were independently assessed by two trained observers (DJ Hunter and DJ Hart). In cases of disagreement, a third adjudicator was used. The intra- and inter-observer reproducibility of the scoring measured on a subgroup of 50 hands had a Kappa statistic of approximately 0.68 for all sites and features.

For the current study, the most recent radiographic and demographic data were used, including cross sectional radiographic data for hip, spine, knee and hand from years 8, 9, 10, and 11 and the age and body mass index (BMI) from the 8th year of the study. All patients were visited at year 8, when the demographic information was collected. Due to the schedule of the radiology department, different joints were assessed in different years (between year 8 and year 11). Total KL score, osteophyte and JSN scores were used as indicators of the total burden of radiographic OA, which was calculated by summing up the individual scores of each joint. Total radiographic scores have been used by researchers in clinical, biomedical, and genetic studies of OA [14,27–29] as an indicator for total burden of OA. In addition, individuals were evaluated for the criteria required for a diagnosis of generalized OA. To this end, joints were defined as being affected by OA if the KL score was ≥2. OA of either the DIP or PIP joint groups was defined as the presence of OA in at least two of the relevant joints. A diagnosis of GOA was based on the definition used by Cooper et al [30]. Fourteen joints or joint groups were considered: the four lumbar joints together with the left and right knee, hip, DIP group, PIP group and thumb CMCs. GOA was defined as the presence of OA in at least five of these 14 joints. Those with fewer than five joints affected were designated as controls.

Genotyping

The samples were genotyped using the Illumina HumanHap610Q array. The normalized intensity data was used by the Illluminus calling algorithm [31] to assign genotypes. No calls were assigned if an individual's most likely genotype was called with a posterior probability threshold of less than 0.95. Sample exclusion criteria were: (i) sample call rate <98%, (ii) heterozygosity across all SNPs ≥2 s.d. from the sample mean; (iii) evidence of non-European ancestry as assessed by PCA comparison with HapMap3 populations; (iv) observed pair-wise IBD probabilities suggestive of sample identity errors; (v). SNP exclusion criteria included (i) Hardy-Weinberg p-value$<10^{-6}$, assessed in a set of unrelated samples; (ii) MAF<1%, assessed in a set of unrelated samples; (iii) SNP call rate <97% (SNPs with MAF≥5%) or < 99% (for 1%≤MAF<5%). For the current study, we retrieved genotype data for all 41 SNPs within the *SMAD3* gene which were available on the array.

Statistics

Since the distribution of the total KL, JSN, and osteophyte scores was skewed, a logarithmic transformation was performed to approximate a normal distribution. Subsequent analyses were performed on the log-transformed values. A linear regression model, testing for an additive genetic model, was used to test the association between each of the 41 candidate SNPs and the total KL, JSN, and osteophyte scores individually. A logistic regression model was used to test the association between each of the 41 SNPs and GOA. Potential confounders such as age and BMI were considered in both models. All SNP associations with $p<0.05$ in the initial analyses were subject to permutation testing in order to control the false positive rate. The permutation method is well established as a robust approach for obtaining empirical significance levels while minimizing Type I errors [32,33], and has been used to correct for multiple testing in genetic association studies [34]. Because of the infinite permutation with our sample size, we used a Monte Carlo permutation procedure and the phenotype labels were reshuffled 10,000 times. The permutation-based p-value was calculated as the proportion of the statistic on all the reshuffled data sets greater than the observed statistic [34]. The significance level was defined as a permutation-based p-value of less than 0.05. All analyses were conducted using STATA/SE 11.2 (Stata Corp, College Station, Texas, USA).

Results

All study subjects were Caucasian females. Radiographic data for spine, hips, knees and hand joints were available for 796, 794, 614, and 687 individuals, respectively. The age and BMI data were available for 843 participants with a mean age of 61.2±5.8 and a mean BMI of 26.7±4.7. Total KL, osteophyte and JSN scores were available for 609, 603, and 607 individuals respectively. As expected, patients with GOA—defined as having 5 or more joints affected—were, on average, older than those with fewer than 5 affected joints, and also had a higher BMI (Table 1). The frequency of subjects with different number of affected joints is presented in Table 2.

Forty-one common SNPs within the *SMAD3* gene were genotyped and passed quality control. They were scattered randomly throughout the *SMAD3* gene, but none were located in exons (Figure 1). The average pairwise R^2 between SNPs was 0.07.

We found that SNP rs3825977 was significantly associated with all phenotypes analyzed, *viz.* total KL, osteophyte and JSN scores. The differences in these traits among individuals with different genotypes are presented in Figures 2, 3, 4. After adjustment for age and BMI, the minor (T) allele of rs3825977—with 20% allele frequency—was associated with a 0.14% increase in log total KL score (95% CI 0.04–0.20, $P_{permutation} = 0.002$). The association is stronger for log total JSN score with $\beta = 0.19$ (95%CI 0.07–0.31, $P_{permutation} = 0.002$) than for log total osteophyte score with $\beta = 0.11$ (95%CI 0.01–0.20, $P_{permutation} = 0.02$). Two other SNPs—rs6494629 and rs2118612—were significant for only total osteophyte score in the univariate analysis but not in a multivariate analysis. All the results of univariate and multivariate linear regression analyses for total KL, osteophyte and JSN scores for all 41 SNPs are presented in Tables S1–S3 in File S1, respectively.

Furthermore, we categorized the study participants into two groups: one with ≥5 joints affected (GOA) and one with <5 joints affected and examined the association of each group with each of the 41 SNPs. We found that the T allele of rs3825977 was significantly associated with a 1.47-fold increased risk of GOA (95% CI 1.02–2.1, $P_{permutation} = 0.046$) after adjustment for age and BMI (Table 3). All results of the associations with each of the 41 SNPs are presented in Table S4 in File S1.

Table 2. Frequency of patients with different number of joints affected.

Number of Joints affected	Frequency (%)
0	43 (7.06%)
1	62 (10.18%)
2	83 (13.63%)
3	93 (15.27%)
4	80 (13.14%)
5	51 (8.37%)
6	64 (10.51%)
7	38 (6.24%)
8	36 (5.91%)
9	22 (3.61%)
10	15 (2.46%)
11	12 (1.97%)
12	9 (1.48%)
13	1 (0.16%)
Total	609 (100%)

Discussion

In the present study we demonstrate a significant association of SNP rs3825977—located in the last intron of *SMAD3*—with the total burden of radiographic OA. This SNP is more strongly associated with total JSN score than with total KL score or osteophyte score, suggesting that the potential mechanism for the association is more likely through cartilage loss rather than osteophyte formation. The same SNP has previously been reported as associated with increased breast cancer risk for *BRCA2* mutation carriers [35]. Although the possible effect of the SNP on *SMAD3* function is still unclear, it is believed that the effects on both breast cancer and generalized OA susceptibility are mediated through the *TGF-β* signaling pathway.

Data on the associations between the *SMAD3* gene and GOA are limited and, to our knowledge, no genetic or genome-wide association study has been performed on GOA. A study by Yao JY, *et al.* [36] was the first to report a connection between *SMAD3* and OA. This paper described a missense mutation located in the linker region of the SMAD3 protein which resulted in an increased expression of matrix metalloproteinase (MMP) 2 and 9 in the serum of one OA mutation carrier compared to MMP expression in other OA patients and in controls. Another study by A. Valdes and colleagues [37] reported the association of a variant in the *SMAD3* gene with hip and knee OA. In that study the frequency of the major (G) allele of rs12901499—located in the first intron of *SMAD3*—was increased in patients undergoing hip or knee

Table 1. Descriptive statistics of the study population.

	GOA (n = 247)	Controls (n = 360)	P-Value
Age	64.21±0.34	58.71±0.3	P<0.0001
BMI	27.50±0.26	26.02±0.2	P<0.0001

Figures are mean ± SD, and Student's T-test was used for the comparison.

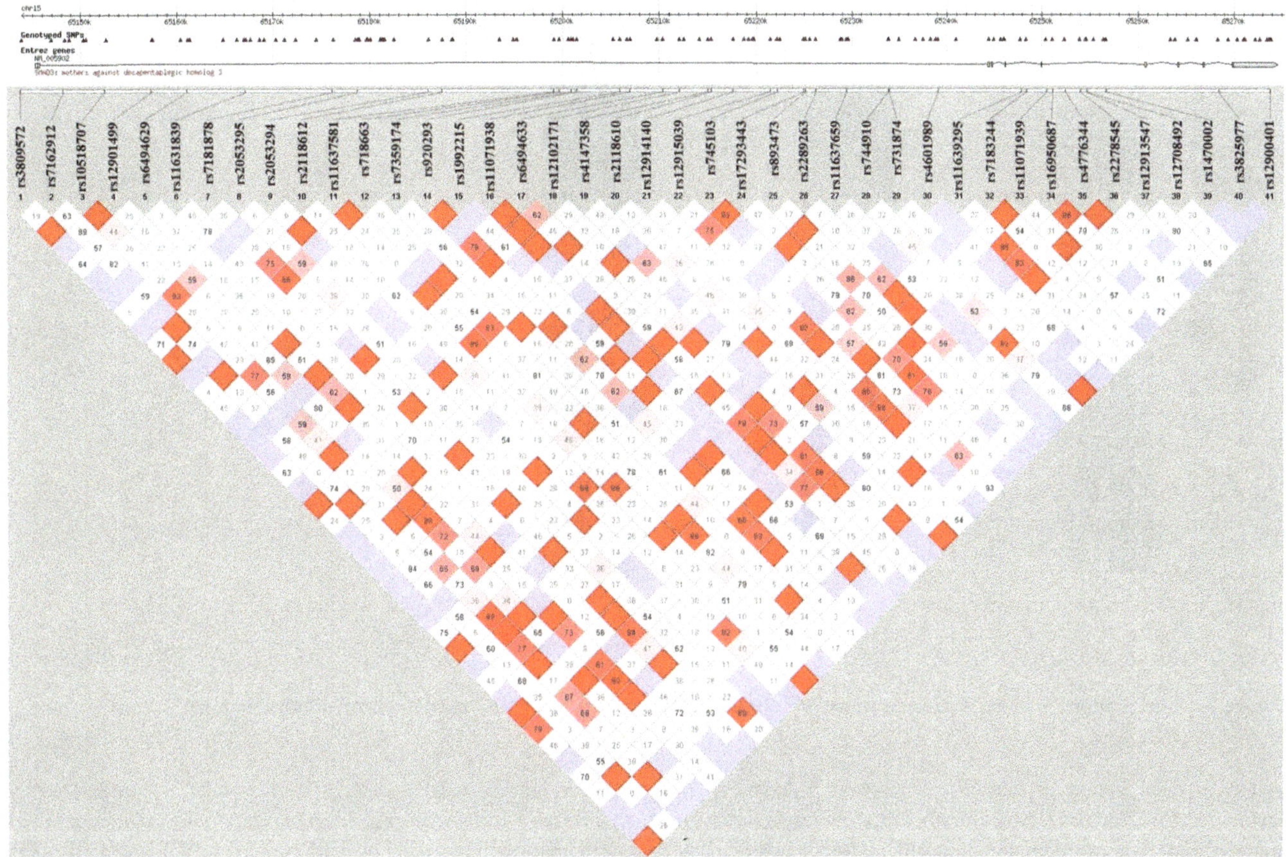

Figure 1. Distribution and LD pattern of 41 genotyped SNPs in SMAD3 gene.

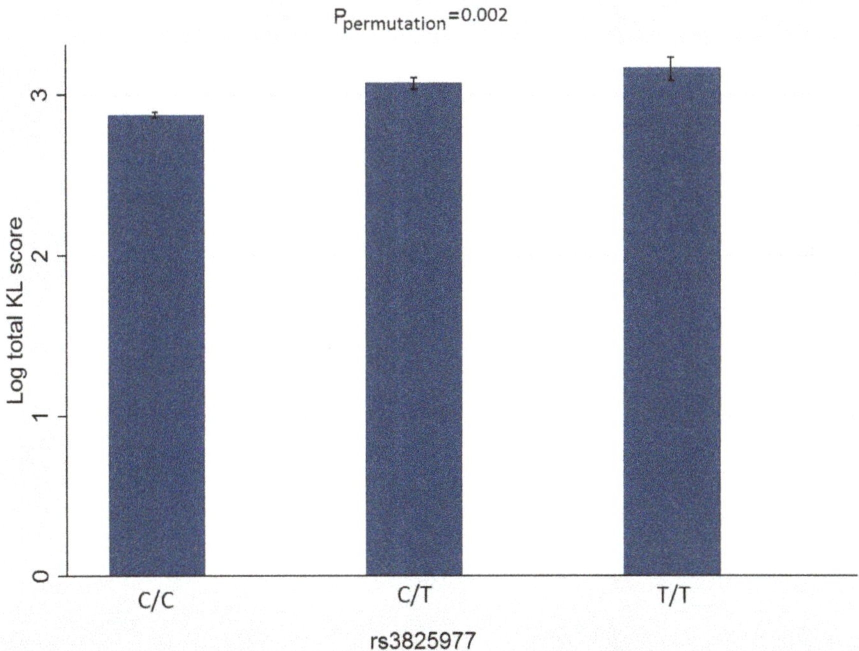

Figure 2. Total KL and each genotype of rs3825977. Error bars indicate Standard Error of the mean.

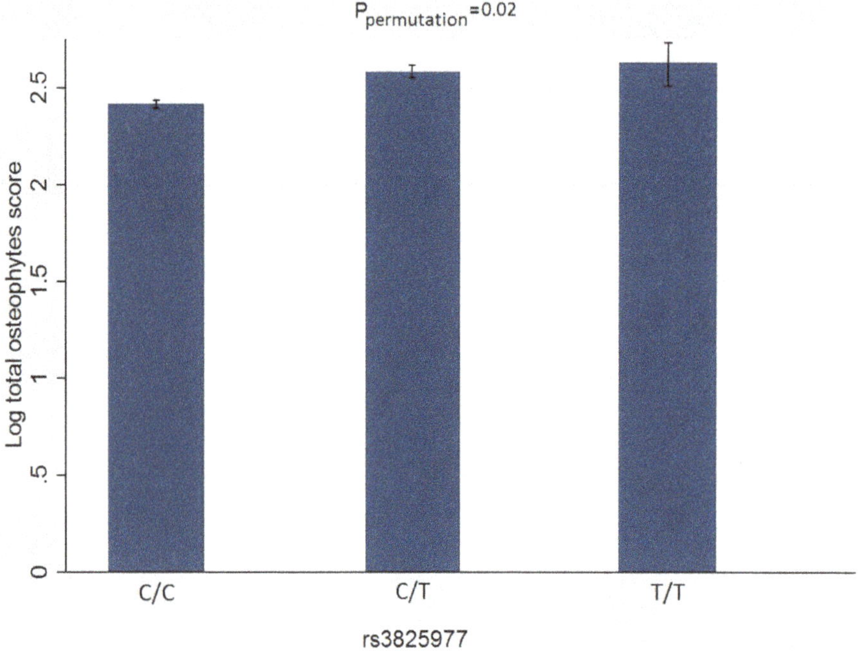

Figure 3. Total osteophyte and each genotype of rs3825977. Error bars indicate Standard Error of the mean.

replacement as compared to controls. A recent study by Jiang Liying *et al.* [38] found this SNP was also associated with hand and knee OA in a northeast Chinese population. However, we did not observe a significant association with rs12901499, which is not in LD with rs3825977 ($R^2 = 0.01$). This may have resulted from the different methods used for the definition and classification of OA in our study and the previous studies which used either end-stage OA (requiring total joint replacement) or symptomatic OA, neither of which is necessarily concordant with radiographic OA [39]. Alternatively, one or both of these SNPs may be non-functional but rather in LD with causal variants in the gene that were not typed in these studies.

Cartilage homeostasis depends on a balance between the catabolic and anabolic activities of chondrocytes being controlled

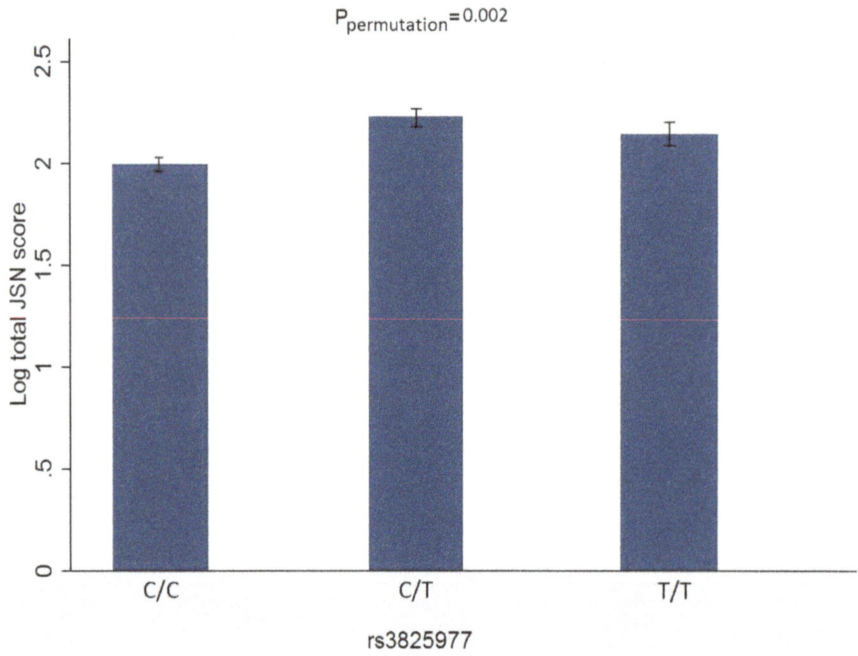

Figure 4. Total JSN and each genotype of rs3825977. Error bars indicate Standard Error of the mean.

Table 3. Association between GOA and rs3825977*.

	Multivariable Analysis			MAF	
Variables	**OR (95% CI)**	**P-value**	$P_{permutation}$	**Cases**	**Controls**
rs3825977 (T vs. C allele)	1.47 (1.02–2.1)	0.037	0.046	0.23	0.17
Age (per year)	1.2 (1.16–1.25)	<0.0001	-	-	-
BMI (per kg/m²)	1.09 (1.04–1.15)	<0.0001	-	-	-

*Logistic regression was used. MAF: Minor allele frequency, OR: Odds Ratio, CI: Confidence interval.

by numerous cytokines and growth factors. *TGF-β* is an important molecule that plays a critical role in the development, growth, maintenance and repair of articular cartilage by modifying the metabolism of the chondrocyte. Deregulation of *TGF-β* signaling and responses have been shown to be involved in OA [20]. The SMAD family proteins, including SMAD3, are important intracellular signals in the *TGF-β* pathway [21]. Another possible mechanism by which SMAD3 acts to maintain cartilage homeostasis is by inducing the expression of type II collagen and repressing *MMP-13*. A recent study by Chen and colleagues [40] showed that *SMAD3* $^{(fl/fl)}$ mice were severely deficient in both type II collagen and aggrecan due to the proteolytic activity of *MMP-13*, which is normally down-regulated by *TGF-β* signals mediated through *SMAD3*.

There are some limitations in the study. All the participants were female, which limits the generalizability. Given its unknown function, it is not clear whether the associated SNP is causal.

Conclusions

We demonstrated that the *SMAD3* gene is associated with the total burden of radiographic OA. As a marker, it has a potential in identifying those with increased risk of OA, thus permitting earlier joint-preserving intervention. It also has potential as a molecular target for developing new OA drugs.

Supporting Information

File S1 Contains the files: Table S1 Univariate and multivariate linear regression for total KL score and each SNP. **Table S2** Univariate and multivariate linear regression for total osteophytes score and each SNP. **Table S3** Univariate and multivariate linear regression for total JSN score and each SNP. **Table S4** Univariate and multivariate logistic regression for GOA and each SNP.
(DOC)

Acknowledgments

We thank all the study participants who made this study possible. Thanks also go to all the staff in the Chingford Study who helped data collection and managing the database. We thank Dr. Roger Green for proofreading the manuscript.

Author Contributions

Conceived and designed the experiments: GZ EAE. Performed the experiments: DH AMV NA TDS. Analyzed the data: EAE GZ YZ. Contributed reagents/materials/analysis tools: GZ EAE AF GM GS PR. Wrote the paper: EAE GZ. Revision: YZ DH AMV AF GM GS PR NA TDS GZ.

References

1. Paitzker K (2003) Pathology of osteoarthritis. In: Osteoarthritis. Edited by K Brandt, M Doherty, L.S. Lohmander, 2nd edn. Oxford: Oxford University Press 49–58.
2. Arden N, Nevitt MC (2006) Osteoarthritis: Epidemiology. Best Practice & Research Clinical Rheumatology Vol. 20, No. 1, pp. 3–25.
3. Arthritis community research & evaluation unit, Toronto Western Research Institute (2010) Prevalence of Arthritis and Rheumatic Diseases around the World, A Growing Burden and Implications for Health Care Needs. Available from: http://www.modelsofcare.ca/pdf/10-02.pdf (last accessed 27 April 2014)
4. Center for disease control and prevention (2010) National Public Health Agenda for Osteoarthritis. Available from: http://www.cdc.gov/arthritis/docs/OAagenda.pdf (last accessed 27 April 2014)
5. Murphy L, Schwartz TA, Helmick CG, Renner JB, Tudor G, et al (2008) Lifetime risk of symptomatic knee osteoarthritis. Arthritis & Rheumatism 59(9):1207–1213
6. Felson DT (2004) An update on the pathogenesis and epidemiology of osteoarthritis. Radiol Clin North Am 42(1):1–9.
7. Tim D Spector, Cicuttini F, Baker J, Loughlin J, Hart D (1996) Genetic influences on osteoarthritis in women: a twin study. BMJ 312: 940–4.
8. Hirsch R, Lethbridge-Cejku M, Hanson R, Scott WW, Reichle R, et al (1998) Familial aggregation of osteoarthritis: data from the Baltimore Longitudinal Study on Aging. Arthritis Rheum 41(7):1227–1232.
9. Riyazi N, Meulenbelt I, Kroon HM, Ronday KH, Le Graverand MH, et al (2005) Evidence for familial aggregation of hand, hip, and spine but not knee osteoarthritis in siblings with multiple joint involvement: the GARP study. Ann Rheum Dis 64(3):438–443.
10. Valdes AM, Spector TD (2011) Genetic epidemiology of hip and knee osteoarthritis. Nat Rev Rheumatol 7(1):23–32.
11. Charcot J (1881) The New Sydenham Society; Clinical lectures on senile and chronic diseases. London 1881.
12. Meulenbelt I (2012) Osteoarthritis year 2011 in review: genetics. Osteoarthritis and Cartilage 20: 218–222.
13. Loughlin J (2011) Genetics of osteoarthritis. Current Opinion in Rheumatology 23(4):479–483.
14. Bijkerk C, Houwing-Duistermaat JJ, Valkenburg HA, Meulenbelt I, Hofman A, et al (1999) Heritabilities of radiologic osteoarthritis in peripheral joints and of disc degeneration of the spine. Arthritis Rheum. 1999 Aug;42(8):1729–35.
15. Van de Laar IM, Oldenburg RA, Pals G, Roos-Hesselink JW, De Graaf BM, et al (2011) Mutations in SMAD3 cause a syndromic form of aortic aneurysms and dissections with early-onset osteoarthritis. Nature Genetics 43: 121e6.
16. Van de Laar IM, Van der Linde D, Oei EH, Bos PK, Bessems JH et al. (2012) Phenotypic spectrum of the SMAD3-related aneurysmseosteoarthritis syndrome. J Med Genet 49: 47–57.
17. Wischmeijer A, Van Laer L, Tortora G, Bolar NA, Van Camp G, et al (2013) Thoracic aortic aneurysm in infancy in aneurysms-osteoarthritis syndrome due to a novel SMAD3 mutation: further delineation of the phenotype. Am J Med Genet A. 161A(5):1028–35.
18. Regalado ES, Guo DC, Villamizar C, Avidan N, Gilchrist D, et al (2011) Exome sequencing identifies SMAD3 mutations as a cause of familial thoracic aortic aneurysm and dissection with intracranial and other arterial aneurysms. Circ Res 109(6):680–6.
19. Hilhorst-Hofstee Y, Scholte AJ, Rijlaarsdam ME, van Haeringen A, Kroft LJ, et al (2013) An unanticipated copy number variant of chromosome 15 disrupting SMAD3 reveals a three-generation family at serious risk for aortic dissection. Clin Genet 83(4):337–44.
20. Finnson KW, Chi Y, Bou-Gharios G, Leask A, Philip A (2012) TGF-b signaling in cartilage homeostasis and osteoarthritis. Front Biosci (Schol Ed) 4: 251–68.
21. Alvarez J, Serra R (2004) Unique and redundant roles of Smad3 in TGF-beta-mediated regulation of long bone development in organ culture. Dev Dyn 230(4):685–99.

22. Chen G, Deng C, Li YP (2012) TGF-β and BMP signaling in osteoblast differentiation and bone formation. Int J Biol Sci 8(2):272–88
23. Yang X, Chen L, Xu X, Li C, Huang C, Deng CX (2001) TGF-beta/Smad3 signals repress chondrocyte hypertrophic differentiation and are required for maintaining articular cartilage. J Cell Biol 2;153(1):35–46.
24. Hart DJ, Spector TD (1993) The relationship of obesity, fat distribution and osteoarthritis in the general population: the Chingford Study. J Rheumatol 20: 331–5.
25. Kellgren JH, Lawrence JS (1963) Atlas of standard radiographs of arthritis; The epidemiology of chronic rheumatism. Oxford: Blackwell Scientific Publications.
26. Burnett S, Hart DJ, Cooper C, Spector TD (1994) A radiographic atlas of osteoarthritis. London: Springer Verlag; 1994.
27. Livshits G, Kato BS, Zhai G, Hart DJ, Hunter D, et al (2007) Genomewide linkage scan of hand osteoarthritis in female twin pairs showing replication of quantitative trait loci on chromosomes 2 and 19. Ann Rheum Dis. 66(5):623–7.
28. Bucsi L, Poór G (1998) Efficacy and tolerability of oral chondroitin sulfate as a symptomatic slow-acting drug for osteoarthritis (SYSADOA) in the treatment of knee osteoarthritis. Osteoarthritis Cartilage. 6 Suppl A:31–6
29. Jordan KM, Syddall HE, Garnero P, Gineyts E, Dennison EM, et al (2006) Urinary CTX-II and glucosyl-galactosyl-pyridinoline are associated with the presence and severity of radiographic knee osteoarthritis in men. Ann Rheum Dis. 65(7):871–7
30. Cooper C, Egger P, Coggon D, Hart DJ, Masud T, et al (1996) Generalized osteoarthritis in women: pattern of joint involvement and approaches to definition for epidemiological studies. J Rheumatol. 23(11):1938–42
31. Teo YY, Inouye M, Small KS, Gwilliam R, Deloukas P, et al (2007) A genotype calling algorithm for the Illumina BeadArray platform. Bioinformatics 15;23(20):2741–6
32. Good P (1994) A practical guide to resampling methods for testing hypotheses. New York: Springer-Verlag
33. Doerge RW, Churchill GA (1996) Permutation tests for multiple loci affecting a quantitative character. Genetics 142: 285–94.
34. Knüppel S, Rohde K, Meidtner K, Drogan D, Holzhütter HG, et al (2013) Evaluation of 41 candidate gene variants for obesity in the EPIC-Potsdam cohort by multi-locus stepwise regression. PLoS ONE 8(7): e68941.
35. Walker LC, Fredericksen ZS, Wang X, Tarrell R, Pankratz VS, et al (2010) Evidence for SMAD3 as a modifier of breast cancer risk in BRCA2 mutation carriers. Breast Cancer Res. 12(6):R102.
36. Yao JY, Wang Y, An J, Mao C, M Hou, et al (2003) Mutations analysis of the SMAD3 gene in human osteoarthritis. European journal of Human Genetics. 11(9):714–7.
37. Valdes AM, Spector TD, Tamm A, Kisand K, Doherty SA, et al (2010) Genetic variation in the SMAD3 gene is associated with hip and knee osteoarthritis. Arthritis and rheumatism 62(8):2347–52.
38. Liying J, Yuchun T, Youcheng W, Yingchen W, Chunyu J, et al (2013) A SMAD3 gene polymorphism is related with osteoarthritis in a Northeast Chinese population. Rheumatology international 33(7), 1763–1768.
39. Hannan MT, Felson DT, Pincus T (2000) Analysis of the discordance between radiographic changes and knee pain in osteoarthritis of the knee. J Rheumatol 27(6):1513–7
40. Chen CG, Thuillier D, Chin EN, Alliston T (2012) Chondrocyte-intrinsic Smad3 represses Runx2-inducible matrix metalloproteinase 13 expression to maintain articular cartilage and prevent osteoarthritis. Arthritis Rheum 64(10):3278–89.

Patients with Severe Radiographic Osteoarthritis Have a Better Prognosis in Physical Functioning after Hip and Knee Replacement

J. Christiaan Keurentjes[1]*, Marta Fiocco[2], Cynthia So-Osman[3], Ron Onstenk[4], Ankie W. M. M. Koopman-Van Gemert[5], Ruud G. Pöll[6], Herman M. Kroon[7], Thea P. M. Vliet Vlieland[1], Rob G. Nelissen[1]

1 Department of Orthopaedic Surgery, Leiden University Medical Center, Leiden, The Netherlands, **2** Department of Medical Statistics and BioInformatics, Leiden University Medical Center, Leiden, The Netherlands, **3** Department of Research and Development, Sanquin Blood Supply South West Region, Leiden, The Netherlands, **4** Department of Orthopaedic Surgery, Groene Hart Hospital, Gouda, The Netherlands, **5** Department of Anaesthesiology, Albert Schweitzer Hospital, Dordrecht, The Netherlands, **6** Department of Orthopaedic Surgery, Slotervaart Hospital, Amsterdam, The Netherlands, **7** Department of Radiology, Leiden University Medical Center, Leiden, The Netherlands

Abstract

Introduction: Although Total Hip and Knee Replacements (THR/TKR) improve Health-Related Quality of Life (HRQoL) at the group level, up to 30% of patients are dissatisfied after surgery due to unfulfilled expectations. We aimed to assess whether the pre-operative radiographic severity of osteoarthritis (OA) is related to the improvement in HRQoL after THR or TKR, both at the population and individual level.

Methods: In this multi-center observational cohort study, HRQoL of OA patients requiring THR or TKR was measured 2 weeks before surgery and at 2–5 years follow-up, using the Short-Form 36 (SF36). Additionally, we measured patient satisfaction on a 11-point Numeric Rating Scale (NRSS). The radiographic severity of OA was classified according to Kellgren and Lawrence (KL) by an independent experienced musculoskeletal radiologist, blinded for the outcome. We compared the mean improvement and probability of a relevant improvement (defined as a patients change score≥Minimal Clinically Important Difference) between patients with mild OA (KL Grade 0–2) and severe OA (KL Grade 3+4), whilst adjusting for confounders.

Results: Severe OA patients improved more and had a higher probability of a relevant improvement in physical functioning after both THR and TKR. For TKR patients with severe OA, larger improvements were found in General Health, Vitality and the Physical Component Summary Scale. The mean NRSS was also higher in severe OA TKR patients.

Discussion: Patients with severe OA have a better prognosis after THR and TKR than patients with mild OA. These findings might help to prevent dissatisfaction after THR and TKR by means of patient selection or expectation management.

Editor: Hamid Reza Baradaran, Tehran University of Medical Sciences, Islamic Republic of Iran

Funding: This study was funded by a grant from the Dutch Arthritis Association (Grant-number: LLP-13). Both the sponsors of the previous trial (ZON-MW, The Netherlands Organization for Health Research and Development; Roche Nederland BV; Sanquin Bloodbank Amsterdam; Haemonetics BV) and the sponsor of the current study (Dutch Arthritis Association) had no role in study design, data collection, data analysis, data interpretation, or writing of the report. The corresponding author had full access to all the data in the study. All authors had final responsibility for the decision to submit for publication.

Competing Interests: The authors have declared that no competing interests exist.

* E-mail: j.c.keurentjes@lumc.nl

Introduction

Total Hip Replacement (THR) and Total Knee Replacement (TKR) are effective surgical interventions, which alleviate pain and improve Health-Related Quality of Life (HRQoL) in patients with hip or knee joint degeneration at the population level. [1] Although on average patients improve markedly after THR or TKR, not all patients benefit from these surgeries. Persistent pain is reported in 9% of THR patients and 20% of TKR patients at long term follow-up. [2] Additionally, up to 30% of patients are dissatisfied after surgery, with higher reported dissatisfaction rates for TKR patients.[3–9] The relatively high dissatisfaction rate is especially worrying, as the therapeutic options are limited in dissatisfied patients after joint replacement. Moreover, given the projected increase in the annual number of THR and TKR performed in the United States, the absolute number of dissatisfied patients is expected to rise. [10].

Unattained expectations of surgery are thought to play an important role in dissatisfaction after joint replacement. [3,4,6,11] In order to successfully manage patient expectations, accurate prediction of the probability of a meaningful improvement for each individual patient is of paramount importance. This probability can be assessed at the individual level using the Minimal Clinically Important Difference (MCID), which is defined as the minimal difference in scores of an outcome measure that is perceived by patients as beneficial or harmful. [12,13]

MCIDs in HRQoL, measured using the Short-Form 36, have been established for THR and TKR.[14–16].

Reports of the effect of the preoperative radiographic severity of osteoarthritis (OA) on the outcome of THR are conflicting: at the population level, Nilsdotter et al showed no effect at one year follow-up, while Meding et al found less postoperative pain at one year follow-up in patients with more preoperative joint space narrowing. [17,18] At the individual level, patients with severe preoperative radiographic OA were more likely to improve in physical functioning. [19] We found no studies addressing the effect of the preoperative radiographic severity of osteoarthritis (OA) on the outcome of TKR.

From a clinical perspective, the preoperative radiographic severity of OA would be a helpful predictor of improvement in HRQoL, as it is both inexpensive and performed routinely for templating purposes. Moreover, the assessment of the severity of preoperative OA could be standardised, whereas this would be more difficult with subjective symptoms such as pain.

We questioned whether the radiographic severity of OA affects the improvement in HRQoL after THR and TKR, both at the population and individual level. Additionally, we questioned whether patient satisfaction with the surgical results differed between patients with mild or severe preoperative radiographical OA.

Methods

We conducted a multi-center follow-up study at the departments of orthopaedic surgery of the Leiden University Medical Center, the Slotervaart hospital in Amsterdam, the Albert Schweitzer hospital in Dordrecht and the Groene Hart hospital in Gouda, the Netherlands, from August 2010 until August 2011. [20] The study was approved by the Medical Ethics Committee of the Leiden University Medical Center and the Medical Ethical Committees of all other participating centers; all patients gave written informed consent (CCMO-Nr: NL29018.058.09; MEC-Nr: P09.189). This study was registered in the Netherlands Trial Register (NTR2190). It concerned the clinical follow-up of a multi-center randomized controlled clinical trial, comparing different blood management modalities in THR and TKR surgery (Netherlands Trial Register: NTR303). In this trial, 2442 primary and revision hip or knee replacements in 2257 patients were included between 2004 and 2009.

All patients who participated in the randomized controlled trial and completed preoperative HRQoL questionnaires, who underwent primary THR of TKR for primary OA and who were alive at the time of inclusion for the present follow-up study were eligible for inclusion. In this study, patients are the subject of interest. Patients who participated more than once in the previous trial, were only allowed to participate once in the current study; the first joint replacement performed in the previous trial was chosen as the index surgery.

Records of the financial administration of all participating centers were checked in order to ascertain that all eligible patients were still alive before being approached. All eligible patients were first sent an invitation letter signed by their treating orthopaedic surgeon, an information brochure and a reply card. Patients who did not respond within 4 weeks after the first invitation were sent another invitation letter. The remaining patients, who did not respond to this second invitation, were contacted by telephone.

Assessments

The assessments of the follow-up study consisted of patient-reported questionnaires, examination of patient records and preoperative radiographs.

Outcomes. HRQoL was measured preoperatively and in the present follow-up study using the SF36, which is translated and validated in the Dutch language. [21,22] The 36 items cover eight domains (physical function, role physical, bodily pain, general health, vitality, social function, role emotional, and mental health), for which a sub-scale score is calculated (100 indicating no symptoms and 0 indicating extreme symptoms). Additionally, these scales are incorporated into two summary measures: a Physical Component Summary (PCS) and Mental Component Summary (MCS).

At the population level, the HRQoL outcome measure was the mean change score, i.e. the mean of each patients postoperative sub-scale score minus their pre-operative sub-scale score). At the individual level, the change scores were used to categorise patients in responders and non-responders, using previously published MCIDs.[14–16] Patients with a change score equal to or larger than the MCID of that particular sub-scale were categorised as a responder; patients whose change score was less than the CID of that particular sub-scale were categorised as non-responders.

Patient satisfaction with the surgical result was measured using an 11-point Numeric Rating Scale of Satisfaction (NRSS; 0 indicating completely dissatisfied, 10 indicating completely satisfied). At the population level, the satisfaction outcome measure was the mean NRSS score. The proportion of patients who achieved a satisfactory outcome (defined as a NRSS>8, according to Brokelman et al [5]) was the satisfaction outcome measure at the individual level.

Exposure. Pre-operative radiographs of the hips (anterior–posterior) and knees (posterior–anterior) were collected from the participating patients' medical records and radiology department. These radiographs were routinely made in each participating center for pre-operative templating purposes. All radiographs were assessed by an experienced musculoskeletal radiologist (HMK), who was blinded for patient characteristics and HRQoL assessments. The method of scoring OA followed that described by Kellgren and Lawrence (KL) (0 indicating no OA, 1 doubtful OA, 2 minimal OA, 3 moderate OA and 4 indicating severe OA). [23] All radiographs were scored twice: both readings were used to establish intra-reader reliability (Intra-Class Correlation hip radiographs: 0.85 (95%CI: 0.82–0.88); Intra-Class Correlation knee radiographs: 0.87 (95%CI: 0.83–0.89)). The second reading was used for further statistical analyses.

As KL grade 0 to 2 and grade 3 and 4 are deemed similar from a clinical perspective, we grouped the severity of pre-operative OA in 2 categories: mild radiographic OA (KL grade 0, 1 or 2) and severe radiographic OA (KL grade 3 or 4).

Potential confounders. Socio-demographic characteristics collected at baseline in the trial included: age at joint replacement and gender. Additionally, the following socio-demographic variables were collected in the questionnaire of the follow-up study: length and weight, in order to calculate the Body Mass Index (BMI) (<25, 25–30, 30–35, >35) and patient reported Charnley classification of co-morbidity (Class A: patients in which the index operated hip or knee are affected only; Class B: patients in which the other hip or knee is affected as well; Class C: patients with a hip or knee replacement and other affected joints and/or a medical condition which affects the patients' ability to ambulate). [24,25].

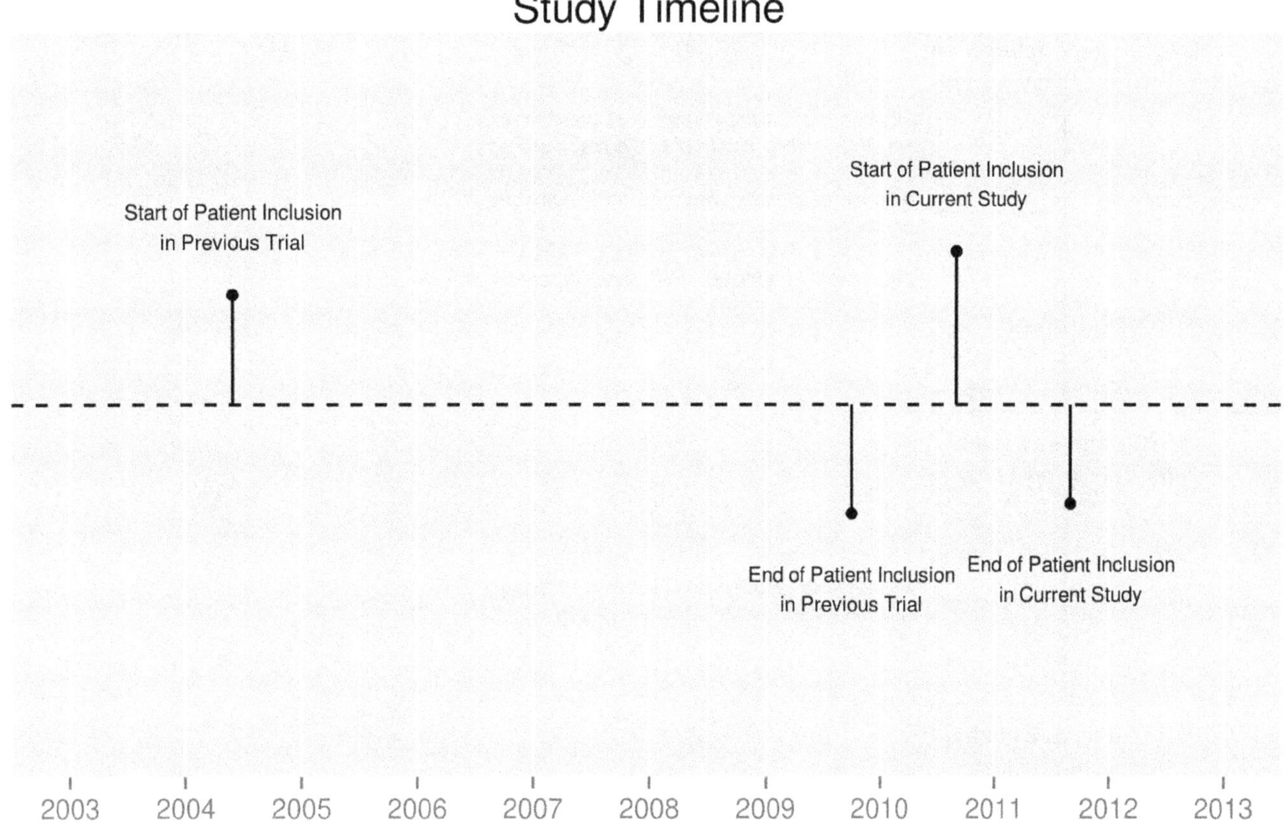

Figure 1. Study Timeline.

Statistical Analysis

We performed descriptive analyses of patients baseline characteristics. In order to investigate the possible extent of self-selection bias, we compared the age at THR or TKR and gender of participants to non-participants.

Patients with missing pre-operative SF36 questionnaires, missing SF36 questionnaires at follow-up or missing pre-operative radiographs were excluded from analyses, as we could not exclude a Missing Not At Random (MNAR) mechanism. Missing values of the Charnley Co-morbidity Classification and BMI were deemed Missing At Random and imputed using Multiple Imputations (MI), in order to improve efficiency of the regression analyses and avert biased regression coefficients. We performed MI (m = 10) using an Expectation-Maximization algorithm, [26] which is implemented in the Amelia 2 package for R. [27,28].

We performed regression analyses in each imputed dataset in order to compare the mean improvement in HRQoL and the probability of achieving a MCID in HRQoL after THR and TKR, between patients with KL grade 0, 1 or 2 and grade 3 or 4. As MCIDs in HRQoL differ between THR patients and TKR patients, we performed all analyses separately for THR and TKR. Possible confounders are age, gender, BMI and poly-articular OA in both THR and TKR patients. We used the Charnley classification as a proxy for poly-articular OA. As the length of follow-up varied considerably, we first stratified our data in quartiles of follow-up length for each imputed dataset. Within each stratum of follow-up length, we performed a multivariate mixed effect linear regression analysis, with the mean improvement in HRQoL and the mean NRSS as the dependent variable, the KL grade and confounders as independent variables and center as a random effect. Stratum-specific mean differences in HRQoL between the KL grades were pooled using inverse variance weighting in order to produce an overall estimate of the mean difference in HRQoL for each imputed data-set. Finally, the $m = 10$ estimates of the mean differences in HRQoL were combined into one estimate, according to Rubin. [29].

Within each stratum of follow-up length, we also performed a multivariate mixed effect logistic regression analysis, with the probability of attaining a MCID in HRQoL and a satisfactory NRSS as the dependent variable, the KL grade and confounders as independent variables and center as a random effect. Stratum-specific odds ratios of attaining a MCID in HRQoL between the KL grades were pooled using inverse variance weighting in order to produce an overall estimate of the odds ratio of attaining a MCID in HRQoL for each imputed data-set. Finally, the $m = 10$ estimates of the mean differences in HRQoL were combined into one estimate, according to Rubin. [29].

All analyses were performed using R, version 2.14.0. [30].

Results

At 2 to 5 years after joint replacement, 723 patients agreed to participate and returned the questionnaires sufficiently completed (participation rate: 46%, figure 1 and 2). Non-participating THR patients were on average 4.32 years older than participants (95%CI: 2.93–5.70 years); Non-participating TKR patients were on average 2.68 years older than participants (95%CI: 1.28–4.09 years). The proportion of males was similar in participants and non-responders. An overview of the patient characteristics is provided in table 1.

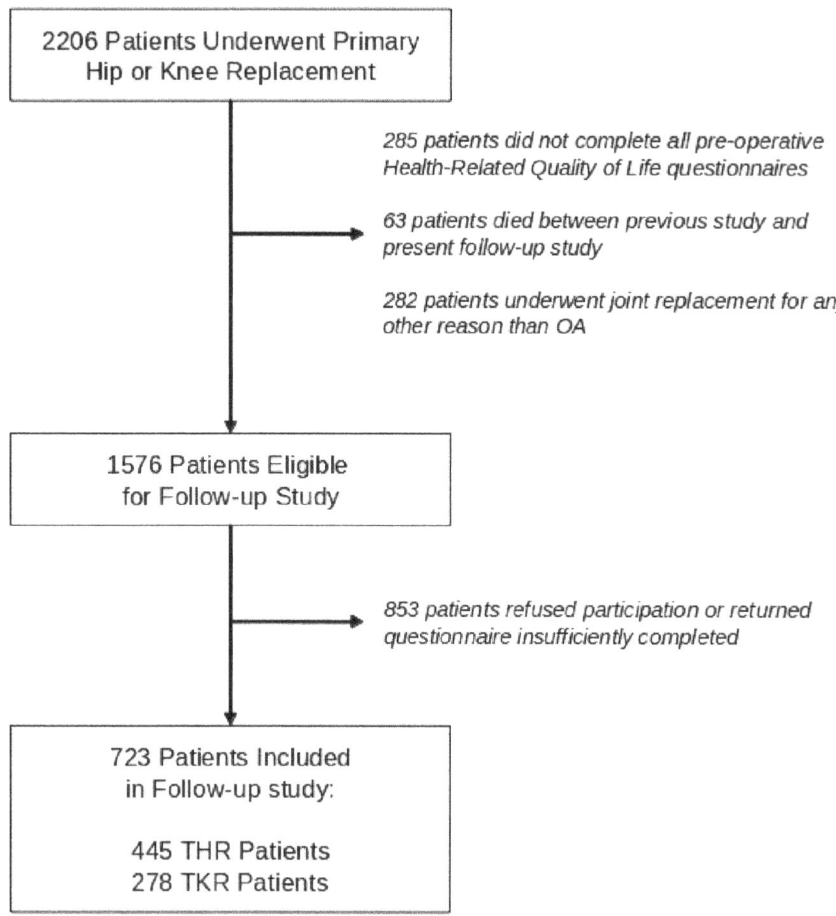
2206 Patients Underwent Primary Hip or Knee Replacement
285 patients did not complete all pre-operative Health-Related Quality of Life questionnaires
63 patients died between previous study and present follow-up study
282 patients underwent joint replacement for any other reason than OA
1576 Patients Eligible for Follow-up Study
853 patients refused participation or returned questionnaire insufficiently completed
723 Patients Included in Follow-up study:
445 THR Patients
278 TKR Patients

Figure 2. Patient Inclusion Flow-chart.

In 13 THR patients and 7 TKR patients, the Charnley classification was missing; in 9 THR patients and 11 TKR patients, the BMI was missing. These missing values were imputed using multiple imputation.

The mean improvement in HRQoL and mean NRSS per KL grade is shown in table 2 for THR patients and table 3 for TKR patients. In THR, patients with severe radiographic OA had a larger improvement in Physical Functioning than patients with mild radiographic OA. The improvement in other domains of HRQoL and the mean NRSS was similar for THR patients of all severities of radiographic OA. In TKR, patients with severe radiographic OA had a larger improvement in Physical functioning than patients with mild radiographic OA. Additionally, patients with severe radiographic OA had a larger improvement in General Health, a larger improvement in the Physical Component Summary Scale and a higher NRSS than patients with mild radiographic OA.

The crude probabilities of achieving a MCID in each dimension of HRQoL are presented in table 4 for THR patients and table 5 for TKR patients. In THR, the probability of achieving a relevant improvement in Physical Functioning was higher in patients with severe radiographic OA than in patients with mild radiographic OA. The probability of achieving a satisfactory outcome was also higher in patients with severe radiographic OA than in patients with mild radiographic OA. The probability of achieving a relevant improvement in other domains of HRQoL was similar for THR patients of all severities of radiographic OA. In TKR, the probability of achieving a relevant improvement in Physical Functioning was higher in patients with severe radiographic OA than in patients with mild radiographic OA. Additionally, the probability of achieving a relevant improvement in General Health and the probability of achieving a satisfactory outcome was also higher in patients with severe radiographic OA than in patients with mild radiographic OA.

Discussion

At the population level, patients with severe radiographic OA improve more in Physical Functioning than patients with mild radiographic OA, both for THR and TKR. At the individual level, THR and TKR patients with severe radiographic OA have a larger probability of a relevant improvement in Physical Functioning than patients with mild radiographic OA. The effects of the preoperative severity of radiographic OA on Physical Functioning are more pronounced in TKR patients than in THR patients. Other domains of HRQoL do not appear to be influenced by the preoperative severity of OA, except General Health and the Physical Component Summary Scale in TKR patients. Additionally, patient satisfaction appears to be better in patients with more severe preoperative radiographic OA.

Limitations of the study include the participation rate and range of follow-up period after joint replacement. Although participation rates of 100% are feasible in small-scaled studies with hard endpoints, [31,32] participation rates in epidemiological studies

Table 1. Patient Characteristics.

Primary THR	Kellgren Grade 0–2	Kellgren Grade 3+4	All Patients
Age at Joint Replacement	65.1 (7.8)	67.4 (8.7)	66.6 (8.5)
Males	23.9%	44.3%	37.5%
Follow-up (years)	2.83 (1.0)	2.79 (0.9)	2.8 (0.93)
Charnley:			
Class A:	25.8%	24.0%	24.6%
Class B:	14.6%	13.7%	14.0%
Class C:	59.6%	62.3%	61.4%
Body Mass Index:			
<25:	29.2%	34.1%	32.5%
25–30:	41.6%	46.4%	44.8%
30–35:	23.6%	16.2%	18.7%
>35:	5.60%	3.40%	4.10%
Primary TKR	**Kellgren Grade 0–2**	**Kellgren Grade 3+4**	**All Patients**
Age at Joint Replacement	65.1 (10.3)	69.5 (8.6)	69.1 (8.9)
Males	31.8%	30.9%	31.0%
Follow-up (years)	3.1 (1.1)	2.79 (0.9)	2.82 (0.93)
Charnley:			
Class A:	4.50%	19.0%	17.5%
Class B:	4.50%	11.4%	10.7%
Class C:	90.9%	69.6%	71.8%
Body Mass Index:			
<25:	33.3%	14.7%	16.3%
25–30:	27.8%	46.7%	45.0%
30–35:	33.3%	21.2%	22.3%
>35:	5.60%	17.4%	16.3%

All values are mean (SD), unless stated otherwise.

Table 2. Improvement in Health-Related Quality of Life and Satisfaction after Hip Replacement: A Comparison Between Patients with Mild to Moderate and Severe Radiographical Pre-Operative Osteoarthritis.

SF36 Sub-Scale	Kellgren Grade 0–2: Mean Improvement (95%CI)	Kellgren Grade 3+4: Mean Improvement (95%CI)	Kellgren Grade 0–2 VS Kellgren Grade 3+4: Mean Adjusted Difference (95%CI)	P-value
Physical Functioning	19.2 (14.2–24.1)	26.2 (22.4–30.0)	8.93 (2.14–15.7)	*0.01*
Role-Physical	36.3 (26.7–45.9)	42.2 (35.4–48.9)	6.39 (−5.89–18.7)	0.31
Bodily Pain	35.9 (30.4–41.3)	36.5 (32.8–40.2)	0.88 (−6.08–7.84)	0.80
General Health	0.60 (−3.50–4.60)	−1.50 (−4.50–1.50)	−0.66 (−5.66–4.34)	0.79
Vitality	9.30 (5.00–13.5)	3.70 (0.80–6.70)	−3.53 (−9.03–1.97)	0.21
Social Functioning	19.4 (13.6–25.2)	14.6 (10.7–18.4)	−4.11 (−11.2–2.97)	0.25
Role Emotional	6.90 (−1.10–14.9)	11.3 (4.70–17.8)	3.11 (−8.22–14.4)	0.59
Mental Health	7.20 (4.00–10.5)	4.60 (2.10–7.10)	−1.80 (−6.13–2.50)	0.41
PCS	10.7 (8.70–12.6)	11.2 (9.90–12.6)	1.94 (−0.57–4.44)	0.13
MCS	1.50 (−0.40–3.40)	−0.50 (−1.80–0.90)	−2.03 (−4.46–0.39)	0.10
NRS Satisfaction	8.5 (8.0–8.9)	8.9 (8.6–9.2)	0.3 (−0.2–0.9)	0.19

Positive values indicate a higher mean improvement in HRQoL after THR in patients with Kellgren Grade 3+4, compared to Grade 0–2.
The mean differences between radiographic severity are adjusted for age, sex, Charnley Comorbidity Classification and BMI and stratified for quartiles of follow-up.

Table 3. Improvement in Health-Related Quality of Life and Satisfaction after Knee Replacement: A Comparison Between Patients with Mild to Moderate and Severe Radiographical Pre-Operative Osteoarthritis.

SF36 Sub-Scale	Kellgren Grade 0–2: Mean Improvement (95%CI)	Kellgren Grade 3+4: Mean Improvement (95%CI)	Kellgren Grade 0–2 VS Kellgren Grade 3+4: Mean Adjusted Difference (95%CI)	P-value
Physical Functioning	−2.10 (−10.5–6.30)	15.1 (11.7–18.5)	19.1 (8.48–29.7)	*<0.001*
Role-Physical	9.10 (−11.9–30.1)	20.6 (−13.5–27.7)	17.4 (−6.32–41.1)	0.15
Bodily Pain	14.5 (3.50–25.5)	25.2 (21.5–29.0)	9.02 (−3.43–21.5)	0.15
General Health	−9.10 (−16.9– −1.30)	−1.50 (−3.80–0.80)	9.23 (1.31–17.2)	*0.02*
Vitality	−5.40 (−13.0–2.30)	1.20 (−1.40–3.80)	8.44 (−0.28–17.2)	0.06
Social Functioning	2.80 (−8.00–13.6)	8.90 (5.40–12.4)	7.44 (−4.18–19.1)	0.21
Role Emotional	4.50 (−17.5–26.6)	5.80 (−0.60–12.1)	8.87 (−11.8–29.6)	0.40
Mental Health	3.40 (−4.00–10.8)	3.00 (0.80–5.10)	0.29 (−6.93–7.50)	0.94
PCS	1.50 (−2.90–6.00)	6.40 (5.10–7.70)	5.64 (1.26–10.0)	*0.01*
MCS	0.10 (−4.30–4.40)	−0.30 (−1.60–1.00)	−0.18 (−4.45–4.10)	0.94
NRS Satisfaction	7.4 (6.1–8.6)	8.2 (7.9–8.6)	1.2 (0.1–2.4)	*0.04*

Positive values indicate a higher mean improvement in HRQoL after THR in patients with Kellgren Grade 3+4, compared to Grade 0–2. The mean differences between radiographic severity are adjusted for age, sex, Charnley Comorbidity Classification and BMI and stratified for quartiles of follow-up.

have been steadily declining in the last 30 years. [33] Even sharper declines have been reported in the past few years. [34] Unfortunately, the participation rate of this study follows this general trend, resulting in a participation rate of 46%. Therefore, we cannot exclude the presence of self-selection bias. In order to limit the extent of this bias, we have sent multiple reminders and have called all patients who did not answer our reminders and who did not return the questionnaire. As incentives, we have included an appealing information brochure in which the primary goals of the follow-up study were explained and a study pen as a small gift. Additionally, patients were urged to participate by their treating physician. However, the participation rate alone does not determine the extent of bias present in any particular study. [34] The difference between participants and non-participants is far more important. [35] As the found differences in demographics were of little clinical relevance, it is unlikely that the study results will be severely biased. Finally, the patient demographics of our study population were similar to those of large-scaled national joint registry studies, regarding age, gender, Charnley classification and BMI. [36,37].

The follow-up period after joint replacement varies between 2 and 5 years. Although a residual effect of follow-up length cannot be excluded, we do not think this is very plausible, as recent evidence suggests that the improvement in HRQoL is sustained up to 5 years after joint replacement surgery. [38,39].

Although joint replacements are highly effective in improving HRQoL at the group level, [1] this is not the case for each individual patient, judging from the relatively high dissatisfaction rates. [40,41] Studying HRQoL at the individual level, using the probability of achieving a clinically important difference as an outcome measure, enables a better prediction of a successful outcome. Moreover, it could provide a helpful way to fine-tune the indication for joint replacement, for which there are no clear cut-off points currently available. [42].

Table 4. Improvement in Health-Related Quality of Life and Satisfaction after Hip Replacement: A Comparison Between Patients with Mild to Moderate and Severe Radiographical Pre-Operative Osteoarthritis.

SF36 Sub-Scale	Kellgren Grade 0–2: Probability of Achieving a MCID (95%CI)	Kellgren Grade 3+4: Probability of Achieving a MCID (95%CI)	Kellgren Grade 0–2 VS Kellgren Grade 3+4: Adjusted Odds Ratio (95%CI)	P-value
Physical Functioning	64/92:69.6% (59.5–78.0)	146/185:78.9% (72.5–84.2)	1.87 (0.97–3.60)	0.06
Role-Physical	55/92:59.8% (49.6–69.2)	124/185:67.0% (60.0–73.4)	1.50 (0.82–2.72)	0.19
Bodily Pain	71/92:77.2% (67.6–84.6)	141/185:76.2% (69.6–81.8)	1.03 (0.52–2.05)	0.93
General Health	62/92:67.4% (57.3–76.1)	117/185:63.2% (56.1–69.9)	0.91 (0.47–1.77)	0.78
Vitality	34/92:37.0% (27.8–47.2)	54/185:29.2% (23.1–36.1)	0.84 (0.46–1.55)	0.58
Social Functioning	42/92:45.7% (35.9–55.8)	80/185:43.2% (36.3–50.4)	0.87 (0.49–1.55)	0.64
Role Emotional	21/92:22.8% (15.4–32.4)	51/185:27.6% (21.6–34.4)	1.01 (0.51–2.01)	0.98
Mental Health	17/92:18.5% (11.9–27.6)	40/185:21.6% (16.3–28.1)	1.26 (0.62–2.58)	0.53
NRS Satisfaction >8	53/92:57.6% (47.4–67.2)	136/185:73.5% (66.7–79.3)	1.95 (1.06–3.59)	*0.03*

Odds Ratios >1 indicate a higher probability of achieving a Minimal Clinically Important Difference in HRQoL after THR in patients with Kellgren Grade 3+4, compared to Grade 0–2.
The odds ratios adjusted for age, sex, Charnley Comorbidity Classification and BMI and stratified for quartiles of follow-up.

Table 5. Improvement in Health-Related Quality of Life and Satisfaction after Knee Replacement: A Comparison Between Patients with Mild to Moderate and Severe Radiographical Pre-Operative Osteoarthritis.

SF36 Sub-Scale	Kellgren Grade 0–2: Probability of Achieving a MCID (95%CI)	Kellgren Grade 3+4: Probability of Achieving a MCID (95%CI)	Kellgren Grade 0–2 VS Kellgren Grade 3+4: Adjusted Odds Ratio (95%CI)	P-value
Physical Functioning	5/22:22.7% (10.1–43.4)	105/191:55.0% (47.9–61.9)	5.44 (1.45–20.3)	*0.01*
Role-Physical	9/22:40.9% (23.3–61.3)	88/191:46.1% (39.2–53.2)	1.46 (0.49–4.32)	0.50
Bodily Pain	15/22:68.2% (47.3–83.6)	136/191:71.2% (64.4–77.2)	1.15 (0.32–4.16)	0.83
General Health	9/22:40.9% (23.3–61.3)	122/191:63.9% (56.9–70.4)	3.56 (1.23–10.4)	*0.02*
Vitality	8/22:36.4% (19.7–57)	86/191:45.0% (38.1–52.1)	1.09 (0.35–3.44)	0.88
Social Functioning	7/22:31.8% (16.4–52.7)	98/191:51.3% (44.3–58.3)	2.84 (0.87–9.32)	0.08
Role Emotional	6/22:27.3% (13.2–48.2)	41/191:21.5% (16.2–27.8)	0.85 (0.26–3.02)	0.85
Mental Health	8/22:36.4% (19.7–57)	79/191:41.4% (34.6–48.4)	2.79 (0.70–11.2)	0.15
NRS Satisfaction >8	9/22:40.9% (23.3–61.3)	116/191:60.7% (53.7–67.4)	2.25 (0.78–6.52)	0.14

Odds Ratios >1 indicate a higher probability of achieving a Minimal Clinically Important Difference in HRQoL after THR in patients with Kellgren Grade 3+4, compared to Grade 0–2.
The odds ratios adjusted for age, sex, Charnley Comorbidity Classification and BMI and stratified for quartiles of follow-up.

Regardless of age, gender, co-morbidity and BMI, we have shown that joint replacement patients with severe preoperative OA have a better prognosis in improvement in Physical Functioning and patient satisfaction with the surgical results. These effects are more pronounced in TKR patients than in THR patients, which might be explained in part by biomechanical factors. The hip joint is a relatively simple ball and socket joint, which is adequately mimicked by a THR. The biomechanical aspects of the knee joint are more difficult to imitate, as the knee is a pivotal hinge joint with 6 degrees of freedom. These degrees of freedom are generally not restored after TKR, which is substantiated in kinematic and kinetic studies. [43] This additional disadvantage of TKR patients who underwent joint replacement for mild radiographic OA is reflected in a smaller increase in Physical Functioning than THR patients who underwent joint replacement for mild radiographic OA. Additionally, the odds of achieving a MCID in Physical Functioning is smaller and the difference in satisfaction is larger.

Clinically, these are promising findings, as dissatisfaction rates are higher in TKR patients than in THR patients. [4,6] Patient satisfaction is thought to be closely related to unfulfilled expectations. Although patient expectations of THR and TKR are similar, recent evidence suggests that THR meets important patient expectations better than TKR. [6,11,44] Our findings could lead to a more fitting expectation management regarding the expected improvement in Physical Functioning, using a single predictor. This improvement in expectation management might lead to higher satisfaction rates.

Plain radiographs have a number of appealing aspects. In the first place, they are inexpensive and easily available, as they are currently a part of the clinical work-up to joint replacement. Secondly, due to the non-invasive character of the test, radiographs are a patient-friendly modality. Finally, they offer a more objective approach to joint complaints. These aspects would make it easy to implement the KL grade in clinical practice, in order to predict HRQoL and satisfaction after joint replacement.

Author Contributions

Conceived and designed the experiments: JCK MF CSO HMK TPMVV RGN. Performed the experiments: JCK RO AWMMKG RGP. Analyzed the data: JCK MF RGN. Contributed reagents/materials/analysis tools: JCK RO AWMMKG RGP RGN. Wrote the paper: JCK MF CSO RO AWMMKG RGP HMK TPMVV RGN.

References

1. Ethgen O, Bruyère O, Richy F, Dardennes C, Reginster J-Y (2004) Health-related quality of life in total hip and total knee arthroplasty. A qualitative and systematic review of the literature. The Journal of bone and joint surgery American volume 86-A: 963–974.
2. Beswick AD, Wylde V, Gooberman-Hill R, Blom A, Dieppe P (2012) What proportion of patients report long-term pain after total hip or knee replacement for osteoarthritis? A systematic review of prospective studies in unselected patients. BMJ open 2: e000435.
3. Gandhi R, Davey JR, Mahomed NN (2008) Predicting patient dissatisfaction following joint replacement surgery. The Journal of rheumatology 35: 2415–2418. doi:10.3899/jrheum.080295.
4. Noble PC, Conditt MA, Cook KF, Mathis KB (2006) The John Insall Award: Patient expectations affect satisfaction with total knee arthroplasty. Clinical orthopaedics and related research 452: 35–43. doi:10.1097/01.blo.0000238825.63648.1e.
5. Brokelman RBG, Van Loon CJM, Rijnberg WJ (2003) Patient versus surgeon satisfaction after total hip arthroplasty. [Miscellaneous Article]. Journal of Bone & Joint Surgery - British Volume 85-B: 495–498.
6. Nilsdotter AK, Toksvig-Larsen S, Roos EM (2009) Knee arthroplasty: are patients' expectations fulfilled? A prospective study of pain and function in 102 patients with 5-year follow-up. Acta orthopaedica 80: 55–61. doi:10.1080/17453670902805007.
7. Lingard EA, Sledge CB, Learmonth ID (2006) PATIENT EXPECTATIONS REGARDING TOTAL KNEE ARTHROPLASTY: DIFFERENCES AMONG THE UNITED STATES, UNITED KINGDOM, AND AUSTRALIA. Journal of Bone & Joint Surgery, American Volume 88: 1201–1207.
8. Garellick G, Malchau H, Herberts P (2000) Survival of hip replacements. A comparison of a randomized trial and a registry. Clinical orthopaedics and related research: 157–167.
9. Baker PN, Van der Meulen JH, Lewsey J, Gregg PJ (2007) The role of pain and function in determining patient satisfaction after total knee replacement. Data from the National Joint Registry for England and Wales. The Journal of bone and joint surgery British volume 89: 893–900. doi:10.1302/0301-620X.89B7.19091.
10. Bini SA, Sidney S, Sorel M (2011) Slowing demand for total joint arthroplasty in a population of 3.2 million. The Journal of arthroplasty 26: 124–128. doi:10.1016/j.arth.2011.03.043.
11. Scott CEH, Bugler KE, Clement ND, Macdonald D, Howie CR, et al. (2012) Patient expectations of arthroplasty of the hip and knee. The Journal of bone and joint surgery British volume 94: 974–981. doi:10.1302/0301-620X.94B7.28219.

12. Jaeschke R, Singer J, Guyatt GH (1989) Measurement of health status. Ascertaining the minimal clinically important difference. Controlled clinical trials 10: 407–415.
13. King MT (2011) A point of minimal important difference (MID): a critique of terminology and methods. Expert review of pharmacoeconomics & outcomes research 11: 171–184. doi:10.1586/erp.11.9.
14. Quintana JM, Escobar A, Bilbao A, Arostegui I, Lafuente I, et al. (2005) Responsiveness and clinically important differences for the WOMAC and SF-36 after hip joint replacement. Osteoarthritis and cartilage/OARS, Osteoarthritis Research Society 13: 1076–1083. doi:10.1016/j.joca.2005.06.012.
15. Escobar A, Quintana JM, Bilbao A, Aróstegui I, Lafuente I, et al. (2007) Responsiveness and clinically important differences for the WOMAC and SF-36 after total knee replacement. Osteoarthritis and cartilage/OARS, Osteoarthritis Research Society 15: 273–280. doi:10.1016/j.joca.2006.09.001.
16. Keurentjes JC, Van Tol F, Fiocco M, Schoones J, Nelissen R (2012) Minimal clinically important differences in health-related quality of life after total hip or knee replacement. Bone and Joint Research 1: 71–77. doi:10.1302/2046-3758.15.2000065.
17. Nilsdotter AK, Aurell Y, Siösteen AK, Lohmander LS, Roos HP (2001) Radiographic stage of osteoarthritis or sex of the patient does not predict one year outcome after total hip arthroplasty. Annals of the rheumatic diseases 60: 228–232.
18. Meding JB, Anderson AR, Faris PM, Keating EM, Ritter MA (2000) Is the preoperative radiograph useful in predicting the outcome of a total hip replacement? Clinical orthopaedics and related research: 156–160.
19. Judge A, Javaid MK, Arden NK, Cushnaghan J, Reading I, et al. (2012) Clinical tool to identify patients who are most likely to achieve long-term improvement in physical function after total hip arthroplasty. Arthritis care & research 64: 881–889. doi:10.1002/acr.21594.
20. Keurentjes JC, Blane D, Bartley M, Keurentjes JJB, Fiocco M, et al. (2013) Socio-Economic Position Has No Effect on Improvement in Health-Related Quality of Life and Patient Satisfaction in Total Hip and Knee Replacement: A Cohort Study. PLoS ONE 8: e56785. doi:10.1371/journal.pone.0056785.
21. Ware JE, Sherbourne CD (1992) The MOS 36-item short-form health survey (SF-36). I. Conceptual framework and item selection. Medical care 30: 473–483.
22. Aaronson NK, Muller M, Cohen PD, Essink-Bot ML, Fekkes M, et al. (1998) Translation, validation, and norming of the Dutch language version of the SF-36 Health Survey in community and chronic disease populations. Journal of clinical epidemiology 51: 1055–1068.
23. KELLGREN JH, LAWRENCE JS (1957) Radiological assessment of osteo-arthrosis. Annals of the rheumatic diseases 16: 494–502.
24. Dunbar MJ, Robertsson O, Ryd L (2004) What's all that noise? The effect of co-morbidity on health outcome questionnaire results after knee arthroplasty. Acta orthopaedica Scandinavica 75: 119–126. doi:10.1080/00016470412331294355.
25. Charnley J (1972) The long-term results of low-friction arthroplasty of the hip performed as a primary intervention. The Journal of bone and joint surgery British volume 54: 61–76.
26. Dempster AP, Laird NM, Rubin DB (1977) Maximum Likelihood Estimation from Incomplete Data Via the EM Algorithm. Journal of the Royal Statistical Association 39: 1–38.
27. Honaker J, King G, Blackwell M (2010) AMELIA II?: A Program for Missing Data. Journal Of Statistical Software 45: 1–53. doi:10.1.1.149.9611.
28. King G, Honaker J, Joseph A, Scheve K (2001) Analyzing Incomplete Political Science Data: An Alternative Algorithm for Multiple Imputation. American Political Science Review 95: 49–69. doi:10.2307/3117628.
29. Rubin DB (1987) Multiple Imputation for Nonresponse in Surveys. Wiley.
30. Team RC (2012) R: A language and environment for statistical computing. Vienna, Austria.: R Foundation for Statistical Computing.
31. Schreurs BW, Keurentjes JC, Gardeniers JWM, Verdonschot N, Slooff TJJH, et al. (2009) Acetabular revision with impacted morsellised cancellous bone grafting and a cemented acetabular component: a 20- to 25-year follow-up. The Journal of bone and joint surgery British volume 91: 1148–1153. doi:10.1302/0301-620X.91B9.21750.
32. Keurentjes JC, Fiocco M, Schreurs BW, Pijls BG, Nouta KA, et al. (2012) Revision surgery is overestimated in hip replacement. Bone and Joint Research 1 : 258–262. doi:10.1302/2046-3758.110.2000104.
33. Hartge P (2006) Participation in population studies. Epidemiology (Cambridge, Mass) 17: 252–254. doi:10.1097/01.ede.0000209441.24307.92.
34. Galea S, Tracy M (2007) Participation rates in epidemiologic studies. Annals of epidemiology 17: 643–653. doi:10.1016/j.annepidem.2007.03.013.
35. Jones J (1996) The effects of non-response on statistical inference. Journal of health & social policy 8: 49–62. doi:10.1300/J045v08n01_05.
36. Malchau HMD, GARELLICK GMD, Eisler TMD, Karrholm JMD, HERBERTS PMD (2005) Presidential guest address: The swedish hip registry: Increasing the sensitivity by patient outcome data. [Article]. Clinical Orthopaedics & Related Research 441: 19–29.
37. Hobbs T (n.d.) TWELVE YEAR REPORT.
38. Ng CY, Ballantyne JA, Brenkel IJ (2007) Quality of life and functional outcome after primary total hip replacement. A five-year follow-up. The Journal of bone and joint surgery British volume 89: 868–873. doi:10.1302/0301-620X.89B7.18482.
39. Bruyère O, Ethgen O, Neuprez A, Zégels B, Gillet P, et al. (2012) Health-related quality of life after total knee or hip replacement for osteoarthritis: a 7-year prospective study. Archives of orthopaedic and trauma surgery.
40. Mancuso CA, Salvati EA, Johanson NA, Peterson MG, Charlson ME (1997) Patients' expectations and satisfaction with total hip arthroplasty. The Journal of arthroplasty 12: 387–396.
41. Vissers MM, De Groot IB, Reijman M, Bussmann JB, Stam HJ, et al. (2010) Functional capacity and actual daily activity do not contribute to patient satisfaction after total knee arthroplasty. BMC musculoskeletal disorders 11: 121. doi:10.1186/1471-2474-11-121.
42. Gossec L, Paternotte S, Bingham CO, Clegg DO, Coste P, et al. (2011) OARSI/OMERACT initiative to define states of severity and indication for joint replacement in hip and knee osteoarthritis. An OMERACT 10 Special Interest Group. The Journal of rheumatology 38: 1765–1769. doi:10.3899/jrheum.110403.
43. Wolterbeek N, Garling EH, Mertens BJ, Nelissen RGHH, Valstar ER (2011) Kinematics and early migration in single-radius mobile- and fixed-bearing total knee prostheses. Clinical biomechanics (Bristol, Avon). doi:10.1016/j.clinbiomech.2011.10.013.
44. De Beer J, Petruccelli D, Adili A, Piccirillo L, Wismer D, et al. (2012) Patient perspective survey of total hip vs total knee arthroplasty surgery. The Journal of arthroplasty 27: 865–9. e1–5.

8

The Identification of CD163 Expressing Phagocytic Chondrocytes in Joint Cartilage and Its Novel Scavenger Role in Cartilage Degradation

Kai Jiao[1], Jing Zhang[1], Mian Zhang[1], Yuying Wei[2], Yaoping Wu[3], Zhong Ying Qiu[1], Jianjun He[1], Yunxin Cao[2], Jintao Hu[2], Han Zhu[3], Li-Na Niu[4], Xu Cao[5], Kun Yang[2]*, Mei-Qing Wang[1]*

1 Department of Oral Anatomy and Physiology and TMD, School of Stomatology, Fourth Military Medical University, Xi'an,China, **2** Department of Immunology, Fourth Military Medical University, Xi'an, China, **3** Department of Orthopedics, Xijing Hospital, Fourth Military Medical University, Xi'an, China, **4** Department of of Prosthodontics, School of Stomatology, Fourth Military Medical University, Xi'an, China, **5** Department of Orthopaedic Surgery, The Johns Hopkins University School of Medicine, Baltimore, Maryland, United States of America

Abstract

Background: Cartilage degradation is a typical characteristic of arthritis. This study examined whether there was a subset of phagocytic chondrocytes that expressed the specific macrophage marker, CD163, and investigated their role in cartilage degradation.

Methods: Cartilage from the knee and temporomandibular joints of Sprague-Dawley rats was harvested. Cartilage degradation was experimentally-induced in rat temporomandibular joints, using published biomechanical dental methods. The expression levels of CD163 and inflammatory factors within cartilage, and the ability of $CD163^+$ chondrocytes to conduct phagocytosis were investigated. Cartilage from the knees of patients with osteoarthritis and normal cartilage from knee amputations was also investigated.

Results: In the experimentally-induced degrading cartilage from temporomandibular joints, phagocytes were capable of engulfing neighboring apoptotic and necrotic cells, and the levels of CD163, TNF-α and MMPs were all increased ($P<0.05$). However, the levels of ACP-1, NO and ROS, which relate to cellular digestion capability were unchanged ($P>0.05$). $CD163^+$ chondrocytes were found in the cartilage mid-zone of temporomandibular joints and knee from healthy, three-week old rats. Furthermore, an increased number of $CD163^+$ chondrocytes with enhanced phagocytic activity were present in $Col\text{-}II^+$ chondrocytes isolated from the degraded cartilage of temporomandibular joints in the eight-week experimental group compared with their age-matched controls. Increased number with enhanced phagocytic activity of $CD163^+$ chondrocytes were also found in isolated $Col\text{-}II^+$ chondrocytes stimulated with TNF-α ($P<0.05$). Mid-zone distribution of $CD163^+$ cells accompanied with increased expression of CD163 and TNF-α were further confirmed in the isolated $Col\text{-}II^+$ chondrocytes from the knee cartilage of human patients with osteoarthritis, in contrast to the controls (both $P<0.05$).

Conclusions: An increased number of $CD163^+$ chondrocytes with enhanced phagocytic activity were discovered within degraded joint cartilage, indicating a role in eliminating degraded tissues. Targeting these cells provides a new strategy for the treatment of arthritis.

Editor: Carmen Infante-Duarte, Charite Universitätsmedizin, Germany

Funding: This work was supported by grants from the National Natural Science Foundation of China (numbers 81271169, 30801315, 30872870). The funders had no role in study design, data collection and analysis, decision to publish, or preparation of the manuscript.

Competing Interests: The authors have declared that no competing interests exist.

* E-mail: yangkunkun@fmmu.edu.cn (KY); mqwang@fmmu.edu.cn (MQW)

These authors contributed equally to this work.

Introduction

Osteoarthritis (OA) is one of the main causes of chronic disability. Moreover, none of the therapies in current use appear to have an obvious impact on impeding or reversing the histopathological progression to advanced OA [1], mainly due to the limited understanding of its pathogenesis. Multiple catabolic factors have been investigated in the context of the breakdown of homeostasis within OA [2]. Recent studies focused on addressing the ability of chondrocytes to repair cartilage in OA, for example, by increasing matrix synthesis [3] in this avascular and alymphatic tissue [4]. At least clinically, OA can be self-limiting, with patients experiencing extended periods without further deterioration in their condition.

Prompt removal of dying cells is crucial for maintaining tissue homeostasis; phagocytosis is the key process in this regard [5]. Mature tissue macrophages form the first line of defense in recognizing and eliminating potential pathogens. The main functions of macrophages include phagocytosis and the production of inflammatory mediators, and these processes are tightly regulated by their surface receptors, which are heterogeneously expressed by mature tissue macrophages [6]. CD163, a member of the scavenger receptor cysteine-rich (SRCR) superfamily (also known as RM3/1, M130, or p155) [7], is one of the most specific surface markers for macrophages that is expressed at high levels in the majority of subpopulations of mature tissue macrophages across species [6,8–11]. Tissue macrophages (for example, in liver, spleen and lymph node) show substantially higher expression of CD163 compared to monocytes [12]. The most well characterized function of CD163 relates to the internalization of the hemoglobin (Hb) - haptoglobin (Hp) complex [13]. CD163 also plays an important role in host defense, in the detection of bacterial infection [8]. Macrophages expressing increased levels of CD163 are found in inflammatory conditions [6,14], and during wound healing [15]. The increased synthesis of CD163 can be indicative of alternative macrophage activation [16].

Chondrocytes are believed to have limited proliferative and regenerative capabilities, dependent on their location within different tissue layers [17]. In arthritic cartilage, there is an increase in the proportion of dead cells or cell debris [18]. The fate of the dead cells and cell debris is unknown, and it is unclear whether there is a role for CD163-mediated phagocytosis within cartilage. Uncovering the mechanisms responsible for removing the cellular debris by phagocytosis within degenerative tissues will facilitate an understanding of the pathogenesis of these complex diseases, such as OA and rheumatoid arthritis (RA), in which tissue homeostasis has broken down. In this study, CD163 expressing ($CD163^{+}$) chondrocytes were identified, for the first time, in healthy knee and temporomandibular joint (TMJ) cartilage from Sprague-Dawley (SD) rats. In addition, an increased percentage of $CD163^{+}$ chondrocytes with enhanced phagocytic activity was observed in the degraded cartilage of TMJs, which was associated with increased expression of tumor tissue necrosis factor alpha (TNF-α) [19–21]. Finally, increased expression of CD163 and TNF-α were confirmed in the knee cartilage from OA patients compared to healthy joints derived from amputees.

Materials and Methods

Sample collection

Female SD rats of three or eight weeks of age were provided by the Animal Center of the Fourth Military Medical University (Xi'an, China). The care of the animals, and all procedures were performed according to institutional guidelines, and were approved by the Ethics Committee of the Fourth Military Medical University. The rats received a standardized diet throughout the procedures, and none of the rats showed any signs of disability. In the experimental (E) groups, biomechanical dental stimulation was applied to the eight-week old female SD rats, as previously described [19–21]. In the sham-treated groups (control groups, C), rats underwent a mock operation procedure with no biomechanical stimulation. TMJs were harvested for morphological observations and for *ex vivo* investigations. The TMJ cartilage of three-week old rats was harvested, and the primary cells were isolated by enzyme digestion of cartilage; these cells were used for the *in vitro* experiments. Knee cartilage from patients with osteoarthritis (OA) or healthy cartilage from patients undergoing knee amputation were collected and investigated by histochemical and immunohistochemical staining and real-time PCR analysis. All patients agreed to the experimental procedures, and provided written informed consent. All procedures were approved by the Ethics Committee of the Fourth Military Medical University. Cartilage was harvested from OA patients aged 59–70 years (including three male patients, aged 53–70 years, mean age 64.3 years, and two female patients, aged 66–70 years, mean age 68 years). Healthy cartilage was harvested from patients undergoing amputations following traumatic traffic-related injuries, but in the absence of injury to the knee joint. Patients were aged 31–44 years (including four male patients aged 31–44 years, mean age 39 years and one female patient, aged 33 years). Additional details are included in the Methods S1.

Tissue preparation for gross-, micro- and ultrastructural observations and immunohistochemistry

Using a dissecting microscope (SZX9, Olympus, Japan) six samples of the most obvious grossly damaged regions of rat TMJ cartilage were examined by transmission electron microscopy (TEM) [19]. Serial midsagittal sections (5 μm-thick) were cut from paraffin-embedded, decalcified TMJ tissue or human knee joint blocks using a microtome. Sections were stained with hematoxylin and eosin (H&E) or toluidine blue for histological assessment [19,20]. TUNEL staining was used for the detection of dead chondrocytes. A standard, three-step, avidin-biotin complex (ABC) immunohistochemical staining protocol or indirect immunofluorescent staining protocol was carried out, as previously reported [20]. The primary antibodies were mouse anti-rat monoclonal CD163 (MCA342R, Serotec Ltd, Oxford, UK, dilution 1:50), mouse anti-human monoclonal CD163 (SC-20066, Santa Cruz, USA, dilution 1:50), and a goat polyclonal TNF-α antibody, which recognizes rat and human TNF-α (sc-1351, Santa Cruz, CA, USA dilution 1:100). Negative controls were incubated with non-immune serum instead of the primary antibody. Five fields at 400× magnification were selected at random, photomicrographs were obtained and the positive cells in each image were counted. Experiments were performed in triplicate.

Tissue preparation for real-time PCR and Western blotting

Total RNA and protein was extracted from control or experimental groups as previously described [19]. Gene expression was analyzed using the Applied Biosystems 7500 Real-Time PCR machine. The amount of target cDNA, relative to GAPDH, was calculated using the formula $2^{-\Delta\Delta Ct}$ [19]. For Western blots, total protein from each group (40 μg) was fractionated by SDS-PAGE and transferred onto a nitrocellulose membrane. The nitrocellulose membrane was blocked with 5% non-fat milk and incubated with the anti-CD163 (1:200) or anti-TNF-α (1:500) antibodies. Signals were revealed by incubation with a horseradish peroxidase-conjugated secondary antibody (1:5000, ZhongShan Goldenbridge Biotechnology, China) and enhanced chemiluminescence detection. Additional details are included in Methods S1.

Chondrocyte isolation

Chondrocytes were isolated from the condylar cartilage of rat TMJs by digestion with 0.25% trypsin (Sigma, St. Louis, MO, USA) for 20 min, followed by 0.2% type II collagenase (Invitrogen, San Diego, CA, USA) for 2–3 h. Cells from human knees were harvested by the same method, except that the duration of digestion with type II collagenase was increased to 9–10 h.

Measurement of the generation of reactive oxygen species (ROS)

Intracellular ROS was detected by means of an oxidation-sensitive fluorescent probe (DCFH-DA). Chondrocytes were collected and washed twice in phosphate-buffered saline (PBS) following incubation with 10 μmol/L DCFH-DA at 37°C for

20 min according to the manufacturer's instructions (Reactive Oxygen Species Assay Kit, Beyotime Institute of Biotechnology, China). DCFH-DA was deacetylated intracellularly by a non-specific esterase, and this product was further oxidized by ROS to the fluorescent compound 2,7-dichlorofluorescein (DCF). DCF fluorescence was detected using a FACSAria flow cytometer (BD Biosciences, San Jose, CA, USA). Thirty thousand events were collected for each sample [22].

Measurement of intracellular nitric oxide (NO) concentration

Chondrocytes were isolated from TMJ condylar cartilage for the measurement of the intracellular levels of NO using the Griess assay according to the protocol of the manufacturer (Total Nitric Oxide Assay Kit, Beyotime Institute of Biotechnology, China) [23].

Collagen-II expressing (Col-II$^+$) cell sorting

Isolated cells from cartilage were incubated at 4°C in 0.1% BSA in PBS for 40 min, incubated with biotin-conjugated Col-II antibody (1 μg/10^6 cells, ab79127, Abcam, UK) at 4°C for 1 h, and washed twice with Dulbecco's PBS (DPBS) containing 5% FBS. Subsequently, cells were incubated with an APC-conjugated secondary antibody (1 μg/10^6 cells, Invitrogen) for 40 min. After thorough washing, cells were resuspended in 0.5 ml DPBS and processed using a FACSAria flow cytometer (BD Biosciences). The sorted primary Col-II$^+$ cells were then used for the testing of the phagocyitc function of CD163$^+$ chondrocytes.

Magnetic sorting of CD163$^+$ cells

CD163 positive (CD163$^+$) cells were selected by the combined use of a mouse anti-rat CD163 primary antibody (1 μg/10^6 cells) and monosized magnetic polystyrene beads (25 μl/1×10^7 cells) pre-coated with human anti-mouse IgG according to the manufacturer's instructions (Dynal 115.31D, Invitrogen). The sorted CD163$^+$ cells were co-cultured with cell debris and were used for the observation of the phagocytosis by living cell workstation. Additional details are described in Methods S1.

Generation of DiO-labeled cell debris and phagocytosis assay

The harvested chondrocyte from rat TMJ cartilage were resuspended at a density of 1×10^6 cells/ml in serum-free Dulbecco's Modified Eagle's medium (DMEM). Then, 5 μl DiO solution (V-22886, Molecular Probes, Inc., USA) was added to 1 ml cell suspension and mixed well by gentle pipetting. After incubation at 37°C for 20 min, the mixture was centrifuged at 1500 rpm for 5 min and then washed twice with warm DMEM. Cell pellets were resuspended in a small amount of media, and frozen at −70°C for 20 min then thawed at 37°C for a further 20 min for ten cycles to yield the DiO-labeled cell debris.

For the phagocytosis assay, the primary Col-II$^+$ cells, at a density of 1×10^6 cells/well, were pre-incubated in DMEM containing 10% fetal bovine serum at 37°C for 48 h, then the cell debris (0.1 ml/well) was added to the wells. The mixture was incubated at 37°C, 5% CO_2 for 48 h in DMEM supplemented with 1% FBS. The rate of phagocytosis of the cell debris was analyzed using the FITC filter of the flow cytometer.

Exogenous TNF-α stimulation

The primary chondrocytes isolated from TMJ cartilage from three-week old SD rats were stimulated for 48 h with vehicle, 10 ng/ml TNF-α alone, or 10 ng/ml TNF-α plus 1 μg/ml CD163 neutralizing antibody (MCA342R, Serotec Ltd.). Following treatment, the cells were harvested for analysis by real-time PCR, flow cytometry and confocal microscopy.

Flow cytometric analysis

Flow cytometry was used to detect the surface expression levels of CD163 and phagocytosis by the Col-II$^+$ cells. Briefly, Col-II$^+$ cells co-cultured with DiO-labeled cartilage debris were incubated at 4°C in 0.1% BSA in PBS, and then incubated with PE-conjugated CD163 antibody (1 μg/10^6 cells, MCA342PE, Serotec Ltd.) at 4°C for 1 h. After washing, the cells were resuspended in 0.5 ml DPBS and analyzed on the flow cytometer.

Confocal microscopy

Cells from joint cartilage that had been co-cultured with DiO-labeled cell debris were fixed with 4% formaldehyde, and incubated overnight at 4°C with the CD163 antibody (MCA342R, Serotec Ltd.). The mixture was then incubated with Cy3-conjugated antibody (1:100, Molecular Probes, Breda, Netherlands) for 1 h, and subsequently with DAPI for 3 min at room temperature. Samples were examined using the green (blue excitation filter, 418 nm), red (green excitation filter, 514 nm) and blue (ultraviolet excitation filter, 418 nm) lasers of the confocal microscope (FV1000, Olympus, Japan). In each field of view, 10 to 15 serial optical z-axis sections (1 μm-thick) were collected using the tri-channel imaging system. Five fields of view at 400× magnification were selected at random, and the total number of CD163$^+$ in each field was counted. In addition, the number of CD163$^+$ cells with FITC-labeled cell debris inside their cell membrane was confirmed by the z-axis scanning (1 μm thick); these were designated phagocytic cells. Experiments were performed in triplicate.

Living cells workstation

The sorted CD163$^+$ chondrocytes were incubated with the DiO-labeled cartilage debris in DMEM at 37°C, 5% CO_2. The living cells workstation recorded a series of images illustrating that the cell debris was undergoing phagocytosis by the CD163$^+$ cells.

Transwell migration assays

An *in vitro* migration assay was performed in 24-well transwell units (Millipore, Merck KGaA, Darmstadt, Germany) with polycarbonate filters (pore size, 8 μm), which were coated on both sides with fibronectin (3 ng/ml, Sigma) [24]. Additional details are described in Methods S1.

Statistical analysis

Statistical analysis was performed using SPSS software, version 11.0 (SPSS, Chicago, IL, USA). All data acquisition and analysis was performed blindly. Quantitative data for control and experimental groups were subjected to one-way ANOVA and Student-Newman-Keuls (SNK-q) post-test. *P*-values of <0.05 were considered to be statistically significant.

Results

Increased number of CD163$^+$ chondrocytes with enhanced phagocytic activity in experimentally-induced, degraded TMJ cartilage

The degradation of TMJ cartilage was induced by our recently reported biomechanical dental stimulation method [19–21]. The induced lesions within the TMJ condyles included dark, unsmooth cartilage surfaces in the 4-week old experimental group and obvious pit lesions in the 8- and 12-week old experimental groups (Figure 1A, arrow). The histological appearance of degraded cartilage, as previously reported [19,20], included fibrillation, and condensed, eosinophilic nuclei, which was accompanied by significantly increased mRNA levels of MMP-3 and -9 (Figure 1B, $P<0.05$) [21]. To explore whether inflammation was involved in the pathogenesis of cartilage degradation, the expression of inflammatory cytokines was investigated. The results showed that increased mRNA expression of TNF-α, but not IL-1, was observed in the experimental groups compared with their age-matched controls (Figure 1B). Since chondrocytes are the only cell type within cartilage and as they remain within various stages of differentiation, we speculated that chondrocytes may take on the role of inflammatory cells within the joint cartilage. In support of this, we found apoptotic and necrotic cells within the mid-zone of degraded TMJ cartilage (Figure 1C, arrowheads), and several of these cells were being engulfed by phagocytic chondrocytes (Figure 1C). The $CD163^+$ cells were located close to the TUNEL-positive dead cells in the mid-zone of the degraded cartilage in the 8-week experimental group, but not in the age-matched controls (Figure 1D). In addition, a significant increase in the mRNA and protein levels of CD163 was found in the 8- and 12-week experimental groups, compared to their age-matched controls. The increase in the expression of TNF-α was already apparent within the 4-week experimental group (Figures 1B and 1E; $P<0.05$).

To confirm the chondrocytic origin of this subset of $CD163^+$ phagocytes in cartilage, type II collagen-expressing ($Col\text{-}II^+$) chondrocytes were isolated from TMJ cartilage of 8-week experimental and control groups. The $CD163^+$ cells constituted approximately 2.2% of the $Col\text{-}II^+$ chondrocytes sorted from condylar cartilage of 8-wk control rats. However, the number of $CD163^+$ cells and their phagocytic activity were significantly higher in the experimental group compared with the age-matched control group (Figure 2A; $P<0.05$). This result was verified by confocal microscopy, where it was observed that the number of $CD163^+$ chondrocytes significantly increased in TMJ cartilage of rats in the 8-week experimental group (Figure 2B; $P<0.05$), irrespective of whether they co-localized with the cell debris. The phagocytic activity of $CD163^+$ chondrocytes was verified by examining serial z-sections, which showed that the cellular debris was located inside the $CD163^+$ cells isolated from TMJ cartilage (Figure 2C). Moreover, this was confirmed by dynamic confocal microscopy showing the DiO-labeled cellular debris undergoing phagocytosis by the sorted $CD163^+$ chondrocytes (Figure 2D; white frame). However, the ability of these phagocytic cells to digest the cellular debris appears limited because no increase in the amount of ROS or nitric oxide (NO) was detected (Figure 2E). In addition, there was no increase in mRNA expression of ACP-1, integrin β1 or integrin α4 (Figure 1B), molecules that play roles in cellular digestion and adhesion, respectively, in isolated chondrocytes from experimental groups compared with their age-matched controls ($P<0.05$).

In addition, immunohistochemical staining showed that $CD163^+$ cells were located in the mid-zone of cartilage in the knees and TMJs of the 3-week old healthy rats (Figure 3A). The $CD163^+$ cells constituted approximately 3.3% of the $Col\text{-}II^+$ cells isolated from TMJ cartilage of 3-week old healthy rats, and approximately 70% of these cells possessed phagocytic activity (Figure 3B).

Taken together, these results indicate the potential capability of the joint cartilage to actively eliminate the degraded tissues by increasing the number of $CD163^+$ chondrocytes and their phagocytic activity.

Exogenous TNF-α increased CD163 expression in primary chondrocytes and promoted migration and phagocytosis

TNF-α is believed to be a critical mediator in the disturbed metabolism and enhanced catabolism of degraded joint cartilage, even in the early stages of cartilage degradation [25]. In chondrocytes, TNF-α alters the expression of many molecules that contribute to cartilage degradation [26]. The results presented here indicate that the expression of TNF-α was increased at the very earliest stages of cartilage degradation, that is, only four weeks after biomechanical dental stimulation. Therefore, we wanted to address whether the increased number of $CD163^+$ chondrocytes and their enhanced phagocytic activity within the degraded cartilage were attributable, at least in part, to the increase in TNF-α. This hypothesis was evaluated in the following *in vitro* studies. Primary chondrocytes, detected as Col-II- and proteoglycan-expressing cells (Figure 4A), were isolated from the TMJ cartilage of three-week old rats, and stimulated by exogenous TNF-α. The primary chondrocytes showed increased mRNA expression of CD163 after 24 and 48 h of TNF-α treatment (Figure 4B; $P<0.05$), and increased percentages of $CD163^+$ cells were observed after 48 h and 72 h of TNF-α treatment (Figures 4C and D; $P<0.05$). In addition, the phagocytic activity of the $CD163^+$ chondrocytes was significantly higher in the TNF-α treatment group compared with the controls ($P<0.05$). The number of phagocytic $CD163^+$ chondrocytes remained at control levels when TNF-α was added in the presence of CD163 neutralizing antibodies (Figures 5A and B; $P>0.05$). The increased number of $CD163^+$ chondrocytes with enhanced phagocytic activity was confirmed by confocal microscopy, and in some cases, the cells co-localized with cellular debris following TNF-α stimulation ($P<0.05$). Once again, this effect could be attenuated to control levels by treatment with a CD163 neutralizing antibody (Figure 6A, arrows and Figure 6B; $P>0.05$). The ability of TNF-α to enhance the phagocytic activity of $CD163^+$ cells was additionally supported by the finding that $CD163^+$ chondrocytes treated with exogenous TNF-α for 24 h showed enhanced migration, which could be attenuated to the level of the control by a TNF-α antibody (Figure 6C).

Collectively, these results demonstrate that there are $CD163^+$ phagocytic chondrocytes in the joint cartilage. Exogenous TNF-α stimulation increased CD163 expression by the primary chondrocytes, and promoted the phagocytic and migratory activities of $CD163^+$ chondrocytes.

Knee cartilage from patients with osteoarthritis showed higher expression of CD163 and TNF-α

CD163 or TNF-α expressing cells were rarely found in amputated, healthy knee cartilage (Figures 7A and B). In contrast, significantly increased numbers of $CD163^+$ and $TNF\text{-}\alpha^+$ cells were observed in the superior mid-zone of knee cartilage from patients with osteoarthritis (OA) (Figures 7A–C; $P<0.05$). In addition, the mRNA expression levels of CD163 and TNF-α were much higher in $Col\text{-}II^+$ chondrocytes isolated from knee cartilage from patients with OA compared with amputees (Figure 7D; $P<0.05$).

Discussion

The current study identified for the first time, a subset of chondrocytes within joint cartilage, characterized as $CD163^+$ phagocytic chondrocytes, which are located at the mid-region, where chondrocytes are generally less differentiated. Osteoarthritis (OA)-like lesions were induced in TMJ cartilage using our previously reported biomechanical dental method [19–21]. Increased numbers of TNF-α expressing chondrocytes, which

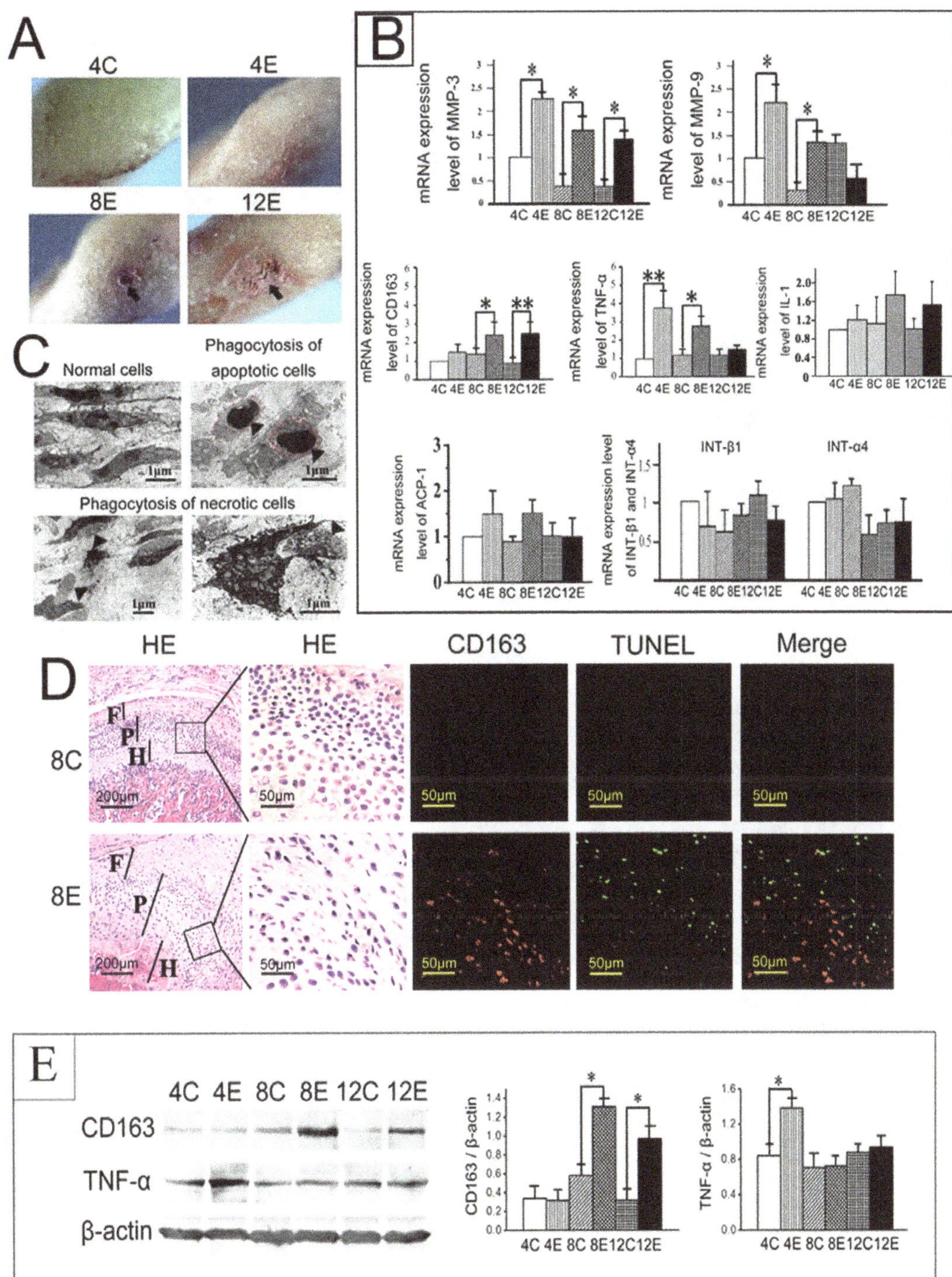

Figure 1. Enhanced phagocytic activity and increased CD163 and TNF-α expression in degraded TMJ cartilage. A: The gross surface morphology of rat temporomandibular joint (TMJ) condyles from control (4C) and experimental (4E, 8E, 12E) groups. Pit lesions are indicated by arrows. B: Comparison of the mRNA levels of MMP-3, MMP-9, CD163, TNF-α, IL-1, ACP-1, integrin-β1 and integrin-α4 in the condylar cartilage of control (C) and experimental (E) groups. C: Transmission electron micrographs of TMJ cartilage from control group (left top panel) and the regions with grossly damaged cartilage from experimental groups (the others panels). The apoptotic (outlined with the red dashed line) and necrotic chondrocytes are shown by arrow heads. Note that within the degraded TMJ cartilage some cells were phagocytizing neighboring apoptotic and necrotic cells. D: Serial sections of condylar cartilage from the 8-week old control (upper panels) and experimental (lower panels) groups, stained with H&E (HE), or co-stained with CD163 and TUNEL. F: fibrous layer; P: proliferative layer; H: hypertrophic layer. E: Comparison of the protein levels of CD163 and TNF-α in the condylar cartilage of control (C) and experimental (E) groups by Western blotting (left panel). Graph representing the quantification of the Western blotting results, normalized to the expression of β-actin. *$P<0.05$, **$P<0.01$. 4C: 4-week old control group; 4E: 4-week old experimental group; 8C: 8-week old control group; 8E: 8-week old experimental group; 12C: 12-week old control group; 12E: 12-week old experimental group.

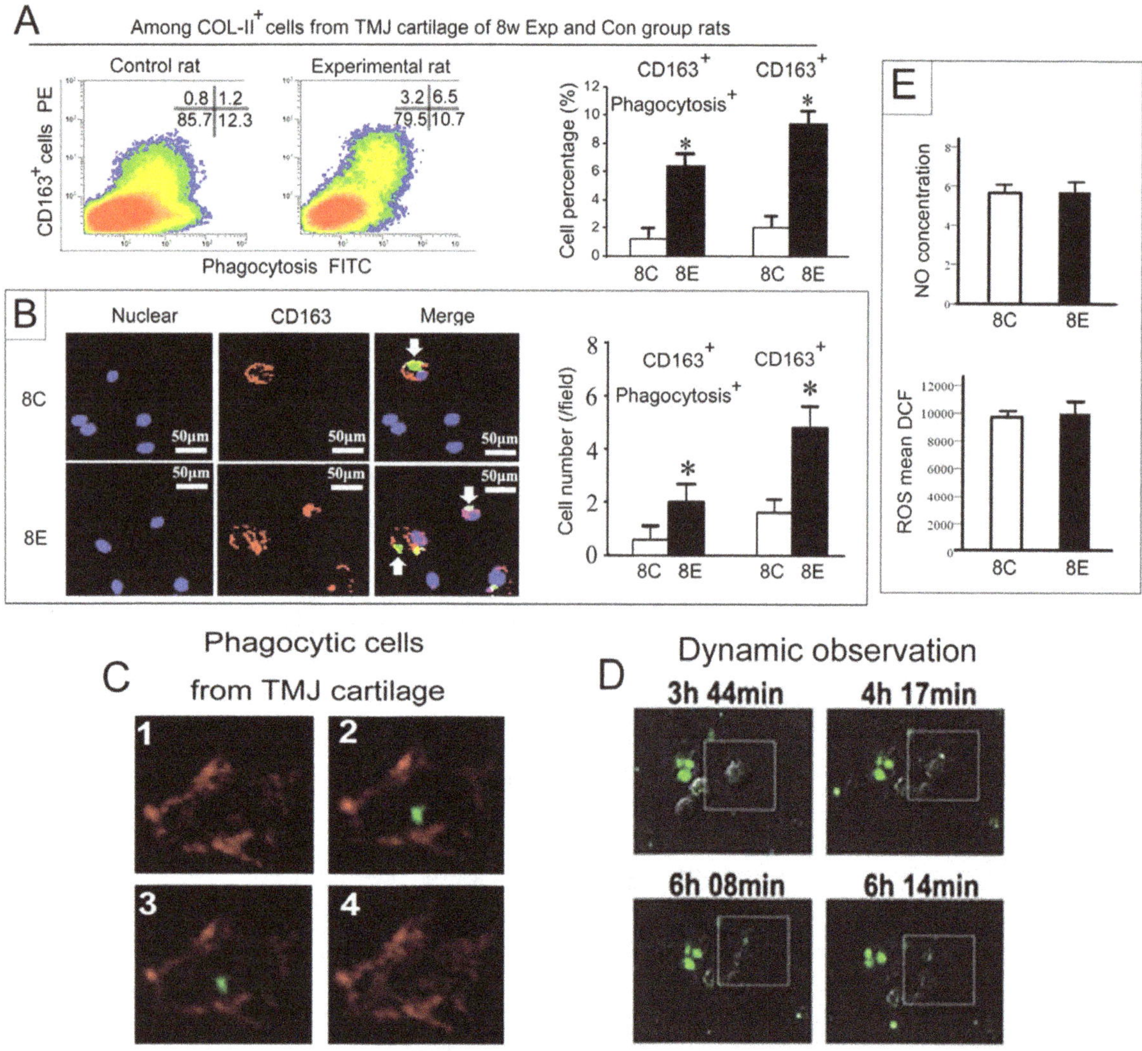

Figure 2. Increase in CD163+ cells with enhanced phagocytic activity in experimentally-induced arthritic cartilage of rat TMJs. A: Flow cytometry analysis and comparison of the percentage of total CD163+ cells and CD163+ cells with phagocytic activity within isolated type II collagen expressing (Col-II+) cells from TMJ cartilage from the 8-week experimental group and their age-matched controls. B: Confocal microscope images of the CD163+ cells and assessment of their phagocytic activity in primary cells isolated from TMJ cartilage. The images reveal an increase in CD163+ cells and enhanced co-localization with the FITC-labeled cell debris in 8-week experimental group compared with the age-matched controls. C: Serial confocal images (1–4) of the primary cells isolated from TMJ cartilage of 3-week old rats co-cultured with DiO-labeled cellular debris. Sections were stained with a CD163 antibody and a Cy3-conjugated secondary antibody. Note that the CD163+ cells showed membrane staining (red) and the cell debris (green) was located inside the cell membrane. D: Dynamic observation of the phagocytic process involving living CD163+ cells sorted from TMJ cartilage engulfing cellular debris. Note that the DiO-labeled debris is undergoing phagocytosis by the CD163+ cell indicated within the white box. E: Comparison of the nitric oxide (NO) concentration and amount of intracellular reactive oxygen species (ROS) in the primary cells isolated from TMJ cartilage from 8-week experimental group and their age-matched controls. $^{*}P<0.05$.

are usually found in degraded cartilage, were observed in these lesions [25,26,27]. In addition, within the OA-like cartilage there were apoptotic and necrotic cells, and an increased percentage of CD163+ chondrocytes with enhanced phagocytic and migratory activities. However, the scavenger function of CD163+ phagocytes within cartilage seems limited due to the restrictions imposed by the dense network of collagen fibrils and proteoglycans that make up articular cartilage. Degradation of the extracellular matrix by an increase in matrix metalloproteinases (MMPs), which is characteristically observed in arthritic cartilage [28–30], could potentially facilitate the mobilization of the CD163+ phagocytes.

TNF-α has been reported to alter the expression of many molecules in chondrocytes that may contribute to the degradation of cartilage [31]. The current results showed that TNF-α treatment increased CD163 expression in chondrocytes and promoted phagocytosis and migration of CD163+ chondrocytes. These studies indicate a novel function for TNF-α within cartilage, which is to stimulate the self-clearing potential of joint cartilage. The increased expression of CD163 was closely correlated with the enhanced phagocytosis observed within the degraded cartilage. Moreover, blocking CD163 expression using neutralizing antibodies largely attenuated the increased phagocytosis of CD163+ chondrocytes stimulated by TNF-α. This indicates that CD163, which is expressed in a subset of chondrocytes, may adopt the role of a scavenger receptor in order to clear the degraded tissue and maintain cartilage homeostasis. This hypothesis is supported by previous studies showing that CD163 acts as an endocytic receptor for both the hemoglobin-haptoglobin complexes and bacteria

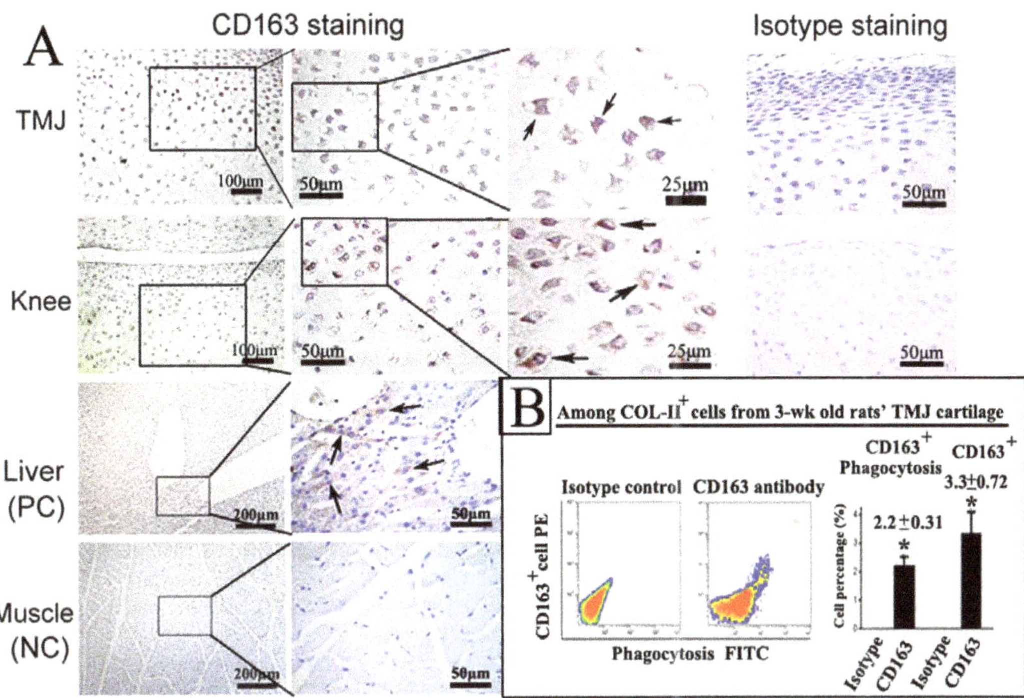

Figure 3. CD163$^+$ chondrocytes in normal joint cartilage of 3-week old rats. A: Immunohistochemical staining of CD163 in cartilage from the TMJ and knee. The CD163$^+$ cells located below the superior zone of the TMJ and knee cartilage, show intense membrane and cytoplasmic staining (arrows). Rat liver and muscle were selected as positive and negative controls, respectively, for the detection of CD163. Membrane staining of CD163$^+$ cells was observed in liver (indicated by arrows), but no CD163$^+$ cells were detected in muscle. As additional controls, TMJ and knee cartilage was also stained with an isotype control antibody. B: Flow cytometric analysis and graphical representation of the percentage of total CD163$^+$ cells and CD163$^+$ cells with phagocytic activity within the Col-II$^+$ cells isolated from TMJ cartilage (n = 3; *$P<0.05$).

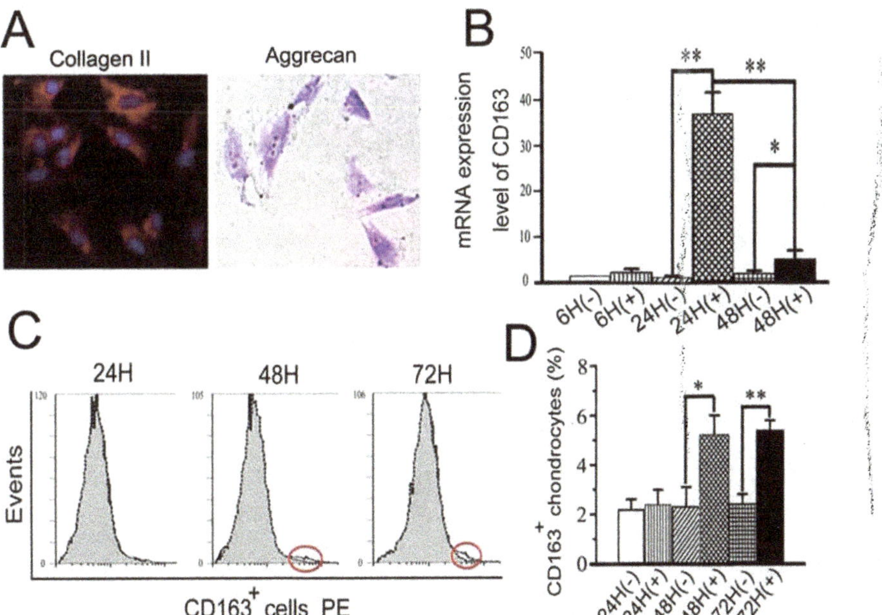

Figure 4. Exogenous TNF-α increased CD163 expression in primary chondrocytes from TMJ cartilage of 3-week old rats. A: The primary cells isolated from TMJ cartilage of 3-week old rats were positive for type II collagen (Col-II) and aggrecan, as detected by immunofluorescence and toluidine blue, respectively (400× magnification). B: A time-course of induction of CD163 mRNA expression in primary cells isolated from TMJ cartilage and treated with 10 ng/ml of TNF-α. C–D: Flow cytometric analysis and graphical representation of the percentage of CD163$^+$ cells within the primary cells isolated from TMJ cartilage and treated with 10 ng/ml of TNF-α.

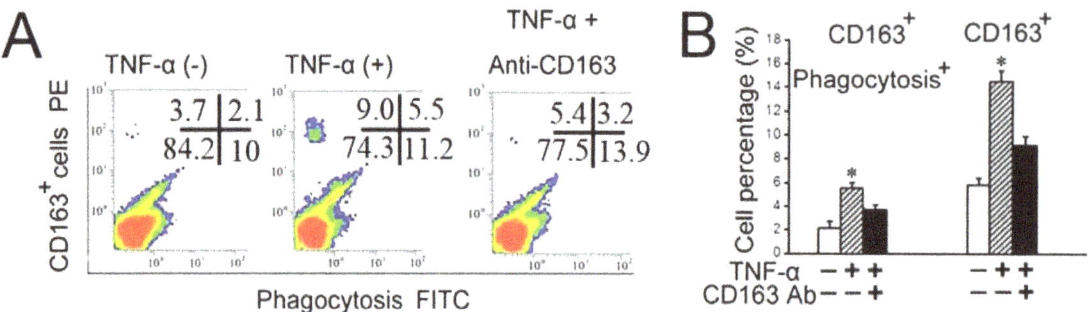

Figure 5. TNF-α increased the phagocytic activity of CD163⁺ cells isolated from 3 week old rat TMJ cartilage. A–B: Flow cytometry analysis (A) and graphical representation (B) of the percentage of total CD163⁺ cells and CD163⁺ cell with phagocytic activity within the primary cells isolated from TMJ cartilage and treated with vehicle, TNF-α alone, or TNF-α and a CD163 neutralizing antibody.

[8,13]. However, further studies are needed to clarify the function of CD163 expressed on the phagocytic chondrocytes. Future experiments could involve the overexpression of CD163 in chondrocytes and a comparison of the difference in phagocytic potential between CD163⁺ and CD163⁻ chondrocytes.

In addition, the CD163⁺ cells constituted approximately 3.3% of the Col-II⁺ chondrocytes isolated from TMJ condylar cartilage, with approximately 70% of the cells possessing the phagocytic activity (Figure 3B). This result suggests that chondrocytes possess an inherent phagocytic/scavenger-like phenotype, which might be a general mechanism for clearing tissue debris arising from different processes within the articular cartilage, such as cartilage development and remodeling, endochondral ossification, and cartilage degradation. In the 8-week control group, the CD163⁺ cells constituted approximately 2.2% of the Col-II⁺ chondrocytes isolated from condylar cartilage (Figure 2A). This low level expression of CD163 in normal TMJ condylar cartilage may explain why the immunohistological staining was absent in the 8-week old group (Figure 1D).

The destruction of the extracellular microenvironment (ECM) facilitates the mobilization of CD163⁺ phagocytic chondrocytes. However, at the same time, this process destroys the environment that maintains the viability of the chondrocytes. This could explain the limited capacity of the CD163⁺ phagocytes to digest cellular debris, although it must be noted that the mRNA analysis was based on the analysis of all cells in the joint cartilage because the

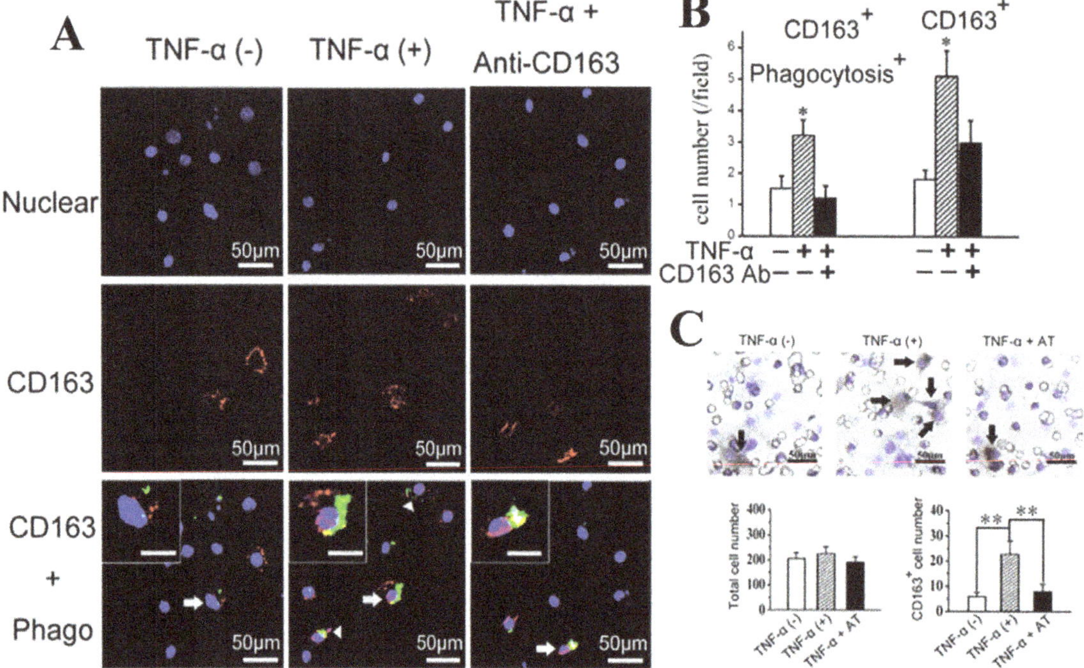

Figure 6. TNF-α increased the phagocytic and migratory activities of CD163⁺ cells isolated from rat TMJ cartilage. A–B: Confocal microscope images (A) and graphical representation (B) of the numbers of CD163⁺ cells and their phagocytic activity within primary cells isolated from TMJ cartilage and treated with vehicle, TNF-α alone, or TNF-α and a CD163 neutralizing antibody. The co-localization of the CD163⁺ cell with DiO-labeled cell debris (arrows), indicates that the cell debris is undergoing phagocytosis by the CD163⁺ cells, as shown in the insets. Bar: 50 μm. C: Transwell assay combined with immunohistochemical staining of CD163 indicates the migratory potential of CD163⁺ cells in response to 10 ng/ml TNF-α, which is impaired in the presence of the TNF-α neutralizing antibody (AT, 1 μg/ml). Arrows indicate the migrating CD163⁺ cells. Five fields were selected at random (at 200× magnification), and the number of CD163⁺ cells and total cells in each image were counted. **$P<0.01$.

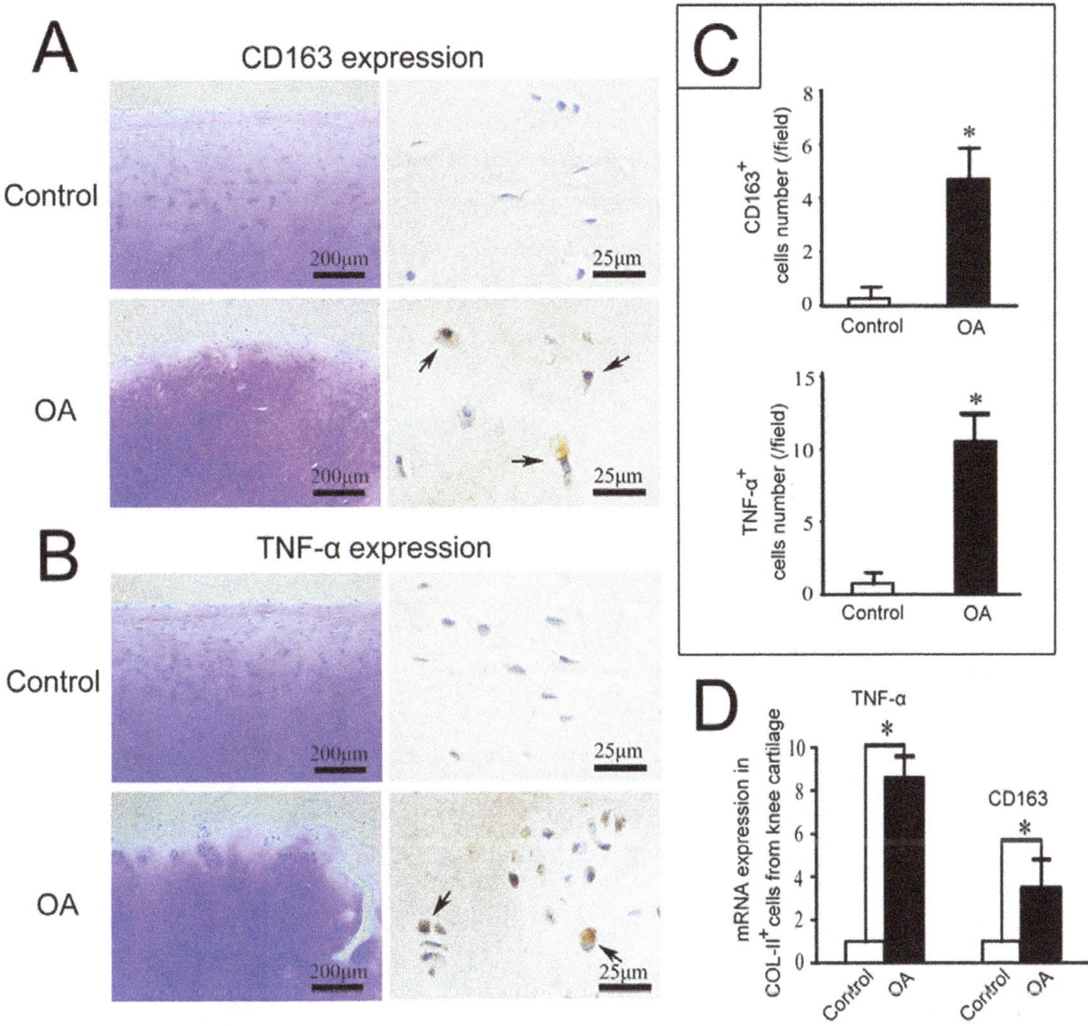

Figure 7. Increased expression of CD163 and TNF-α in knee cartilage from osteoarthritis patients. A and B: Toluidine blue and immunohistochemical staining of CD163 and TNF-α. C: Quantification of $CD163^+$ and TNF-α^+ cells from immunohistochemistry samples comparing the knee cartilage from patients with osteoarthritis (OA) or amputees (control). D: Comparison of the mRNA levels of TNF-α and CD163 in Col-II^+ cells isolated from knee cartilage from OA patients or amputees (control). *$P<0.05$.

limited number of $CD163^+$ cells within cartilage precluded the functional analysis of this specific cellular subset. The paradox is obvious: there is a requirement for degradation of the ECM to facilitate the mobilization of $CD163^+$ phagocytes. However, ECM is needed to maintain phagocyte viability. The increased phagocytosis but limited digestion capability of this cell population within degraded cartilage may sensitize them to cell death leading to the secretion of additional inflammatory cytokines, and resulting in the progressive degradation of cartilage in arthritis.

One previous *in vitro* study using flow cytometry showed that approximately 90% of chondrocytes could phagocytose FITC-latex particles [32]. However, our pilot study performing the same experiments showed that the FITC-latex particles stick easily to the surfaces of the chondrocytes, causing false positive results (data not shown). Therefore, in the present study, DiO-labeled cell debris was used to evaluate phagocytosis. In order to exclude false results caused by non-specific adhesion, the cells were thoroughly washed prior to analysis by flow cytometry. In addition, the confocal serial z-section scans together with the images from the living cells workstation verified the phagocytic activity of $CD163^+$ chondrocytes. Owing to these efforts, we have successfully identified an increase in the phagocytic activity of $CD163^+$ chondrocytes from degraded cartilage of 8-week old experimental rats compared with controls, as well as in chondrocytes stimulated by TNF-α. Notably, in the present study, the percentage of CD163 negative phagocytic chondrocytes was consistently maintained at about 10% (Figure 2 and Figure 5A), irrespective of any treatment, suggesting that this phagocytic cell population within cartilage may not be as responsive to abnormal stimuli as the $CD163^+$ phagocytic chondrocytes.

Increased expression of TNF-α and CD163 was observed in cartilage from OA patients compared with healthy cartilage, providing evidence that chondrocytes might undergo transdifferentiation to adopt a scavenger role. However, the gender and age difference between the two study groups should also be taken into consideration. Further clinical studies to clarify the observed difference are therefore needed, within individuals of the same gender and across a similar age distribution.

In summary, we have identified a new subset of chondrocytes, the $CD163^+$ phagocytes, in joint cartilage. The results presented in this study provide new insights into the function of the chondrocytes, namely the scavenger function of CD163$^+$ phagocytic chondrocytes in joint cartilage. During the early stages of cartilage degradation, some phagocytic chondrocytes appear to be capable of migrating to and clearing the degraded tissue, and therefore may have the potential to prevent further tissue damage. However, in the presence of continued stimulation, this scavenger capability would be overridden and the disease would progress. The dual role of cartilage ECM, providing cellular nutrition whilst restricting the mobilization of the defensive cartilage-resident phagocytes, offers insights for the management of OA. The therapeutic approach would require the effective elimination of the damaged tissue without extensive matrix degradation in order to provide a nutritional environment for the functional phagocytes in cartilage. Therefore, one future therapeutic strategy for arthritis could be to degrade the extracellular matrix at the early stages of the disease whilst providing cellular nutrition in homogenate form to the cartilage.

Author Contributions

Important suggestions on the experimental design and critical comments on the manuscript: XC. Conceived and designed the experiments: MQW KY. Performed the experiments: KJ JZ MZ Y. Wei. Analyzed the data: YC J.Hu LNN ZYQ. Contributed reagents/materials/analysis tools: HZ Y. Wu J. He. Wrote the paper: KJ MQW KY.

References

1. Hunter DJ (2011) Pharmacologic therapy for osteoarthritis—the era of disease modification 7:13–22.
2. Heinegard D, Saxne T (2011) The role of the cartilage matrix in osteoarthritis. Nat Rev Rheumatol 7:50–6.
3. Sampson ER, Hilton MJ, Tian Y, Chen D, Schwarz EM, et al. (2011) Teriparatide as a chondroregenerative therapy for injury-induced osteoarthritis. Sci Transl Med 3:101–93.
4. Umlauf D, Frank S, Pap T, Bertrand J (2010) Cartilage biology, pathology, and repair. Cell Mol Life Sci 67:4197–211.
5. Elliott MR, Ravichandran KS (2010) Clearance of apoptotic cells: implications in health and disease. J Cell Biol 189:1059–70.
6. Polfliet MM, Fabriek BO, Daniels WP, Dijkstra CD, van den Berg TK (2006) The rat macrophage scavenger receptor CD163: expression, regulation and role in inflammatory mediator production. Immunobiology 211:419–25.
7. Hogger P, Dreier J, Droste A, Buck F, Sorg C (1998) Identification of the integral membrane protein RM3/1 on human monocytes as a glucocorticoid-inducible member of the scavenger receptor cysteine-rich family (CD163). J Immunol 161:1883–90.
8. Fabriek BO, van Bruggen R, Deng DM, Ligtenberg AJ, Nazmi K, et al. (2009) The macrophage scavenger receptor CD163 functions as an innate immune sensor for bacteria. Blood 113:887–92.
9. Lau SK, Chu PG, Weiss LM (2004) CD163: a specific marker of macrophages in paraffin-embedded tissue samples. Am J Clin Pathol 122:794–801.
10. Law SK, Micklem KJ, Shaw JM, Zhang XP, Dong Y, et al. (1993) A new macrophage differentiation antigen which is a member of the scavenger receptor superfamily. Eur J Immunol 23:2320–5.
11. Maniecki MB, Etzerodt A, Moestrup SK, Moller HJ, Graversen JH (2011) Comparative assessment of the recognition of domain-specific CD163 monoclonal antibodies in human monocytes explains wide discrepancy in reported levels of cellular surface CD163 expression. Immunobiology 216:882–90.
12. Sanchez C, Domenech N, Vazquez J, Alonso F, Ezquerra A, et al. (1999) The porcine 2A10 antigen is homologous to human CD163 and related to macrophage differentiation. J Immunol 162:5230–7.
13. Kristiansen M, Graversen JH, Jacobsen C, Sonne O, Hoffman HJ, et al. (2001) Identification of the haemoglobin scavenger receptor. Nature 409:198–201.
14. Zwadlo G, Voegeli R, Osthoff KS, Sorg C (1987) A monoclonal antibody to a novel differentiation antigen on human macrophages associated with the down-regulatory phase of the inflammatory process. Exp Cell Biol 55:295–304.
15. Goerdt S, Bhardwaj R, Sorg C (1993) Inducible expression of MS-1 high-molecular-weight protein by endothelial cells of continuous origin and by dendritic cells/macrophages in vivo and in vitro. Am J Pathol 142:1409–22.
16. Gordon S (2003) Alternative activation of macrophages. Nat Rev Immunol 3:23–35.
17. Lotz MK, Otsuki S, Grogan SP, Sah R, Terkeltaub R, et al. (2010) Cartilage cell clusters. Arthritis Rheum 62:2206–18.
18. Yatsugi N, Tsukazaki T, Osaki M, Koji T, Yamashita S, et al. (2000) Apoptosis of articular chondrocytes in rheumatoid arthritis and osteoarthritis: correlation of apoptosis with degree of cartilage destruction and expression of apoptosis-related proteins of p53 and c-myc. J Orthop Sci 5:150–6.
19. Jiao K, Niu LN, Wang MQ, Dai J, Yu SB, et al. (2011) Subchondral bone loss following orthodontically induced cartilage degradation in the mandibular condyles of rats. Bone 48:362–71.
20. Jiao K, Wang MQ, Niu LN, Dai J, Yu SB, et al. (2009) Death and proliferation of chondrocytes in the degraded mandibular condylar cartilage of rats induced by experimentally created disordered occlusion. Apoptosis 14:22–30.
21. Wang GW, Wang MQ, Wang XJ, Yu SB, Liu XD, et al. (2010) Changes in the expression of MMP-3, MMP-9, TIMP-1 and aggrecan in the condylar cartilage of rats induced by experimentally created disordered occlusion. Arch Oral Biol 55:887–95.
22. Ye J, Li J, Yu Y, Wei Q, Deng W, et al. (2010) L-carnitine attenuates oxidant injury in HK-2 cells via ROS-mitochondria pathway. Regul Pept 161:58–66.
23. Ling Y, Ye X, Ji H, Zhang YH, Lai YS, et al. (2010) Synthesis and evaluation of nitric oxide-releasing derivatives of farnesylthiosalicylic acid as anti-tumor agents. Bioorg Med Chem 18:3448–56.
24. Chang C, Lauffenburger DA, Morales TI (2003) Motile chondrocytes from newborn calf: migration properties and synthesis of collagen II. Osteoarthritis Cartilage 11:603–12.
25. Kapoor M, Martel-Pelletier J, Lajeunesse D, Pelletier JP, Fahmi H (2011) Role of proinflammatory cytokines in the pathophysiology of osteoarthritis. Nat Rev Rheumatol 7:33–42.
26. Abramson SB, Yazici Y (2006) Biologics in development for rheumatoid arthritis: relevance to osteoarthritis. Adv Drug Deliv Rev 58:212–25.
27. Arend WP, Dayer JM (1990) Cytokines and cytokine inhibitors or antagonists in rheumatoid arthritis. Arthritis Rheum 33:305–15.
28. Bigg HF, Rowan AD (2001) The inhibition of metalloproteinases as a therapeutic target in rheumatoid arthritis and osteoarthritis. Curr Opin Pharmacol 1:314–20.
29. Heinegard D, Saxne T (2011) The role of the cartilage matrix in osteoarthritis. Nat Rev Rheumatol 7:50–6.
30. Martel-Pelletier J, Welsch DJ, Pelletier JP (2001) Metalloproteases and inhibitors in arthritic diseases. Best Pract Res Clin Rheumatol 15:805–29.
31. Cho TJ, Lehmann W, Edgar C, Sadeghi C, Hou A, et al. (2003) Tumor necrosis factor alpha activation of the apoptotic cascade in murine articular chondrocytes is associated with the induction of metalloproteinases and specific pro-resorptive factors. Arthritis Rheum 48:2845–54.
32. Castillo EC, Kouri JB (2004) A new role for chondrocytes as non-professional phagocytes. An in vitro study. Microsc Res Tech 64:269–8.

9

Efficacy of Tai Chi on Pain, Stiffness and Function in Patients with Osteoarthritis

Jun-Hong Yan[1]◑, Wan-Jie Gu[2]◑, Jian Sun[1], Wen-Xiao Zhang[1], Bao-Wei Li[1], Lei Pan[3]*

1 Department of Clinical Medical Technology, Affiliated Hospital of Binzhou Medical College, Binzhou, PR China, **2** Department of Anaesthesiology, The First Affiliated Hospital, Guangxi Medical University, Nanning, Guangxi, PR China, **3** Department of Internal Medicine, The First Affiliated Hospital, Guangzhou Medical College, Guangzhou, PR China

Abstract

Background: Whether Tai Chi benefits patients with osteoarthritis remains controversial. We performed a meta-analysis to assess the effectiveness of Tai Chi exercise for pain, stiffness, and physical function in patients with osteoarthritis.

Methods: A computerized search of PubMed and Embase (up to Sept 2012) was performed to identify relevant studies. The outcome measures were pain, stiffness, and physical function. Two investigators identified eligible studies and extracted data independently. The quality of the included studies was assessed by the Jadad score. Standard mean differences (SMDs) and 95% confidence intervals (CIs) were calculated and pooled using a random effects model. The change in outcomes from baseline was compared to the minimum clinically important difference.

Results: A total of seven randomized controlled trials involving 348 patients with osteoarthritis met the inclusion criteria. The mean Jadad score was 3.6. The pooled SMD was −0.45 (95% CI −0.70−−0.20, P = 0.0005) for pain, −0.31 (95% CI −0.60−−0.02, P = 0.04) for stiffness, and −0.61 (95% CI −0.85−−0.37, P<0.00001) for physical function. A change of 32.2–36.4% in the outcomes was greater than the minimum clinically important difference.

Conclusions: Twelve-week Tai Chi is beneficial for improving arthritic symptoms and physical function in patients with osteoarthritis and should be included in rehabilitation programs. However, the evidence may be limited by potential biases; thus, larger scale randomized controlled trials are needed to confirm the current findings and investigate the long-term effects of Tai Chi.

Editor: Steve Milanese, University of South Australia, Australia

Funding: The authors have no support or funding to report.

Competing Interests: The authors have declared that no competing interests exist.

* E-mail: zypl781102@163.com

◑ These authors contributed equally to this work.

Introduction

Osteoarthritis (OA) is a leading cause of musculoskeletal pain and disability [1,2]. OA is one of the most frequent causes of pain, loss of function, and disability in adults in Western countries, occurring in the majority of people over 65 years of age and in roughly 80% of those over 75 years of age [3]. No cure is currently available for OA and treatment options include primarily pharmacological or surgical treatment [4]. Taking into account the increasing prevalence of OA and associated disability, social, and economic costs, the American College of Rheumatology has developed guidelines for non-pharmacological therapy including exercise, education, physical therapy, and relatively low costs for OA [5,6]. However, despite the potential benefits of exercise, very few OA patients participate in regular physical activity [7]. Tai Chi (TC) was developed in the 17th century in China. TC is a low-impact physical activity with slow and gentle movements associated with health benefits, including increased flexibility and lower extremity muscle strength, improved fitness and cardiovascular health, better gait, balance, functional performance, and arthritic symptoms, for a variety of conditions, including OA [8–11].

Some published clinical trials of TC in patients with OA have shown inconsistent results for pain, stiffness, and physical function [11–15]. To the best of our knowledge, the previous systematic review (SR) suggested that the evidence is insufficient to support TC reduction of pain or improvement of physical function [16], and the latest SR suggested that TC may be effective for controlling pain and improving physical function in patients with knee OA [17]. Unfortunately, the latter SR included a randomized controlled trial (RCT) [18] that was withdrawn due to fraud, and lacked two RCTs that can be pooled to perform a meta-analysis. Therefore, we performed an updated meta-analysis to critically assess the effects of TC on pain, stiffness, and physical function in patients with OA.

Methods

Data Sources and Searches

A computerized search was performed in the PubMed and Embase databases (up to Sept 2012) for original research articles

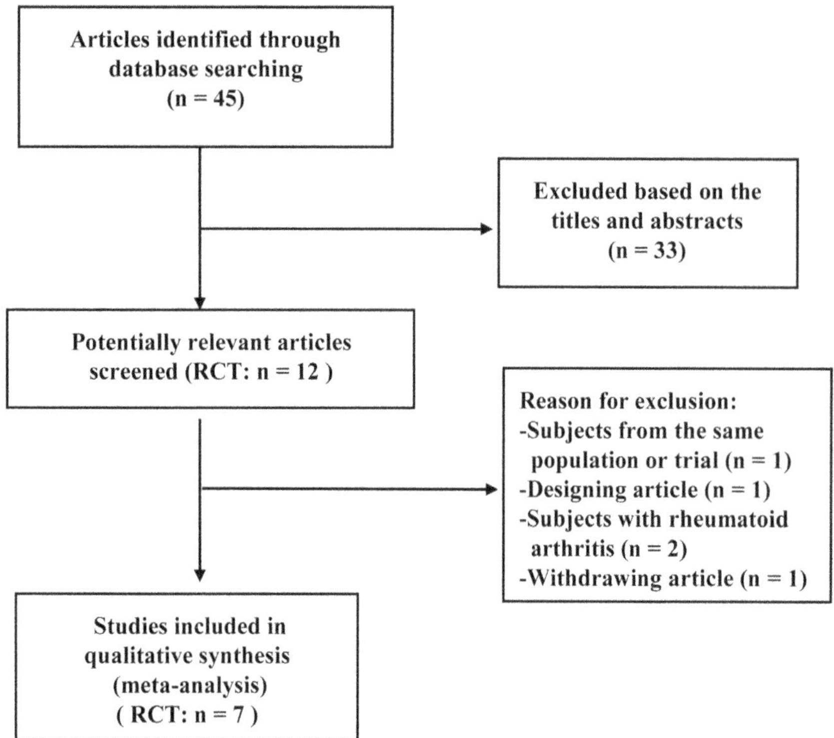

Figure 1. Search strategy and flow chart for this meta-analysis. RCT: randomized controlled trial.

using the following keywords: *(taiji OR taichi OR taiji chuan OR taichi qigong) AND (osteoarthritis OR osteoarthrosis OR OA OR degenerative arthritis OR degenerative arthritides)*. The search was limited to human subjects. No language restriction was imposed. Bibliographies of all potentially relevant studies, identified relevant articles (including unpublished studies, meta-analyses, a follow-up from reference lists of relevant articles, and personal contact with experts in this field), and international guidelines were searched by hand.

The following selection criteria were applied: (i) population, patients diagnosed with OA localized in any joints according to American College of Rheumatology criteria; (ii) intervention, Tai Chi, TaiJi Chuan, or Tai Chi Qigong with or without other treatment; (iii) comparison intervention, any type of control; (iv) outcome measures, pain, stiffness, and function assessed by Western Ontario and McMaster Universities Osteoarthritis Index (WOMAC); and (v) study design, RCT. Higher WOMAC scores indicate greater pain, stiffness, or physical disability.

Data Extraction and Quality Assessment

For each study, we recorded the first author, year of publication, sample size, OA site, intervention duration and frequency, exercise time, intervention in the control population, and outcomes, including intergroup differences. To assess eligibility, the data and trial quality information were extracted from the papers selected for inclusion in the meta-analysis independently by two investigators (J Sun and WJ Gu). Extracted data were entered into a standardized Excel file and checked by a third investigator (JH Yan). Any disagreements were resolved by discussion and consensus. The outcome measures were pain, stiffness, and physical function.

The methodological quality of each trial was evaluated using the Jadad scale [19]. The scale consists of three items describing randomization (0–2 points), blinding (0–2 points), and dropouts and withdrawals (0–1 points) in RCTs. A score of 1 is given for each of the points described. Another point is obtained when the method of randomization and/or blinding is given and is appropriate; when it is inappropriate a point is deducted. Thus, the quality scale ranges from 0 to 5 points and higher scores indicate better reporting. The studies are considered to be of low quality if the Jadad score is ≤ 2 and high quality if the score is ≥ 3 [20]. This study followed the Preferred Reporting Items for Systematic Reviews and Meta-Analyses (PRISMA) statement [21].

Data Analysis

All data were combined using Revman 5.1.0 (http://ims.cochrane.org/revman). For continuous outcomes, a mean difference was calculated using the standard mean difference (SMD) because the WOMAC scale measured the outcomes on different subscales: pain subscale (7–35 points, 0–500 mm and 0–100 mm), stiffness subscale (2–10 points, 0–200 mm), and physical function subscale (17–85 points, 0–1700 mm and 0–100 mm). Higher WOMAC scores indicate greater pain, stiffness, or physical disability. The SMDs were estimated from each study with the associated 95% confidence intervals (CIs) and pooled across studies using a random effects model [22]. Heterogeneity across studies was tested using the I^2 statistic, a quantitative measure of inconsistency across studies. Studies with an I^2 of 25% to 50% were considered to have low heterogeneity, I^2 of 50% to 75% was considered moderate heterogeneity, and $I^2>75\%$ was considered high heterogeneity [23]. If $I^2>50\%$, potential sources of heterogeneity were identified by sensitivity analyses conducted by omitting one study in each turn and investigating the influence of a single study on the overall pooled estimate. A subgroup analysis was conducted based on different durations. Potential publication bias was assessed by visually inspecting of the Begg funnel plots. $P<0.05$ was considered significant.

Table 1. Characteristics of randomized controlled trials included in the meta-analysis.

Study, year	Patients No. (M/F); OA site	Age, Mean, yrs (I/C)	Study group (n)	Intervention (Tai Chi) group				Control group	Study design/Jadad score
				Duration (weeks)/ Exercise Time	Frequency	Outcomes (WOMAC)	Intergroup differences	Intervention	
Adler 2007 [28]	14 (1/13); Hip or knee	70.8/72.8	Tai Chi (8); Control (6)	10/60 min	Once weekly	Pain	NS	Nonphysical recreational activity (Bingo)	RCT/3
Brismee et al., 2007 [12]	41 (7/34); Knee	70.8/68.8	Tai Chi (22); Control (19)	12/40 min	Three times weekly for 6 weeks plus homebased Tai Chi for 6 weeks	Pain Stiffness Function	NS P<0.05 P<0.05	Attention control program	Single-blind, RCT/4
Fransen et al., 2007 [26]	97 (25/72); Hip or knee	70.8/69.6	Tai Chi (56); Control (41)	12/60 min	Twice a week	Pain Function	NS P<0.05	Waiting list	Double-blind, RCT/4
Lee et al., 2009 [27]	44 (3/41); Knee	70.2/66.9	Tai Chi (29); Control (15)	8/60 min	Twice a week	Pain Stiffness Function	P<0.05 NS NS	Waiting list	Single-blind, RCT/4
Song et al., 2003 [11]	43 (0/43); Knee	64.8/62.5	Tai Chi (22); Control (21)	12/60 min	Three times a week	Pain Stiffness	P<0.05 P<0.05	Routine treatment	RCT/3
Song et al., 2009 [24]	69(0/69); Knee	62.36/59.94	Tai Chi (30); Control (39)	24/60 min	Twice weekly for the first 3 weeks and once weekly for the next weeks	Pain Stiffness Function	NS NS P<0.05	Self-help programme	RCT/3
Wang et al., 2009 [25]	40 (10/30); Knee	63.0/68.0	Tai Chi (20); Control (20)	12/60 min	Twice a week	Pain Stiffness Function	P<0.05 P<0.05 NS	Wellness education and stretching	Single-blind, RCT/4

Note: M/F: Male/Female; OA: osteoarthritis; I/C: Intervention/Control; WOMAC: Western Ontario and McMaster Universities Osteoarthritis Index; NS: not significant; RCT: randomized controlled trial.

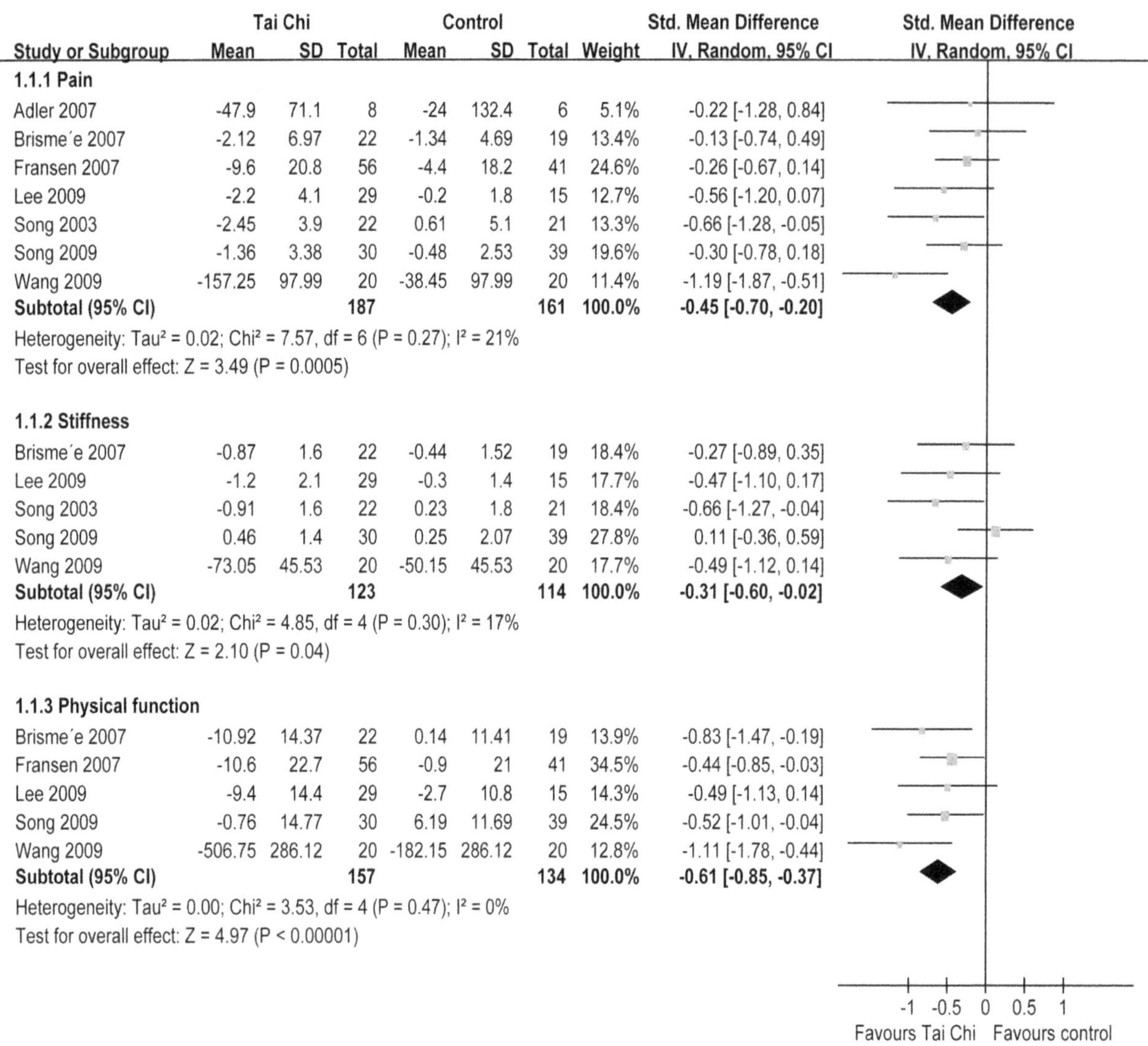

Tai Chi
Control
Std. Mean Difference
Std. Mean Difference
Study or Subgroup Mean SD Total Mean SD Total Weight IV, Random, 95% CI
IV, Random, 95% CI
1.1.1 Pain
Adler 2007 -47.9 71.1 8 -24 132.4 6 5.1% -0.22 [-1.28, 0.84]
Brisme'e 2007 -2.12 6.97 22 -1.34 4.69 19 13.4% -0.13 [-0.74, 0.49]
Fransen 2007 -9.6 20.8 56 -4.4 18.2 41 24.6% -0.26 [-0.67, 0.14]
Lee 2009 -2.2 4.1 29 -0.2 1.8 15 12.7% -0.56 [-1.20, 0.07]
Song 2003 -2.45 3.9 22 0.61 5.1 21 13.3% -0.66 [-1.28, -0.05]
Song 2009 -1.36 3.38 30 -0.48 2.53 39 19.6% -0.30 [-0.78, 0.18]
Wang 2009 -157.25 97.99 20 -38.45 97.99 20 11.4% -1.19 [-1.87, -0.51]
Subtotal (95% CI) 187 161 100.0% -0.45 [-0.70, -0.20]
Heterogeneity: Tau² = 0.02; Chi² = 7.57, df = 6 (P = 0.27); I² = 21%
Test for overall effect: Z = 3.49 (P = 0.0005)
1.1.2 Stiffness
Brisme'e 2007 -0.87 1.6 22 -0.44 1.52 19 18.4% -0.27 [-0.89, 0.35]
Lee 2009 -1.2 2.1 29 -0.3 1.4 15 17.7% -0.47 [-1.10, 0.17]
Song 2003 -0.91 1.6 22 0.23 1.8 21 18.4% -0.66 [-1.27, -0.04]
Song 2009 0.46 1.4 30 0.25 2.07 39 27.8% 0.11 [-0.36, 0.59]
Wang 2009 -73.05 45.53 20 -50.15 45.53 20 17.7% -0.49 [-1.12, 0.14]
Subtotal (95% CI) 123 114 100.0% -0.31 [-0.60, -0.02]
Heterogeneity: Tau² = 0.02; Chi² = 4.85, df = 4 (P = 0.30); I² = 17%
Test for overall effect: Z = 2.10 (P = 0.04)
1.1.3 Physical function
Brisme'e 2007 -10.92 14.37 22 0.14 11.41 19 13.9% -0.83 [-1.47, -0.19]
Fransen 2007 -10.6 22.7 56 -0.9 21 41 34.5% -0.44 [-0.85, -0.03]
Lee 2009 -9.4 14.4 29 -2.7 10.8 15 14.3% -0.49 [-1.13, 0.14]
Song 2009 -0.76 14.77 30 6.19 11.69 39 24.5% -0.52 [-1.01, -0.04]
Wang 2009 -506.75 286.12 20 -182.15 286.12 20 12.8% -1.11 [-1.78, -0.44]
Subtotal (95% CI) 157 134 100.0% -0.61 [-0.85, -0.37]
Heterogeneity: Tau² = 0.00; Chi² = 3.53, df = 4 (P = 0.47); I² = 0%
Test for overall effect: Z = 4.97 (P < 0.00001)
-1 -0.5 0 0.5 1
Favours Tai Chi Favours control

Figure 2. A Forest plot of the meta-analyses of RCTs comparing Tai Chi group with control group for change in pain, stiffness and physical function. Each block represents a study and the area of each block is proportional to the precision of the mean treatment effect in that study. The horizontal line represents each study's 95% confidence interval (CI) for the treatment effect. The centre of the diamond is the average treatment effect across studies, and the width of the diamond denotes its 95% CI.

Results

Search Results

The initial search yielded 45 relevant publications, of which 33 were excluded for duplicate studies and various reasons (reviews, non-randomized studies, or not relevant to our analysis) on the basis of the titles and abstracts (Figure 1). Twelve potentially relevant studies were identified for full-text analysis, but one RCT was excluded because of designing type (a protocol article) and two RCTs were excluded because it included subjects with rheumatoid arthritis. As the outcome measures of two RCTs resulted from the same population or trial, one RCT was withdrawn [18]. Finally, seven RCTs were selected for this meta-analysis, one published in Korean [24] and six published in English [11,12,25–28].

Study Characteristics

The main characteristics of the seven RCTs included in the meta-analysis are presented in Table 1. The studies were published between 2003 and 2009. The sample size of the trials ranged from 14 to 97 (total 348, 46 males and 302 females). All patients were elderly. The OA site was primarily the knee; thus, participates mainly referred to patients with knee OA. Follow-up ranged from 8 to 24 weeks and exercise time lasted 40–60 min. Two investigators (L Pan and WJ Gu) agreed on every item of the Jadad score. The mean Jadad score for the studies was 3.6 (range 3–4).

Meta-analysis of Outcome Measures

All seven RCTs reported pain [11,12,24–28]. The aggregated results of these studies suggest that TC is associated with significantly reduced pain (SMD = −0.45, 95% CI −0.77–−0.20, P = 0.0005, P for heterogeneity = 0.27, $I^2 = 21\%$) (Figure 2). Subgroup analyses were conducted based on different duration: >12 weeks (18–24 weeks), <12 weeks (8–10 weeks), and 12 weeks. For duration >12 weeks, TC did not significantly reduce pain (SMD = −0.17, 95% CI −0.56–0.23, P = 0.41, P for

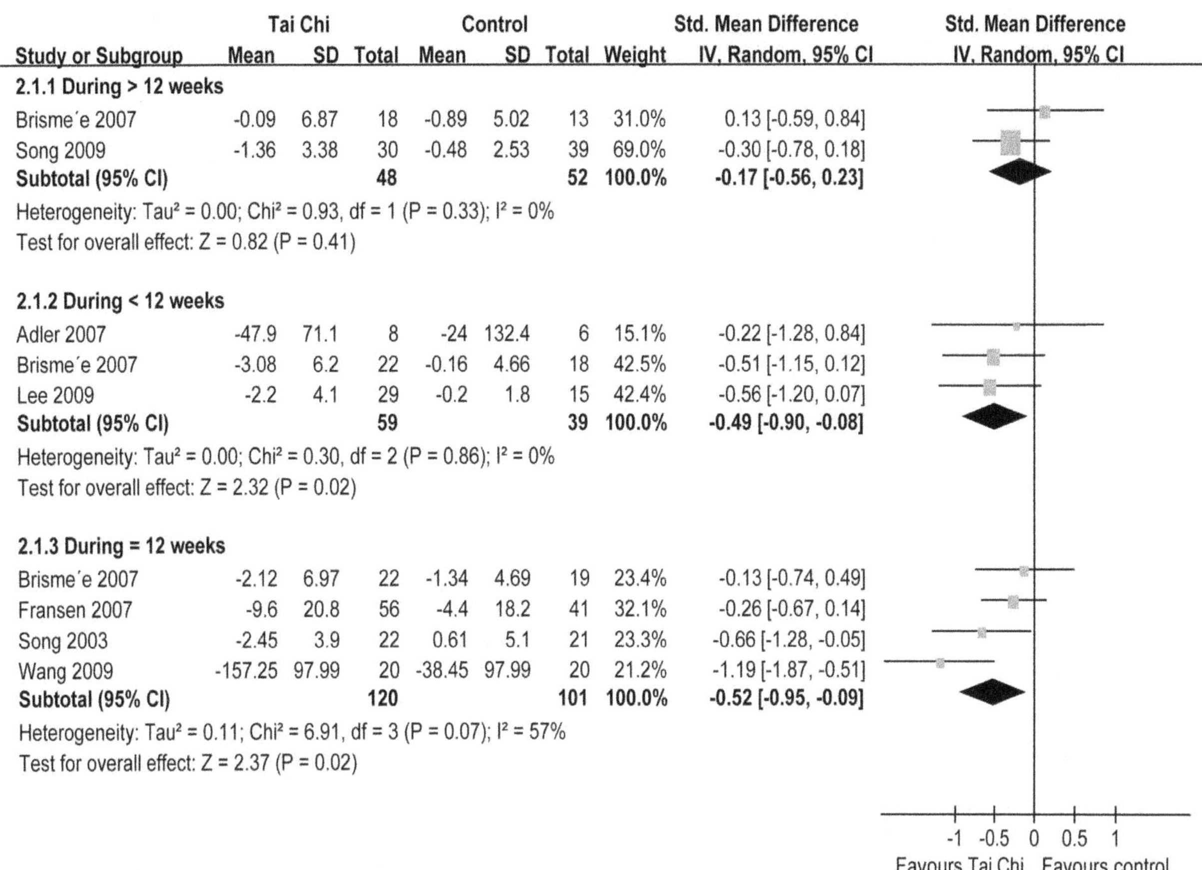

Tai Chi
Control
Std. Mean Difference
Std. Mean Difference
Study or Subgroup Mean SD Total Mean SD Total Weight IV, Random, 95% CI
IV, Random, 95% CI
2.1.1 During > 12 weeks
Brisme'e 2007 -0.09 6.87 18 -0.89 5.02 13 31.0% 0.13 [-0.59, 0.84]
Song 2009 -1.36 3.38 30 -0.48 2.53 39 69.0% -0.30 [-0.78, 0.18]
Subtotal (95% CI) 48 52 100.0% -0.17 [-0.56, 0.23]
Heterogeneity: Tau² = 0.00; Chi² = 0.93, df = 1 (P = 0.33); I² = 0%
Test for overall effect: Z = 0.82 (P = 0.41)
2.1.2 During < 12 weeks
Adler 2007 -47.9 71.1 8 -24 132.4 6 15.1% -0.22 [-1.28, 0.84]
Brisme'e 2007 -3.08 6.2 22 -0.16 4.66 18 42.5% -0.51 [-1.15, 0.12]
Lee 2009 -2.2 4.1 29 -0.2 1.8 15 42.4% -0.56 [-1.20, 0.07]
Subtotal (95% CI) 59 39 100.0% -0.49 [-0.90, -0.08]
Heterogeneity: Tau² = 0.00; Chi² = 0.30, df = 2 (P = 0.86); I² = 0%
Test for overall effect: Z = 2.32 (P = 0.02)
2.1.3 During = 12 weeks
Brisme'e 2007 -2.12 6.97 22 -1.34 4.69 19 23.4% -0.13 [-0.74, 0.49]
Fransen 2007 -9.6 20.8 56 -4.4 18.2 41 32.1% -0.26 [-0.67, 0.14]
Song 2003 -2.45 3.9 22 0.61 5.1 21 23.3% -0.66 [-1.28, -0.05]
Wang 2009 -157.25 97.99 20 -38.45 97.99 20 21.2% -1.19 [-1.87, -0.51]
Subtotal (95% CI) 120 101 100.0% -0.52 [-0.95, -0.09]
Heterogeneity: Tau² = 0.11; Chi² = 6.91, df = 3 (P = 0.07); I² = 57%
Test for overall effect: Z = 2.37 (P = 0.02)
-1 -0.5 0 0.5 1
Favours Tai Chi Favours control

Figure 3. A Forest plot of the subgroup analyses of RCTs comparing Tai Chi group with control group for change in pain.

heterogeneity = 0.33, $I^2 = 0\%$); duration <12 weeks, TC significantly reduced pain (SMD = −0.49, 95% CI −0.90- −0.08, P = 0.02, P for heterogeneity = 0.86, $I^2 = 0\%$); and duration = 12 weeks, TC significantly reduced pain (SMD = −0.52, 95% CI −0.95–−0.09, P = 0.02, P for heterogeneity = 0.07, $I^2 = 57\%$) (Figure 3).

Five RCTs reported stiffness [11,12,24,25,27]. The aggregated results of these studies suggest that TC is associated with significantly reduced stiffness (SMD = −0.31, 95% CI −0.60–−0.02, P = 0.04, P for heterogeneity = 0.30, $I^2 = 17\%$) (Figure 2). In the subgroup analyses, TC did not reduce stiffness for duration >12 weeks (SMD = 0.13, 95% CI −0.26–0.53, P = 0.51, P for heterogeneity = 0.89, $I^2 = 0\%$) or duration <12 weeks (SMD = −0.40, 95% CI −0.85–0.04, P = 0.08, P for heterogeneity = 0.77, $I^2 = 0\%$), but for duration = 12 weeks, TC significantly reduced stiffness (SMD = −0.47, 95% CI −0.83–−0.12, P = 0.01, P for heterogeneity = 0.68, $I^2 = 0\%$) (Figure 4).

Five RCTs reported physical function [12,24–27]. The aggregated results of these studies suggest that TC significantly improves physical function (SMD = −0.61, 95% CI −0.85–−0.37, P<0.00001, P for heterogeneity = 0.47, $I^2 = 0\%$) (Figure 2). In the subgroup analyses, for duration >12 weeks, TC improved physical function (SMD = −0.45, 95% CI −0.85–−0.04, P = 0.03, P for heterogeneity = 0.57, $I^2 = 0\%$); duration <12 weeks, TC significantly improved physical function (SMD = −0.71, 95% CI −1.16–−0.25, P = 0.002, P for heterogeneity = 0.34, $I^2 = 0\%$); and duration = 12 weeks, TC significantly improved physical function (SMD = −0.72, 95% CI −1.12–−0.31, P = 0.0005, P for heterogeneity = 0.21, $I^2 = 37\%$) (Figure 5).

In addition, we performed a funnel plot for pain, stiffness, and physical function, which included 7 RCTs, 5 RCTs, and 5 RCTs, respectively. However, the limiting RCTs make it difficult to interpret the result of publication bias (Figure 6). Finally, the changes in the outcomes from baseline for pain, stiffness, and physical function were 34.0%, 36.4%, and 32.2%, respectively.

Discussion

The major purpose of this meta-analysis was to update and critically evaluate the effects of TC training on arthritic symptoms and physical function in older patients with OA. Our meta-analysis suggests that 12-week TC significantly improves pain, stiffness, and physical function in patients with knee OA, which indicates that TC has benefits in the management of OA and should be available in rehabilitation programs as an alternative approach for patients with knee OA.

The primary goals in the management of OA are currently to alleviate arthritic symptoms, including pain and stiffness, maintain or improve joint mobility and quality of life, increase muscle strength, and minimize the disabling effects of OA [29,30]. Rehabilitation is regarded as an effective non-pharmaceutical therapy in the management of OA [31]. However, very few OA patients participate in any type of rehabilitation for fear of falling and exacerbating arthritic symptoms, which results in deconditioning and loss of physical function [32]. Even those who participate in a rehabilitation program show poor adherence [33]. For individuals with OA, rehabilitation intervention should be pursued cautiously because general exercise can apply either

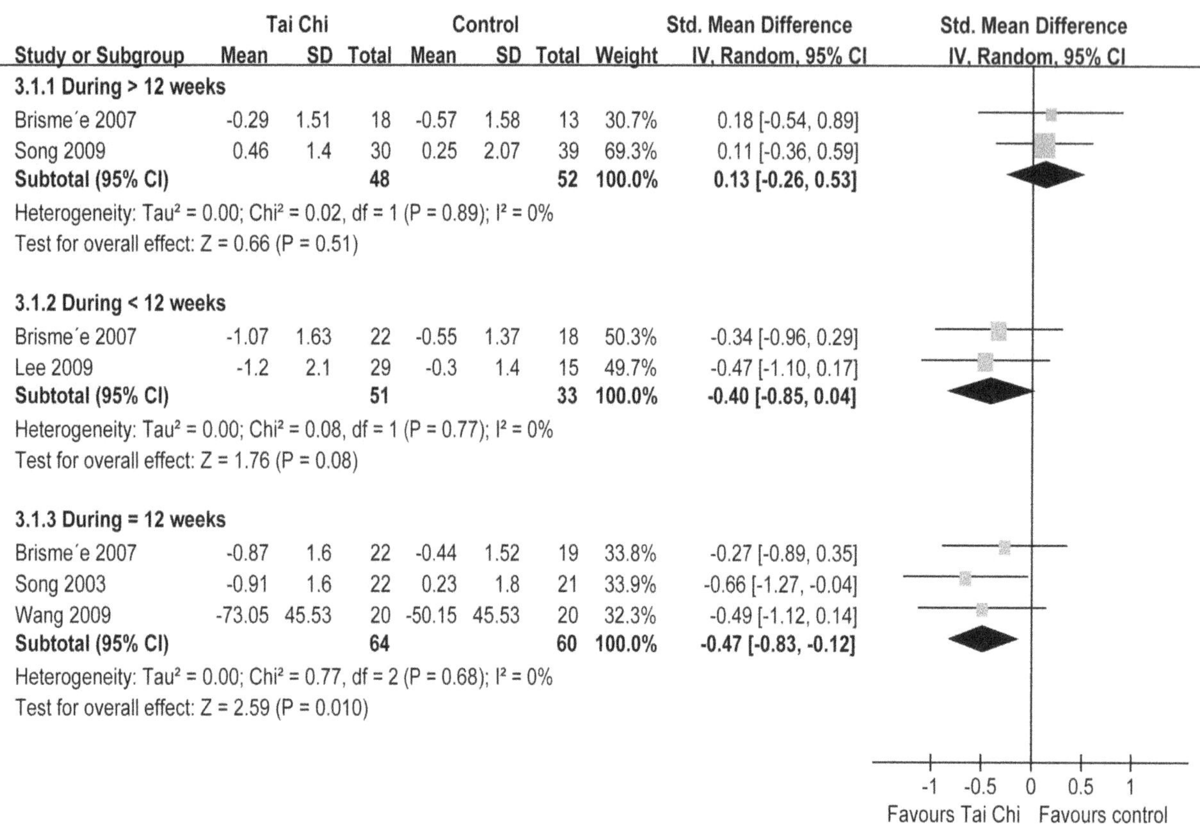

Tai Chi
Control
Std. Mean Difference
Std. Mean Difference
Study or Subgroup Mean SD Total Mean SD Total Weight IV, Random, 95% CI
IV, Random, 95% CI
3.1.1 During > 12 weeks
Brisme´e 2007 -0.29 1.51 18 -0.57 1.58 13 30.7% 0.18 [-0.54, 0.89]
Song 2009 0.46 1.4 30 0.25 2.07 39 69.3% 0.11 [-0.36, 0.59]
Subtotal (95% CI) 48 52 100.0% 0.13 [-0.26, 0.53]
Heterogeneity: Tau² = 0.00; Chi² = 0.02, df = 1 (P = 0.89); I² = 0%
Test for overall effect: Z = 0.66 (P = 0.51)
3.1.2 During < 12 weeks
Brisme´e 2007 -1.07 1.63 22 -0.55 1.37 18 50.3% -0.34 [-0.96, 0.29]
Lee 2009 -1.2 2.1 29 -0.3 1.4 15 49.7% -0.47 [-1.10, 0.17]
Subtotal (95% CI) 51 33 100.0% -0.40 [-0.85, 0.04]
Heterogeneity: Tau² = 0.00; Chi² = 0.08, df = 1 (P = 0.77); I² = 0%
Test for overall effect: Z = 1.76 (P = 0.08)
3.1.3 During = 12 weeks
Brisme´e 2007 -0.87 1.6 22 -0.44 1.52 19 33.8% -0.27 [-0.89, 0.35]
Song 2003 -0.91 1.6 22 0.23 1.8 21 33.9% -0.66 [-1.27, -0.04]
Wang 2009 -73.05 45.53 20 -50.15 45.53 20 32.3% -0.49 [-1.12, 0.14]
Subtotal (95% CI) 64 60 100.0% -0.47 [-0.83, -0.12]
Heterogeneity: Tau² = 0.00; Chi² = 0.77, df = 2 (P = 0.68); I² = 0%
Test for overall effect: Z = 2.59 (P = 0.010)
-1 -0.5 0 0.5 1
Favours Tai Chi Favours control

Figure 4. A Forest plot of the subgroup analyses of RCTs comparing Tai Chi group with control group for change in stiffness.

injurious or beneficial effects on the joints. Recent studies have evaluated the role of TC, which enhances balance, strength, flexibility, and self-efficacy, and decreases pain and stiffness in various patients with chronic conditions. TC is a potential option for the management of OA and is superior to other forms of rehabilitation for elders because it involves a series of gentle fluid movements reputedly good for maintaining mobility and gradually improves muscle strength and range of motion without exacerbating arthritic symptoms [34]. Growing evidence suggests that TC may reduce arthritic symptoms and/or improve physical function in patients with OA [14,27,29]. However, other trials failed to investigate these positive effects and were unable to draw a positive conclusion [17,28,32].

Our results showed that 12-week TC is effective at reducing pain and stiffness and improving physical function in patients with knee OA. Subgroup analyses suggested that 8–10 weeks of short-term TC can significantly improve pain and physical function, and 18–24 weeks of TC improves physical function. Theoretically, TC could be more effective over the long-term, but the positive effects of 12-week TC were not sustained after 6–12 weeks duration, which is consistent with previous findings [12]. This change with the long-term TC exercise is interesting, but additional studies are needed to investigate the long-term effects of TC in patients with knee OA. In addition, most of the patients in the RCTs included in our study were elderly females and the OA site was primarily the knee, which is consistent with the current epidemiology of OA [3].

Recent efforts have suggested a minimal clinically important difference (MCID) for WOMAC scores from both pharmacological and rehabilitation trials. Changes of 20–25% in the WOMAC score are considered to be clinically relevant [35], but the most recent study suggested that a 16–18% reduction in the WOMAC score is associated with the MCID and should be appropriate for use in the interpretation of clinical studies, as well as in clinical care [36]. Our results indicate that a reduction of 32.2–36.4% from baseline was greater than the MCID of 16–18% or 20–25%, which suggests that TC has beneficial effects on pain, stiffness, and physical function in patients with knee OA.

Our results are similar to the latest SR [17]. In detail, this previous SR showed that TC may be effective at controlling pain and improving physical function in patients with knee OA. However, the authors did not compare their results with the MCID because the results were difficult to compare quantitatively due to the use of different assessment measures for evaluating outcomes. Therefore, we pooled the outcome measures (e.g., pain, stiffness, and function) assessed by the same WOMAC score in order to compare the results with the MCID. Our results indicate the presence of sufficient clinical evidence of reduced pain and stiffness and improved physical function.

The possible mechanisms responsible for the beneficial effects of TC that differ from other forms of exercise are still unclear. TC harmonizes yin-yang and promotes homeostasis between body and mind. TC is a lower intensity exercise of flowing circular movements, balance and weight shifting, deep breathing regulation and meditation, and visualization, and focuses on internal awareness [37,38]. TC encourages patients to move fluidly with less strain, and improved joint stability and decreased joint pain may be beneficial for patients with knee OA. In addition, the movement characteristics of slowness, quietness, and stillness inherent to TC and its steady rhythm and slow movements aid in relaxation and offer beneficial changes in symptoms and mood, which may promote psychological well-being and positively

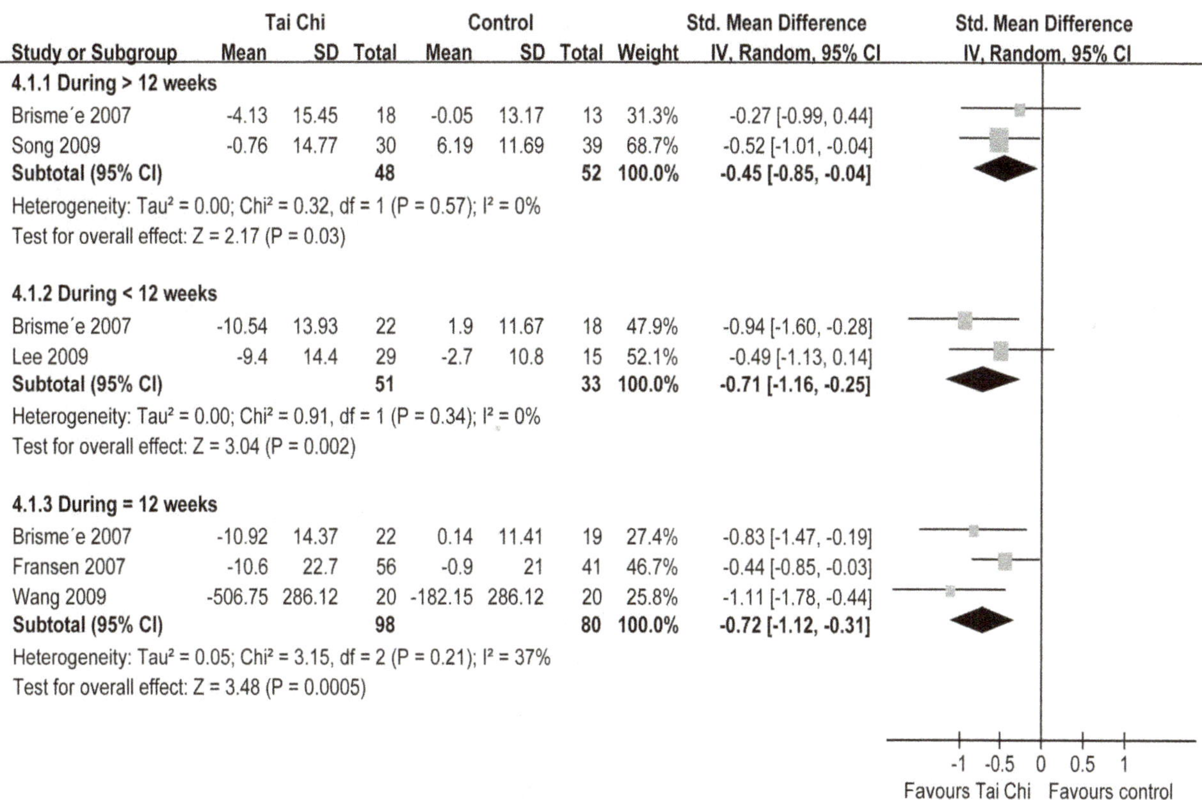

Study or Subgroup	Tai Chi Mean	Tai Chi SD	Tai Chi Total	Control Mean	Control SD	Control Total	Weight	Std. Mean Difference IV, Random, 95% CI
4.1.1 During > 12 weeks								
Brisme´e 2007	-4.13	15.45	18	-0.05	13.17	13	31.3%	-0.27 [-0.99, 0.44]
Song 2009	-0.76	14.77	30	6.19	11.69	39	68.7%	-0.52 [-1.01, -0.04]
Subtotal (95% CI)			**48**			**52**	**100.0%**	**-0.45 [-0.85, -0.04]**
Heterogeneity: Tau² = 0.00; Chi² = 0.32, df = 1 (P = 0.57); I² = 0%								
Test for overall effect: Z = 2.17 (P = 0.03)								
4.1.2 During < 12 weeks								
Brisme´e 2007	-10.54	13.93	22	1.9	11.67	18	47.9%	-0.94 [-1.60, -0.28]
Lee 2009	-9.4	14.4	29	-2.7	10.8	15	52.1%	-0.49 [-1.13, 0.14]
Subtotal (95% CI)			**51**			**33**	**100.0%**	**-0.71 [-1.16, -0.25]**
Heterogeneity: Tau² = 0.00; Chi² = 0.91, df = 1 (P = 0.34); I² = 0%								
Test for overall effect: Z = 3.04 (P = 0.002)								
4.1.3 During = 12 weeks								
Brisme´e 2007	-10.92	14.37	22	0.14	11.41	19	27.4%	-0.83 [-1.47, -0.19]
Fransen 2007	-10.6	22.7	56	-0.9	21	41	46.7%	-0.44 [-0.85, -0.03]
Wang 2009	-506.75	286.12	20	-182.15	286.12	20	25.8%	-1.11 [-1.78, -0.44]
Subtotal (95% CI)			**98**			**80**	**100.0%**	**-0.72 [-1.12, -0.31]**
Heterogeneity: Tau² = 0.05; Chi² = 3.15, df = 2 (P = 0.21); I² = 37%								
Test for overall effect: Z = 3.48 (P = 0.0005)								

Figure 5. A Forest plot of the subgroup analyses of RCTs comparing Tai Chi group with control group for change in physical function.

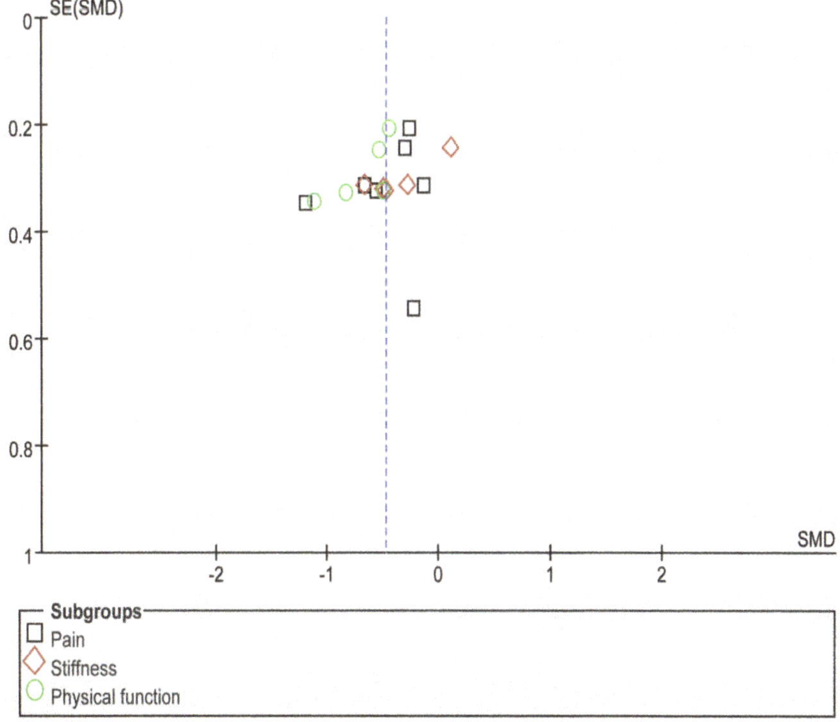

Figure 6. A Funnel plot for pain, stiffness, and physical function.

influence chronic pain in patients with knee OA [39]. Therefore, the nature of TC and the multiple potential effects on the body and mind that differ from other conventional exercise may account for these beneficial effects; however, further studies are needed to better understand the benefits, mechanisms, and role of TC in the prevention and management of OA.

We found that most studies lacked other objective outcome measures, including exercise performance (e.g., 6-min walk distance), quality of life, body mass index, muscle strength, immune function, and survival, which would result in more reliable and convincing evidence of the effects of TC in patients with OA. Furthermore, comparing TC with general forms of exercise, such as jogging and motion or flexibility exercises, would be better, but this method has not seen much use in clinical research. Therefore, focusing on these additional interesting clues may be useful for future research on the topic. In addition, future researchers should attempt to understand the relationships among impairment, functional limitations, and disability.

Finally, we found no significant side effects or adverse events associated with TC, and participants had relatively high adherence in most studies, indicating that TC is safe and has satisfactory compliance. Given no special setting, no additional costs, independence from weather conditions, and multiple benefits to the body, TC should be an alternative to other exercise training and be incorporated into rehabilitation programs as a potential non-pharmacological treatment for patients with OA.

This study had numerous limitations. First, our analysis is based on seven RCTs, all of which had a small sample size. Overestimation of the treatment effect is more likely in smaller trials compared to larger trials. Although we performed a funnel plot for the outcomes, the limiting RCTs make it difficult to interpret the result of publication bias. Moreover, a major limitation of our subgroup analyses is that some (<12 and >12 weeks) are based only on 2 to 3 studies; thus, the conclusions about the duration of TC exercise should be interpreted with caution. Next, the targeted population varied greatly (e.g., patients of different gender, ethnicity, and duration of OA). The adopted TC protocols differed. These factors may have a potential impact on our results. Finally, some missing and unpublished data may lead to bias.

In summary, the positive findings of this study suggest that 12-week TC has beneficial effects on the management of knee OA, including reduced pain and stiffness and improved physical function. As an alternative, effective, inexpensive, and accessible approach, TC should be available in rehabilitation programs. However, given the heterogeneity among study designs and small RCTs, additional larger scale RCTs are needed to substantiate the current findings and investigate the long-term effects of TC in patients with knee OA.

Author Contributions

Performed the literature search and the data extraction: JHY WJG JS WXZ BWL. Responsible for the final approval of the version to be published: JHY WJG JS WXZ BWL LP. Conceived and designed the experiments: LP. Performed the experiments: JHY WJG JS WXZ BWL. Analyzed the data: LP JHY WJG JS WXZ BWL. Wrote the paper: LP JHY WJG JS WXZ BWL.

References

1. Katz JD, Nayyar G (2009) Introduction: arthritis and myositis. Ann N Y Acad Sci 1154: 3–9.
2. Bennell KL, Hinman RS (2011) A review of the clinical evidence for exercise in osteoarthritis of the hip and knee. J Sci Med Sport 14: 4–9.
3. Arden N, Nevitt MC (2006) Osteoarthritis: epidemiology. Best Pract Res Clin Rheumatol 20: 3–25.
4. Hochberg MC (2010) Opportunities for the prevention of osteoarthritis. Semin Arthritis Rheum 39: 321–322.
5. (2000) Recommendations for the medical management of osteoarthritis of the hip and knee: 2000 update. American College of Rheumatology Subcommittee on Osteoarthritis Guidelines. Arthritis Rheum 43: 1905–1915.
6. Richmond J, Hunter D, Irrgang J, Jones MH, Snyder-Mackler L, et al. (2010) American Academy of Orthopaedic Surgeons clinical practice guideline on the treatment of osteoarthritis (OA) of the knee. J Bone Joint Surg Am 92: 990–993.
7. Gecht MR, Connell KJ, Sinacore JM, Prohaska TR (1996) A survey of exercise beliefs and exercise habits among people with arthritis. Arthritis Care Res 9: 82–88.
8. Ramachandran AK, Rosengren KS, Yang Y, Hsiao-Wecksler ET (2007) Effect of Tai Chi on gait and obstacle crossing behaviors in middle-aged adults. Gait Posture 26: 248–255.
9. Faber MJ, Bosscher RJ, Chin APMJ, van Wieringen PC (2006) Effects of exercise programs on falls and mobility in frail and pre-frail older adults: A multicenter randomized controlled trial. Arch Phys Med Rehabil 87: 885–896.
10. Pan L, Yan JH, Guo YZ, Yan JH (2013) Effects of Tai Chi training on exercise capacity and quality of life in patients with chronic heart failure: a meta-analysis. Eur J Heart Fail 15:316–323.
11. Song R, Lee EO, Lam P, Bae SC (2003) Effects of tai chi exercise on pain, balance, muscle strength, and perceived difficulties in physical functioning in older women with osteoarthritis: a randomized clinical trial. J Rheumatol 30: 2039–2044.
12. Brismee JM, Paige RL, Chyu MC, Boatright JD, Hagar JM, et al. (2007) Group and home-based tai chi in elderly subjects with knee osteoarthritis: a randomized controlled trial. Clin Rehabil 21: 99–111.
13. Song R, Lee EO, Lam P, Bae SC (2007) Effects of a Sun-style Tai Chi exercise on arthritic symptoms, motivation and the performance of health behaviors in women with osteoarthritis. Taehan Kanho Hakhoe Chi 37: 249–256.
14. Hartman CA, Manos TM, Winter C, Hartman DM, Li B, et al. (2000) Effects of T'ai Chi training on function and quality of life indicators in older adults with osteoarthritis. J Am Geriatr Soc 48: 1553–1559.
15. Lee HY (2006) [Comparison of effects among Tai-Chi exercise, aquatic exercise, and a self-help program for patients with knee osteoarthritis]. Taehan Kanho Hakhoe Chi 36: 571–580.
16. Lee MS, Pittler MH, Ernst E (2008) Tai chi for osteoarthritis: a systematic review. Clin Rheumatol 27: 211–218.
17. Kang JW, Lee MS, Posadzki P, Ernst E (2011) T'ai chi for the treatment of osteoarthritis: a systematic review and meta-analysis. BMJ Open 1: e000035.
18. Ni GX, Song L, Yu B, Huang CH, Lin JH (2010) Tai chi improves physical function in older Chinese women with knee osteoarthritis. J Clin Rheumatol 16: 64–67.
19. Jadad AR, Moore RA, Carroll D, Jenkinson C, Reynolds DJ, et al. (1996) Assessing the quality of reports of randomized clinical trials: is blinding necessary? Control Clin Trials 17: 1–12.
20. Kjaergard LL, Villumsen J, Gluud C (2001) Reported methodologic quality and discrepancies between large and small randomized trials in meta-analyses. Ann Intern Med 135: 982–989.
21. Liberati A, Altman DG, Tetzlaff J, Mulrow C, Gotzsche PC, et al. (2009) The PRISMA statement for reporting systematic reviews and meta-analyses of studies that evaluate healthcare interventions: explanation and elaboration. BMJ 339: b2700.
22. DerSimonian R, Laird N (1986) Meta-analysis in clinical trials. Control Clin Trials 7: 177–188.
23. Higgins JP, Thompson SG, Deeks JJ, Altman DG (2003) Measuring inconsistency in meta-analyses. BMJ 327: 557–560.
24. Song R, Eom A, Lee EO, Lam P, Bae SC (2009) [Effects of tai chi combined with self-help program on arthritic symptoms and fear of falling in women with osteoarthritis]. J Muscle Joint Health 16:46–54.
25. Wang C, Schmid CH, Hibberd PL, Kalish R, Roubenoff R, et al. (2009) Tai Chi is effective in treating knee osteoarthritis: a randomized controlled trial. Arthritis Rheum 61: 1545–1553.
26. Fransen M, Nairn L, Winstanley J, Lam P, Edmonds J (2007) Physical activity for osteoarthritis management: a randomized controlled clinical trial evaluating hydrotherapy or Tai Chi classes. Arthritis Rheum 57: 407–414.
27. Lee HJ, Park HJ, Chae Y, Kim SY, Kim SN, et al. (2009) Tai Chi Qigong for the quality of life of patients with knee osteoarthritis: a pilot, randomized, waiting list controlled trial. Clin Rehabil 23: 504–511.
28. Adler PA (2007) The effects of tai chi on pain and function in older adults with osteoarthritis. PhD dissertation. Frances Payne Bolton School of Nursing, Case Western Reserve University, Ohio.

29. Chyu MC, von Bergen V, Brismee JM, Zhang Y, Yeh JK, et al. (2011) Complementary and alternative exercises for management of osteoarthritis. Arthritis 2011: 364319.
30. Hawker GA, Mian S, Bednis K, Stanaitis I (2011) Osteoarthritis year 2010 in review: non-pharmacologic therapy. Osteoarthritis Cartilage 19: 366–374.
31. Sayre EC, Li LC, Kopec JA, Esdaile JM, Bar S, et al. (2010) The effect of disease site (knee, hip, hand, foot, lower back or neck) on employment reduction due to osteoarthritis. PLoS One 5: e10470.
32. Manninen P, Riihimaki H, Heliovaara M, Suomalainen O (2001) Physical exercise and risk of severe knee osteoarthritis requiring arthroplasty. Rheumatology (Oxford) 40: 432–437.
33. Munro JF, Nicholl JP, Brazier JE, Davey R, Cochrane T (2004) Cost effectiveness of a community based exercise programme in over 65 year olds: cluster randomised trial. J Epidemiol Community Health 58: 1004–1010.
34. Zhou DH (1982) Preventive geriatrics: an overview from traditional Chinese medicine. Am J Chin Med 10: 32–39.
35. Barr S, Bellamy N, Buchanan WW, Chalmers A, Ford PM, et al. (1994) A comparative study of signal versus aggregate methods of outcome measurement based on the WOMAC Osteoarthritis Index. Western Ontario and McMaster Universities Osteoarthritis Index. J Rheumatol 21: 2106–2112.
36. Hmamouchi I, Allali F, Tahiri L, Khazzani H, Mansouri LE, et al. (2012) Clinically important improvement in the WOMAC and predictor factors for response to non-specific non-steroidal anti-inflammatory drugs in osteoarthritic patients: a prospective study. BMC Res Notes 5: 58.
37. Gatts S (2008) A Tai Chi Chuan training model to improve balance control in older adults. Curr Aging Sci 1: 68–70.
38. Guan H, Koceja DM (2011) Effects of long-term tai chi practice on balance and H-reflex characteristics. Am J Chin Med 39: 251–260.
39. Yocum DE, Castro WL, Cornett M (2000) Exercise, education, and behavioral modification as alternative therapy for pain and stress in rheumatic disease. Rheum Dis Clin North Am 26: 145–159, x–xi.

10

Progression of Cartilage Degradation, Bone Resorption and Pain in Rat Temporomandibular Joint Osteoarthritis Induced by Injection of Iodoacetate

Xue-Dong Wang[1], Xiao-Xing Kou[1], Dan-Qing He[1], Min-Min Zeng[1], Zhen Meng[2], Rui-Yun Bi[2], Yan Liu[1], Jie-Ni Zhang[1], Ye-Hua Gan[2]*, Yan-Heng Zhou[1]*

1 Department of Orthodontics, Peking University School and Hospital of Stomatology, Beijing, China, **2** Center for Temporomandibular Disorders and Orofacial Pain, Peking University School and Hospital of Stomatology, Beijing, China

Abstract

Background: Osteoarthritis (OA) is an important subtype of temporomandibular disorders. A simple and reproducible animal model that mimics the histopathologic changes, both in the cartilage and subchondral bone, and clinical symptoms of temporomandibular joint osteoarthritis (TMJOA) would help in our understanding of its process and underlying mechanism.

Objective: To explore whether injection of monosodium iodoacetate (MIA) into the upper compartment of rat TMJ could induce OA-like lesions.

Methods: Female rats were injected with varied doses of MIA into the upper compartment and observed for up to 12 weeks. Histologic, radiographic, behavioral, and molecular changes in the TMJ were evaluated by light and electron microscopy, MicroCT scanning, head withdrawal threshold test, real-time PCR, immunohistochemistry, and TUNEL assay.

Results: The intermediate zone of the disc loosened by 1 day post-MIA injection and thinned thereafter. Injection of an MIA dose of 0.5 mg or higher induced typical OA-like lesions in the TMJ within 4 weeks. Condylar destruction presented in a time-dependent manner, including chondrocyte apoptosis in the early stages, subsequent cartilage matrix disorganization and subchondral bone erosion, fibrosis, subchondral bone sclerosis, and osteophyte formation in the late stages. Nociceptive responses increased in the early stages, corresponding to severe synovitis. Furthermore, chondrocyte apoptosis and an imbalance between anabolism and catabolism of cartilage and subchondral bone might account for the condylar destruction.

Conclusions: Multi-level data demonstrated a reliable and convenient rat model of TMJOA could be induced by MIA injection into the upper compartment. The model might facilitate TMJOA related researches.

Editor: Andre Van Wijnen, University of Massachusetts Medical, United States of America

Funding: This project is supported by the National Natural Science Foundation of China (Grant No. 81070849) and China International Science and Technology Cooperation (Grant No. 2010DFB32980). The funders had no role in study design, data collection and analysis, decision to publish, or preparation of the manuscript.

Competing Interests: The authors have declared that no competing interests exist.

* E-mail: kqyehuagan@bjmu.edu.cn (YHG); yanhengzhou@gmail.com (YHZ)

Introduction

Temporomandibular joint osteoarthritis (TMJOA) is an important subtype of temporomandibular disorders (TMD) [1,2] and is especially common in female patients with severe pain and dysfunction of the temporomandibular joint (TMJ) [3,4]. OA is characterized by a progressive degradation of cartilage, subchondral bone remodeling, synovitis, and chronic pain [3,5,6].

However, the process of TMJOA remains obscure. Chondrocyte death due to either apoptosis or necrosis is assumed to be a central feature in the degeneration of osteoarthritic cartilage and to contribute to the development of clinical or experimental OA [7,8]. Resorption and abrasion of condylar subchondral bone are unique in TMJOA, which usually shows no typical pannus in the synovium whereas rheumatoid arthritis does [3]. Therefore, a proper animal model may provide a useful way to understand the pathogenesis of TMJOA and to evaluate potential therapeutic interventions [9].

Thus far, several methods have attempted to create animal models of TMJOA, including surgical [10], mechanical [11], drug-inducing [12,13], and spontaneously occurring methods [14]. Due to the limited availability of special animal species, slow progression of the disease, and complicated operations, the use of spontaneous or surgical-induced methods was limited [13,15]. In addition, the lack of progressive changes led to a number of drug-induced models being merely models of cartilage damage rather than OA [9]. A simple and reproducible animal model of

TMJOA that mimics the histopathologic changes both in cartilage and subchondral bone, as well as clinical symptoms, is still needed.

Intra-articular injection of monosodium iodoacetate (MIA) to induce OA-like lesions is widely used to induce knee OA [16,17,18,19,20,21]. MIA mainly inhibits the activity of glyceraldehyde-3-phosphate dehydrogenase leading to apoptosis of chondrocytes [18,20,22]. The MIA-induced OA model has the great advantage of easy modulation of the progression and severity of the articular lesions by modification of MIA concentration [19]. Although a few studies have attempted to induce OA-like lesions in rabbit TMJ by MIA injection into the lower compartment with or without surgical assistance [13,23,24], it is important to explore whether MIA could induce OA-like lesions in the rat TMJ, since rats are one of the most widely used species in experimental research and drug toxicology testing [15]. The TMJ is partitioned by a disc, which forms a larger upper and smaller lower compartment. Agent injection into the lower compartment is a difficult procedure both in humans and animals because of its limited space [25], whereas injection into the upper compartment, even in rats, is technically and manually preferable, and has often been used previously [26,27,28].

The question then arises as to whether MIA injection into the upper compartment of the rat TMJ can be used to create a comprehensive OA model. To address this question, investigations at the histopathologic, radiographic, molecular, and noceiceptive behavioral levels were performed in this study to examine whether injection of MIA into the upper compartment of the rat TMJ could induce OA-like lesions in the entire joint.

Materials and Methods

Ethics Statement

With the approval of the Peking University Institutional Animal Care and Use Committee (NO: LA2012-59), all rats were housed under controlled temperatures in a 12 h light/dark cycle with easy access to food and water.

Induction of TMJOA

A total of 72 female Sprague-Dawley rats (180–200 g) were randomly assigned to either the experimental (n = 42) or control (n = 30) groups. The experimental schedule is illustrated in Fig. 1A. TMJOA was induced by injection of MIA (Sigma, Saint Louis, USA) dissolved in 50 µL saline into the upper compartment of bilateral TMJs using a 27-gauge 0.5-inch needle without surgical assistance. We first confirmed the injection site by injection of 50 µL dye into the upper compartment (Fig. 1B).

Dose Course

Various doses of MIA (0.05, 0.1, 0.5, 1, or 2 mg) were injected into the upper compartment of bilateral TMJs of rats in five experimental groups (n = 3/group), while 50 µL saline was injected into TMJs of rats in the control group (n = 3). All rats were sacrificed on day 28 post-injection to validate the adequate dose of MIA for further observations (**Fig. 1A**).

Time Course

After the dose course test, 0.5 mg MIA (minimum effective dose) or saline was injected into TMJs and rats were sacrificed on days 1, 3, 7, 14, 28, 56, or 84 post-injection (n = 3/group) (**Fig. 1A**).

To determine gene expression profiles during the induction of TMJOA, an additional 12 rats, divided into two groups (n = 6/group), were injected with 0.5 mg MIA or saline and sacrificed on day 14 post-injection.

Head Withdrawal Threshold (HWT) Measurements

The nociceptive behavior of animals was assessed based on the HWT as described previously [27]. HWT measurements were performed pre-MIA/saline injection and on days 1, 3, 7, 14, 21, 28, 35, and 42 post-injection (**Fig. 1A**). The HWT was calculated as a mean value per joint of 3 rats/group.

Tissue Harvesting

All rats were sacrificed by pentobarbital overdose. For histopathology, the TMJs of two rats in each group were removed bilaterally *en bloc*, fixed in 4% paraformaldehyde, and demineralized in 15% EDTA. For radiographic examination, the bilateral condyles of one rat in each group were dissected.

For real-time PCR analysis, the condyle heads of six rats in each group (0.5 mg MIA for 2 weeks or control) were dissected. Bilateral condyle heads of each rat were pooled for sufficient RNA extraction owing to the difficulty of isolating and acquiring enough cartilage from the small condylar head of rat and the reason that both the cartilage and subchondral bone were affected by MIA.

Scanning Electron Microscopy (SEM) and Transmission Electron Microscopy (TEM)

TMJ discs and condylar cartilage were dissected from the rats on day 1 post-injection (n = 3/group). SEM and TEM were performed as described previously [29]. Briefly, the samples were fixed with 2.5% fluteraldehyde solution and 1% osmium tetroxide (Sigma). For SEM, the disc section was produced by tearing through the intermediate zone. For TEM, the intermediate zone of the disc or condylar cartilage was embedded in epoxy resin. Ultrathin sections (100 nm) were stained with lead citrate and uranyl acetate.

Histopathologic Staining

Paraffin-embedded TMJ blocs were sagittally cut in serial sections at a 5-µm thickness. Sections were stained with hematoxylin and eosin (HE) for routine histological evaluation. Safranin O-fast green (S.O) and Toluidine blue (TB) stains were used to evaluate proteoglycans in the cartilage matrix [18].

MicroCT Examination

Radiographs of condyles were obtained with a high-resolution MicroCT system (Inveon, Siemens, Germany). The specimens were scanned at 60 kV, 300 µA, and 8.5 µm-effective pixel size. The images were analyzed using software provided by the manufacturer. All sagittal images were captured using the same parameters: Ct = −550; W = 550.

Real-time PCR

Total RNA was isolated from the condylar heads containing cartilage and subchondral bone using TRIzol reagent (Invitrogen, Carlsbad, USA) according to the manufacturer' s instructions. The condylar heads were ground into powder in liquid nitrogen using a cryogenic grinder (6770 Freezer/Mill, SPEX SamplePrep, NJ, USA). Reverse transcription were performed with an iScript cDNA synthesis kit (Bio-Rad) in 20 µl reaction volume containing 1 µg of total RNA as described previously [27,30]. Real-time PCR was performed with Power SYBR Green PCR Master Mix (Applied Biosystems) using a 7500 real-time PCR System (Applied Biosystems). The amplification specificity was confirmed by melting curve. The sequences of primers for rat β-actin [31], Collagen I and Aggrecan [32], Collagen II [33], ADAMTS5 (aggrecanase-2) [34], Tissue Inhibitors of Metalloproteinase (TIMP)2 [35], TNFα [36], Bax, Fas, FasL, Caspase2, Caspase3,

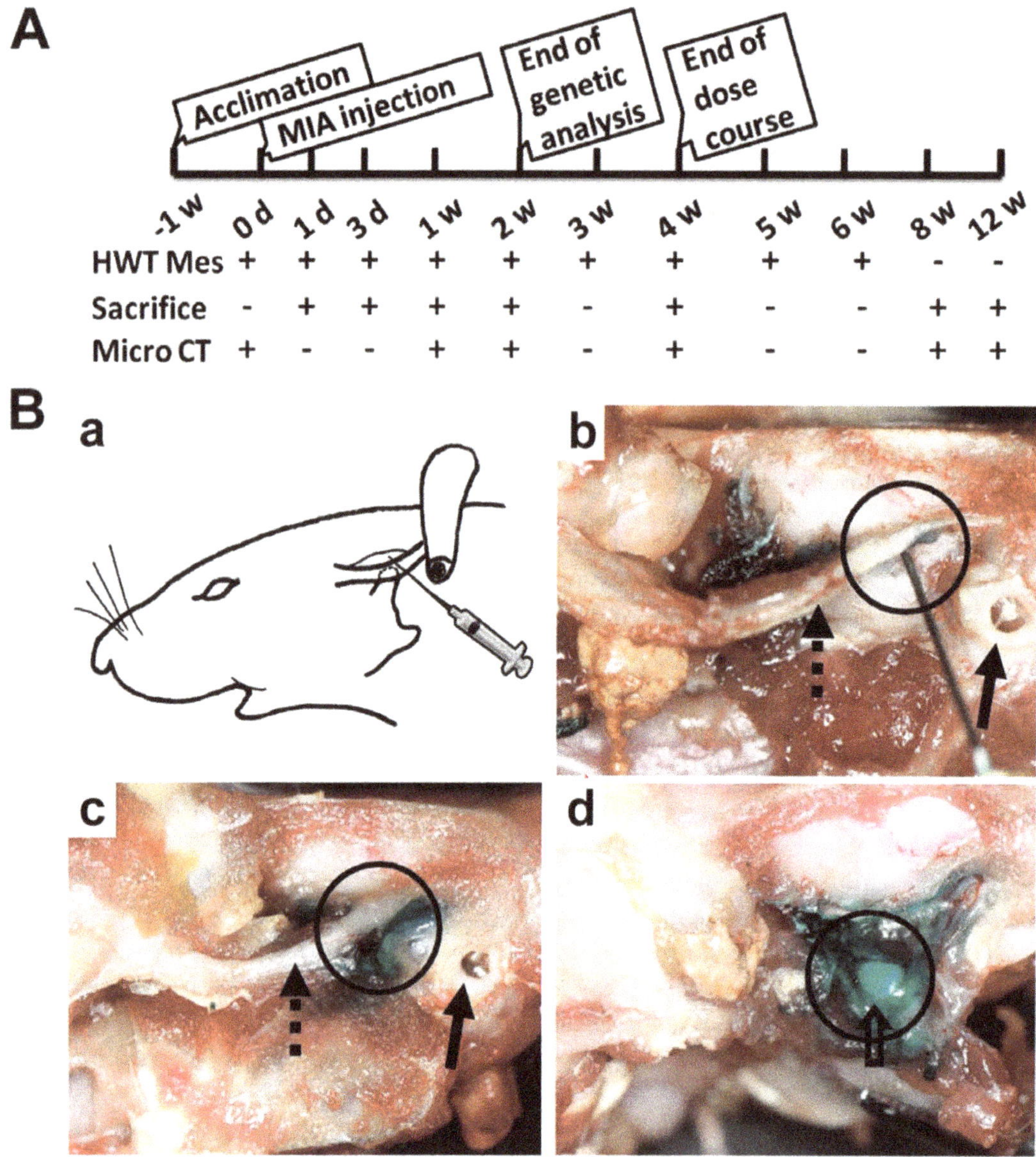

Figure 1. Outline of experimental design and confirmation of injection site into upper compartment of rat TMJ. A: Outline of experimental design. B: Photograph of dye (fast green solution) injection into the upper compartment of the left TMJ. (a). Needle insertion was 5 mm anterior to the external auditory canal. (b). Dissection showed that the needle was right under the root of the zygoma (dotted arrow), anterior of the external auditory canal (arrow), stopped at the temporal fossa, and was located in the upper compartment (black circle). (c). 50 μL dye was injected. (d). Opening the capsule revealed that the dye was restricted to the upper compartment of the TMJ (disc and condyle: hollow arrow).

Caspase8, and Caspase9 [37], and alfa-smooth muscle actin (α-SMA) [38] were all previously described and their efficiency was confirmed by sequencing their conventional PCR products. The primers for rat Matrix Metalloproteinase (MMP)3 (sense: 5′-ACCTATTCCTGGTTGCTG-3′; anti-sense: 5′-GGTCTGTGGAGGACTTGTA-3′), MMP13 (sense: 5′-CTGACCTGG- GATTTCCAAAA-3′; anti-sense: 5′-ACACGTGGTTCCCTGAGAAG-3′), TIMP1 (sense: 5′-CCTCTGGCATCCTCTTGT-3′; anti-sense: 5′-TTGATCT-CATAACGC- TGGT-3′), and Proliferating Cell Nuclear Antigen (PCNA) (sense: 5′-CCAGGG- CTCCATCCTGAA-3′; anti-sense: 5′-CCCAGCAGGCCTCATTGAT-3′) were designed with Primer Premier Version 5.0 software and their efficiency was confirmed by sequencing their conventional PCR products.

Terminal Deoxynucleotidyl Transferase dUTP nick end Labeling (TUNEL) Assay

Apoptosis was examined *in situ* using a TUNEL assay according to the manufacturer's instructions (Roche, Mannheim, Germany). Briefly, sections were deparaffinized, rehydrated, pretreated with protease K (10 μg/ml, Sigma) for 20 min, and blocked with 3% bovine serum albumin for 20 min at room temperature. The sections were incubated with TUNEL reaction mixture for 1 h at 37°C and covered with fluorescence mounting medium (Zhongshan-Golden-Bridge-Biotechnology, Beijing). Confocal microscopic images were acquired using a Zeiss laser-scanning microscope (LSM 510).

Immunohistochemical (IHC) Staining

IHC staining was performed with a two-step detection kit (Zhongshan-Golden-Bridge-Biotechnology) as described previously [27]. The primary antibodies were MMP3 (Abcam, 1:100 dilution), caspase3 (Cell Signaling Technology, 1:1000 dilution), and α-SMA (Abcam 1:100 dilution).

Statistical Analysis

Statistical analysis was performed using SPSS version 11.0 for Windows. All data were presented as mean ± SEM. Following confirmation of normal data distribution, all data between the experimental and control groups were analyzed using Student's t tests with P values <0.05 considered to be statistically significant.

Results

Confirmation of Injection into Upper Compartment

To confirm the injection site in the upper compartment of the TMJ, one rat was preliminarily dissected after injection of fast green solution into the upper compartment. The needle was inserted right under the root of the zygoma, beneath the temporal fossa into the upper compartment. The green stained region was mainly limited to the upper compartment (Fig. 1B).

Ultrastructural Changes in Disc

To determine whether MIA injected into the upper compartment of the TMJ could diffuse into the lower compartment, the ultrastructure of the TMJ disc was evaluated by SEM and TEM 1 day after injection of MIA or saline (Fig. 2). SEM showed that the surface of the disc in the control group was furrowed and covered by an evenly distributed gelatinous layer, whereas the intermediate zone of the disc in the MIA group lost these features and presented a limited region with a thinner and smooth surface surrounded by areas with a rough and uneven surface. From the section view of the intermediate zone, disc cells in the control group inserted into the collagen fibrils, whereas the disc cells in the MIA group were crimpled and rounded, detached from the surrounding collagen fibrils (Fig. 2A).

TEM showed that the disc cells of the intermediate zone in the control group were surrounded by a dense, collagenous extracellular matrix (ECM) and the cell junction was tight, with ovoid-shaped mitochondria around the nucleus. However, the disc cells in the MIA group underwent morphological changes, including cell shrinkage, condensation of the cytoplasm and nucleus, cell membrane detachment from the surrounding collagen fibrils, and loosened cell junctions accompanied by the disrupted ECM. Some cells even presented features of apoptosis, such as chromatin compaction, swelling mitochondria, and vacuolar degeneration (Fig. 2B).

Dose-dependent Histopathologic Changes in TMJ

To understand the effects of MIA on the TMJ, the morphology of the TMJ was examined for 4 weeks after injection with saline or increasing doses of MIA (Fig. 3A). In the control TMJ, HE staining showed that the condylar cartilage was a regular alignment of multilayer chondrocytes. S.O and TB staining showed that the hypertrophic layer was stained red and metachromatically purple, respectively, indicating abundant proteoglycans in the condylar cartilage. In the 0.05 mg MIA group, HE staining showed that the condylar cartilage was slightly decreased in cell number and thickness as compared with the control. S.O and TB staining showed slight decreases in cartilage proteoglycans. In the 0.1 mg MIA group, discontinuousness of the hypertrophic layer with peripheral cartilage thickening was observed. However, in the 0.5 mg group, HE staining showed severe discontinuity of the four-layer cartilage, regional loss of chondrocytes, peripheral proliferation and clustering of chondrocytes, a disorganized matrix network, horizontal clefts, and subchondral bone resorption with adjacent bone marrow filled with fibroblast-like cells. TB and S.O staining showed severe loss of staining in irregularly arranged chondrocytes and enhanced staining at the periphery. In the 1 mg and 2 mg MIA groups, complete loss of chondrocytes, severe thinning of cartilage, and subchondral bone erosion were evident in the lesion, but without peripheral clustering of chondrocytes and thickening of the cartilage. Typical OA-like destruction of the cartilage and erosion of the subchondral bone were observed in the 0.5 mg MIA group [39]. Therefore, 0.5 mg was defined as the minimum effective dose of MIA for induction of typical OA-like lesions in the rat TMJ.

Time-dependent Histopathologic Changes in TMJ

To further characterize the development of OA, the major structures of the TMJ were evaluated after injection of 0.5 mg MIA at different time points for up to 12 weeks (Fig. 3B, C).

With regard to the condyle, chondrocytes disappeared following MIA induction and the matrix was less stained within the proliferative zone in the anterior and central areas of the condyle corresponding to the load-bearing region. Additionally, scattered cells with nuclear condensation were evident after 3 days. Loss of chondrocytes in all of the cartilage layers with no matrix staining was observed by 1 week. In addition to the above features, regional osteolysis and peripheral chondrocyte proliferation with deep matrix staining were observed by 2 weeks. By 4 weeks, typical OA-like lesions were observed, as described for the 0.5 mg MIA group in the dose course. By 8 weeks, fibrosis in the lesions was evident and the subchondral bone was developing sclerosis. By 12 weeks, the condylar lesions were fully repaired by sclerotic subchondral bone and thin cartilage with disorganized chondrocytes. These changes over the 12-week period were not due to aging effects when compared with the control group. (Fig. 3B).

Time-dependent changes, including synovitis, disc thinning, and the destruction of temporal fossa cartilage following MIA induction, are shown in Fig. 3C. Massive fibrin-like exudates were observed in the upper compartments of TMJs in the experimental group by 3 days to 1 week after MIA injection, but not in the control group. Abundant proliferative villi consisting of multi-layer synovial lining cells and apparent infiltrated mononucleated cells were present in the upper compartment by 2 weeks. The synovial villi decreased and became smaller by 4 weeks and nearly disappeared by 12 weeks. Chondrocytes were almost lost in the cartilage of the temporal fossa and intermediate zone of the disc by 3 days after MIA injection. Until 2 weeks,there were almost no further changes in the disc and temporal fossa. From 4 weeks to 12 weeks, the disc and the cartilage of the temporal fossa became thinner, but the subchondral bone of the temporal fossa remained intact and no disc perforation was observed.

Radiographic Changes in Subchondral Bone

To fully understand the changes in the subchondral bone after MIA-injection (0.5 mg/joint), radiographic changes in the condyle were evaluated by MicroCT scanning (Fig. 4A). On sagittal images, the bone surface of the control condyle was smooth and continuous, whereas the bone surface of the anterior and central areas of the condyle was discontinuous by 1 week after MIA injection. Multi-erosions, characterized by translucency disrupting the bone surface of the load bearing areas, grew deeper and more extensive with obvious defects from 2 to 4 weeks. By 8 weeks, the

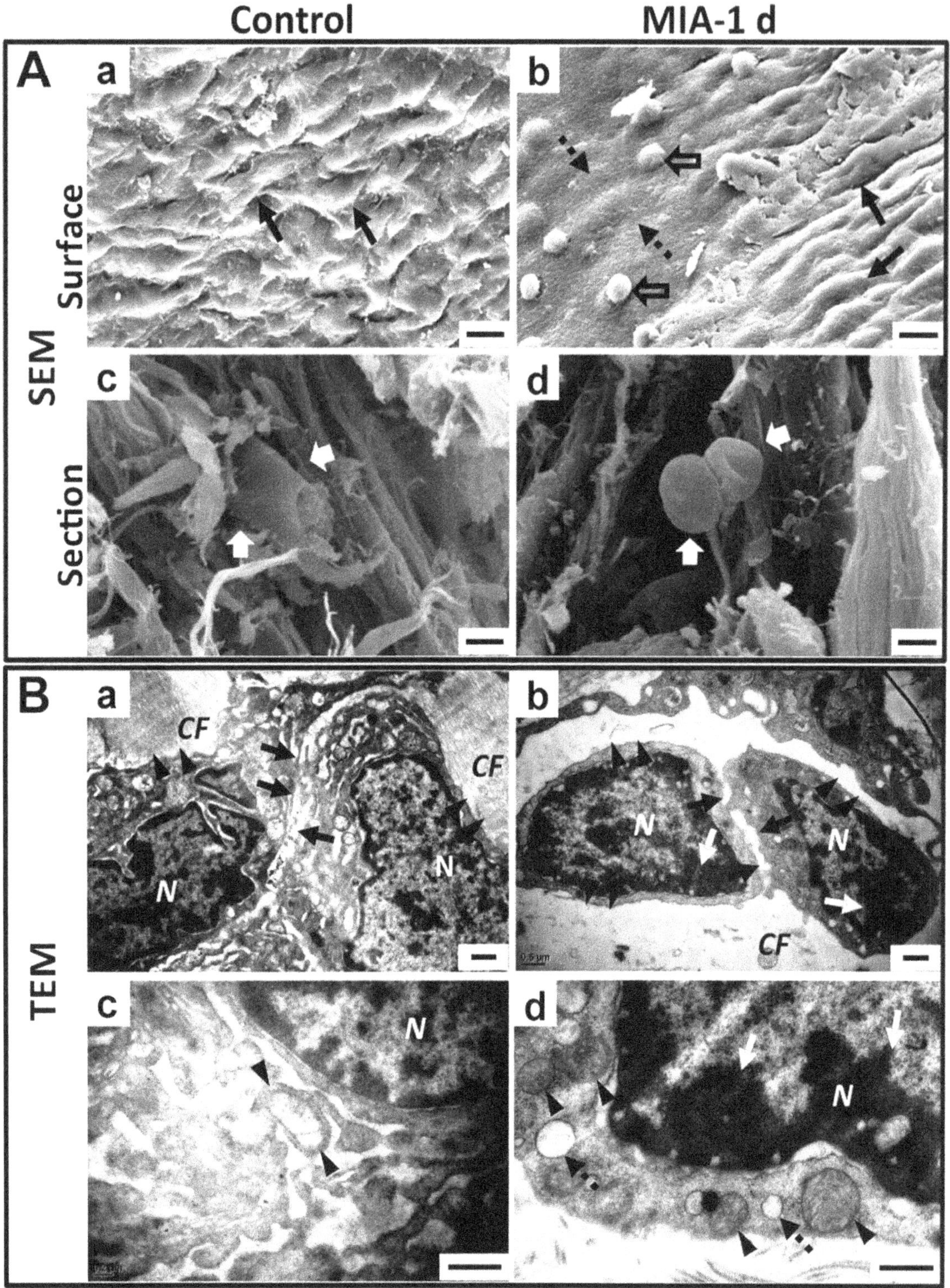

Figure 2. Ultrastructural changes in disc 1 day after MIA injection into upper compartment of TMJ. A. SEM view of the disc. (a). The furrowed surface (arrow) of the control joint. (b). The surface 1 day after MIA treatment, showing regional flattening in the intermediate zone (dotted arrow) with residual gelatin condensed to a mass (hollow arrow), surrounded by an area with a rough and uneven surface (arrow). (c). Section view of the control disc showed the disc cells studded in the collagen fibrils (white arrow). (d). Section view of the disc of the MIA-treated group showed that disc cells were crimpled and detached from the collagen fibrils (white arrow). B. TEM view of the intermediate zone of the disc. (a). Cells in the control disc were closely attached to the collagen fibrils (arrowhead) and cell junctions were tight (arrow). (b). The cells in the MIA-treated disc were shrunken with condensed chromatin (white arrow), detached from the disrupted ECM (arrowhead), and had loose cell junctions (arrow). (c). Mitochondria were regularly tubular-shaped (arrow) around the nuclei in the control disc. (d). Chromatin compaction (white arrow), swollen mitochondria (arrowhead), and vacuolar degeneration (dotted arrow) were observed in the disc cells 1 day after MIA treatment. (CF: collagen fibers; N: nucleus; Bar = 50 μm in A-a, b; Bar = 20 μm in A-c, d; Bar = 0.5 μm in B).

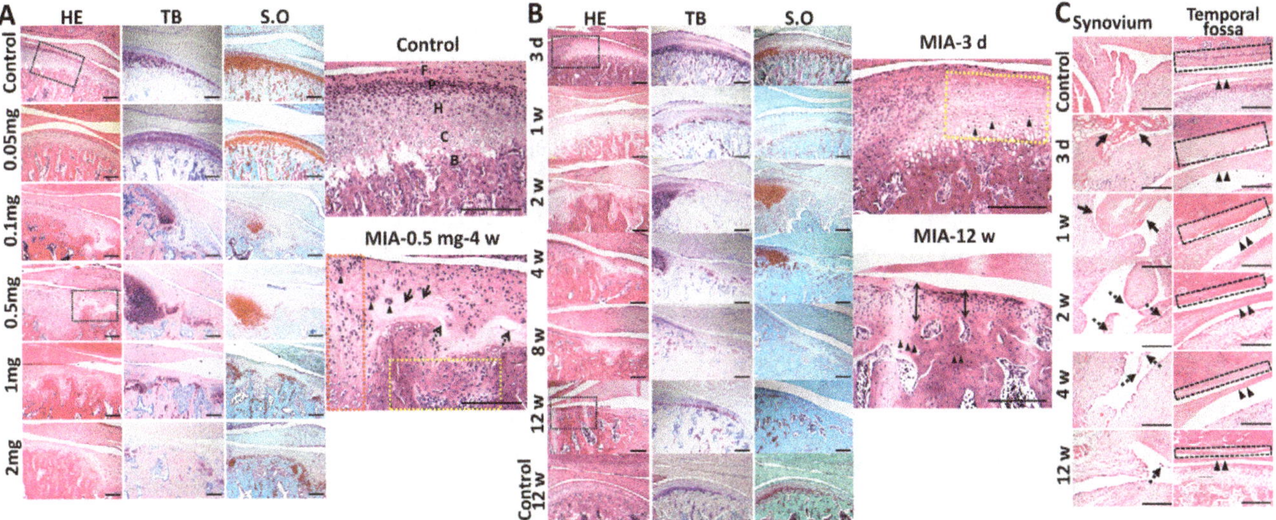

Figure 3. Dose- and time-dependent histopathologic changes in TMJ tissues. TMJ was sectioned in saggital for HE, TB and S.O staining. A. Dose course (0.05 mg, 0.1 mg, 0.5 mg, 1 mg, 2mg per joint) of MIA 4 weeks post-injection. Black frames are magnified. Condylar cartilage in the controls stained purple blue by TB and red by S.O; (F: fibrous layer; P: proliferative layer; H: hypertrophy layer; C: calcified layer; B: subchondral bone.). Typical OA-like lesion induced by 0.5 mg MIA, including regional loss of chondrocytes (arrow), chondrocyte cluster formation (arrowhead), horizontal cleft (dotted arrow), peripheral chondrocyte proliferation (red frame), and subchondral bone erosion with adjacent bone marrow full of fibroblast-like cells (yellow frame). Lesions staining by TB and S.O was uneven. (Bar = 200 μm) B. Time-dependent changes in the condyle following MIA injection (0.5 mg/joint; 3 days to 12 weeks). Black frames were magnified. After three days, chondrocytes in the anterior and central areas of the cartilage were lightly stained with nuclear condensation (arrowhead). At 12 weeks, thin cartilage (double arrow) and sclerotic subchondral bone (arrowhead) replaced the lesion. (Bar = 200 μm) C. Time-dependent changes in the synovium, disc, and temporal fossa following MIA injection. Time-dependent changes in synovitis (fibrin-like exudates: arrow; proliferative villi of the synovium: dotted arrow), hypo-cellular change and thinning of the disc (arrowhead), and destruction of temporal fossa cartilage (black frame) following MIA induction are shown. (Bar = 300 μm).

bone surrounding the lesion became sclerotic. By 12 weeks, the lesion was replaced with smooth but sclerotic bone. Osteophytes began to present from 4 weeks until 12 weeks after MIA injection.

Hyperalgesia of TMJ after Induction of TMJOA

To understand the relationship between the nociceptive response and histopathological changes, the HWT was measured at different time points after MIA injection (0.5 mg/joint). (Fig. 4B). The HWT significantly decreased 24 h after MIA injection ($P<0.01$), remained at a decreased level until 3 weeks ($P<0.05$), but then gradually recovered to baseline by 4 weeks, as compared with the control group.

Induction of Condylar Chondrocyte Apoptosis

To understand the mechanism underlying MIA-induced chondrocyte loss in the condylar cartilage, TEM examinations and a TUNEL assay were performed following MIA injection (0.5 mg/joint). TEM showed that the chondrocytes in the control group were polygonal with abundant mitochondria and endoplasmic reticulum, whereas chondrocytes in the group treated with MIA showed typical apoptotic features, including cell shrinkage, nuclear condensation, vacuolar degeneration, and apoptotic bodies, after 1 day (Fig. 5A). Three days after MIA injection, TUNEL-positive chondrocytes were observed diffusely in the area corresponding to the region with HE unstained nuclei, but not in the control group. However, 1 week after MIA injection, the TUNEL positive chondrocytes almost disappeared in the same region due to the extreme loss of chondrocytes as shown by HE staining (Fig. 5B).

Expression of Metabolism and Apoptosis Related Genes of Condyle after MIA Injection

To further understand the molecular events underlying condylar destruction following MIA induction (0.5 mg/joint), the expressions of genes related to the metabolism of cartilage and bone and apoptosis were examined from the condylar head contain both cartilage and subchondral bone by real-time PCR and IHC 2 weeks after MIA injection. As compared with the control group, mRNA expression of main matrix components, including aggrecan and collagen I and II, were significantly downregulated. However, mRNA expression of the matrix degrading proteases MMP3, MMP13, and ADAMTS5 were significantly upregulated in the MIA group. In contrast, TIMP2, but not TIMP1, was correspondingly downregulated (Fig. 6A). MIA induction resulted in a significant increase in the expression of the proapoptotic genes of the death receptor family, such as Fas, FasL, caspase8, caspase3, and BAX, but not caspase2 and caspase9 (Fig. 6B). PCNA and α-SMA, markers of proliferation and fibrosis [40,41], respectively, were also upregulated in the MIA group (Fig. 6B). Moreover, IHC showed that MMP3 was mainly expressed in the hypertrophic layer in the control cartilage, but diffuse staining of MMP3 was observed in the chondrocytes adjacent to the lesion. Stronger staining of caspase3 was observed diffusely in the proliferative and hypertrophic layers adjacent to the lesion as compared with the control group. Expression of α-SMA was mainly in the hypertrophic chondrocytes in the control group, whereas it was enhanced in the chondrocytes of the proliferative and hypertrophic layers adjacent to the OA-like lesion by 4 weeks after MIA injection (Fig. 6C).

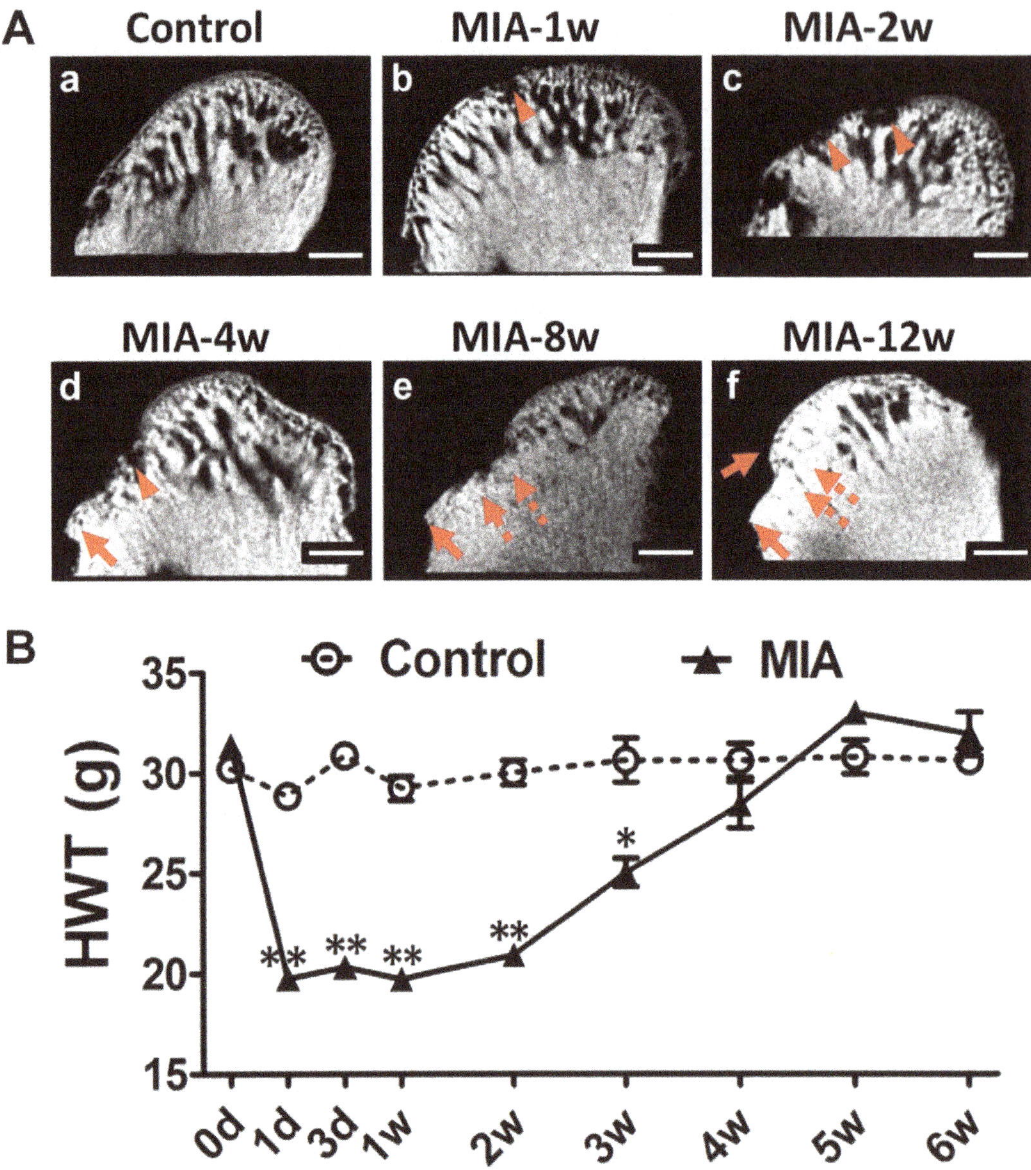

Figure 4. Time-dependent radiographic changes in condylar subchondral bone and nociceptive responses following MIA injection (0.5 mg/joint). A. Representative images of the condyle by MicroCT scanning with a sagittal section view demonstrated. (a). Control condyle showed intact subchondral bone with a smooth, continuous surface. (b). Regional loss of surface bone (arrowhead) occurred in the frontal bevel of the condyle by 1 week. (c). Multiple erosions of subchondral bone (arrowhead) were observed by 2 weeks. (d). Erosion in the subchondral bone grew deeper and was much more extensive with obvious defects (arrowhead) and osteophyte formation (arrow) by 4 weeks. (e and f). Sclerotic changes (dotted arrow) and osteophytes (arrow) were evident by 8 weeks and 12 weeks. (Bar = 300 μm) B. Changes in animal nociceptive response after MIA injection into TMJ. The HWT was significantly decreased in the first 3 weeks after MIA injection, but gradually recovered to control levels from 4 weeks post-injection. All data were presented as mean ± SEM. (n = 3; $^{**}P<0.01$; $^{*}P<0.05$).

Discussion

In this study, we provided multi-level data to show that a comprehensive rat model of TMJOA could be successfully established through MIA injection into the upper compartment of the TMJ. First, electron microscopy showed that the intermediate zone of the disc loosened to facilitate the diffusion of MIA into the lower compartment. Second, histopathologic analysis illustrated that typical OA-like lesions in the TMJ, including degenerative changes in the condyle, disc, and temporal fossa, as well as synovitis, were induced by MIA in a dose- and time-dependent manner. Third, subchondral bone destruction, which is characteristic of the early stage of OA, and sclerosis, which is seen during the later stage of OA, were observed by MicroCT scanning. Fourth, the molecular analysis revealed that chondrocytic apoptosis and the imbalance between the anabolism and catabolism of cartilage and subchondral bone might account for the advanced condylar destruction following MIA induction. Fifth, nociceptive responses increased in the early stages corresponding to the presence of synovitis. To the best of our knowledge, this is the first report to demonstrate that MIA can effectively induce typical OA-like lesions in the TMJ of a rodent species.

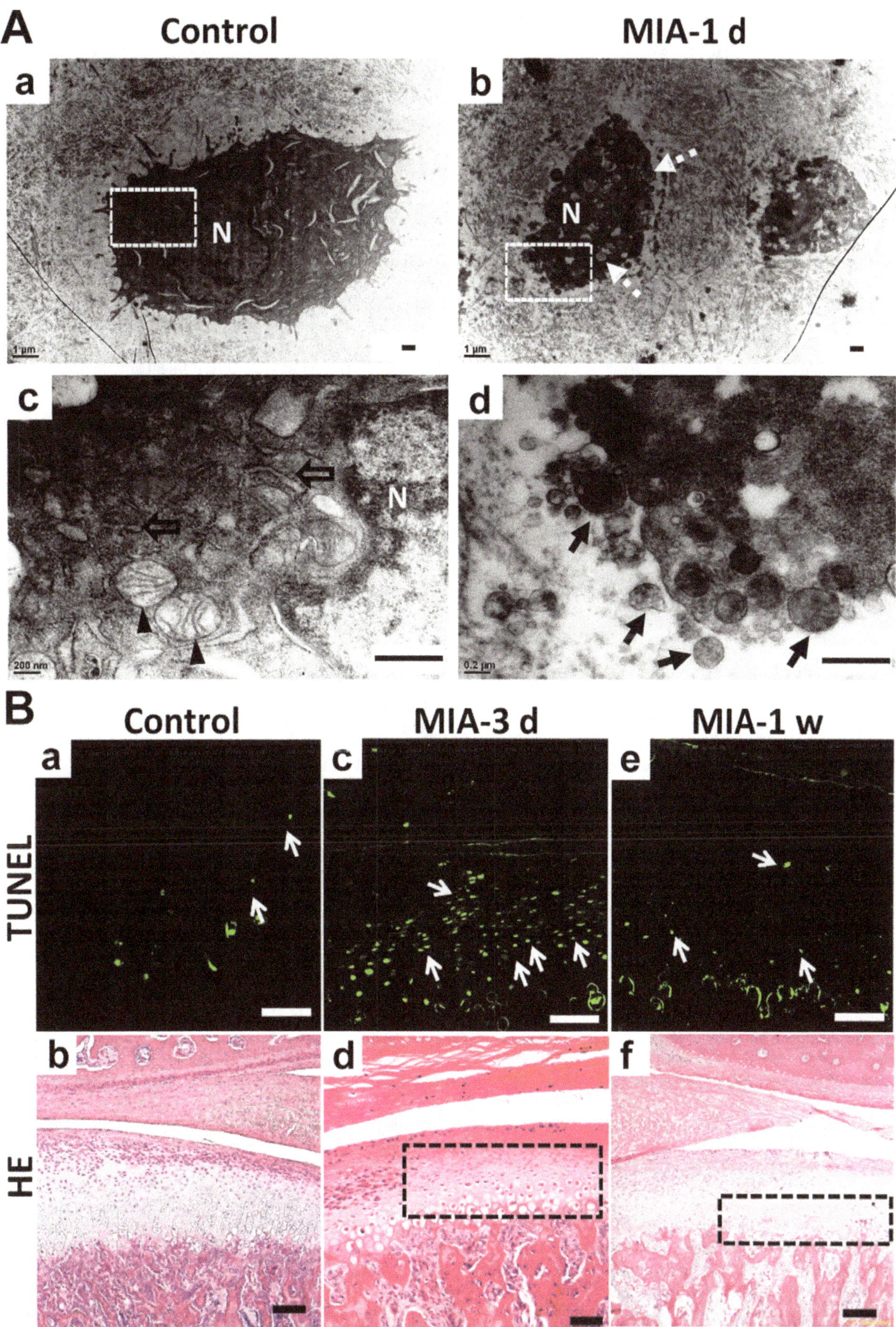
A
Control
MIA-1 d
a
b
c
d
N
1 µm
200 nm
0.2 µm
B
Control
MIA-3 d
MIA-1 w
TUNEL
HE
e
f

Figure 5. Apoptosis of chondrocytes in condyle after MIA treatment. A. TEM view of condylar chondrocytes. (a). The chondrocytes in the control group were polygonal. (b). Chondrocytes treated by MIA were shrunken with vacuolar degeneration after 1 day (dotted arrow). (c). Magnified photograph of the white frame in (a). Abundant mitochondria (arrowhead) and endoplasmic reticulum (hollow arrow) were observed around the nuclei (N) in the control chondrocyte. (d). Magnified photograph of the white frame in (b). Apoptotic bodies (black arrow) were observed in the chondrocyte following MIA induction. (Bar = 0.5 μm) B. Comparison of TUNEL assay and HE staining results. (a) There were few apoptotic chondrocytes (arrow) in the control group and the corresponding HE staining shown in (b). (c). Diffuse apoptotic chondrocytes were observed in the region corresponding to the lightly stained area with nuclear condensation of HE staining (black frame in d) at 3 days post-MIA injection. The TUNEL positive chondrocytes almost disappeared (e) due to the extreme loss of chondrocytes as shown by HE staining (black frame in f) at 1 week. (Bar = 80 μm).

The histopathologic features of MIA-induced lesions in the rat TMJ were similar to that of TMJOA. The present study revealed a typical time- and dose-dependent degeneration of TMJ tissues, showing the progress of cartilage degradation, erosion, osteophyte formation, and sclerosis in the subchondral bone, synovitis, and thinning in the disc and temporal surface. The current results are similar to the previous description of TMJOA [2]. The lesions were specifically limited to the load-bearing areas of the condyle. Although MIA was injected into the upper compartment and should have a more direct action on the surface of the temporal fossa than on the condyle, the destruction of condylar cartilage and subchondral bone was more severe than that of the temporal fossa. This feature is similar to the clinical and experimental observations that the condyle is active and undergoes greater destruction and remodeling [42,43,44]. Interestingly, the disc did not prevent MIA from penetrating into the lower compartment. In as little as 24 h the disc cells underwent apoptotic changes, such as cell body shrinkage and mitochondrial breakage, accompanied by disruptive ECM and loosened junctions between cells and between cells and the ECM. These changes facilitated the penetration of MIA through the disc to the lower compartment after injection into the upper compartment.

The radiographic findings of MIA-induced lesions in the rat TMJ were similar to that of TMJOA. The typical clinical radiographic findings for the condyle are erosion, sclerosis, and osteophytes [3]. All of these features could also be observed with MicroCT in our MIA-induced rat TMJOA model. Moreover, the radiographic features of our TMJOA model corresponded well to the histopathologic changes. Therefore, this MIA model provides detailed histopathologic changes for the corresponding radiographic changes. In addition, this model can also be used for in vivo radiographic analysis of subchondral bone to understand the pathogenesis of TMJOA, as it already known for knee OA [17].

Nociceptive responses of MIA-induced TMJOA corresponded to the observed histopathologic changes. Pain is one of the predominant clinical features of OA and it may arise from the soft tissues around the joint or the subchondral bone undergoing destruction [45]. Therefore, a successful animal model of OA should have appropriate nociceptive responses corresponding to its histopathologic changes. The HWT is usually used evaluating TMJ nociceptive responses and is inversely associated with TMJ inflammation and pain [26]. We observed that TMJ hyperalgesia corresponded to the observed histological and radiographic changes in the MIA-induced TMJOA. Specifically, the hyperalgesia of TMJ in the first week after MIA injection could be mainly inflammatory response, whereas in the 2–4 weeks after MIA injection, the hyperalgesia could well correspond to the subsequent pronounced destruction of condylar cartilage and subchondral bone erosion. When the synovitis was alleviated and cartilage damage was repaired by fibrous tissue and the subchondral bone underwent a sclerotic change, the nociceptive responses correspondingly returned to baseline. This was consistent with known clinical features. For example, patients often experience severe pain during the active destructive phase of TMJOA with synovitis [46] and feel alleviation over time [47,48]. However, the hyperalgesia in our TMJOA model recovered to the control level within 6 weeks, whereas last-long hyperalgesia was observed in the MIA-induced knee joint OA model [49]. Although the reasons for this difference are unknown, it might be related to the difference in the degree of cartilage damage induced by MIA in different joints, since the same dose of MIA induces more severe cartilage loss in the knee joint than in the TMJ [49]. It might also be related to the properties of the different types of cartilage, i.e., the TMJ is covered with fibrocartilage and the knee joint with hyaline cartilage. Since the hyperalgesia of the TMJ correspondingly reflected the degree of lesions induced by MIA, our results also suggested that MIA-induced TMJOA can be used for evaluating osteoarthritic pain in the TMJ.

MIA induced TMJOA through chondrocyte apoptosis and the disturbance of cartilage and subchondral bone metabolism. MIA could sensitively induce chondrocyte apoptosis as early as 1 day after MIA injection and condylar apoptosis reached a peak on day 3, leading to hypocellular changes in the cartilage and disc. Chondrocyte apoptosis in the early stages could be an important initiator of cartilage degeneration. Genes of the death receptor family, such as Fas and FasL, have been reported to be related to chondrocyte apoptosis [50,51,52]. Gene expression of the death receptor family and IHC staining of caspase3 further showed that the apoptotic process appeared to be caspase-dependent. This is consistent with previous studies of OA in the knee [18,22] and discectomy-induced TMJOA [53]. In addition, cartilage degeneration also results from the imbalance between anabolism and catabolism due to increased matrix degrading proteases and decreased synthesis of matrix [54]. Although the genes expression was evaluated from the condylar head containing both cartilage and subchondral bone, the results showed that the catabolic genes MMP3, MMP13, and ADAMTS5 were elevated in the condylar head, whereas the anabolic genes aggrecan and collagen I and II were decreased in the condylar head. The observed changes in gene expression were similar to previous reports of experimental OA or clinical OA [55,56]. Therefore, MIA-induced imbalances in gene expression with regard to cartilage metabolism and subchondral bone could also be an important factor contributing to condylar deterioration.

The present model of TMJOA has advantages and disadvantages. Lack of severe histopathologic changes associated with TMJOA, such as vertical splitting in the cartilage, exposure of subchondral bone, and disc perforation, could be one of the disadvantages for MIA-induced TMJOA model. In contrast, advantages include the signs of reconstruction, including hypertrophic reactions in the cartilage surrounding lesions, fibrous restoration as represented by α-SMA [41] overexpression in the proliferative cells, and hypertrophy of the chondrocyte layer at 4 weeks post-MIA injection. In addition, sclerosis of subchondral bone and osteophyte formation were observed in the later stages, which mimics the typical clinical features [42]. Lesion repair following MIA injection was also reported in a rabbit model [13,23]. TMJOA is a self-limiting disease and reconstruction plays

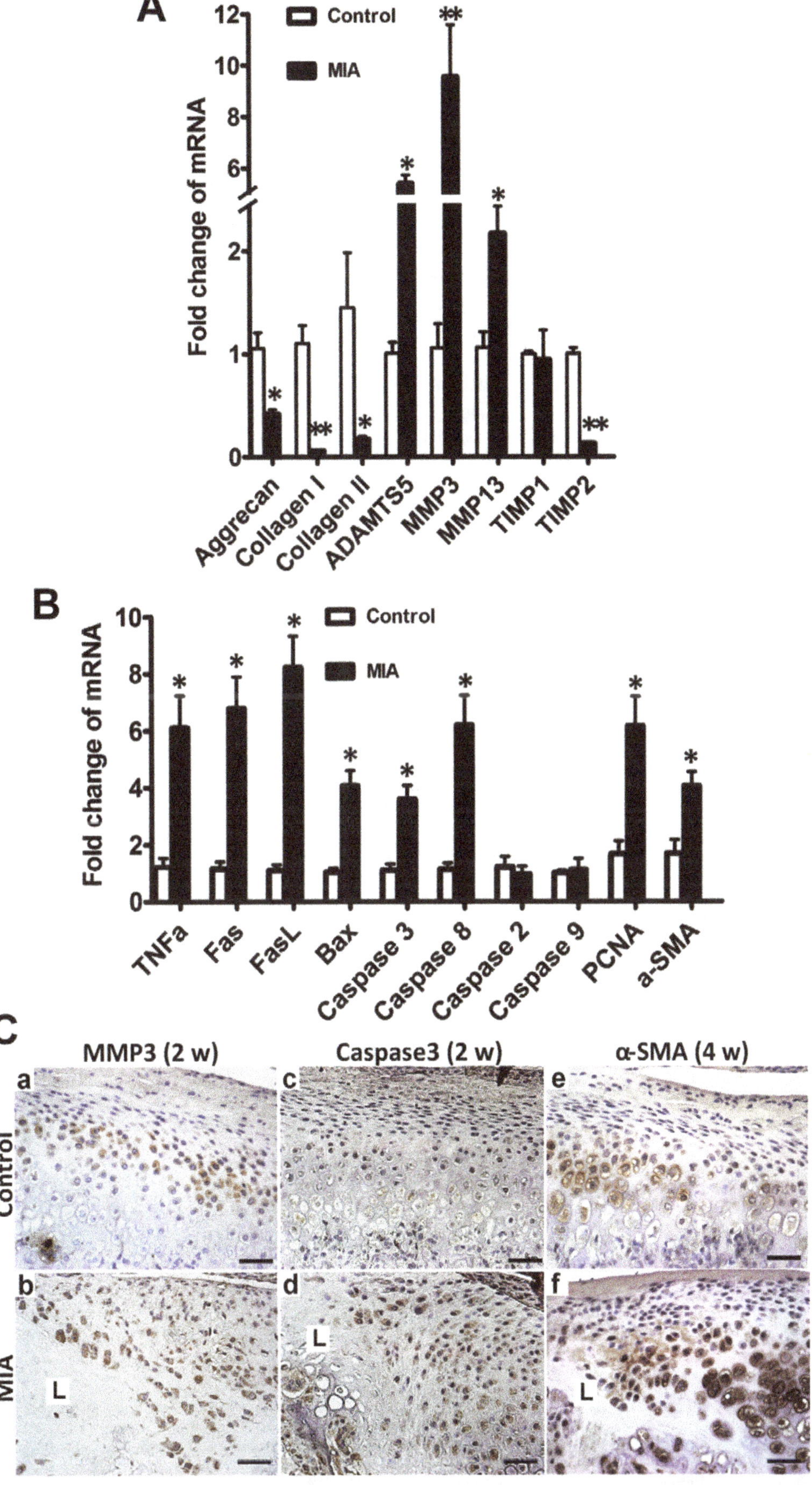
A
Control
MIA
Fold change of mRNA
Aggrecan
Collagen I
Collagen II
ADAMTS5
MMP3
MMP13
TIMP1
TIMP2
B
Control
MIA
Fold change of mRNA
TNFa
Fas
FasL
Bax
Caspase 3
Caspase 8
Caspase 2
Caspase 9
PCNA
a-SMA
C
MMP3 (2 w)
Caspase3 (2 w)
α-SMA (4 w)
Control
MIA
a
b
c
d
e
f
L

Figure 6. Changes in gene and protein expression in condyle following MIA injection were evaluated by real-time PCR and IHC, respectively. A. Two weeks after MIA injection, anabolism-associated aggrecan and collagen I and II were downregulated compared with the control group. Catabolism-associated MMP3, MMP13, and ADAMTS5 were upregulated and TIMP2, but not TIMP1, was correspondingly downregulated. B. Two weeks after MIA (0.5 mg) injection, apoptosis-associated genes of the death receptor family, such as, TNFα, Fas, FasL, caspase8, caspase3, and BAX, but not caspase2 and caspase9, were significantly elevated in the MIA injection group; PCNA and α-SMA, representing proliferation and fibrous restoration, respectively, were upregulated (mean ± SEM; n = 6; $^{**}P<0.01$; $^{*}P<0.05$). C. There were very few chondrocytes left in the lesion labeled as L 2 weeks after MIA (0.5 mg) injection. MMP3 was mainly expressed in the hypertrophic layer in the control cartilage (a). Diffuse staining of MMP3 was observed in the chondrocytes adjacent to the lesion (L) at 2 weeks (b). Caspase3 was rarely expressed in the control cartilage (c). Enhanced staining of caspase3 was observed in the proliferative and hypertrophic layers adjacent to the lesion (L) at 2 weeks (d). Expression of α-SMA was mainly in the hypertrophic chondrocytes in the control group (e). Stronger staining of α-SMA was observed adjacent to the lesion (L) at 4 weeks (f). (Bar = 40 μm).

an important role [2]. However, reconstruction is rarely seen in TMJOA models induced by methods other than MIA. Although several animal models of TMJOA have been established, our multi-level data suggest that the present rat model accurately mimicked most of the clinical features of TMJOA.

In conclusion, the present study demonstrated a reliable and simple rat model of TMJOA induced by intra-articular injection of MIA into the upper compartment. The histopathologic, radiographic, behavioral, and molecular changes of this model will help us to understand the progression of TMJOA and to facilitate future TMJOA-associated researches.

Acknowledgments

We would like to thank Professor Yan Gao for the assistance with histopathologic evaluation.

Author Contributions

Conceived and designed the experiments: XDW XXK YHG YHZ. Performed the experiments: XDW XXK MMZ DQH ZM RYB YL JNZ. Analyzed the data: XDW XXK YHG YHZ. Contributed reagents/ materials/analysis tools: XDW XXK YHG YHZ. Wrote the paper: XDW YHG YHZ.

References

1. Dworkin SF, LeResche L (1992) Research diagnostic criteria for temporomandibular disorders: review, criteria, examinations and specifications, critique. J Craniomandib Disord 6: 301–355.
2. Zarb GA, Carlsson GE (1999) Temporomandibular disorders: osteoarthritis. J Orofac Pain 13: 295–306.
3. Israel HA, Diamond B, Saed-Nejad F, Ratcliffe A (1998) Osteoarthritis and synovitis as major pathoses of the temporomandibular joint: comparison of clinical diagnosis with arthroscopic morphology. J Oral Maxillofac Surg 56: 1023–1027; discussion 1028.
4. Stegenga B, de Bont LG, Boering G (1989) Osteoarthrosis as the cause of craniomandibular pain and dysfunction: a unifying concept. J Oral Maxillofac Surg 47: 249–256.
5. Karsdal MA, Leeming DJ, Dam EB, Henriksen K, Alexandersen P, et al. (2008) Should subchondral bone turnover be targeted when treating osteoarthritis? Osteoarthritis Cartilage 16: 638–646.
6. Stegenga B (2001) Osteoarthritis of the temporomandibular joint organ and its relationship to disc displacement. J Orofac Pain 15: 193–205.
7. Imirzalioglu P, Uckan S, Guler N, Haberal A, Uckan D (2009) Synovial apoptosis in temporomandibular joint disc displacement without reduction. Oral Surg Oral Med Oral Pathol Oral Radiol Endod 108: 693–698.
8. Aigner T, Kim HA (2002) Apoptosis and cellular vitality: issues in osteoarthritic cartilage degeneration. Arthritis Rheum 46: 1986–1996.
9. Brandt KD (2002) Animal models of osteoarthritis. Biorheology 39: 221–235.
10. Meng J, Ma X, Ma D, Xu C (2005) Microarray analysis of differential gene expression in temporomandibular joint condylar cartilage after experimentally induced osteoarthritis. Osteoarthritis Cartilage 13: 1115–1125.
11. Fujisawa T, Kuboki T, Kasai T, Sonoyama W, Kojima S, et al. (2003) A repetitive, steady mouth opening induced an osteoarthritis-like lesion in the rabbit temporomandibular joint. J Dent Res 82: 731–735.
12. Xinmin Y, Jian H (2005) Treatment of temporomandibular joint osteoarthritis with viscosupplementation and arthrocentesis on rabbit model. Oral Surg Oral Med Oral Pathol Oral Radiol Endod 100: e35–38.
13. Cledes G, Felizardo R, Foucart JM, Carpentier P (2006) Validation of a chemical osteoarthritis model in rabbit temporomandibular joint: a compliment to biomechanical models. Int J Oral Maxillofac Surg 35: 1026–1033.
14. Wadhwa S, Embree MC, Kilts T, Young MF, Ameye LG (2005) Accelerated osteoarthritis in the temporomandibular joint of biglycan/fibromodulin double-deficient mice. Osteoarthritis Cartilage 13: 817–827.
15. Bendele AM (2001) Animal models of osteoarthritis. J Musculoskelet Neuronal Interact 1: 363–376.
16. Schuelert N, Zhang C, Mogg AJ, Broad LM, Hepburn DL, et al. (2010) Paradoxical effects of the cannabinoid CB2 receptor agonist GW405833 on rat osteoarthritic knee joint pain. Osteoarthritis Cartilage 18: 1536–1543.
17. Mohan G, Perilli E, Kuliwaba JS, Humphries JM, Parkinson IH, et al. (2011) Application of in vivo micro-computed tomography in the temporal characterisation of subchondral bone architecture in a rat model of low-dose monosodium iodoacetate induced osteoarthritis. Arthritis Res Ther 13: R210.
18. Bar-Yehuda S, Rath-Wolfson L, Del Valle L, Ochaion A, Cohen S, et al. (2009) Induction of an antiinflammatory effect and prevention of cartilage damage in rat knee osteoarthritis by CF101 treatment. Arthritis Rheum 60: 3061–3071.
19. Guingamp C, Gegout-Pottie P, Philippe L, Terlain B, Netter P, et al. (1997) Mono-iodoacetate-induced experimental osteoarthritis: a dose-response study of loss of mobility, morphology, and biochemistry. Arthritis Rheum 40: 1670–1679.
20. Kalbhen DA (1987) Chemical model of osteoarthritis–a pharmacological evaluation. J Rheumatol 14 Spec No: 130–131.
21. Nam J, Perera P, Liu J, Rath B, Deschner J, et al. (2011) Sequential alterations in catabolic and anabolic gene expression parallel pathological changes during progression of monoiodoacetate-induced arthritis. PLoS One 6: e24320.
22. Grossin L, Cournil-Henrionnet C, Pinzano A, Gaborit N, Dumas D, et al. (2006) Gene transfer with HSP 70 in rat chondrocytes confers cytoprotection in vitro and during experimental osteoarthritis. FASEB J 20: 65–75.
23. Guler N, Kurkcu M, Duygu G, Cam B (2011) Sodium iodoacetate induced osteoarthrosis model in rabbit temporomandibular joint: CT and histological study (Part I). Int J Oral Maxillofac Surg.
24. Duygu G, Guler N, Cam B, Kurkcu M (2011) The effects of high molecular weight hyaluronic acid (Hylan G-F 20) on experimentally induced temporomandibular joint osteoartrosis: part II. Int J Oral Maxillofac Surg.
25. Li C, Zhang Y, Lv J, Shi Z (2012) Inferior or double joint spaces injection versus superior joint space injection for temporomandibular disorders: a systematic review and meta-analysis. J Oral Maxillofac Surg 70: 37–44.
26. Ren K (1999) An improved method for assessing mechanical allodynia in the rat. Physiol Behav 67: 711–716.
27. Wu YW, Bi YP, Kou XX, Xu W, Ma LQ, et al. (2010) 17-Beta-estradiol enhanced allodynia of inflammatory temporomandibular joint through upregulation of hippocampal TRPV1 in ovariectomized rats. J Neurosci 30: 8710–8719.
28. Wang XD, Kou XX, Mao JJ, Gan YH, Zhou YH (2012) Sustained Inflammation Induces Degeneration of the Temporomandibular Joint. J Dent Res.
29. Liu Y, Mai S, Li N, Yiu CK, Mao J, et al. (2011) Differences between top-down and bottom-up approaches in mineralizing thick, partially demineralized collagen scaffolds. Acta Biomater 7: 1742–1751.
30. Kou XX, Wu YW, Ding Y, Hao T, Bi RY, et al. (2011) 17beta-estradiol aggravates temporomandibular joint inflammation through the NF-kappaB pathway in ovariectomized rats. Arthritis Rheum 63: 1888–1897.
31. Tian YF, Zhang PB, Xiao XL, Zhang JS, Zhao JJ, et al. (2007) The quantification of ADAMTS expression in an animal model of cerebral ischemia using real-time PCR. Acta Anaesthesiol Scand 51: 158–164.
32. Wang XD, Kou XX, Mao JJ, Gan YH, Zhou YH (2012) Sustained inflammation induces degeneration of the temporomandibular joint. J Dent Res 91: 499–505.
33. Kinkel MD, Horton WE (2003) Coordinate down-regulation of cartilage matrix gene expression in Bcl-2 deficient chondrocytes is associated with decreased SOX9 expression and decreased mRNA stability. Journal of Cellular Biochemistry 88: 941–953.
34. Bao JP, Chen WP, Feng J, Hu PF, Shi ZL, et al. (2010) Leptin plays a catabolic role on articular cartilage. Molecular Biology Reports 37: 3265–3272.
35. Deschner J, Rath-Deschner B, Agarwal S (2006) Regulation of matrix metalloproteinase expression by dynamic tensile strain in rat fibrochondrocytes. Osteoarthritis and Cartilage 14: 264–272.

36. Rioja I, Bush KA, Buckton JB, Dickson MC, Life PF (2004) Joint cytokine quantification in two rodent arthritis models: kinetics of expression, correlation of mRNA and protein levels and response to prednisolone treatment. Clin Exp Immunol 137: 65–73.
37. Kijima K, Toyosawa K, Yasuba M, Matsuoka N, Adachi T, et al. (2004) Gene expression analysis of the rat testis after treatment with di(2-ethylhexyl) phthalate using cDNA microarray and real-time RT-PCR. Toxicology and Applied Pharmacology 200: 103–110.
38. Gao Y, Deng J, Yu XF, Yang DL, Gong QH, et al. (2011) Ginsenoside Rg1 inhibits vascular intimal hyperplasia in balloon-injured rat carotid artery by down-regulation of extracellular signal-regulated kinase 2. Journal of Ethnopharmacology 138: 472–478.
39. Dijkgraaf LC, de Bont LG, Boering G, Liem RS (1995) The structure, biochemistry, and metabolism of osteoarthritic cartilage: a review of the literature. J Oral Maxillofac Surg 53: 1182–1192.
40. Darby IA, Hewitson TD (2007) Fibroblast differentiation in wound healing and fibrosis. Int Rev Cytol 257: 143–179.
41. Lee CH, Shah B, Moioli EK, Mao JJ (2010) CTGF directs fibroblast differentiation from human mesenchymal stem/stromal cells and defines connective tissue healing in a rodent injury model. J Clin Invest 120: 3340–3349.
42. Shen G, Darendeliler MA (2005) The adaptive remodeling of condylar cartilage--a transition from chondrogenesis to osteogenesis. J Dent Res 84: 691–699.
43. Gruber HE, Gregg J (2003) Subchondral bone resorption in temporomandibular joint disorders. Cells Tissues Organs 174: 17–25.
44. Beek M, Koolstra JH, van Ruijven LJ, van Eijden TM (2001) Three-dimensional finite element analysis of the cartilaginous structures in the human temporomandibular joint. J Dent Res 80: 1913–1918.
45. Tanaka E, Detamore MS, Mercuri LG (2008) Degenerative disorders of the temporomandibular joint: etiology, diagnosis, and treatment. J Dent Res 87: 296–307.
46. Takahashi T, Nagai H, Seki H, Fukuda M (1999) Relationship between joint effusion, joint pain, and protein levels in joint lavage fluid of patients with internal derangement and osteoarthritis of the temporomandibular joint. J Oral Maxillofac Surg 57: 1187–1193; discussion 1193–1184.
47. Schmitter M, Wacker K, Pritsch M, Giannakopoulos NN, Klose C, et al. (2010) Preliminary longitudinal report on symptom outcomes in symptomatic and asymptomatic women with imaging evidence of temporomandibular joint arthritic changes. Int J Prosthodont 23: 544–551.
48. Campos MI, Campos PS, Cangussu MC, Guimaraes RC, Line SR (2008) Analysis of magnetic resonance imaging characteristics and pain in temporomandibular joints with and without degenerative changes of the condyle. Int J Oral Maxillofac Surg 37: 529–534.
49. Im HJ, Kim JS, Li X, Kotwal N, Sumner DR, et al. (2010) Alteration of sensory neurons and spinal response to an experimental osteoarthritis pain model. Arthritis Rheum 62: 2995–3005.
50. Hashimoto S, Setareh M, Ochs RL, Lotz M (1997) Fas/Fas ligand expression and induction of apoptosis in chondrocytes. Arthritis Rheum 40: 1749–1755.
51. Chagin AS, Karimian E, Zaman F, Takigawa M, Chrysis D, et al. (2007) Tamoxifen induces permanent growth arrest through selective induction of apoptosis in growth plate chondrocytes in cultured rat metatarsal bones. Bone 40: 1415–1424.
52. Nakamura T, Imai Y, Matsumoto T, Sato S, Takeuchi K, et al. (2007) Estrogen prevents bone loss via estrogen receptor alpha and induction of Fas ligand in osteoclasts. Cell 130: 811–823.
53. Kouri-Flores JB, Abbud-Lozoya KA, Roja-Morales L (2002) Kinetics of the ultrastructural changes in apoptotic chondrocytes from an osteoarthrosis rat model: a window of comparison to the cellular mechanism of apoptosis in human chondrocytes. Ultrastruct Pathol 26: 33–40.
54. Berenbaum F (2004) Signaling transduction: target in osteoarthritis. Curr Opin Rheumatol 16: 616–622.
55. Baragi VM, Becher G, Bendele AM, Biesinger R, Bluhm H, et al. (2009) A new class of potent matrix metalloproteinase 13 inhibitors for potential treatment of osteoarthritis: Evidence of histologic and clinical efficacy without musculoskeletal toxicity in rat models. Arthritis Rheum 60: 2008–2018.
56. Sandy JD, Verscharen C (2001) Analysis of aggrecan in human knee cartilage and synovial fluid indicates that aggrecanase (ADAMTS) activity is responsible for the catabolic turnover and loss of whole aggrecan whereas other protease activity is required for C-terminal processing in vivo. Biochem J 358: 615–626.

11

High Resolution T1ρ Mapping of *In Vivo* Human Knee Cartilage at 7T

Anup Singh[1,2]*, Mohammad Haris[1,3], Kejia Cai[1,4], Feliks Kogan[1], Hari Hariharan[1], Ravinder Reddy[1]

1 CMROI, Department of Radiology, University of Pennsylvania, Philadelphia, Pennsylvania, United States of America, **2** Center for Biomedical Engineering, Indian Institute of Technology Delhi, Delhi, India, **3** Research Branch, Sidra Medical and Research Center, Doha, Qatar, **4** Radiology, University of Illinois at Chicago, Chicago, Illinois, United States of America

Abstract

Purpose: Spin lattice relaxation time in rotating frame (T1ρ) mapping of human knee cartilage has shown promise in detecting biochemical changes during osteoarthritis. Due to higher field strength, MRI at 7T has advantages in term of SNR compared to clinical MR scanners and this can be used to increase in image resolution. Objective of current study was to evaluate the feasibility of high resolution T1ρ mapping of *in vivo* human knee cartilage at 7T MR scanner.

Materials and Methods: In this study we have used a T1ρ prepared GRE pulse sequence for obtaining high resolution (in plan resolution $=0.2\ mm^2$) T1ρ MRI of human knee cartilage at 7T. The effect of a global and localized reference frequency and reference voltage setting on B_0, B_1 and T1ρ maps in cartilage was evaluated. Test-retest reliability results of T1ρ values from asymptomatic subjects as well as T1ρ maps from abnormal cartilage of two human subjects are presented. These results are compared with T1ρ MRI data obtained from 3T.

Results: Our approach enabled acquisition of 3D-T1ρ data within allowed SAR limits at 7T. SNR of cartilage on T1ρ weighted images was greater than 90. Off-resonance effects present in the cartilage B_0, B_1 and T1ρ maps obtained using global shim and reference frequency and voltage setting, were reduced by the proposed localized reference frequency and voltage setting. T1ρ values of cartilage obtained with the localized approach were reproducible. Abnormal knee cartilage showed elevated T1ρ values in affected regions. T1ρ values at 7T were significantly lower ($p<0.05$) compared to those obtained at 3T.

Conclusion: In summary, by using proposed localized frequency and voltage setting approach, high-resolution 3D-T1ρ maps of *in vivo* human knee cartilage can be obtained in clinically acceptable scan times (<30 min) and SAR constraints, which provides the ability to characterize cartilage molecular integrity.

Editor: Amir A. Zadpoor, Delft University of Technology (TUDelft), Netherlands

Funding: This work was performed at an NIH-NIBIB supported Biomedical Technology Research Center (P41EB015893) and was supported by NIAMS grant NIH-R01AR45404. The funders had no role in study design, data collection and analysis, decision to publish, or preparation of the manuscript.

Competing Interests: The authors have declared that no competing interests exist.

* E-mail: anups.minhas@gmail.com

Introduction

Cartilage is a thin tissue with a thickness varying between 1 and 6 mm [1] and consists of multiple zones, particularly superficial, transitional or middle and deep zones. The superficial zone is the thinnest with a relative thickness of ~10-20% and the deep zone is thickest with a thickness of ~50–60% of the total cartilage thickness. It has been reported that Osteoarthritis (OA) starts in the superficial zone with loss of proteoglycans [2–4]. High resolution MRI is always desirable for better characterization of focal aberrations in cartilage molecular integrity. Recent anatomical imaging studies on musculoskeletal system at 7T whole body MRI scanner have already shown around two fold expected SNR advantage compared to 3T [5–7].

Spin lattice relaxation time in rotating frame (T1ρ) MRI [8] measurements have been used to explore incipient molecular changes associated with OA. Several T1ρ mapping studies of very high resolution in *ex vivo* cartilage tissue have shown exquisite cartilage classification [9–11]. T1ρ mapping has been used to characterize *in vivo* human articular cartilage at clinical MR field strengths (1.5 T and 3T) [9,12–22]. At clinical field strengths (1.5 T and 3T), planar resolution of *in vivo* 3D-T1ρ maps has been limited due to a combination of issues related to adequate SNR, appropriate RF coils and scanning time constraints.

T1ρ MRI of knee cartilage at 7T is also expected to have same SNR advantage compared to 3T and to provide better classification of cartilage regional integrity during OA. The SNR gain can be exploited for obtaining higher resolution T1ρ mapping at 7T. However, $T_{1\rho}$ MRI at 7T is challenging due to increase in specific absorption ratio (SAR) and B_0 and B_1 field inhomogeneity effects.

In this study, for the first time, we have obtained high resolution 3D-T1ρ weighted data and maps from human knee cartilage at 7T. A localized frequency and reference voltage setting approach for reducing off resonance effects is presented. The B_0 and B_1 field inhomogeneity maps of knee cartilage are obtained and SNR of human knee cartilage is computed from articular cartilage of all the subjects. Reproducibility of $T_{1\rho}$ values in cartilage of asymptomatic subjects is tested. Finally, $T_{1\rho}$ data from abnormal knee cartilage of two human subjects is presented. $T_{1\rho}$ values of articular cartilage from healthy human subjects obtained from 7T are compared with those obtained at a 3T clinical scanner. Advantages and challenges of implementing $T_{1\rho}$ mapping at 7T are outlined.

Methods and Materials

Ethics Statement

All Studies were conducted under an approved Institutional Review Board protocol of the University of Pennsylvania. Written informed consent from each volunteer was obtained after explaining the study protocol.

Subjects, MRI Scanner and Coil Information

Eight healthy volunteers (20–35 Y), one volunteer (44 Y) with a previously diagnosed with meniscal tear and cartilage pathology and one volunteer with knee pain (62 Y) underwent T1ρ MRI of knee at a whole body 7T scanner (Magnetom 7 Tesla, Siemens-Healthcare, Erlangen, Germany) using a CP Transmit/28 channel receive array knee coil (inner diameter = 15.4 to 18 cm, Quality Electrodynamics, Mayfield Village, OH). Subjects were scanned for either one or both knees. Some of the healthy subjects were scanned 3 to 4 times for optimization of protocol and evaluating field inhomogeneity effects.

T1ρ Pulse Sequence

A modified T1ρ pulse sequence based on previously reported sequence [17,23], consisting of a B_1 and B_0 compensated T1ρ preparation pulse cluster [17] followed by a chemical shift selective fat saturation pulse and a segmented radiofrequency spoiled gradient echo with multiple shots readout acquisition with centric phase encoding order was used (Figure 1).

MRI Data Acquisition Procedure

T1ρ imaging protocol for knee cartilage consists of following steps. A tri-plane GRE localizer scans (~0.5 min.); global shimming and center frequency and transmit voltage setting (~1 min.); 3D structural image acquisition with isotropic voxel (0.6×0.6×0.6 mm^3) used for guiding selection of T1ρ imaging slices (~4 min); reference frequency and voltage were set corresponding to a small volume covering patellar cartilage using localized stimulated echo acquisition mode (STEAM) single voxel spectra (SVS) (~2 min); 3D-T1ρ data in axial orientation for patellar cartilage (~8 min); reference frequency and voltage were set corresponding to a small volume covering femoral and tibial cartilages using SVS (~2 min); 3D-T1ρ data in coronal orientation for femoral and tibial cartilages (~8 min).

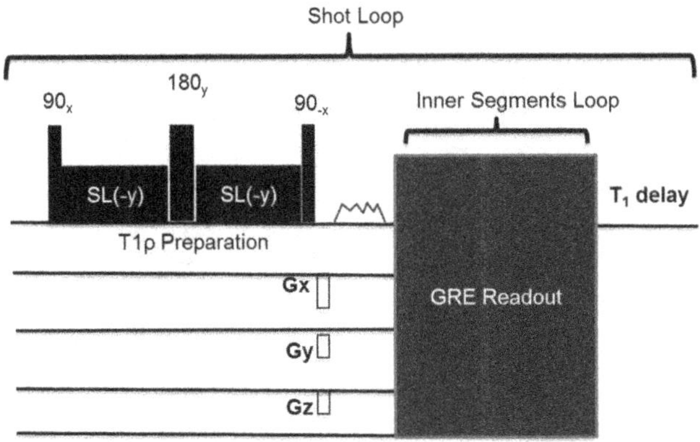

Figure 1. Single shot pulse sequence diagram of T1ρ MRI. T1ρ pulse sequence consist of a B_1 and B_0 compensated T1ρ preparation pulse cluster, crusher gradients, chemical shift selective fat saturation pulse, a gradient echo readout acquisition with centric phase encoding order and T1 recovery delay.

T1ρ MRI Data Protocol

3D T1ρ imaging was performed with spin lock pulse amplitude B_{1sl} = 500 Hz, spin lock times (TSL) = 0, 10, 20, 30, 40 ms and with imaging parameters: TR/TE = 9.7/4.9 ms, flip angle = 10°, FOV = 140×140×30 mm^3, matrix size = 448×224×10, number of averages = 1, number of shots per slice encode = 2 and a shot TR of 5 seconds. Scan time for one set of 3D-T1ρ data (slices = 10 and TSLs = 5) was 8.3 min. Two sets of T1ρ data were acquired, one in axial orientation (for patellar cartilage) and another in the coronal orientation (for weight-bearing femoral and tibial cartilage). Since higher resolution were required mainly along cartilage thickness, data were acquired with 50% phase encode resolution and the phase encoding directions were set as 'right to left' for both scans.

B_0 and B_1 Data Protocol

For obtaining field inhomogeneity information on knee cartilage, B_0 and B_1 field maps were obtained for five healthy volunteers. For B_0 map, we acquired WASSR data [24,25] with following parameters: saturation B_1 = 20 Hz and saturation duration = 200 ms, saturation frequency offset range = −0.8 to 0.8 ppm with step size of 0.1 ppm, TR/TE = 7.8/3.9 ms, flip angle = 10°, FOV = 140×140×30 mm^3, matrix size = 256×128×10, number of averages = 1, number of shots per slice encode = 1 and a shot TR of 5 seconds. For B_1 field map, flip crush sequence with two flip angles 30 and 60 degree was used.

Reproducibility Study Procedure

For reproducibility studies, knee was positioned in the approximately same place and orientation inside the coil by using foam pads. In addition, we used "ImScribe" software tool (written in Matlab) that allows reproducible selection of the same anatomical FOV in Siemens MRI. The program is written in Matlab and requires the installation of the SPM software toolbox. In this study, we have used affine transformation based registration in ImScribe tool. 3D structural imaging data from two scans and a localizer slice from first scan were used as an input in Imscribe software for obtaining same location during 2nd scan. T1ρ data from the healthy subjects (n = 8) were obtained at two time points (different days, within 1 month period).

T1ρ MRI Data at 3T

For comparison of T1ρ values, we also acquired T1ρ MRI data from six of the healthy volunteers with the same imaging sequence parameters in a 3T clinical scanner (Tim-Trio, Siemens-Healthcare, Erlangen, Germany) using a quadrature-spiral-bird-cage transmit/8 channel receive Knee Coil (inner diameter = 15.4 to 18 cm, In-Vivo, Gainesville, FL).

Reference Voltage Calculation Using STEAM

The signal from SVS STEAM sequence with identical flip angles (α) for three pulses is proportional to $\sin^3(\alpha)$. Flip angle α is directly proportional to reference voltage setting in the Siemens

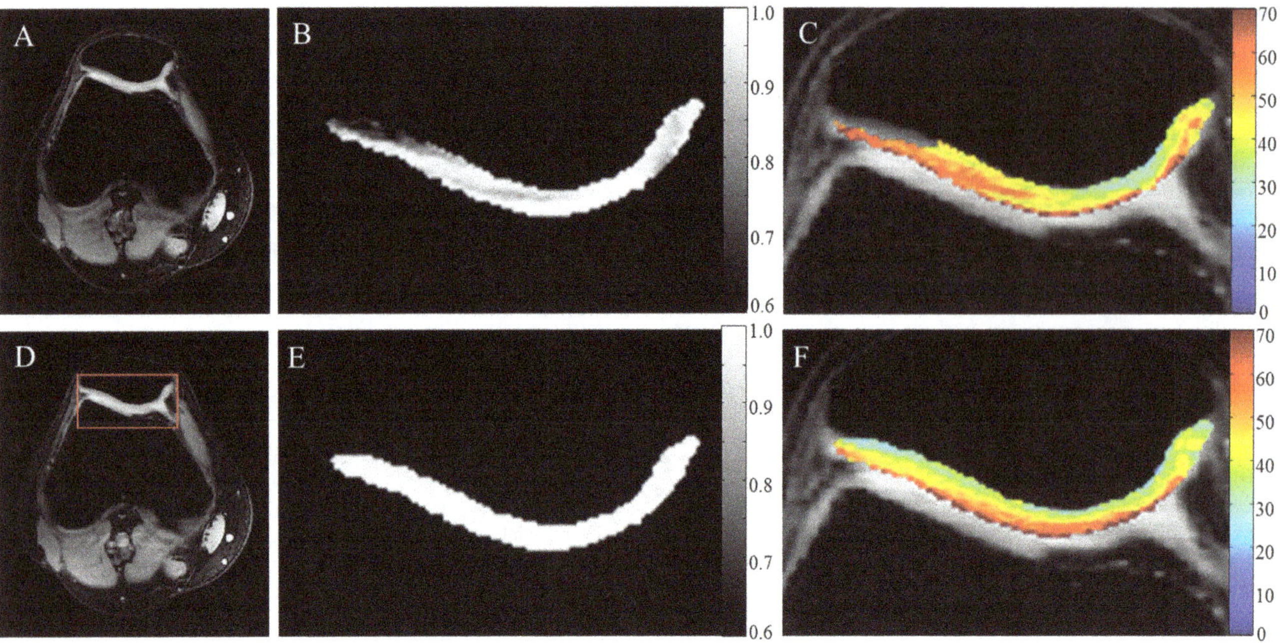

Figure 2. Off-resonance effect on T1ρ mapping. Top row contains anatomical image (A), goodness of fit (R^2) map (B) and T1ρ map (C) corresponding to global volume reference frequency and voltage. Bottom row contains anatomical image (D), R^2 map (E) and T1ρ map (F) corresponding to local volume (rectangular box on anatomical image) around patellar cartilage based reference frequency and voltage. Note that pixels on cartilage with $R^2<0.8$ are not displayed on final map.

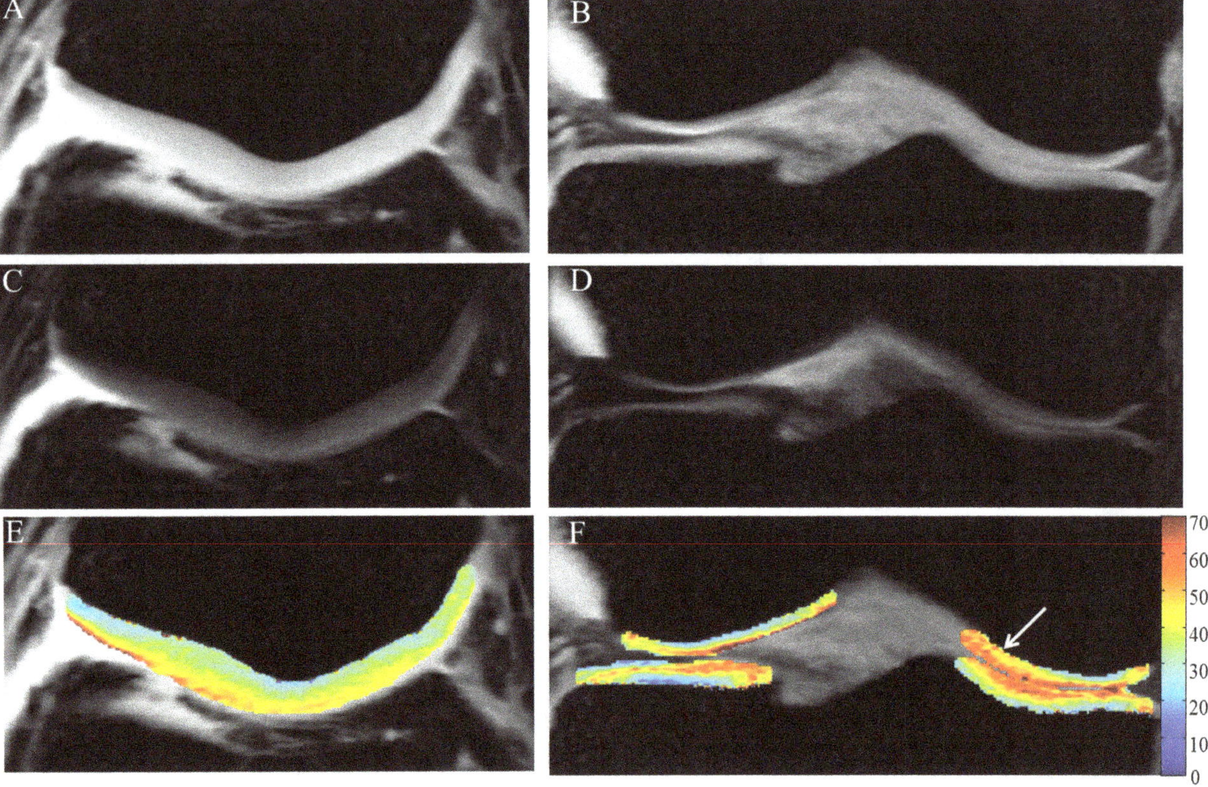

Figure 3. High resolution T1ρ maps of articular cartilage. First column images show patellar cartilage in axial orientation and 2nd column images show femoral and tibial cartilage in coronal orientation of a healthy volunteer at 7T. First row (A&B) contain high resolution anatomical images (TSL = 0), 2nd row (C&D) contain high resolution T1ρ-weighted images corresponding to TSL = 40 ms and 3rd row contain high resolution T1ρ (ms) maps of cartilage overlaid on anatomical images. Arrow indicates the medial side femoral cartilage with reduced contrast among different layers due to magic angle effect. Note that these are cropped images.

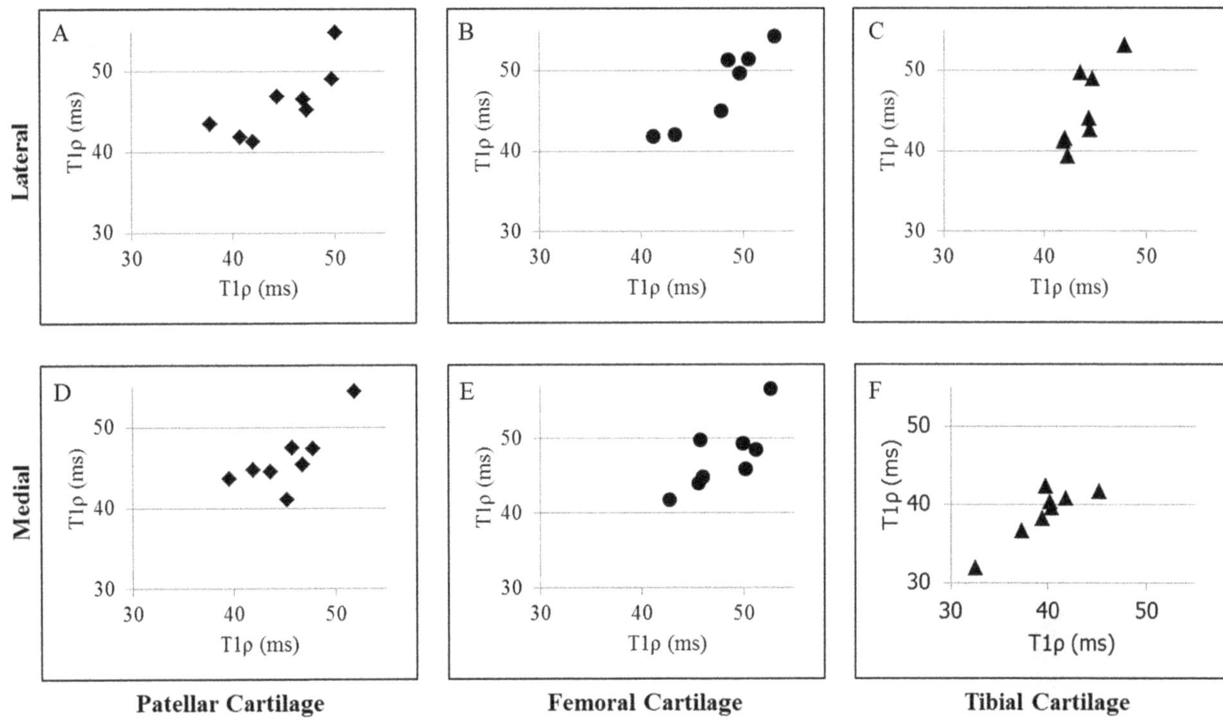

Figure 4. Scatter plots of test-retest data of T1ρ values in different cartilage facets for 8 subjects at 7T.

scanner, which corresponds to a peak B_1 of 11.77 μT. We calculated the flip angle corresponding to a preset reference voltage (x) from maximum of water signals obtained with two spectra acquired with a reference voltage of x (S_1) and 2x (S_2), using the formula as: $\alpha = \cos^{-1}\left(\frac{S_2}{8S_1}\right)^{\frac{1}{3}}$. Final reference voltage (V) is calculated using expression: $V = x \times \left(\frac{\Pi}{2\alpha}\right)$.

Image Processing

MRI data were processed using Image-J software [26] and in-house written programs in MATLAB. Data were pre-processed for motion correction using rigid body registration followed by segmentation of cartilage sections. 3D T1ρ data sets corresponding to each TSL (>0) were registered automatically with respect to TSL = 0 ms data. T1ρ-weighted (T1ρ-W) images corresponding to a TSL = 20 ms were used for generating 3D cartilage mask using manual segmentation of cartilage. Cartilage sections in 3D cartilage mask were further subdivided into medial and lateral sides and into three zones, deep, middle and superficial, by a semi-automatic segmentation program. This program requires the user input for medial and lateral side selection and it divides a 3D mask of cartilage into three regions (zones) using morphological operations. This division is just an approximation to expected cartilage division mentioned in the 'Introduction'.

SNR Calculations

The SNR of T1ρ-W images on cartilage was obtained, as a ratio of average value of a region of interest (ROI) on cartilage and standard deviation (s.d.) of an ROI in background noise[27], from T1ρ-W images. A factor of 0.655 was also multiplied to SNR for accounting Rician noise distribution in MRI magnitude images [27]. An ROI on the cartilage of central slice of T1ρ –W data and four ROIs in background noise of same slice were drawn and SNR of cartilage was computed with respect to each of these background noise ROIs. Final SNR was computed as an average of these four SNR. Average values and standard deviations were computed for multiple segmented sections. B_0 and B_1 (B_{1rel}) maps were generated using previously described procedure in [24,25] and [25]respectively.

T1ρ Mapping

The T1ρ-W data corresponding to different TSLs were fitted voxel-wise to a mono-exponential decay expression, $S(TSL) = S(0) \times e^{\left(-\frac{TSL}{T1\rho}\right)}$, for computing T1ρ values. Goodness of fit parameter (R^2) was also computed. In the current study, the T1ρ-W image corresponding to a TSL = 0 ms was used as a base or anatomical image. T1ρ maps were color overlaid on the base image.

Statistical Analysis

Mean and s.d of T1ρ values in different cartilage facets were computed. For test-retest reliability experiment, Intraclass correlation (ICC) coefficient along with 95% confident interval was computed using SPSS (Version 20). ICC with p value less that 0.05 was considered as statistically significant. In addition, Pearson correlation coefficient and coefficient of variations were also computed. Student's t-test was used to evaluate significance of difference of T1ρ values in medial vs lateral side of cartilage at 7T. T1ρ values at 3T and 7T were also compared using t-test.

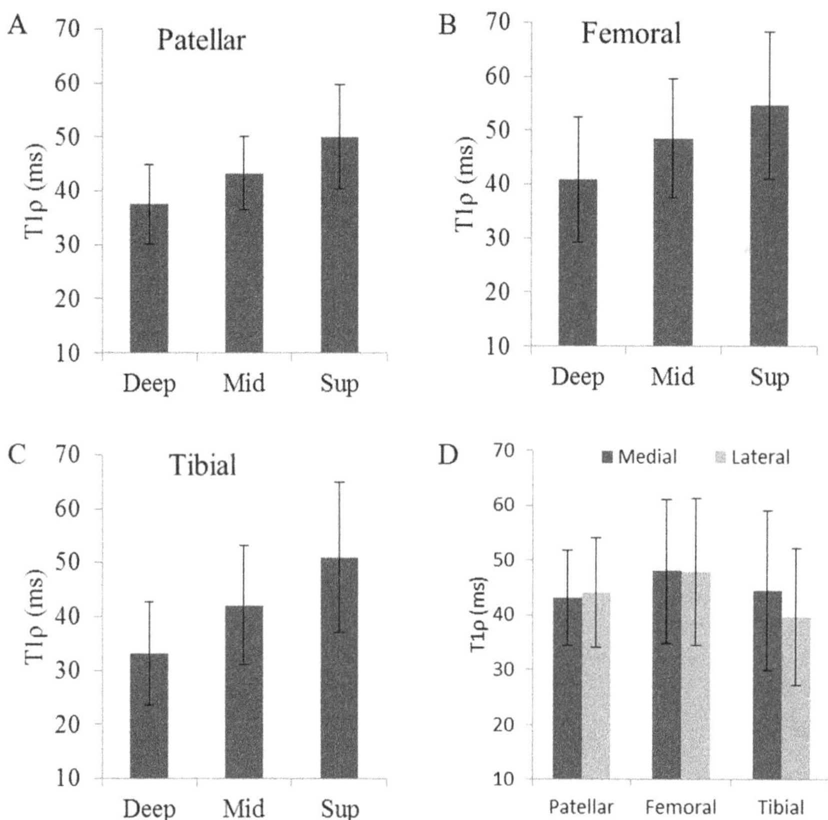

Figure 5. Bar plots represents T1ρ analysis of knee cartilage at 7T. T1ρ values from deep, middle and superficial zones of patellar, femoral and tibial cartilage are shown in Fig (A, B, C). T1ρ values from medial and lateral side of cartilage are shown in Fig. D.

Results

SAR during T1ρ MRI

In this study, SAR was well within the scanner set limits in all the experiments. Moreover, none of the volunteers reported any heating discomfort during study.

Reference Frequency Offset

In the current study, reference frequency obtained using a SVS covering patellar cartilage region at 7T was typically offset from the reference frequency obtained from scanner prescan by around 139±26 Hz (mean ± s.d.) in different experiments. For femoral and tibial cartilage this offset in frequency was 7±31 Hz (mean ± s.d.). After localized reference frequency setting, the offset variations obtained from B_0 field maps across cartilage were around 0±30 Hz (mean ± s.d.).

Reference Voltage Offset

Reference voltages obtained using SVS on different facets of articular cartilage and those obtained using scanner prescan were similar (within 6% difference). B_{1rel} map obtained after localized voltage setting showed a value of 1.0±0.1 (mean ± s.d.) on cartilage.

SNR of T1ρ-W Images

The SNR of base images (In plane resolution = 0.2 mm^2) on the cartilage averaged over all the subjects were ~240, while the lowest SNR of T1ρ-weighted images (TSL = 40 ms) on the cartilage were ~90 at 7T.

Effect of SVS vs Scanner Prescan Based Reference Frequency and Voltage on T1ρ Mapping

Quality of exponential fitting for T1ρ maps at 7T obtained using SVS based reference frequency and voltage were better compared to those obtained using scanner prescan as can be seen

Table 1. Intra class correlation (ICC) coefficient values for test-retest reliability experiment along with 95% CI in open brackets.

Cartilage	Patellar	Femoral	Tibial
Lateral	0.87(0.38, 0.97)	0.86(0.23, 0.97)	0.93(0.69, 0.99)
Medial	0.88(0.47, 0.98)	0.96(0.81, 0.99)	0.73(−0.3, 0.95)

ICC coefficients were statistically significant ($p<0.05$) for all the cartilage facets.

Table 2. Pearson correlation coefficient values for test-retest reliability experiment for medial and lateral sides of different cartilage facets.

Cartilage	Patellar	Femoral	Tibial
Lateral	0.87	0.86	0.93
Medial	0.88	0.96	0.73

Correlation coefficients were statistically significant ($p<0.05$) for all the cartilage facets.

from corresponding R^2 maps (Fig. 2B and 2E). Actual T1ρ map obtained with scanner prescan set reference frequency seems to show elevated T1ρ values in middle and deep zone of healthy cartilage as pointed by arrow on Fig. 2C. In all the experiments, localized reference and voltage setting approach resulted in R^2 value greater than 0.9 for all the voxels in the cartilage and hence improved the reliability of high resolution T1ρ mapping.

T1ρ Data from Healthy Subject

T1ρ-W and T1ρ maps from articular cartilage of a healthy subject are shown in Fig.3. T1ρ values in most of the cartilage are higher in the superficial zone compared to the deep zone. This trend of T1ρ values from deep to superficial zone is maintained in most of the cartilage, except in a few regions where contrast among the layers disappears (as pointed out by arrow in Fig. 3E-F). This phenomenon has been characterized due to the magic angle effect, which decouples dipolar-dipolar interaction of collagen and eliminates contrast between layers [9].

Reproducibility of T1ρ Mapping

Scatter plot (Fig. 4) show T1ρ values in test-retest experiment. ICC coefficients, along with 95% CI, for test-retest reliability of T1ρ measurements in different facets of cartilage are reported in Table 1. ICC coefficients in all the facets of cartilage are statistically significant ($p<0.05$). Note that 95% CI in some facets are quite wide (Table 1). A high Pearson correlation coefficient was observed for test-retest reliability experiment (Table 2). Average coefficient of variation was under 5% in all the cartilage facets for test-retest experiment (Table 3).

T1ρ Analysis

T1ρ values in different facets of cartilage are shown in Fig. 5. T1ρ values were higher in superficial zones compared to middle and deep zones. For the data presented in current study, no significant difference was observed between medial and lateral sides of cartilage.

T1ρ Analysis at 3T vs 7T

Average T1ρ values at 7T were lower (~15%) compared to those obtained at 3T (Table 4). This difference was statistically significant ($p<0.05$) based upon t-test.

T1ρ Data from Patients

Edema in femur bone and pathology in meniscus are clearly visible on high resolution anatomical image of a patient with knee injury (Fig. 6A). On the T1ρ-W image (Fig. 6B) signal intensity of femoral cartilage near femur bone edema is higher. In the medial femoral cartilage there is a clear elevation of T1ρ values in a focal region (Fig. 6C). Average T1ρ values in this focal ROI is 113 ms which is more than double compared to normal cartilage. Femoral cartilage thickness in this region is ~1.5 mm. In addition, an unidentified pathology on femoral cartilage is clearly visible as a dark line on anatomical image (pointed by dotted white arrow on Fig. 6A). This pathology is observed on femoral cartilage of three consecutive slices. Results from another subject with abnormal patellar knee cartilage also showed elevated T1ρ values in the cartilage particularly in the three focal regions on patellar cartilage (Fig. 7).

Discussion

In this study we have presented an approach for obtaining reliable high resolution 3D-T1ρ mapping of human knee cartilage at 7T MRI.

The effects of B_0 and B_1 inhomogeneities during spin-locking increased at 7T due to increase in field inhomogeneity. Offsets induced by B_0 inhomogeneity results in off-resonance spin locking effects that produce inaccurate T1ρ maps. As such, a spin-echo based T1ρ pulse cluster is expected to mitigate B_0-field inhomogeneity based artifacts, provided that the B_1 field is homogenous. Because of B_1 inhomogeneity in cartilage at 7T, spin echo based T1ρ pulse cluster may not be efficient in removing such artifacts. In this study, after global shimming, reference frequency and reference voltage from a local volume around cartilage was performed using localized SVS. With this approach, these field inhomogeneity artifacts were reduced significantly and reliable T1ρ maps of knee cartilage were obtained.

Standard Siemens scanner prescan uses a 10 mm axial slice at the isocenter of the magnet to set the reference frequency and voltage. In this study, femoral/tibial cartilage is located closer to isocenter than patellar cartilage. Hence the difference between SVS based reference frequency and scanner prescan based reference frequency was small, while in patellar cartilage this difference was higher. Scanner prescan based reference frequency

Table 3. Coefficient variation (mean ± s.d.) values (%) for test-retest reliability experiment for medial and lateral sides of different cartilage facets.

Cartilage	Patellar	Femoral	Tibial
Lateral	3.6±2.4	3.5±2.2	2.5±1.9
Medial	3.5±3.2	2.3±1.6	4.3±3.2

Table 4. Analysis of T1ρ values (ms) for human knee cartilage (n = 6) at 3T and 7T.

	Patellar	Femoral	Tibial
3T	50.5±2.4	49.3±3.4	47.2±2.1
7T	43.9±2.9	47.3±3.5	41.2±0.8

Values are reported as mean±s.d. calculated over all subjects data.

setting leads to bigger off resonance effects in the T1ρ weighted images and results in erroneous T1ρ estimation.

Entire 3D-T1ρ imaging protocol as described in the method section can be run under 30 min with an in-plane resolution of 0.2 mm^2. In this study we have presented T1ρ results using linear fitting approach only due to computing time efficiency. As such for some data sets we have compared T1ρ maps obtained using linear and non-linear fitting approaches. Due to high SNR of the T1ρ data in the current study, both approaches provided similar T1ρ values.

T1ρ values of femoral cartilage on the medial side of the patient with a meniscal tear are much higher compared to average T1ρ values from healthy cartilage. Since the femoral cartilage thickness in this region is ~1.5 mm, higher resolution images and maps provided better classification of this focal region. Moreover, there is fluid in between the femoral and tibial cartilage in certain regions which have been segmented out. In the case of lower resolution, effects of partial voluming of cartilage with this free fluid would be increased and could confound interpretation of results. Although, free water suppression could reduce this problem to some extent it can also affect the cartilage signal differently in different zones. High resolution T1ρ mapping is essential in detecting changes in cartilage in such situations.

The main focus of our projects has been T1ρ imaging of patellar, femoral and tibial cartilages. In the current study, we have acquired separate data in axial and coronal orientations, as in our ongoing studies at lower field scanners. The main advantage of acquiring data in this mode is that we can reduce phase resolution without affecting the resolution along the thickness of the cartilage by setting the phase encoding direction as right-to-left. The overall

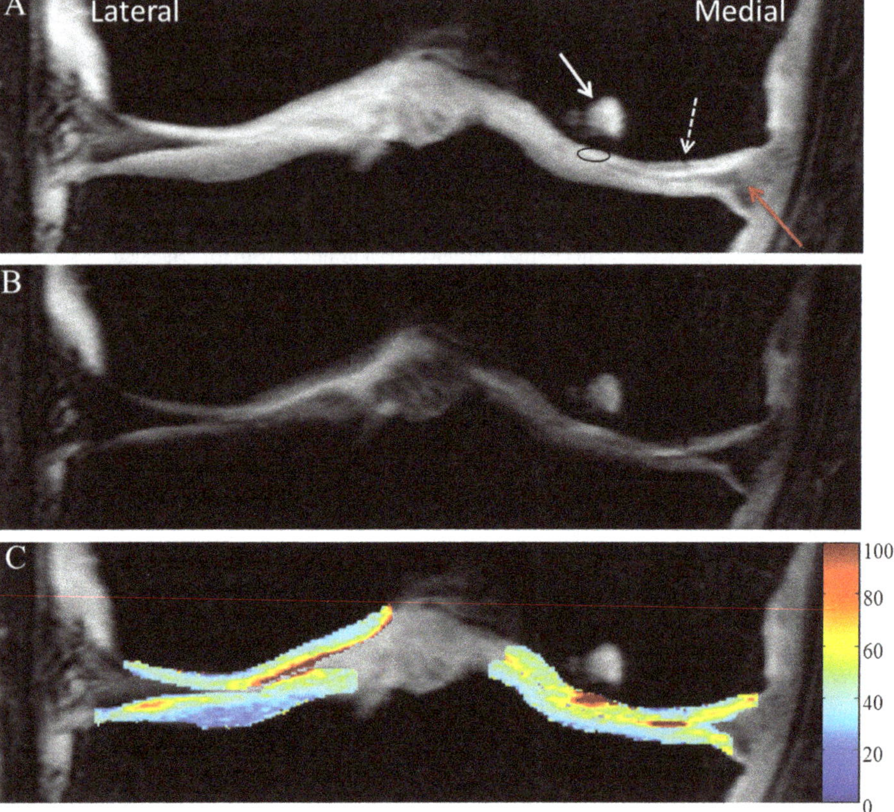

Figure 6. High resolution data from volunteer with meniscal tear and femoral cartilage pathology in medial side. Fig A represents anatomical image, Fig B represents T1ρ-weighted image corresponding to TSL = 40 ms and Fig C contain T1ρ (ms) map of femoral and tibial cartilages overlaid on anatomical image. The red arrow on anatomical image points to meniscal tear, the solid white arrow points to edema in femur and the dotted white arrow points to an unidentified pathology in cartilage. In the focal ROI (on anatomical image), mean T1ρ value is = 113 ms. T1ρ values >300 ms are threshold to zero. Color scale was adjusted to highlight focal region on femoral cartilage with high T1ρ values. Note that only cropped images are shown.

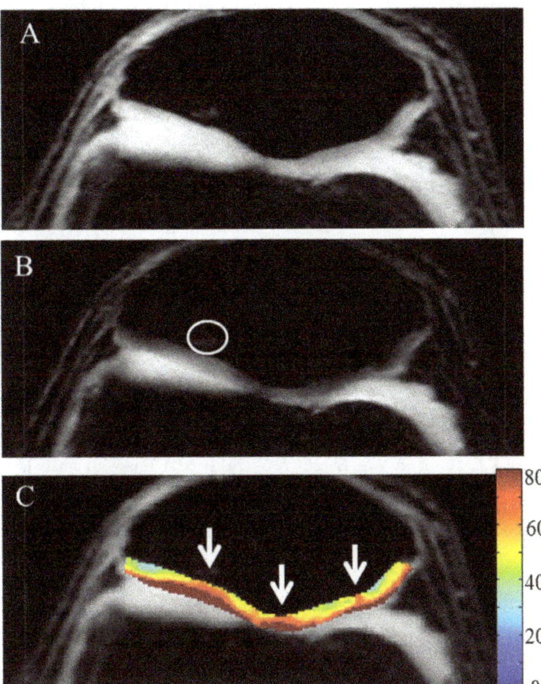

Figure 7. High resolution images from volunteer with abnormal patellar cartilage. Fig A represents anatomical image, Fig B represents T1ρ-weighted image corresponding to TSL =40 ms and Fig C contain T1ρ (ms) map of patellar cartilages overlaid on anatomical image. Circular ROI on Fig.B encircles edema in bone. White arrows on Fig.C point to abnormal cartilage regions. Color scale was adjusted to highlight abnormal region on cartilage with high T1ρ values. Note that only cropped images are shown.

scan time for sagittal orientation for covering patellar cartilage and weight-bearing femoral/tibial cartilage together, will require much longer scan times.

When using a GRE readout, T1 recovery process can mix with T1ρ preparation and can alter actual T1ρ values. For minimizing this effect we have used a centric encoding scheme and 2 shots. Inclusion of more shots may further reduce this effect but requires a longer scanning time.

Main source of contrast between cartilage layers is the dipolar-dipolar interaction of collagens. "Magic angle effects" can mitigate dipolar-dipolar interaction and hence reduce contrast between layers. This phenomenon was observed in some parts of cartilage where T1ρ contrast between deep and superficial zones was reduced substantially. Magic angle effects can interfere with interpretation of T1ρ values in cartilage. Alternatively, dipolar-dipolar interaction based effects can be mitigated using a high power spin lock (>1000 Hz); however, this is limited in human studies by SAR constraints.

Although in this study we demonstrated the T1ρ maps with 0.2 mm^2 in plane resolution, it is possible to obtain even higher resolution images (<0.1 mm^2), albeit with increased scan time that may be prohibitively too long to be useful for human studies. Therefore, the resolution of T1ρ maps in this study has to be traded for the scan-time savings.

In this study, we have used maximum TSL of 40 ms so that all the T1ρ experiments run under allowed systems SAR limits. Since T1ρ values in the healthy cartilage were below 60 ms, TSLs range used in the current study is sufficient to provide accurate estimation of T1ρ values. In case of increased T1ρ values as observed during cartilage pathology, estimation of T1ρ values may not be accurate due to limited TSLs range.

Reduction in T1ρ values at 7T compared to at 3T could be due to the increase in both chemical exchange based and dipolar-dipolar interaction based effects at 7T compared to 3T. By using higher spin lock power (>1000 Hz), these effects can be decoupled. However, spin lock power used in the current study is not sufficient to completely decouple these effects and this could have resulted in lower T1ρ values at 7T compared to 3T.

In this study, we have exploited the experimental high SNR ≥90 at 7T for obtaining high resolution 3D T1ρ maps of human knee cartilage. Due to around two fold increase in SNR from 3T to 7T, obtaining same resolution 3D T1ρ data with similar SNR at 3T, it would require around four times increase in scan time compared to 7T. Note that we have not compared the SNR at 7T with 3T due to the difference in the coils used in this study.

In conclusion, in the current study, we have demonstrated the feasibility of reliable T1ρ mapping and SNR advantage at 7T MRI was exploited to obtain high-resolution T1ρ maps of *in vivo* human knee cartilage in a clinically relevant scan times and SAR constraints. Feasibility of T1ρ MRI at 7T provides the ability to characterize spatial abnormalities in cartilage molecular integrity.

Acknowledgments

The authors acknowledge Mr. Sidyarth Garimall and Mr. Ben Hendler for help in data processing; Dr Walter W Witschey, Dr. Ari Borthakur, Dr. Mark Elliot, Mr. Mathew Fenty and Mr. Mathew Sochor for technical support and discussions;

Author Contributions

Conceived and designed the experiments: AS HH RR. Performed the experiments: AS MH KC FK. Analyzed the data: AS MH KC FK. Contributed reagents/materials/analysis tools: AS MH KC FK. Wrote the paper: AS MH KC FK HH RR. Designed the software used in analysis: AS.

References

1. Cohen ZA, McCarthy DM, Kwak SD, Legrand P, Fogarasi F, et al. (1999) Knee cartilage topography, thickness, and contact areas from MRI: in-vitro calibration and in-vivo measurements. Osteoarthritis Cartilage 7: 95–109.
2. Saarakkala S, Julkunen P, Kiviranta P, Makitalo J, Jurvelin JS, et al. (2010) Depth-wise progression of osteoarthritis in human articular cartilage: investigation of composition, structure and biomechanics. Osteoarthritis Cartilage 18: 73–81.
3. Blanco FJ, Guitian R, Vazquez-Martul E, de Toro FJ, Galdo F (1998) Osteoarthritis chondrocytes die by apoptosis. A possible pathway for osteoarthritis pathology. Arthritis Rheum 41: 284–289.
4. Young AA, McLennan S, Smith MM, Smith SM, Cake MA, et al. (2006) Proteoglycan 4 downregulation in a sheep meniscectomy model of early osteoarthritis. Arthritis Res Ther 8: R41.
5. Pakin SK, Cavalcanti C, La Rocca R, Schweitzer ME, Regatte RR (2006) Ultra-high-field MRI of knee joint at 7.0 T: preliminary experience. Acad Radiol 13: 1135–1142.
6. Chang G, Wiggins GC, Xia D, Lattanzi R, Madelin G, et al. (2012) Comparison of a 28-channel receive array coil and quadrature volume coil for morphologic imaging and T2 mapping of knee cartilage at 7T. J Magn Reson Imaging 35: 441–448.
7. Regatte RR, Schweitzer ME (2007) Ultra-high-field MRI of the musculoskeletal system at 7.0 T. J Magn Reson Imaging 25: 262–269.
8. Redfield AG (1955) Nuclear Magnetic Resonance Saturation and Rotary Saturation in Solids. Physical Review 98: 13.
9. Akella SV, Regatte RR, Wheaton AJ, Borthakur A, Reddy R (2004) Reduction of residual dipolar interaction in cartilage by spin-lock technique. Magn Reson Med 52: 1103–1109.

10. Wheaton AJ, Dodge GR, Elliott DM, Nicoll SB, Reddy R (2005) Quantification of cartilage biomechanical and biochemical properties via T1rho magnetic resonance imaging. Magn Reson Med 54: 1087–1093.
11. Wang N, Xia Y (2012) Orientational dependent sensitivities of T2 and T1rho towards trypsin degradation and Gd-DTPA2- presence in bovine nasal cartilage. MAGMA 25: 297–304.
12. Borthakur A, Wheaton AJ, Gougoutas AJ, Akella SV, Regatte RR, et al. (2004) In vivo measurement of T1rho dispersion in the human brain at 1.5 tesla. J Magn Reson Imaging 19: 403–409.
13. Regatte RR, Akella SV, Wheaton AJ, Lech G, Borthakur A, et al. (2004) 3D-T1rho-relaxation mapping of articular cartilage: in vivo assessment of early degenerative changes in symptomatic osteoarthritic subjects. Acad Radiol 11: 741–749.
14. Wheaton AJ, Borthakur A, Kneeland JB, Regatte RR, Akella SV, et al. (2004) In vivo quantification of T1rho using a multislice spin-lock pulse sequence. Magn Reson Med 52: 1453–1458.
15. Pakin SK, Schweitzer ME, Regatte RR (2006) 3D-T1rho quantitation of patellar cartilage at 3.0 T. J Magn Reson Imaging 24: 1357–1363.
16. Li X, Benjamin Ma C, Link TM, Castillo DD, Blumenkrantz G, et al. (2007) In vivo T(1rho) and T(2) mapping of articular cartilage in osteoarthritis of the knee using 3T MRI. Osteoarthritis Cartilage 15: 789–797.
17. Witschey WR, 2nd, Borthakur A, Elliott MA, Mellon E, Niyogi S, et al. (2007) Artifacts in T1 rho-weighted imaging: compensation for B(1) and B(0) field imperfections. J Magn Reson 186: 75–85.
18. Witschey WR, Borthakur A, Elliott MA, Mellon E, Niyogi S, et al. (2007) Compensation for spin-lock artifacts using an off-resonance rotary echo in T1rhooff-weighted imaging. Magn Reson Med 57: 2–7.
19. Witschey WR, Borthakur A, Elliott MA, Fenty M, Sochor MA, et al. (2008) T1rho-prepared balanced gradient echo for rapid 3D T1rho MRI. J Magn Reson Imaging 28: 744–754.
20. Witschey WR, Borthakur A, Elliott MA, Magland J, McArdle EL, et al. (2009) Spin-locked balanced steady-state free-precession (slSSFP). Magn Reson Med 62: 993–1001.
21. Witschey WR, Borthakur A, Fenty M, Kneeland BJ, Lonner JH, et al. (2010) T1rho MRI quantification of arthroscopically confirmed cartilage degeneration. Magn Reson Med 63: 1376–1382.
22. Goto H, Iwama Y, Fujii M, Aoyama N, Kubo S, et al. (2012) A preliminary study of the T1rho values of normal knee cartilage using 3T-MRI. Eur J Radiol 81: e796–803.
23. Borthakur A, Wheaton A, Charagundla SR, Shapiro EM, Regatte RR, et al. (2003) Three-dimensional T1rho-weighted MRI at 1.5 Tesla. J Magn Reson Imaging 17: 730–736.
24. Kim M, Gillen J, Landman BA, Zhou J, van Zijl PC (2009) Water saturation shift referencing (WASSR) for chemical exchange saturation transfer (CEST) experiments. Magn Reson Med 61: 1441–1450.
25. Singh A, Haris M, Cai K, Kassey VB, Kogan F, et al. (2012) Chemical exchange saturation transfer magnetic resonance imaging of human knee cartilage at 3T and 7T. Magn Reson Med 68: 588–594.
26. Schneider CA, Rasband WS, Eliceiri KW (2012) NIH Image to ImageJ: 25 years of image analysis. Nat Methods 9: 671–675.
27. Firbank MJ, Coulthard A, Harrison RM, Williams ED (1999) A comparison of two methods for measuring the signal to noise ratio on MR images. Phys Med Biol 44: N261–264.

12

Antagonism of Bradykinin B2 Receptor Prevents Inflammatory Responses in Human Endothelial Cells by Quenching the NF-kB Pathway Activation

Erika Terzuoli[1], Stefania Meini[2], Paola Cucchi[2], Claudio Catalani[2], Cecilia Cialdai[2], Carlo Alberto Maggi[2], Antonio Giachetti[1], Marina Ziche[1]*, Sandra Donnini[1]*

1 Department of Life Sciences, University of Siena, Siena, Italy, **2** Pharmacology Department, Menarini Ricerche S.p.A, Florence, Italy

Abstract

Background: Bradykinin (BK) induces angiogenesis by promoting vessel permeability, growth and remodeling. This study aimed to demonstrate that the B2R antagonist, fasitibant, inhibits the BK pro-angiogenic effects.

Methodology: We assesed the ability of fasibitant to antagonize the BK stimulation of cultured human cells (HUVEC) and circulating pro-angiogenic cells (PACs), in producing cell permeability (paracellular flux), migration and pseocapillary formation. The latter parameter was studied in vitro (matrigel assay) and in vivo in mice (matrigel plug) and in rat model of experimental osteoarthritis (OA). We also evaluated NF-κB activation in cultured cells by measuring its nuclear translocation and its downstream effectors such as the proangiogenic ciclooxygenase-2 (COX-2), prostaglandin E-2 and vascular endothelial growth factor (VEGF).

Principal findings: HUVEC, exposed to BK (1–10 μM), showed increased permeability, disassembly of adherens and tight-junction, increased cell migration, and pseudocapillaries formation. We observed a significant increase of vessel density in the matrigel assay in mice and in rats OA model. Importantly, B2R stimulation elicited, both in HUVEC and PACs, NF-κB activation, leading to COX-2 overexpression, enhanced prostaglandin E-2 production. and VEGF output. The BK/NF-κB axis, and the ensuing amplification of inflammatory/angiogenic responses were fully prevented by fasitibant as well as by IKK VII, an NF-κB. Inhibitor.

Conclusion: This work illustrates the role of the endothelium in the inflammation provoked by the BK/NF-κB axis. It also demonstates that B2R blockade by the antaogonist fasibitant, abolishes both the initial stimulus and its amplification, strongly attenuating the propagation of inflammation.

Editor: Costanza Emanueli, University of Bristol, United Kingdom

Funding: Menarini Ricerche S.p.A. provided, in part, the resources for the study. Erika Terzuoli was supported by a fellowship from the Fondazione Italiana per la Ricerca sul Cancro (FIRC). No additional external funding was received for this study. The funders had no role in study design, data collection and analysis, decision to publish, or preparation of the manuscript.

Competing Interests: Stefania Meini, Paola Cucchi, Claudio Catalani, Cecilia Cialdai and Carlo Alberto Maggi are employed by Menarini Ricerche S.p.A. who provided, in part, the resources for the study. There are no patents, products in development or marketed products to declare. This does not alter the authors' adherence to all the PLOS ONE policies on sharing data and materials, as detailed online in the guide for authors.

* E-mail: sandra.donnini@unisi.it (SD); marina.ziche@unisi.it (MZ)

Introduction

The inflammation elicited by bradykinin (BK) through the B1 and B2 receptors (B1R, B2R) recapitules the cardinal signs of an inflammatory response as it induces: vascular permeability, hyperthermia, oedema, pain and neo-vessel formation (angiogenesis) [1–7]. More recently, BK has been described to be involved in the pathogenesis of degenerative joint diseases, such as the knee osteoarthritis [8–10]. During the osteoarthritis process, chronic inflammation promotes the imbalance of metabolic and degradative signals. BK, through the B2R, contributes to the chronic inflammatory response in the knee osteoarhritis, activating different cells, including synovial cells or chondrocytes, and inducing the release of pro-inflammatory cytokines, as well as the products of ciclooxygenase (COX) and lipooxygenase (LOX) [10,11]. Several peptide and non-peptide B2R antagonists have been synthesised [12,13]. Icatibant, a peptide compound, is one of the first B2R antagonists synthesised, now approved for the therapy of hereditary angio-oedema attacks [7,14]. Recently, the non-peptide B2R antagonist fasitibant (formerly MEN16132) showed a remarkably high affinity and antagonist potency toward B2R in different species, including humans [15–18]. In preclinical models of inflammation and pain, including osteoarthritis, fasitibant was effective and long lasting in blocking both exogenous and endogenous BK [19–22]. The compound is now undergoing a phase II clinical study in knee osteoarthritis patients (ClinicalTrials.gov: NCT01091116).

Angiogenesis plays a pivotal role in the advancement of inflammatory diseases progression, including osteoarthritis, as a source of inflammatory cells, cytokine and protease activity [23].

Vascular growth both in the synovium and at the osteochondral junction have been associated with osteoarthritis, which is characterized by synovitis and progressive cartilage degeneration, thus novel therapies capable to limit angiogenesis, besides inflammation and pain, might be a desirable target [24,25]. Notably, in the progression of osteoarthritis, the benefits of agents that suppress neovascularization has been very impressive, providing a solid rationale for pursuing anti-angiogenesis strategies in patients affected by chronic inflammatory diseases [26]. Of relevance to this study are recent reports describing the role of the kallikrein/bradykinin system, through the B2R in the recruitment of circulating pro-angiogenic cells, a process which leads to tissue vascularization [27].

BK is known to induce angiogenesis by activating endothelial cells, and promoting vessel permeability, growth and remodeling [28,1,4,5]. The present study aimed to demonstrate that the B2R antagonist, fasitibant, inhibits the BK pro-angiogenic effects, both in *in vitro* and *in vivo* studies. Moreover, we provide evidence that, in endothelial cells and in circulating proangiogenic cells (PACs), BK activates the pro-inflammatory NF-κB transcriptional factor, which, in turn, promotes the overexpression of a wide array of inflammatory genes (e.g. interleukins, chemokines, COX-2, MMPs). As a measure of the functional NF-κB activation, we assessed the COX-2/prostaglandin E-2 (PGE-2) pathway, because of their established role as pro-inflammatory and pro-angiogenic signals. We demonstrate that fasitibant abolished pro-angiogenic effects by suppressing the B2R-dependent BK-induced NF-κB transcription factor activation.

Results

HUVEC Express B2 but not B1 Receptors

In order to evaluate the anti-angiogenic activity exerted by fasitibant on cultured human umbelical venular endothelial cells, HUVEC, first, we assessed the presence of the BK receptors, B1 and B2, by measuring their respective mRNA and protein expression (Fig. 1A and B). The B2R was revealed in terms of messenger (Fig. 1A) and protein, and it was not modulated by the presence of BK (Fig. 1B and Fig. S1). The B1R was undetectable in HUVEC (Fig. 1A), either in basal condition (0.1% FCS) after BK or 10% FCS stimulation (Fig. S1).

Fasitibant Prevents Changes in Permeability, and Adherens and Tight-junction Signals Induced by BK

Endothelial permeability, a common histopatological marker of inflammation, is also a typical response to several angiogenic factors [29]. In a model of *in vitro* endothelial permeability, BK produced a significant increase of paracellular flux of fluorescent-conjugated dextran, which was time- and concentration-dependent (Fig. 1C). Cotreatment of HUVEC with BK (10 μM) and fasitibant (1 μM), abolished the BK-induced paracellular flux increase, restoring the flux to control level (Fig. 1D). A lower fasitibant concentration (0.1 μM) produced a non-significant inhibition (data not shown).

In a condition of *in vitro* confluence, cells regulate permeability through the expression of cell-type-specific transmembrane adhesion proteins, such as vascular endothelial-cadherin (VEC), at adherens junctions, and zonula occludens-1 (ZO-1), at tight junctions. Consistent with its permeability effects, BK drastically reduced the typical pattern of fluorescence localization of either VEC (Fig. 2A, panel b vs. panel a and Fig. S2 A) or ZO-1 (Fig. 2B, panel b vs. panel a and Fig. S2 A) at the cell-cell contacts, as shown by the white arrows in panels a vs. b in both Figs. 2A and B. Fasitibant restored the cytoskeletal organization of both molecules (Fig. 2A, panel d, and Fig. 2B, panel d). Further analysis of VEC expression by immunofluorescence at a lower magnification (20X) clearly depicts the dramatic reduction of adherens junction in response to BK (Fig. 2C, panel b vs. a) contrasting with that of fasitibant treatment (Fig. 2C, panel d vs. b).

It is known that VEC expression decreases β-catenin phosphorylation/translocation into the nucleus [30]. Consistent with the observed disassembly of VEC, BK (1 or 10 μM) increased cytoplamic β-catenin phosphorylation, an effect fully reversed by fasitibant (Fig. 2D, compare lane 5 and 6 vs. 2 and 3, Fig. S2 B for quantification).

These observations clearly indicate that fasitibant prevents BK-induced permeability by counteracting the disassembly of adherens and tight junction.

Fasitibant Inhibits BK-induced Angiogenesis

BK promotes angiogenesis by directly stimulating endothelial cell (EC) growth and migration [4]. In HUVEC, BK induced both a concentration-dependent cell proliferation (measured by the incorporation of BrdU) and migration (measured by the wound healing assay), with a maximal effect at 1 μM (data not shown). Fasitibant (1 μM) co-incubated with BK (1 μM), suppressed its effects (Fig. S3 A and B, Fig. S3 C for wound healing assay quantification). Further, the anti-angiogenic effect of fasitibant was evident also in a 3D differentiation model. When plated in a thin layer of matrigel and stimulated with BK, HUVEC organized in a network of pseudocapillary tubes that invaded the gel (Fig. 3A, panel b vs. a). Fasitibant co-treatment reduced the number of pseudocapillary in terms of completed circles (Fig. 3A, panel d vs. b and Fig. 3B for quantification). Similarly, BK promoted pseudocapillary sprouting in a microcarrier-beads-HUVEC model (Fig. S4 A and B for quantification). Fasitibant co-treatment abolished the cellular sprouting, affecting not only the number and length of BK-induced sproutings, (Fig. S4 A, panel d vs. b, and B for quantification), but reducing ($p<0.001$) capillary diameter (Fig. S4 C, panels b vs. a, and D for quantification).

To further test the anti-angiogenic activity of the B2R antagonist, we used the Matrigel implant assay. Matrigel plugs, both with BK alone or in presence of fasitibant, were injected subcutaneously in mice and harvested after 10 days. Implants containing BK showed several branched structures throughout the implant (Fig. 3C, panel b). Conversely, in implants in which BK and fasitibant were concomitantly administered, angiogenesis was markedly reduced (Fig. 3C panel d vs. b). Quantitative analysis of viable/functioning vessels by hemoglobin determination revealed that BK (10 μM) produced a 2.3-fold increase in blood content compared with control (Fig. 3D), whereas administration of fasitibant (1 μM) reduced vessel density by 50% (Fig. 3D). All together the results demonstrate that the B2R antagonist impairs BK-dependent endothelial cell activation and angiogenesis.

Angiogenesis and Progenitor Hematopoietic Cells in Experimental Osteoarthritis in Rats: Effect of B2R Antagonism

We assessed the relevance of fasitibant on angiogenic process in a model of experimental (intra-articular administration of monosodium iodoacetate, MIA) osteoarthritis in rats. In this model, we observed a marked infiltration of inflammatory cells with dearrengment of synovial tissue structure, as evaluated by hematoxylin and eosin staining, which was reduced by simultaneus fasitibant administration (Fig. 4A). Moreover, MIA administrationin produced a significant increase of vessel

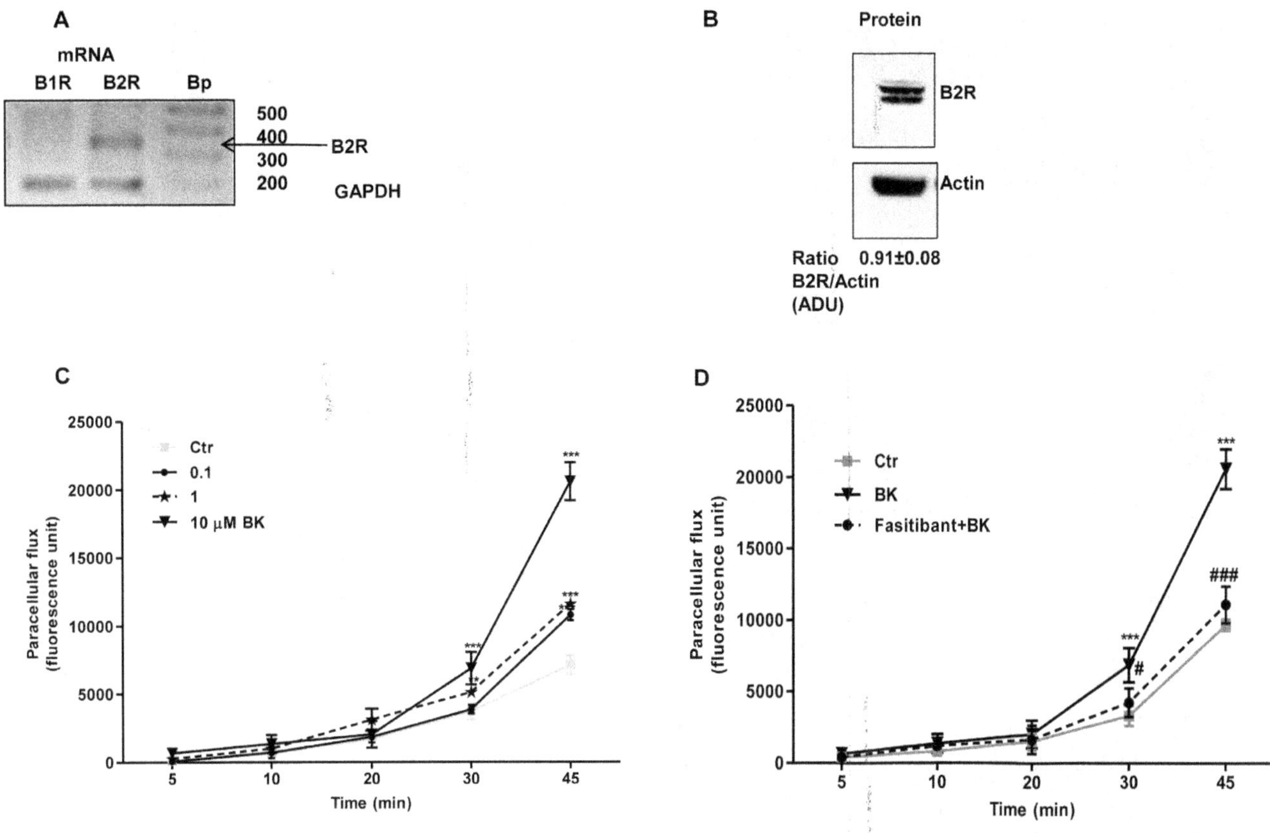

Figure 1. B2R stimulation promotes changes of cell permeability. (A) mRNA expression for B1 and B2 receptors, (B2R mRNA is approximately 339 pb) and (B) western blot analysis of B2 receptor in HUVEC. (Experiments are run three time; n = 3). (C) Permeability in HUVEC monolayer was detected as passage of fluorescence-coniugated FITC-Dextran from upper to lower compartments (Numbers represent mean ± SEM of three experiments run in triplicate; n = 3); ***p<0.001, **p<0.01, *p<0.05 compared to untreated cells (D). Fasitibant (1 μM), prevents the enhanced permeability, n = 3; ***p<0.001 compared to untreated cells #p<0.05, ###p<0.001 to BK-treated cells.

density, evidenced by CD31 staining (Fig. 4B panel b vs. panel a, and Fig. 4C, p<0.01). The co-treatment with fasitibant significantly reduced the number of vessels (Fig. 4B, panel d, and Fig. 4C), demonstrating anti-angiogenic properties. Next, measurements of VEGF levels in synovial fluids (Fig. 4D), showed significantly higher levels in MIA treated rats (640±26 pg/ml) compared to control (490±29 pg/ml, p<0.001, Fig. 4D). Fasitibant, significantly reduced VEGF levels (520±15 pg/ml, P<0.01, Fig. 4D).

A number of reports support the notion that circulating proangiogenic cells (PACs) foster angiogenesis in selected diseases, including osteoarthritis [26]. Indeed we found a significant enrichment of progenitor cells, evidenced by CD133 staining and localised around the vessels, in the MIA treated rats (Fig. 4E panel b vs. panel a), that was reduced by concomitant administration of fasitibant (Fig. 4E, panel d).

BK Activates the NF-κB-signaling Pathway Producing a Persistent Activation of Human Endothelial Cells

Next, to learn how the acute and short lived inflammatory responses elicited by BK in the human endothelium would lead to a chronic endothelial activation, a condition sufficient to promote the degenerative pathologies of the joints [31], we studied the transcription factor NF-κB, a master regulator for the inflammatory cascade. We therefore examined NF-κB translocation from the cytoplasm into the nucleus, a fundamental index of NF-κB gene transcriptional activation, using western blot analysis for anti-p65 NF-κB antibody. BK stimulated NF-κB translocation rapidly, as its presence in the nucleus was detectable as early as 5 min, persisting up to 30 min following BK (Fig. 5A, Fig. S5 A for quantification). Importantly, the B2R antagonist prevented the nuclear translocation of the transcription factor (15 min), and the ensuing activation of the inflammatory pathways, evaluated by western blot and immunofluorescence (Fig. 5B and C, Fig. S5 B for quantification).

NF-κB activation entails overexpression of a number of genes and their pro-inflammatory products (e.g. cytokines, MMPs, COX-2) which promote a chronic type of inflammation and further stimulate the endothelium to form neo-vessels. In this work on human endothelium we focused on inducible enzymes of the arachidonic acid pathway, i.e. COX-2 and mPGES-1, because their product, PGE-2, is widely recognized as an important factor in fostering pathological angiogenesis [32]. We observed that BK induced a consistent biphasic over-expression of COX-2 (at 1 and at 6 hrs following BK exposure) and of mPGES-1 (Fig. 6A and B). The enhanced expression of these synthetic enzymes yielded a nearly twofold increase of PGE-2 production (Fig. 6C). Simultaneous incubation of HUVEC with BK and fasitibant reduced the overexpression of both COX-2 and mPGES-1 (Fig. 6D), and significantly attenuated the PGE-2 output (Fig. 6E; p<0.001). The level of PGE-2 production in the endothelium greatly influenced its functions, such as migration and pseudocapillary formation, which were enhanced by BK exposure, and conversely inhibited by fasibitant. Similarly, the IKK inhibitor VII (0.2 μM), nearly

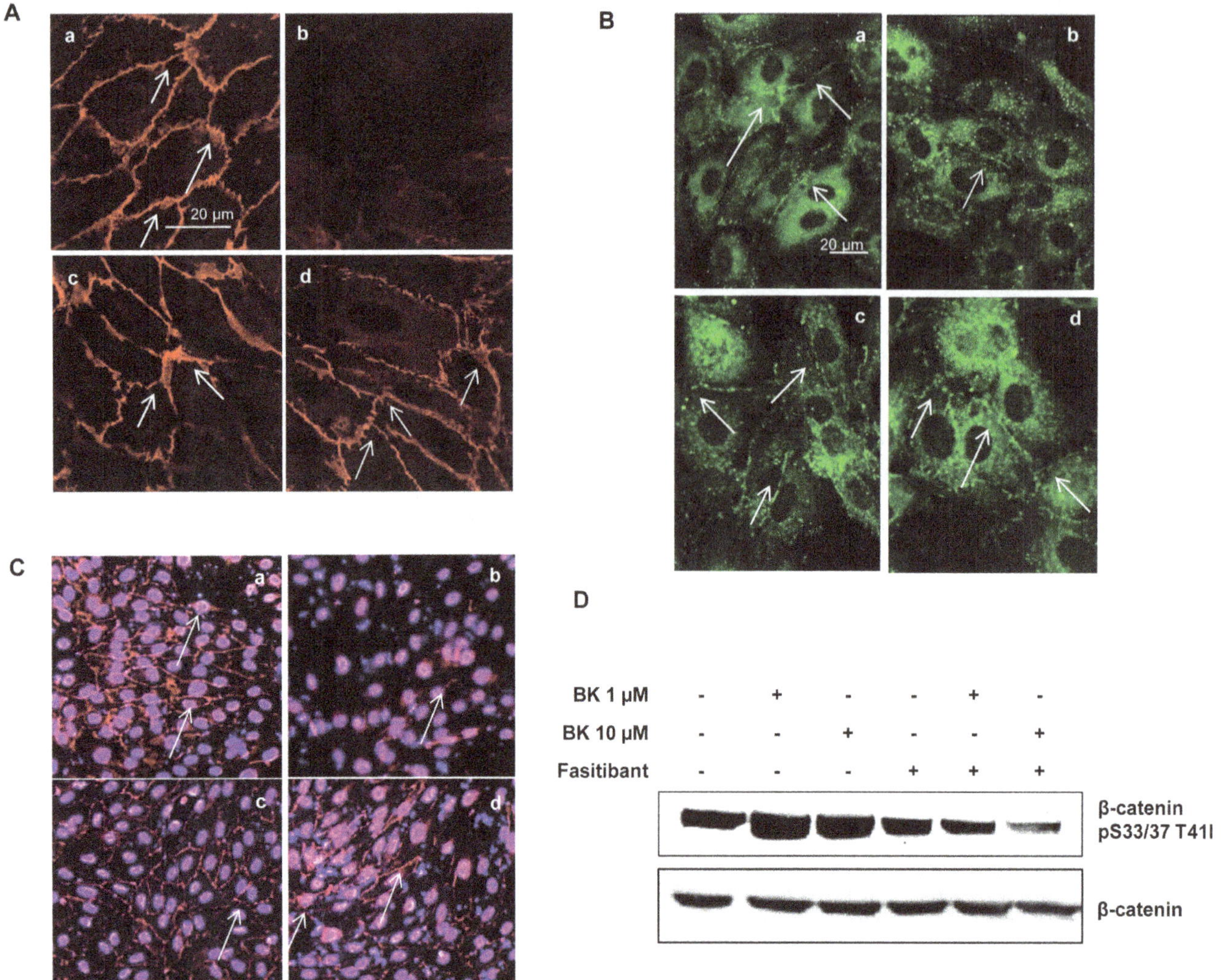

Figure 2. BK-induced changes of endothelial junctions signals are blocked by fasitibant in HUVEC. (A) Confocal analysis of VEC expression (white arrowheads) in 0.1% FBS (a), BK (1 µM) (b), fasitibant (1 µM) (c), fasitibant+BK (d). (B–C) ZO-1 (60 X) and VEC (20 X) expression (white arrowheads), evaluated by immunofluorescence analysis, in 0.1% FBS (a), BK (1 µM) (b), fasitibant (1 µM) (c), fasitibant+BK (d). Bar = 20 µM. (D) Cytoplamic β-catenin phosphorylation, (western blot), in cells treated with BK (1 or 10 µM) with/without fasitibant (1 µM). Gels representative of three experiments; n = 3.

suppressed the BK-induced COX-2 overexpression (Fig. 6F) and affected also the formation pseudocapillaries in matrigel (Fig. 6G, panel d versus panel b).

Interestingly, we found similar results in PACs (Fig. 7). PACs expressed B2R (Fig. S6), and BK induced NF-kB activation, evaluated as nuclear translocation and phosphorylation of p65, COX-2 expression and PGE-2 production (Fig. 7A–D), which were reduced by treatment with fasitibant (0.1 µM), or IKK inhibitor VII (0.2 µM).

All together these results demonstrate that BK, the initial stimulus for the activation of the NF-κB pathway, has important consequences for the human endothelium as it amplifies the inflammatory response by involving enhanced expression of genes and their pro-inflammatory products. These results also clerly show that blockade of the initial stimulus through kinin B2 receptor blockade by fasitibant abolishes the BK/NF-κB axis and prevents the progression of inflammation.

Discussion

This work delineates the profile of a novel selective B2R antagonist, fasitibant, in blocking the BK-induced activation of vascular endothelium. Fasitibant binds to the human B2R exhibiting a sub-nanomolar affinity, similar to that of the peptidic antagonist icatibant (pK_i 10.1–10.5), whereas in virtue of its dissociation-rate remarkably slower [33] fasitibant displays a significantly higher functional potency in blocking BK induced responses (pK_B values 10.3 and 8.5 for fasitibant and icatibant, respectively) [15]. Moreover, fasitibant, in an *in vivo* model of osteoarthritis, has been shown to reduce oedema, to possess a long lasting pain-relieving activity, and to lower the output of BK and prostanoids in the joint [21].

Because oedema formation is associated with an increased leakage from the blood vessel of the joint, its is likely that the compound opposes the effect of BK on the endothelial cells lining these vessels. Indeed, this work demonstrates that fasitibant antagonizes the activation of endothelial cells induced by BK,

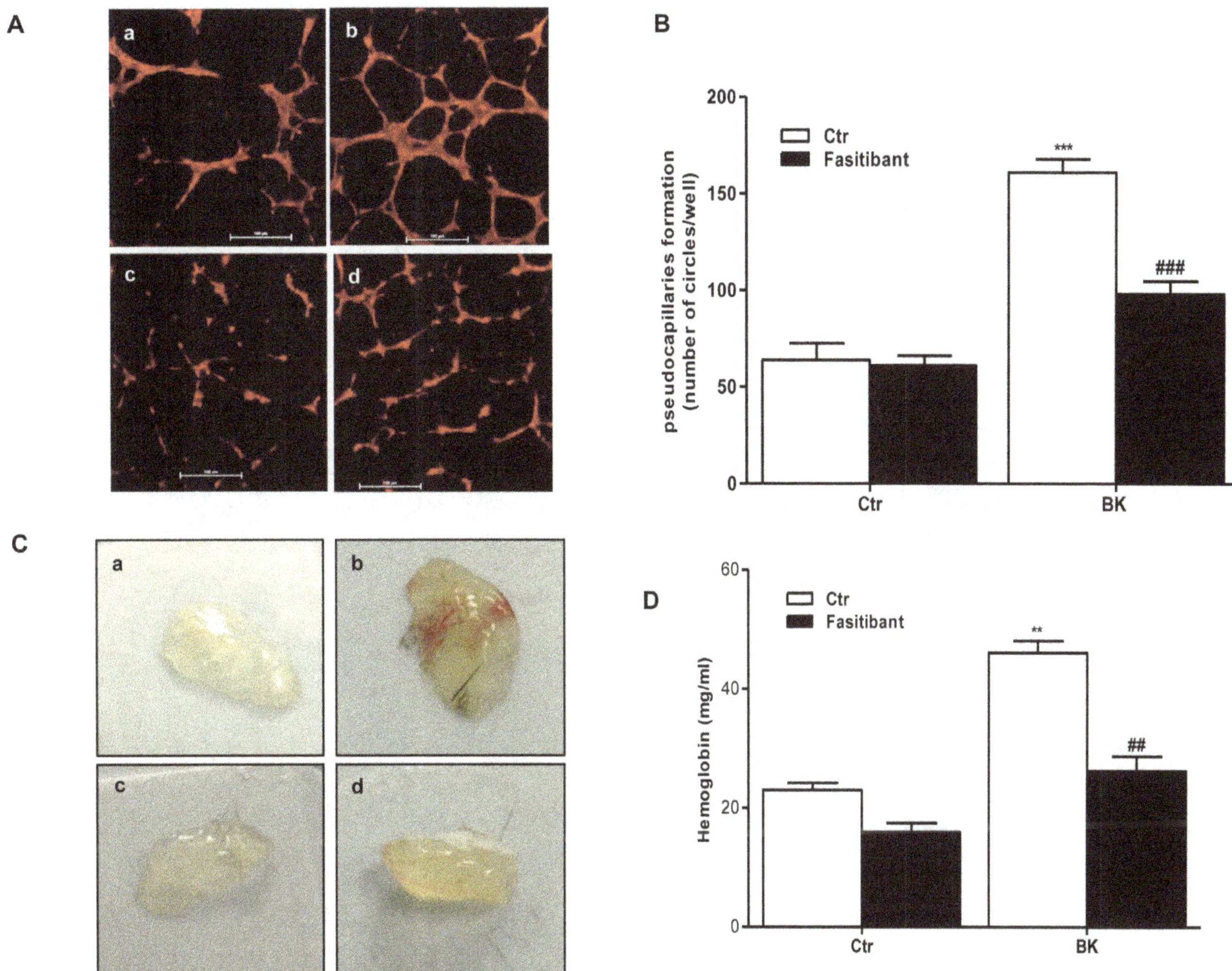

Figure 3. B2R blockade reduces BK-induced angiogenesis. (A) Representative pictures of pseudocapillaries formation in Matrigel from HUVEC in 0.1% FBS (a), exposed to BK (1 µM) (b), to fasitibant (1 µM) (c), to fasitibant+BK (d), observed 12 hrs after cell seeding. (B). Quantification of pseudocapillaries obtained by counting numbers of complete circles/well; Numbers represent mean ± SEM of three experiments run in triplicate. (C) BK induces vascularization in subcutaneously-injected Matrigel implants in mice. panel a: none, b: BK, c: fasitibant and d: fasitibant+BK. (D) Quantitative analysis of hemoglobin/angiogenesis in implants. For each condition (n = 6), the means ± SD are shown. **p<0.01, compared to untreated cells; ##P<0.01 to BK-treated cells.

abolishing the massive increase of microvascular permeability. Similarly, fasitibant preventes the BK-induced changes of endothelial signals indicative of faulty membrane, i.e. the VE-cadherin (VEC) and zonula occludens (ZO)-1 proteins and β-catenin phosphorylation. Thus, blockade of the B2R preserves the charateristic barrier function of the endothelium, by preventing the disorganization of the adherens and tight junctions *in face of* injurious stimuli, and exerts a tight control on the efflux rate.

A major finding concerns the BK ability to activate the trancription factor NF-κB, as evidenced by its translocation toward the cell nucleus, an event which occurs within minutes from BK addition to endothelial cells. NF-κB, a pivotal regulator of inflammation [34,35], in its transcriptional role, subserves a wide repertoire of inflammatory genes (cytokines, growth factors, enzymes). The delayed overexpression of COX-2 and overproduction of PGE-2, observed in HUVEC challenged with BK, represent a clear functional evidence of the involvement of the NF-kB in gene regulation. Thus, it appears that BK functions as the initial trigger for a robust chronic inflammatory response sustained by a wide variety of inflammatory genes and mediators.

Notably, fasibitant application to endothelial cells aborted the NF-κB nuclear translocation, therefore inhibiting the functional sequelae of its activation. Similarly, IKK VII, an inhibitor of NF-κB, prevented endothelial functions related to its active state.

Thus, these results delineate distinct, but overlapping phases of the inflammatory response to BK in the endothelium. An acute one, possibly involving fast signals, such as VEC and ZO-1 disassembling, with phoshorylation of beta catenin, and NF-κB translocation, followed by a chronic phase, involving gene transcription and protein synthesis initiated by NF-κB transcriptional activity. This amplification mechanism of local and short-lived signals, such as that of BK, exhaustively reviewed by Pober and Sessa [31], is crucial for the evolution of inflammation. Antagonism of B2R, completely suppresses this progression.

The endothelium, activated through B2 receptor stimulation and by the NF-κB cascade products, exibits the typical angiogenic phenotype, as shown by the abundant sprouting of new capillaries

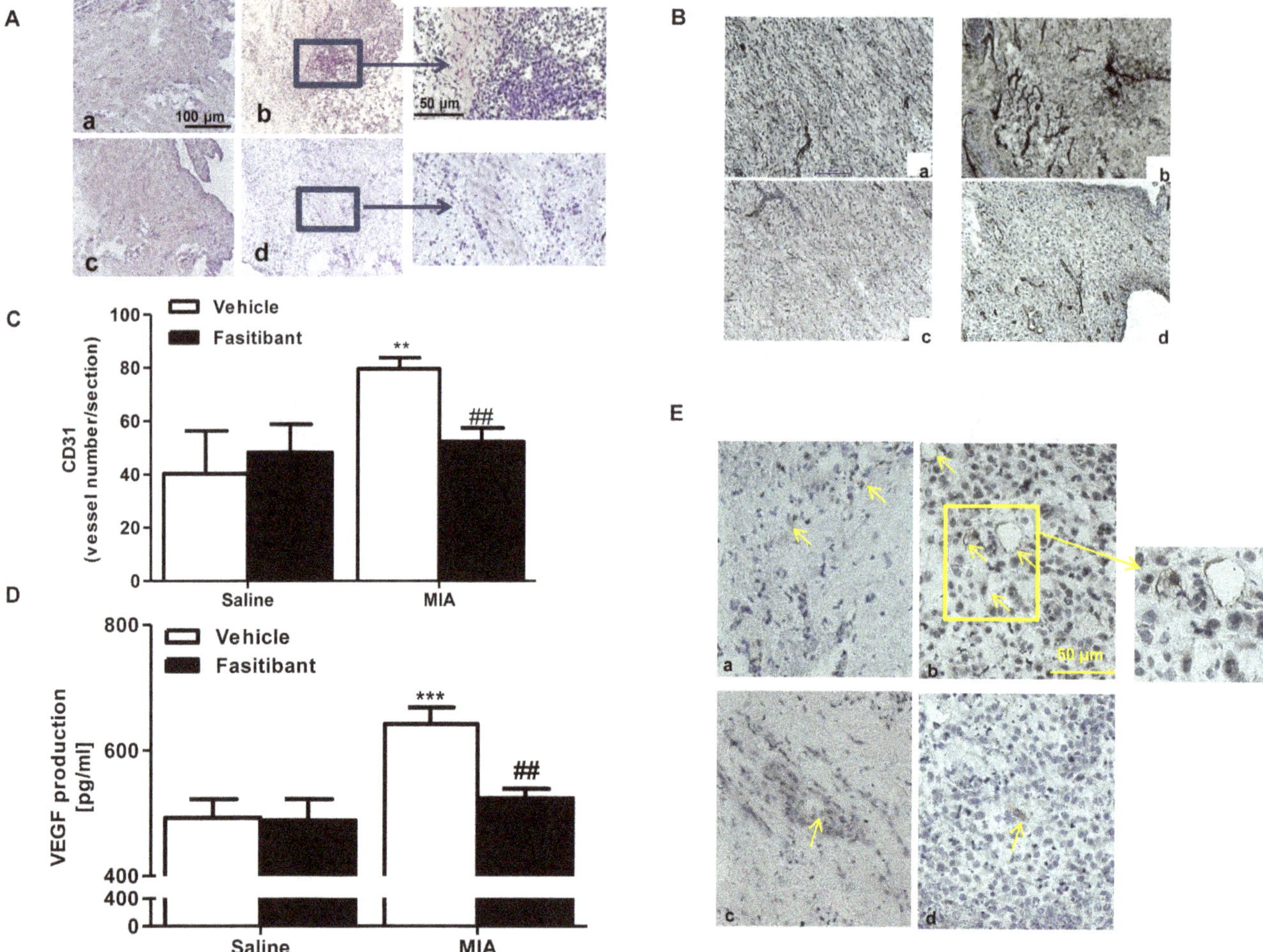

Figure 4. Effect of fasitibant on angiogenesis and circulating proangiogenic cells in experimental osteoarthritis in rats. (A) Representative images of hematoxylin/eosin staining (20 X) in synovial tissue from rats after intra articular injection of: saline (a), MIA (b), fasitibant with saline (c) or MIA with fasitibant, as described in Materials and Methods. Bar = 100 µM. Inset at higher magnification (40 X). Bar = 50 µM. (B–C) Representative images and quantification of CD-31 staining (40 X) in rats as described in A; Bar = 50 µM; quantification of CD-31 was performed counting 10 random field/section for slides; each slide has four sections. Data represent vessels counted for section in synovial tissue **P<0.01 compared to saline; ##P<0.01 compared to MIA. (D) ELISA immunoassay for VEGF in synovial fluids of rats treated as described in A. ***P<0.001 compared to saline; ##P<0.01 to MIA. (E) Representative images of CD-133 staining in rats as described in A; Bar = 50 µM. Inset at higher magnification (40 X).

observed in this work in various *in vitro* and *in vivo* assays. This effect was preceeded by growth and enhanced motility of endothelial cells. Particularly significant were the results *in vivo* on the matrigel plug, which illustrate the invasion of blood capillaries of the plug under BK challenge and their suppression provided by fasibitant.

We also reproduced these effects in the in vivo experimental model of OA [21]. Indeed, treatment with MIA induced a marked inflammatory response in the rat joint, characterized by enhanced microvessel density and enrichment of circulating proangiogenic cells (PACs). In vitro, in cultured PACs, again we observed the BK mediated amplification of the inflammatory response, as shown by NF-kB activation and COX-2-PGE-2 pathway activation. All these effects were blocked by fasitibant aplication. Corroborating these findings, a recent report shows the stringent requirement for NF-κB activation in the process of arteriogenesis [36].

In conclusion this work illustrates that blockade of the B2 receptor by a selective antagonist, prevents the acute inflammatory responses of the vascular endothelium, and aborts the ensuing amplification through the NF-κB pathway, and its propagation associated to pathological angiogenesis.

Methods

Reagents

Reagents were as follows: BK, 40 kDa FITC-Dextran, hyaluronidase, arachidonic acid (AA) anti-Mouse IgG FITC, anti-Rabbit IgG TRICT, anti-B2 receptor, and anti-β-actin (Sigma Chemical); anti-COX-2 and anti-mPGES-1 (Cayman Chemicals); IKK inhibitor VII, anti-p65 and anti CD31 (Millipore); anti-ZO-1 (BD Transduction); anti-p-β catenin (Ser33, 37/Thr41) and anti-β catenin (Cell Signaling); anti VE-Cadherin (e-Bioscience); anti-H2A (Santa Cruz), anti-phospho-p65 (Bioss); anti-CD133 (Boster Immunoleader). Fasitibant ((4*S*)-4-amino-5-{4-[4-(2,4-dichloro-3-{[(2,4-dimethylquinolin-8-yl) oxy]methyl}benzenesulfonamido)oxane-4-carbonyl]piperazin-1-yl}-*N*,*N*,*N*-trimethyl-5-oxopentan-1-aminium chloride dihydrochloride or MEN16132) (batch number

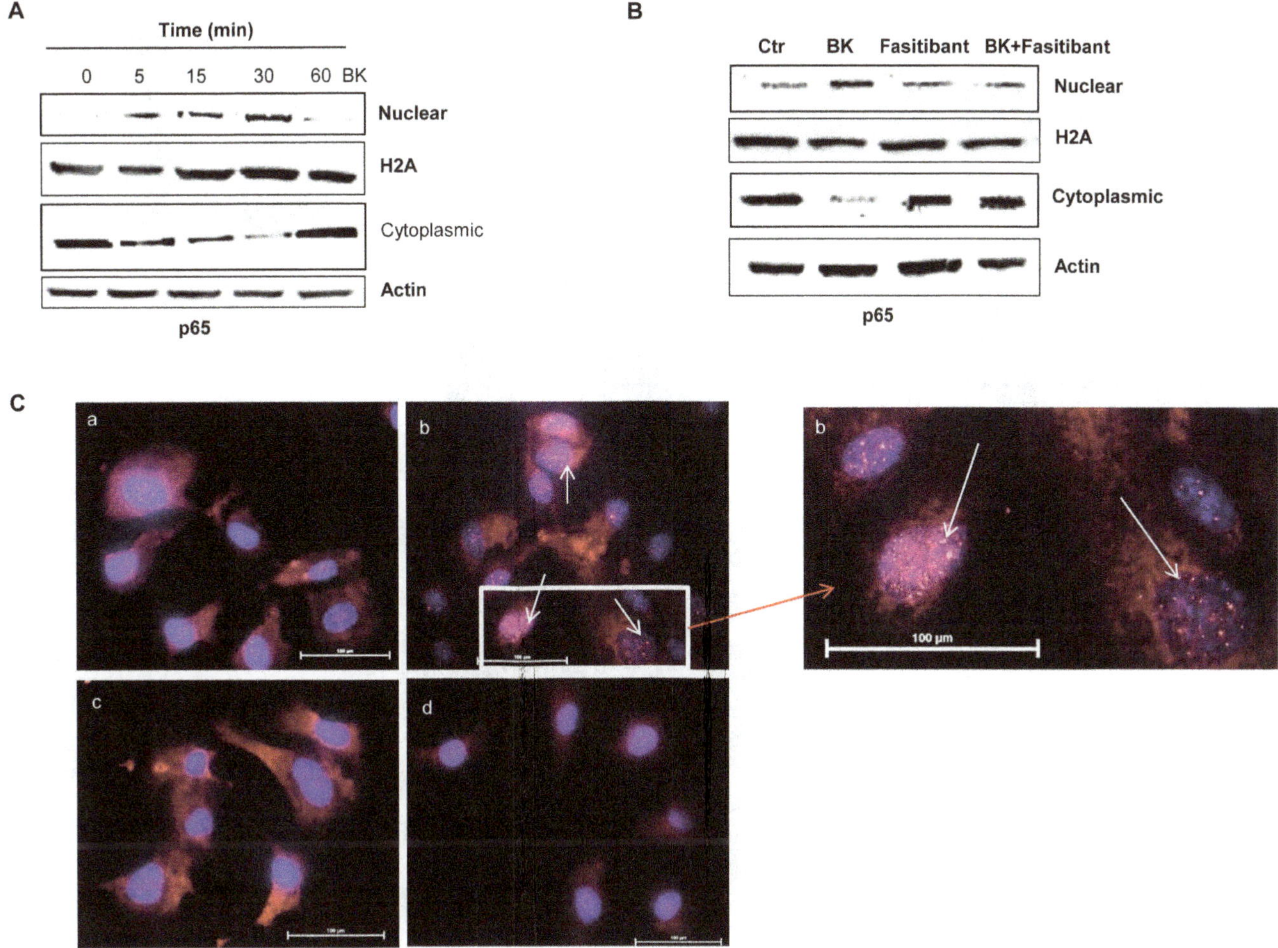

Figure 5. BK stimulates translocation/activation of NF-κB in HUVEC. (A) NF-κB translocation following BK (1 µM) exposure for the indicated times, (B) or following exposure to BK (1 µM, 30 min) in presence/absence of fasitibant (1 µM). Gel are representative of three experiments. (C) Immunofluorescence analysis (40 X) of NF-κB translocation in HUVEC in 0.1% FBS (a), BK (1 µM) (b), fasitibant (1 µM,) (c), fasitibant+BK (d). Inset at higher magnification. Bar = 100 µM.

2010/02), was synthesized in Menarini Ricerche, (Chemistry Development Department, Pisa, Italy).

Cell Culture

Human Umbilical cord vein endothelial cells (HUVEC) were from Cambrex and were maintained in basal EGM-2 and 10% FBS (Hyclone). Cells were split 1:3 twice a week, and used until they reached passage 7. Primary human hematopoietic-proangiogenic cells (PACs, CD133+ and CD34+ cells) isolated from human bone marrow, were from Lonza (2M-102), and were maintained in IMDM and 15% FBS. Cells were split 1:2 once a week, and used until they reached passage 5.

RT-PCR

Bradykinin 1 and 2 receptors mRNA expression were measured through differential RT-PCR. Cells were maintained for 24 hrs in 0.1%, 10% FBS or treated with BK (1 µM) and total RNA was obtained using RNA mini kit (Qiagen). RNA (0.5 µg) was reverse transcribed using a RT-PCR kit (Applied Biosystems). Differential RT-PCR was carried out by using the following primers [37]: B2R (339 bp) 5′-GTCCATGGCCGGATGCGCGG-3′ (sense), 5′-CGATGCAGCGTATCCAGGAAGGTGC-3′ (antisense); B1R (437 bp) 5′-GGCAGAAATCTACCTGGCCAACC-3′ (sense), 5′GCCAGTGGTAGGAGGAAACCCAG-3′ (antisense). Results were normalized with GAPDH (196 bp) 5′-CCATGGA-GAAGGCTGGGG-3′ (sense) and 5′-CAAAGTTGTCATG-GATGACC-3′ (antisense).

Western Blot

3×10^5 cells (HUVEC) or 1.5×10^5 cells (PACs) were plated in 6 or 3 cm diameter dishes, respectively. After 24 h, cells were exposed to 0.1% FBS or BK in presence/absence of fasitibant or IKK inhibitor VII. Cells were scraped in a lysis buffer containing 50 mM Tris HCl (pH 7.4), 150 mM NaCl, 1 mM EGTA, 10 mM NaF, 1% Triton and 1% protease inhibitor cocktail. To prepare the nuclear fractions, 8×10^5 cells were plated in 10 cm diameter dishes. After 24 h, cells were exposed to 0.1% FBS (Control condition) or BK in presence/absence of fasitibant. Cells were then suspended in extraction buffer containing (in mM) 10 HEPES, 1 DTT, 10 KCl, 50 NaF, 0.1 EDTA, 0.1 EGTA, 1 Na_3VO_4, 0.5 PMSF and 0.1 NP-40 at 4°C, homogenized, and centrifuged at 1,000 *g* for 10 min to separate the nuclei. The supernatant was centrifuged at 13,000 *g* for 15 min three times to yield the cytosolic fraction. The nuclear fraction was lysed in buffer containing (in mM) 20 HEPES, 1 EDTA, 1 EGTA and 0.5 PMSF and stored in −80°C before use.

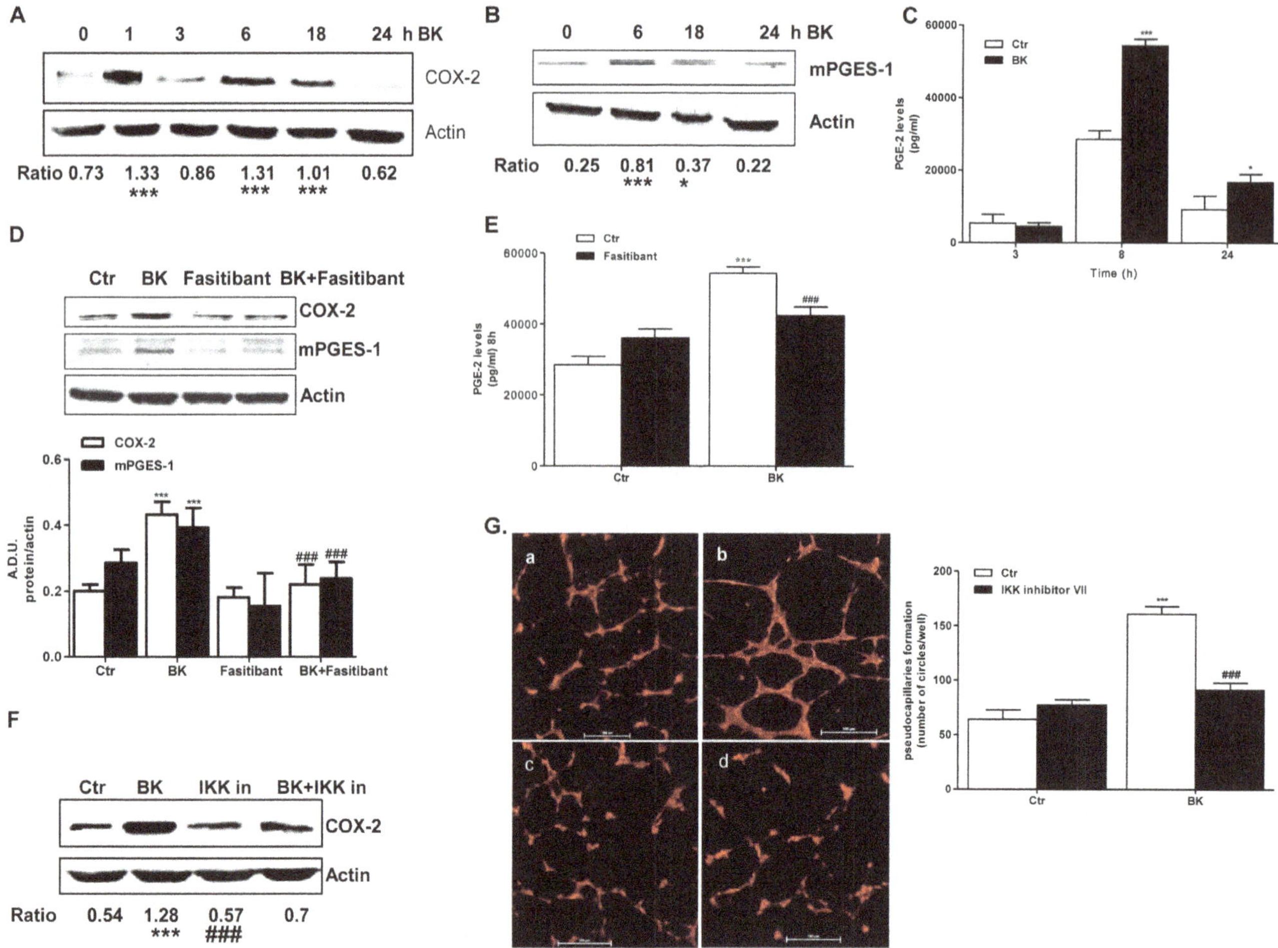

Figure 6. Fasitibant suppresses BK-induced COX-2 signaling. (A–B) COX-2 and mPGES-1 expression (western blot) in HUVEC treated with BK (1 μM) for the indicated times. Gels are representative of three experiments. The ratio between COX-2 or mPGES-1 over actin is reported. *p<0.05, ***p<0.001, compared to untreated cells. (C) PGE-2 release in the conditioned medium of HUVEC treated with BK (1 μM) for the indicated times. All PGE-2 release experiments in this paper were performed in archidonic acid pre-treated cells. Numbers represent mean ± SEM of three experiments. *p<0.05, ***p<0.001, compared to untreated cells; (D) COX-2 and mPGES-1 expression in HUVEC treated with BK (1 μM, 6 hrs) with/without fasitibant (1 μM). Gels are representative of three experiments. Graphs represent the optical densities related to the ratio between COX-2 or mPGES-1 over actin. A.D.U. (arbitrary density unit), numbers represent mean ± SD of three experiments ***p<0.001, compared to untreated cells; ###P<0.001 to BK-treated cells. (E) PGE-2 release from HUVEC treated with BK (1 μM) in presence/absence of fasitibant (1 μM), for 8 hrs; Numbers represent mean ± SEM of three experiments. ***p<0.001, compared to untreated cells; ###P<0.001 to BK-treated cells; (F) COX-2 expression (western blot) in HUVEC pretreated for 30 min with IKK inhibitor VII (0.2 μM), and treated with BK (1 μM, 6 hrs). Gel is representative of three experiments. The ratio between COX-2 over actin is reported. ***p<0.001 compared to untreated cells; ###P<0.001 to BK-treated cells. (G) Representative pictures and quantification of pseudocapillary formation in Matrigel by HUVEC exposed to 0.1% FBS (panel a), BK (1 μM, panel b), IKK inhibitor VII (0.2 μM, panel c) with or without BK (1 μM, panel d), observed at 12 hrs after cell seeding. Quantification was obtained as above, ***p<0.001, compared to untreated cells; ###P<0.001 to BK-treated cells. Numbers represent mean ± SEM of three experiments.

Equal amounts (50 μg) of protein were separated by SDS-PAGE onto a gradient 4–12% gel and transferred to a nitrocellulose membrane. The membranes were blocked (1 h) in a solution of 5% (wt/vol) milk and then incubated overnight at 4°C with the primary antibodies: anti-B2 Receptor, anti- p-β catenin (Ser33, 37/Thr41), anti-COX-2, anti-phospho-p65 and anti-p65 (each 1:1000) or anti mPGES-1 (1:200) and normalized for β-Actin (1:10,000), H2A (1:1000, for nuclear fraction) or β catenin (1:1000). After 1 hr incubation in a secondary antibody anti IgG HRP (diluted 1:2500, Promega), the immunoreaction were revealed by chemioluminescence.

Permeability

HUVEC were seeded at 1×10^5 on collagen-coated insert membranes (Corning) with 0.4 μm diameter pores, and the inserts were placed in a 12 multiwell plate, for 48 h. Monolayers were treated with BK (0.1–1–10 μM) with/without fasitibant (0.1–1–10 μM), then a 40 kDa FITC-Dextran (10 μM), was added on top of cells, allowing the fluorescent molecules to pass through the cell monolayer. The extent of permeability was determined in a time range (0–45 min) by measuring the fluorescence in a plate reader (Tecan), at 485/535 nm, excitation/emission, respectively. Arbitrary values were plotted against time.

Immunofluorescence

Cells were cultured on coverslips, treated with BK 1 or 10 μM in presence/absence of fasitibant and then fixed in paraformaldheyde 4% or cold acetone (5 min), washed in PBS and incubated with BSA 3% (45 min). Cells were then incubated for 16 hrs with anti- ZO-1 (1:50) or anti-p65 (1:40) or anti-VE-cadherin (1:60)

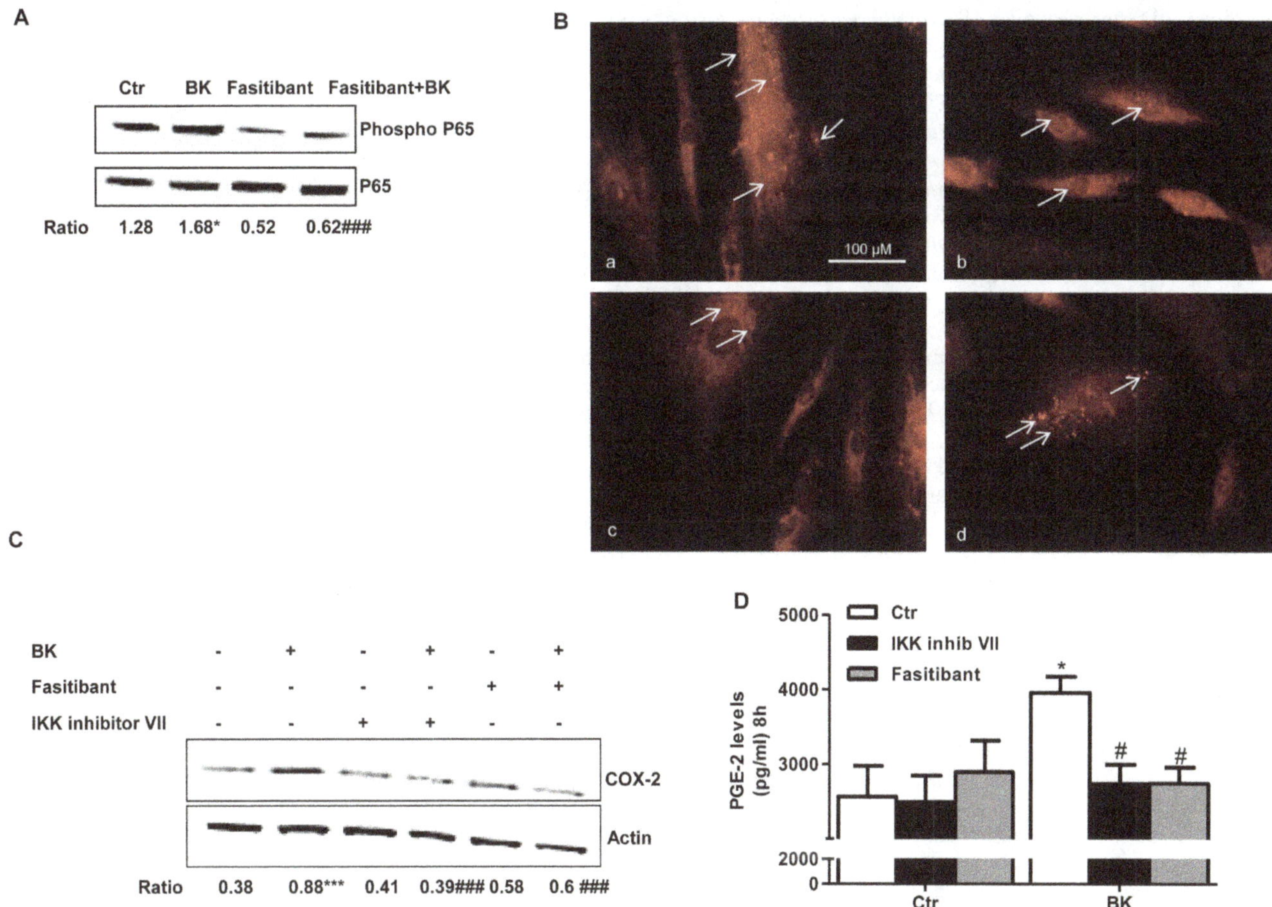

Figure 7. BK stimulates translocation/phosphorylation of NF-κB in circulating proangiogenic cells. (A) p65 (NF-κB) phosphorylation following exposure to BK (1 μM, 15 min) in presence/absence of fasitibant (0.1 μM). Gel are representative of three experiments. The ratio between p-p65 over p65 is reported. *p<0.05 compared to untreated cells; ###P<0.001 to BK-treated cells. (B) Immunofluorescence (40 X) of NF-κB translocation in PACs in 0.1% FBS (a), BK (1 μM) (b), fasitibant (0.1 μM,) (c), fasitibant+BK (d). Bar = 100 μM. (C) COX-2 expression in human hematopoietic progenitor cells pretreated for 30 min with IKK inhibitor VII (0.2 μM) or with fasitibant (0.1 μM), and treated with BK (1 μM, 6 hrs). Gel is representative of three experiments. The ratio between COX-2 over actin is reported. ***p<0.001 compared to untreated cells; ###P<0.001 to BK-treated cells. (D) PGE-2 release from PACs treated with BK (1 μM) in presence/absence of fasitibant (0.1 μM) or IKK inhibitor VII (0.2 μM), for 8 hrs. Numbers represent mean ± SEM of three experiments. *p<0.01, compared to untreated cells; #P<0.01 to BK-treated cells.

antibodies, in PBS containing 0.5% BSA. After incubation with the secondary antibody anti-Mouse IgG FITC (ZO-1) or anti-Rabbit IgG TRICT, (p65 and VE-cadherin) (1 h), cells were washed and the coverslips mounted with Mowioll 4–88 (Calbiochem) and images of cells were taken using a Nikon Eclipse TE 300 inverted microscope by a digital camera and NIS Element software (for ZO-1, VE-cadherin and p65, images at 20–60 X magnification) or using a confocal microscope Zeiss LSM700 (VE-cadherin, at 60 X magnification).

BrDU Labeling Assay

Cell proliferation was determined by 5-bromo-2′-deoxy-uridine (BrdU) incorporation using a colorimetric ELISA according to the manufacturer's instructions (Roche). Briefly, 1.5×10^3 cells were seeded in 96 multiplate. After 24 hrs cells were incubated with BK (0.1–1–10 μM) in the presence/absence of fasitibant (0.1–1 μM) for 10 hrs. BrdU was added during the late stage (4 h) of incubation. Stained cells were counted with a light microscope (Nikon Eclipse E400) at 20 X magnification. Data are reported as BrdU labeled cell/well.

Wound Assay

Endothelial cells were seeded into 24-well plates (1×10^5 cells/well) and incubated for 24 h to grow into a confluent monolayer. Then, the monolayer was scraped using a sterile 20–200 μl micropipette tip to create a wound of ±1 mm width. The cells were washed twice with PBS and fresh medium containing test substances (BK: 0.1–1–10 μM, with/without fasitibant 1 μM) was added with ARA-C (2.5 μg/ml) to inhibit cell proliferation. Images of the wound in each well were acquired from 0 to 12 hrs under a phase contrast microscope at 20 X magnification. Results are expressed as area of migrated cells, 12 h vs. time 0. After 12 h, the cells were stained with Hoechst 33342, and images were obtained using as described above.

In vitro Angiogenesis Model

HUVEC were pre-treated with IKK inhibitor VII (0.2 μM for 30 min) and then exposed to BK (1 μM) or treated with fasitibant (1 μM) in presence/absence of BK. Cells were then plated onto a thin layer (300 μl) of basement membrane matrix (Matrigel; BD Biosciences) in 24-well plates at 6×10^4 cells/well in EBM. After 12 h, the medium was removed and the cells were fixed, and stained using DY554 phalloidin (Thermo Fisher Scientific) for F-actin. Images of cells were obtained as reported above. Quantification of tubular structures and photomicrographs were performed as previously described [38].

Sprouting Formation *in vitro*

Cytodex microcarrier beads (500 mg) (Sigma) were swollen in 100 µl PBS (2 h) and then autoclaved (121°C, 20 min). 3×10^5 HUVEC were seeded onto 1.000 cytodex microcarrier beads in 0.5 ml of EGM, 20% FBS. The mixture was incubated at 37°C to allow cell attachment and shaken every 30 min for 6 h. The HUVEC-coated beads were washed in serum free medium and added to 2.5 mg/ml fibrinogen solution. 15 µl of mixture were plated in 12 well plate in the presence of thrombin allowing the polymerization at room temperature. The gel was maintained with medium supplemented with 1% FBS. HUVEC, were treated with BK in presence/absence of fasitibant. Experiment was maintained for 4 days. Data are reported as quantification of total length of pseudocapillary like structures.

In vivo Matrigel Angiogenesis Assay

This study was carried out in strict accordance with the recommendations in the Guide for the Care and Use of Laboratory Animals of the University of Siena (Polo Scientifico San Miniato). The protocol was approved by the Committee on the Ethics of Animal Experiments of the Azienda Ospedaliera Universitaria Senese (Permit Number: D-08032010). Further, all procedures were carried out in accordance with the Italian law (Legislative Decree no. 116, 27 January 1992), which acknowledges the European Directive 86/609/EEC. Injection of matrigel was performed without anesthesia, and all efforts were made to minimize suffering. Mice were sacrified with carbon dioxyde.

Similarly, for the Osteoarthritis assay (see below), all animal care and experimental procedures were conducted in compliance with the principles and guidelines of the European Union (2010/63/UE) and the Italian government regulations, and approved by the ethical committee of Menarini Ricerche.

C57 black mice (20–25 g) were kept in temperature- and humidity-controlled rooms (22°C, 50%) with lights on from 07:00 to 19:00, water and food available ad libitum. BK and fasitibant were diluted in Matrigel (Becton Dickinson, growth factors and phenol red-free) on ice to a final concentration of 1 µg/ml and 1 µM, respectively. C57/B6J mice (12 week old) were subcutaneously injected in the dorsal midline region with 0.5 ml of Matrigel alone or with Matrigel containing the stimuli. After 10 days mice were euthanized and implants harvested. Plugs were resuspended in 1 ml of Drabkin's solution for 18 h at 4°C. Hemoglobin concentration was determined by absorbance at 540 nm and compared with a standard curve (Sigma).

Induction of Osteoarthritis in Rats

Osteoarthritis was induced by intra-articular (i.ar.) injection of monosodium iodoacetate (MIA) solution in the knee joint [21,22]. Male rats (Wistar, 250–280 g, Harlan laboratories) were divided in 4 groups (five animal for group), anesthetized with pentobarbital (40 mg/kg, 3 ml/kg i.p.) and treated with a single i.ar. injection of saline (control, 25 µl), MIA (1 mg/25 µl), fasitibant (10 µg/25), or MIA+fasitibant into the joint space of both knees. I.ar. injections were performed through the intrapatellar ligament after shaving the skin, and was followed by a gentle flexion of the knee. Solutions were prepared under sterile conditions and injected by using a 50-µl Hamilton microliter syringe with a 6-mm, 27-gauge needle that was inserted into the joint for approximately 2 to 3 mm. After three days, animals were anesthetized with urethane (1.2 g/kg, i.p.): synovial fluid was washed out from right knee and the synovial capsule obtained from the left knee. The synovial fluid washing was performed with 100 µl of saline, and the recovered volume centrifuged (5 min at 4°C at 10,000 g) and conserved at −80°C for VEGF and PGE-2 measurements. The synovial capsule was embedded in Tissue-Tek O.C.T. (Sakura, San Marcos, USA), for histology. The doses of MIA and fasitibant were selected on the basis of previous experiments [21,22].

Immunohistochemical Analysis

Six-µm-thick cryostat sections from tissue samples were processed for immunohistochemical and hematoxylin and eosin staining. For histopathological analysis of CD31 or CD133 we used hematoxylin and immunohistochemical staining. After inactivating of endogenous peroxidase activity and blocking of cross-reactivity with 3% BSA the sections were incubated at 4°C for 18 h with a diluted solution of CD31 (1:120, Millipore) or CD133 (1:70, Boster immunoleader). Location of the primary antibodies was achieved by subsequent application of a biotin-conjugated antiprimary antibody, a streptavidin-peroxidase and diaminobenzidine (Sigma). The staining was developed using a commercial immunoperoxidase staining kit following the manufacturer's instruction (the biotin–streptavidin complex method, Millipore). The slides were counter-stained with hematoxylin. Negative controls were established by replacing the primary antibody with PBS. Specific staining for CD31 or CD133 was categorized as either positive or negative based on the presence of brown-color staining. Images were analyzed using Nikon Eclypse T200 (20x magnification). Quantification of CD31 was performed counting 10 random field/section for slides.

Immuno-assays for VEGF

Quantification of rat VEGF in the synovial fluid was determined by ELISA using a Rat Quantikine kit (R&D System). Synovial fluid diluted (1:5) in the standard diluents, was treated with hyaluronidase (600 U) for 1 h at 37°C on a shaker before measurements and assayed as indicated in manufacturer's instructions. Results are expressed as pg/ml.

PGE-2 EIA Kit

PGE-2 was measured by an EIA kit (ENZO lifetech). Cells were exposed to BK (3, 8 or 24 h) in presence/absence of fasitibant and treated with 10 µM arachidonic acid (AA). Cell culture supernatants were assayed at a final dilution of 1:10. PACs were exposed to BK (8 h) in presence/absence of fasitibant and treated with 10 µM arachidonic acid (AA); cell culture supernatant was assayed as indicated in manufacturer's instructions. PGE-2 was expressed as [pg/ml], normalized to total protein concentration.

Data Analysis and Statistical Procedures

Results are either representative or average of at least three independent experiments done in triplicate. Statistical analysis was performed using ANOVA test, Bonferroni test and t test for unpaired data (Prism, GraphPad). $P<0.05$ was considered statistically significant.

Supporting Information

Figure S1 BK stimulation does not change BR1 or BR2 mRNA expression. (A) mRNA expression for B1 and B2 receptors in HUVEC treated with 0.1% FBS (first lane), 10% FBS (second lane) or BK (1 µM, third lane). The ratio between B2R over GAPDH is reported.

Figure S2 BK-induced changes of endothelial junctions signals and β-catenin phosphorylation are blocked by fasitibant in HUVEC. (A) Graphs represent the percentage of positive cells for VEC (leftt graph) or ZO-1 (right graph) immunofluorescence. (B) Graphs represent the optical densities related to the ratio between phospho-β catenin over β catenin. A.D.U. (arbitrary density unit), **p<0.01 and ***p<0.001 versus control, ###p<0.001 versus BK. Numbers represent mean ± SD of three experiments.

Figure S3 Fasitibant impairs endothelial cell growth and migration. (A) Cells were exposed to BK (1 μM), or to BK in presence/absence of fasitibant (0.1–1 μM) for 10 hrs and growth was evaluated by BrdU incorporation. Data are reported as cell number counted/well. Numbers represent mean ± SEM of three experiments run in triplicate. (B) Scratch wound healing assay on HUVEC treated with 0.1% FBS (a), BK (1 μM) (b), fasitibant (1 μM) (c), fasitibant+BK (d). (C) Quantification of cell migration was reported as area of migrated cells. ***p<0.001, compared to untreated cells; ###p<0.001 to BK-treated cells. Numbers represent mean ± SEM of three experiments run in triplicate.

Figure S4 BK-induced angiogenesis *in vitro* is reduced by B2R blockade. (A) Representative pictures of microcarrier-HUVEC in 0.1% FBS (a), exposed to BK (1 μM) (b), to fasitibant (1 μM) (c), to fasitibant+BK (d). (B) Quantification of sprouting lenght (μm); Numbers represent mean ± SEM of three experiments run in triplicate. ***p<0.001, compared to untreated cells; ###p<0.001 to BK-treated cells. (C) Representative pictures of capillary structures (diameter) in microcarrier-HUVEC treated with BK (1 μM, panel a) in presence/absence of fasitibant (1 μM, panel b). (D) Quantificationof sprouting diameter (μm); Numbers represent mean ± SEM of three experiments run in triplicate. ***p<0.001, compared to untreated cells; ###p<0.001 to BK-treated cells.

Figure S5 BK stimulates translocation/activation of NF-κB in HUVEC. (A–B) Graphs represent the optical densities related to the ratio between nuclear p65 over H2A, or cytoplasmic p65 over actin. A.D.U. (arbitrary density unit), numbers represent mean ± SD of three experiments. (A) Comparison between: cytoplasmic vs. nuclear fraction at time: 0 p<0.001, 30 min p<0.05, 60 min p<0.001; BK treatment vs. ctr in nuclear or cytoplasmic fraction at time:5 min p<0.001, 15 min p<0.001 and 30 min p<0.001. (B) Comparison between: cytoplasmic vs. nuclear fraction in control (0.1% FBS) condition p<0.001; BK treatment vs. ctr in nuclear or cytoplasmic fraction p<0.001, co-treatment between fasitibant and BK vs. BK p<0.001.

Figure S6 B2R expression in human circulating proangiogenic cells. Western blot analysis of B2 receptor in human circulating proangiogenic cells treated with 0.1% FBS (Ctr) or BK (1 μM) for 24 h. (Experiments are run three time; n = 3). The ratio between B2R over actin is reported.

Author Contributions

Conceived and designed the experiments: ET SM MZ AG SD. Performed the experiments: ET PC C. Catalani C. Caldai. Analyzed the data: ET SM AG MZ SD. Contributed reagents/materials/analysis tools: SM PC C. Catalani CAM. Wrote the paper: ET AG MZ SD.

References

1. Orsenigo F, Giampietro C, Ferrari A, Corada M, Galaup A, et al (2012) Phosphorylation of VE-cadherin is modulated by haemodynamic forces and contributes to the regulation of vascular permeability in vivo. Nat Commun 3: 1208.
2. Shaw OM, Harper JL (2011) Bradykinin receptor 2 extends inflammatory cell recruitment in a model of acute gouty arthritis. Biochem Biophys Res Commun 416: 266–9.
3. Wieczorek M, Pilyawskaya A, Burkard M, Zuzack JS, Jones SW, et al (1997). Bradykinin Antagonists in human systems: correlation between receptor binding, calcium signalling in isolated cells, and functional activity in isolated ileum. Biochemical Pharmacology 54: 283–291.
4. Morbidelli L, Parenti A, Giovannelli L, Granger HJ, Ledda F, et al (1998) B1 receptor involvement in the effect of bradykinin on venular endothelial cell proliferation and potentiation of FGF-2 effects. Br J Pharmacol 124: 1286–1292.
5. Parenti A, Morbidelli L, Ledda F, Granger HJ, Ziche M (2001) The bradykinin/B1 receptor promotes angiogenesis by up-regulation of endogenous FGF-2 in endothelium via the nitric oxide synthase pathway. FASEB J 15: 1487–98.
6. Cao T, Brain SD, Khodr B, Khalil Z (2002) B1 and B2 antagonists and bradykinin-induced blood flow in rat skin inflammation. Inflamm Res 51: 295–9.
7. Bas M (2012) Clinical efficacy of icatibant in the treatment of acute hereditary angioedema during the FAST-3 trial. Expert Rev Clin Immunol 8: 707–17.
8. Bond AP, Lemon M, Dieppe PA, Bhoola KD (1997) Generation of kinins in synovial fluid from patients with arthropathy. Immunopharmacol 36: 209–216.
9. Meini S, Maggi CA (2008) Knee osteoarthritis: a role for bradykinin? Inflamm Res 57: 351–61.
10. Bellucci F, Cucchi P, Catalani C, Giuliani S, Meini S, et al (2009) Novel effects mediated by bradykinin and pharmacological characterization of bradykinin B2 receptor antagonism in human synovial fibroblasts. Br J Pharmacol 158: 1996–2004.
11. Meini S, Cucchi P, Catalani C, Bellucci F, Giuliani S, et al (2011a) Bradykinin and B(2) receptor antagonism in rat and human articular chondrocytes. Br J Pharmacol 162: 611–622.
12. Leeb-Lundberg LM, Marceau F, Muller-Esterl W, Pettibone DJ, Zuraw BL (2005) International union of pharmacology XLV. Classification of the kinin receptor family: from molecular mechanisms to pathophysiological consequences. Pharmacol Rev 57: 27–77.
13. Fincham CI, Bressan A, Paris M, Rossi C, Fattori D (2009) Bradykinin receptor antagonists-a review of the patent literature 2005–2008. Expert Opin Ther Pat 19: 919–41.
14. Charignon D, Späth P, Martin L, Drouet C (2012) Icatibant, the bradykinin B2 receptor antagonist with target to the interconnected kinin systems. Expert Opin Pharmacother 13: 2233–47.
15. Cucchi P, Meini S, Bressan A, Catalani C, Bellucci F, et al (2005) MEN16132, a novel potent and selective nonpeptide antagonist for the human bradykinin B2 receptor. In vitro pharmacology and molecular characterization. Eur J Pharmacol 528:7–16.
16. Meini S, Cucchi P, Bellucci F, Catalani C, Giuliani S, et al (2007) Comparative antagonist pharmacology at the native mouse bradykinin B2 receptor: radioligand binding and smooth muscle contractility studies. Br J Pharmacol 150: 313–20.
17. Meini S, Cucchi P, Catalani C, Bellucci F, Giuliani S, P etal (2009) Pharmacological characterization of the bradykinin B2 receptor antagonist MEN16132 in rat in vitro bioassays. Eur J Pharmacol 615: 10–6.
18. Meini S, Cucchi P, Catalani C, Bellucci F, Santicioli P, et al (2010) Radioligand binding characterization of the bradykinin B(2) receptor in the rabbit and pig ileal smooth muscle. Eur J Pharmacol 635: 34–9.
19. Valenti C, Cialdai C, Giuliani S, Tramontana M, Quartara L, et al (2008) MEN16132, a kinin B2 receptor antagonist, prevents the endogenous bradykinin effects in guinea-pig airways. Eur J Pharmacol 579: 350–6.
20. Valenti C, Giuliani S, Cialdai C, Tramontana M, Maggi CA (2010) Anti-inflammatory synergy of MEN16132, a kinin B2 receptor antagonist, and dexamethasone in carrageenan-induced knee joint arthritis in rats. Br J Pharmacol 161: 1616–27.
21. Cialdai C, Giuliani S, Valenti C, Tramontana M, Maggi CA (2009) Effect of Intra-articular4-(S)-amino-5-(4-{4-[2,4-dichloro-3-(2,4-dimethyl-8-quinolyloxy-methyl)phenylsulfo namido]-tetrahydro-2H-4-pyranylcarbonyl} piperazino)-5-oxopentyl](trimethyl)ammonium chloride hydrochloride (MEN16132), a kinin B2 receptor antagonist, on nociceptive response in monosodium iodoacetate-induced experimental osteoarthritis in rats. J Pharmacol Exp Ther 331: 1025–32.
22. Gomis A, Meini S, Miralles A, Valenti C, Giuliani S, et al, (2013) Blockade of nociceptive sensory afferent activity of the rat knee joint by the bradykinin B2 receptor antagonist fasitibant. Osteoarthritis Cartilage 21: 1346–1354.
23. Walsh DA, Haywood L (2001) Angiogenesis: a therapeutic target in arthritis. Curr Opin Investig Drugs 2: 1054–63.

24. Haywood L, McWilliams DF, Pearson CI, Gill SE, Ganesan A, et al (2003) Inflammation and angiogenesis in osteoarthritis. Arthritis Rheum 48: 2173–7.
25. Walsh DA, Bonnet CS, Turner EL, Wilson D, Situ M, et al (2007) Angiogenesis in the synovium and at the osteochondral junction in osteoarthritis. Osteoarthritis Cartilage 15: 743–51.
26. Carmeliet P, Jain RK (2000) Angiogenesis in cancer and other diseases. Nature 407: 249–57.
27. Spinetti G, Fortunato O, Cordella D, Portararo P, Kränkel N, et al (2011) Tissue kallikrein is essential for invasive capacity of circulating proangiogenic cells. Circ Res 108: 284–93.
28. Frimm Cde, Sun Y, Weber KT (1996) Wound healing following myocardial infarction in the rat: role for bradykinin and prostaglandins. J. Mol. Cell Cardiol. 28: 1279–1285.
29. Weis SM, Cheresh DA (2005) Pathophysiological consequences of VEGF-induced vascular permeability. Nature 437: 497–504.
30. Taddei A, Giampietro C, Conti A, Orsenigo F, Breviario F, et al (2008) Endothelial adherens junctions control tight junctions by VE-cadherin-mediated upregulation of claudin-5. Nat Cell Biol 10: 923–34.
31. Pober JS, Sessa WC (2007) Evolving functions of endothelial cells in inflammation. Nat Rev Immunol 7: 803–15.
32. Finetti F, Donnini S, Giachetti A, Morbidelli L, Ziche M (2009) Prostaglandin E(2) primes the angiogenic switch via a synergic interaction with the fibroblast growth factor-2 pathway. Circ Res 105: 657–66.
33. Meini S, Bellucci F, Catalani C, Cucchi P, Giolitti A, et al (2011b) Comparison of the molecular interactions of two antagonists, MEN16132 or icatibant, at the human kinin B2 receptor. Br J Pharmacol 162: 1202–1212.
34. Barnes PJ, Karin M (1997) Nuclear factor-kappa B: a pivotal transcription factor in chronic inflammatory diseases. N Engl J Med 336: 1066–1071.
35. Tak PP, Firestein GS (2001) NF-kappa B: a key role in inflammatory diseases. J Clin Invest 107: 7–11.
36. Tirziu D, Jaba IM, Yu P, Larrivée B, Coon BG, et al (2012) Endothelial nuclear factor-κB-dependent regulation of arteriogenesis and branching. Circulation 126: 2589–600.
37. Wohlfart P, Dedio J, Wirth K, Schölkens BA, Wiemer G (1997) Different B1 kinin receptor expression and pharmacology in endothelial cells of different origins and species. J Pharmacol Exp Ther 280: 1109–16.
38. Donnini S, Solito R, Cetti E, Corti F, Giachetti A, et al (2010) Abeta peptides accelerate the senescence of endothelial cells in vitro and in vivo, impairing angiogenesis. FASEB J 24: 2385–95.

13

The CCL2/CCR2 Axis Enhances Vascular Cell Adhesion Molecule-1 Expression in Human Synovial Fibroblasts

Yu-Min Lin[1,2], Chin-Jung Hsu[3,4], Yuan-Ya Liao[5], Ming-Chih Chou[1]*, Chih-Hsin Tang[6,7]*

1 Institute of Medicine, Chung Shan Medical University, Taichung, Taiwan, 2 Department of Orthopedic Surgery, Taichung Veterans General Hospital, Taichung, Taiwan, 3 School of Chinese Medicine, China Medical University, Taichung, Taiwan, 4 Department of Orthopaedics, China Medical University Hospital, Taichung, Taiwan, 5 Department of Surgery, Chung Shan Medical University Hospital, Taichung, Taiwan, 6 Department of Pharmacology, School of Medicine, China Medical University, Taichung, Taiwan, 7 Graduate Institute of Basic Medical Science, China Medical University, Taichung, Taiwan

Abstract

Background: Chemokine ligand 2 (CCL2), also known as monocyte chemoattractant protein-1 (MCP-1), belongs to the CC chemokine family that is associated with the disease status and outcomes of osteoarthritis (OA). Here, we investigated the intracellular signaling pathways involved in CCL2-induced vascular cell adhesion molecule-1 (VCAM-1) expression in human OA synovial fibroblasts (OASFs).

Methodology/Principal Findings: Stimulation of OASFs with CCL2 induced VCAM-1 expression. CCL2-mediated VCAM-1 expression was attenuated by CCR2 inhibitor (RS102895), PKCδ inhibitor (rottlerin), p38MAPK inhibitor (SB203580), and AP-1 inhibitors (curcumin and tanshinone IIA). Stimulation of cells with CCL2 increased PKCδ and p38MAPK activation. Treatment of OASFs with CCL2 also increased the c-Jun phosphorylation and c-Jun binding to the AP-1 element on the VCAM-1 promoter. Moreover, CCL2-mediated CCR2, PKCδ, p38MAPK, and AP-1 pathway promoted the adhesion of monocytes to the OASFs monolayer.

Conclusions/Significance: Our results suggest that CCL2 increases VCAM-1 expression in human OASFs via the CCR2, PKCδ, p38MAPK, c-Jun, and AP-1 signaling pathway. The CCL2-induced VCAM-1 expression promoted monocytes adhesion to human OASFs.

Editor: Sebastian Grundmann, University Hospital Freiburg, Germany

Funding: This work was supported by grants from the National Science Council of Taiwan (NSC99-2320 B 039 003 MY3 and NSC100-2320-B-039-028-MY3). The funders had no role in study design, data collection and analysis, decision to publish, or preparation of the manuscript.

Competing Interests: The authors have declared that no competing interests exist.

* E-mail: chtang@mail.cmu.edu.tw (CHT); cshe032@csh.org.tw (MCC)

Introduction

Osteoarthritis (OA) is a chronic joint disorder characterized by slow progressive degeneration of articular cartilage, subchondral bone alteration, and variable secondary synovial inflammation. In response to macrophage-derived proinflammatory cytokines such as interleukin (IL)-1β and tumor necrosis factor-α (TNF-α), OA synovial fibroblasts (OASFs) produce chemokines that promote inflammation, neovascularization, and cartilage degradation via activation of matrix-degrading enzymes such as matrix metalloproteinases (MMPs) [1,2]. Although the pathogenesis of the disease remains elusive, there is increasing evidence indicating that mononuclear cells migration plays an important role in the perpetuation of inflammation in synovium [3,4]. Adhesion and infiltration of mononuclear cells to inflammatory sites are regulated by adhesion molecules, such as vascular adhesion molecule-1 (VCAM-1) [5,6].

Cell adhesion molecules are transmembranes glycoprotein that mediates cell-cell and cell-extracellular matrix interactions. VCAM-1 has recently emerged as a highly significant predictor of the risk of OA [7,8]. Up-regulation of VCAM-1 has been shown in the synovial lining of OA patients by immunohistochemical staining and in cultured human OASFs by Western blotting [7,8]. Reducing the levels of VCAM-1 in synovial fluid may suppress the inflammatory response in knee OA [9]. VCAM-1 is involved in the process of infiltration of synovium with mononuclear cells leading to the initiation and progression of the disease. However, the molecular mechanisms by which cytokines induce VCAM-1 expression in human OASFs remain unclear.

Chemokines are low molecular weight secretory proteins that can regulate the chemotaxis and metabolic activity of specific leukocyte subsets. Monocyte chemoattractant protein 1 (MCP-1)/chemokine ligand 2 (CCL2), a ligand of CCR2, is chemotactic for monocyte/macrophages and activated T cells [10,11]. It was reported that the levels of CCL2 are increased in the blood, synovial fluid, and synovial tissue of patients with OA and rheumatoid arthritis (RA) [12,13]. Injection of CCL2 into rabbit joints resulted in marked macrophage infiltration in the affected joint [14]. Treatment with CCL2 antagonist before disease onset in an MRL/lpr mouse model of arthritis was shown to prevent the onset of arthritis [15]. These data suggest that CCL2 plays an important role during OA pathogenesis.

Although the roles of cytokines and adhesion molecules in polymorphonuclear cells adhesion to endothelial cells have been described in detail, little is known about the mechanisms underlying the interaction between monocytes and human OASFs. Previous studies have shown that CCL2 plays important role in OA pathogenesis [16,17]. In the present study, we explored the possible intracellular signaling pathways involved in CCL2-induced VCAM-1 expression in human OASFs. The results show that CCL2 activates the CCR2 receptor which in turn activates protein kinase Cδ (PKCδ), p38MAPK, and AP-1 signaling pathway, leading to the upregulation of VCAM-1 expression. The increased VCAM-1 expression correlates with enhanced adhesion of monocytes to CCL2-stimulated OASFs.

Materials and Methods

Materials

Protein A/G beads; anti-mouse and anti-rabbit IgG-conjugated horseradish peroxidase; rabbit polyclonal antibodies specific for PKCδ, p38MAPK, p-p38MAPK(Tyr182) (sc-7973), c-Jun, p-c-Jun(Ser73) (sc-16311-R), and β-actin; and siRNA against PKCδ and c-Jun were purchased from Santa Cruz Biotechnology (Santa Cruz, CA, USA). Rabbit polyclonal antibody specific for PKCδ phosphorylated at Tyr^{331} was purchased from Cell Signaling and Neuroscience (Danvers, MA, USA). Rottlerin, GF109203X, SB203580, curcumin, and tanshinone IIA were purchased from Calbiochem (San Diego, CA, USA). Recombinant human CCL2 was purchased from R&D Systems (Minneapolis, MN, USA). The p38MAPK dominant negative mutant was provided by Dr. J. Han (University of Texas South-western Medical Center, Dallas, TX). All other chemicals were obtained from Sigma-Aldrich (St. Louis, MO, USA).

Cell Cultures

The study protocol was approved by the Institutional Review Board of China Medical University Hospital, and all subjects gave informed written consent before enrollment. Human synovial fibroblasts were isolated using collagenase treatment of synovial tissues obtained from knee replacement surgeries of 33 patients with OA and 15 samples of normal synovial tissues obtained at arthroscopy from trauma/joint derangement. The synovial fluid concentration of CCL2 was measured with an enzyme-linked immunosorbent assay (ELISA) according to the protocol provided by the manufacturer (Human CCL2 ELISA kit; R&D systems, Minneapolis, MN). OASFs were isolated, cultured, and characterized as previously described [18,19]. Experiments were performed using cells from passages 3 to 6.

THP-1, a human leukemia cell line of monocyte/macrophage lineage, was obtained from American Type Culture Collection (Manassas, VA, USA) and grown in RPMI-1640 medium with 10% fetal bovine serum.

Quantitative Real-time PCR

Total RNA was extracted from OASFs using a TRIzol kit (MDBio Inc., Taipei, Taiwan). The reverse transcription reaction was performed using 2 μg of total RNA that was reverse transcribed into cDNA using oligo (dT) primer [20,21]. The quantitative real-time PCR (qPCR) analysis was carried out using Taqman® one-step PCR Master Mix (Applied Biosystems, Foster City, CA). cDNA templates (2 μl) were added per 25-μl reaction with sequence-specific primers and Taqman® probes. Sequences for all target gene primers and probes were purchased commercially (β-actin was used as internal control) (Applied Biosystems). The qPCR assays were carried out in triplicate on an StepOnePlus sequence detection system. The cycling conditions involved 10-min polymerase activation at 95°C, followed by 40 cycles at 95°C for 15 s and 60°C for 60 s. The threshold was set above the non-template control background and within the linear phase of the target gene amplification to calculate the cycle number at which the transcript was detected (denoted CT). Reactions were normalized to copies of β-actin mRNA within the same sample using the $-\Delta\Delta CT$ method. The levels of mRNA are expressed as the fold change in expression level compared with that of controls.

Western Blot Analysis

Cellular lysates were prepared as described previously [22,23]. Proteins (30 μg) were resolved on SDS-PAGE and transferred to immobilon polyvinyldifluoride (PVDF) membranes. The blots were blocked with 4% BSA for 1 h at room temperature and then probed with rabbit anti-human antibodies against PKCδ, VCAM-1, p38MAPK, or p-p38MAPK (β-actin was used as loading control) (1:1000) for 1 h at room temperature. After three washes, the blots were subsequently incubated with donkey anti-rabbit peroxidase-conjugated secondary antibody (1:1000) for 1 h at room temperature. The blots were visualized by enhanced chemiluminescence with Kodak X-OMAT LS film (Eastman Kodak, Rochester, NY).

Flow Cytometry Analysis

Human synovial fibroblasts were plated in six-well dishes. The cells were then washed with PBS and detached with trypsin at 37°C. Cells were fixed for 10 min in PBS containing 1% paraformaldehyde. After being rinsed in PBS, the cells were incubated with mouse anti-human antibody against VCAM-1 (1:100) for 1 h at 4°C. Cells were then washed again and incubated with fluorescein isothiocyanate-conjugated goat anti-mouse secondary IgG (1:100; Leinco Technologies Inc., St. Louis, MO, USA) for 45 min (Isogenic control antibody was used to detect the background fluorescence) and analyzed by flow cytometry using FACS Calibur (10000 cells were collected for each experiment) and CellQuest software (BD Biosciences).

Transfection of siRNAs

ON-TARGETplus siRNA of PKCδ, c-Jun, and control were purchased from Dharmacon Research (Lafayette, CO). Transient transfection of siRNAs was carried out using Lipofectamine 2000 transfection reagent. siRNA (100 nM) was formulated with Lipofectamine 2000 transfection reagent according to the manufacturer's instruction.

Cell Adhesion Assay

THP-1 cells were labeled with BCECF-AM (10 μM) at 37°C for 1 h in RPMI-1640 medium and subsequently washed by centrifugation. OASFs grown on glass coverslips were incubated with CCL2 for 6 h. Confluent CCL2-treated OASFs were incubated with THP-1 cells (2×10^6 cells/ml) at 37°C for 1 h. Non-adherent THP-1 cells were then removed and gently washed with PBS. The number of adherent THP-1 cells was counted in four randomly chosen fields per well at 200X high power using a fluorescence microscope (Zeiss, Axiovert 200 M).

Chromatin Immunoprecipitation Assay

Chromatin immunoprecipitation analysis was performed as described previously [24]. DNA immunoprecipitated by anti-c-Jun antibody was purified. The DNA was then extracted with phenol-chloroform. The purified DNA pellet was subjected to PCR, and PCR products were resolved using 1.5% agarose gel electrophoresis and visualized by UV light. The primer 5′-CGGTTAAATCTCACAGCCCA-3′ and the reverse primer 5′-TTCTCTTACAAGAGAAAGGA-3′ (−403 to −30; contain AP-

1 binding site). The forward primer 5′-CCAATGGGGGAGA-TAGACCT-3′) and the reverse primer 5′-ACCGCAAACC-CAGTTAAAAA-3′ (−1015 to −775; dose not contain AP-1 binding site) (MDBio Inc., Taipei, Taiwan) were specifically designed to correspond to the VCAM-1 promoter region [24].

Statistics

The values reported are means ± S.E. Statistical comparisons between two samples were performed using Student's *t*-test. Statistical comparisons of more than two groups were performed using one-way analysis of variance (ANOVA) with Bonferroni's *post-hoc* test. In all cases, $p<0.05$ was considered significant.

Results

CCL2 Induces VCAM-1 Expression in Human Synovial Fibroblasts

CCL2 has been shown to play important role in OA pathogenesis [16,17]. Therefore, we wanted to examine human synovial fibroblast tissues for the expression of the CCL2 by using ELISA. Concentrations of CCL2 in synovial fluid were significantly higher in patients with OA than in controls (Fig. 1A). The medium from OASFs showed significant expression of CCL2, which was higher than that in medium from normal SFs (Fig. 1B). Next, we directly applied CCL2 in OASFs and examined the expression of VCAM-1 (an important regulator that promotes monocytes adhesion to endothelial cells). Treatment of OASFs with CCL2 (3–30 ng/ml) for 24 h induced mRNA and cell surface VCAM-1 expression in a concentration-dependent manner, as shown by qPCR and flow cytometry (Fig. 1C&D). In addition, CCL2 also increased VCAM-1 protein expression dose-dependently (Fig. 1E). These data indicate that CCL2 increases VCAM-1 expression in human OASFs.

The CCL2/CCR2 Axis Promotes VCAM-1 Expression in Human Synovial Fibroblasts

Previous studies have shown CCL2 affects cell function through binding to cell surface CCR2 or CCR4 receptor [25,26]. Pretreatment of cells with CCR2 inhibitor RS102895 but not CCR4 inhibitor C0214 abrogated the CCL2-induced mRNA and cell surface VCAM-1 expression (Fig. 2A&B). In addition, RS102895 but not C0124 blocked the CCL2-increased protein expression of VCMA-1 (Fig. 2C). These results indicate that CCL2 induced VCAM-1 expression through CCR2 receptor in human OASFs.

The PKCδ and p38MAPK Signaling Pathways are Involved in CCL2-mediated Increase of VCAM-1 Expression

PKC has been shown to play an important role in the cellular functions modulated by several stimuli [27,28]. To determine whether PKC isoforms were involved in CCL2 triggered VCAM-1 expression, OASFs were pretreated with either GF109203X, a pan-PKC inhibitor, or rottlerin, a selective PKCδ inhibitor [29] for 30 min and then incubated with CCL2 for 24 h. As shown in Figure 3A–C, pretreatment with GF109203X and rottlerin reduced CCL2-induced VCAM-1 expression, suggesting that PKCδ may play a role in CCL2-induced VCAM-1 production in OASFs. Transfection of cells with PKCδ siRNA also reduced CCL2-induced VCAM-1 expression (Fig. 3D&E). We then directly measured PKCδ phosphorylation in response to CCL2 and found that stimulation of OASFs led to a significant increase in phosphorylation of PKCδ (Fig. 3F). Pretreatment of cells with RS102895 blocked the CCL2-induced PKCδ phosphorylation (Fig. 3G). Taken together, these results indicate that the CCR2 and PKCδ-dependent pathway is involved in CCL2-induced VCAM-1 expression.

PKCδ-dependent p38MAPK activation is involved in the regulation of VCAM-1 expression [30]. Therefore, we wanted to examine whether CCL2 stimulation enhanced p38MAPK activation in human OASFs. Pretreatment of cells for 30 min with p38 inhibitor SB203580 reduced CCL2-induced VCAM-1 expression (Fig. 4A–C). On the other hand, SB203580 did not affect the basal level of VCAM-1 expression (Fig. 4C; lower panel). In addition, transfection of cells with dominant-negative mutant of p38MAPK also reduced CCL2-mediated VCAM-1 up-regulation (Fig. 4D&E). Furthermore, stimulation of OASFs with CCL2 induced the phosphorylation of p38 in a time-dependent manner (Fig. 4F). Pretreatment of cells with RS102895 and rottlerin blocked the CCL2-induced p38MAPK phosphorylation (Fig. 4G). It has been reported that p38MAPK, ERK, and JNK mediate CCL2 signaling [31,32]. However, pretreatment of OASFs with ERK inhibitor PD98059 and JNK inhibitor SP600125 only slightly reduced CCL2-increased VCAM-1 mRNA expression (Fig. 4A). Therefore, p38MAPK may be more important than ERK and JNK in CCL2-mediated VCAM-1 expression. Based on these results, it appears that CCL2 acts through a signaling pathway involving the CCR2, PKCδ, and p38MAPK to enhance VCAM-1 expression in human OASFs.

AP-1 is Involved in the CCL2-mediated Increase of VCAM-1 Expression

AP-1 is a transcription factor that plays a crucial role in immune and inflammatory responses. It have been reported that the VCAM-1 promoter includes binding sites for AP-1 [33]. Therefore, we examined the effect of CCL2 on AP-1 transcriptional activation. Pretreatment of cells for 30 min with AP-1 inhibitors (curcumin and tanshinone IIA) inhibited CCL2-induced VCAM-1 expression (Fig. 5A–C). AP-1 activation was further evaluated by analyzing the c-Jun phosphorylation as well as by a chromatin immunoprecipitation assay. Transfection of OASFs with c-Jun siRNA reduced CCL2-mediated increase of VCAM-1 expression (Fig. 5D&E). Stimulation of cells with CCL2 increased c-Jun phosphorylation (Fig. 5F). Pretreatment of cells with RS102895, rottlerin, and SB203580 reduced the CCL2-induced c-Jun phosphorylation (Fig. 6A).

The *in vivo* recruitment of c-Jun to the VCAM-1 promoter (−403 to −30) was assessed via chromatin immunoprecipitation assay [24]. *In vivo* binding of c-Jun to the AP-1 element of the VCAM-1 promoter occurred after CCL2 stimulation (Fig. 6B). The binding of c-Jun to the AP-1 element by CCL2 was attenuated by RS102895, rottlerin, and SB203580 (Fig. 6B). On the other hand, CCL2 stimulation did not increase the binding activity of c-Jun to the VCAM-1 promoter without AP-1 binding site (Fig. 6B). These results indicate that CCL2-induced VCAM-1 expression was mediated through the CCR2, PKCδ, p38MAPK, and AP-1 pathway in human OASFs.

CCL2 Promotes Monocytes Adhesion through the CCR2, PKCδ, p38MAPK, and AP-1 Pathway

Next, we wanted to measure the monocytes adhesion to OASFs after treatment with CCL2. The adhesion assay was carried out using THP-1 as a monocyte model. Treatment of OASFs with CCL2 enhanced the adhesion between OASFs and THP-1 cells dose-dependently (Fig. 6C&E). In order to determine whether CCR2, PKCδ, p38MAPK, and AP-1 pathway can induce monocytes to adhere to OASFs monolayer, we pretreated of OASFs with RS102895, rottlerin, SB203580, and tanshinone IIA

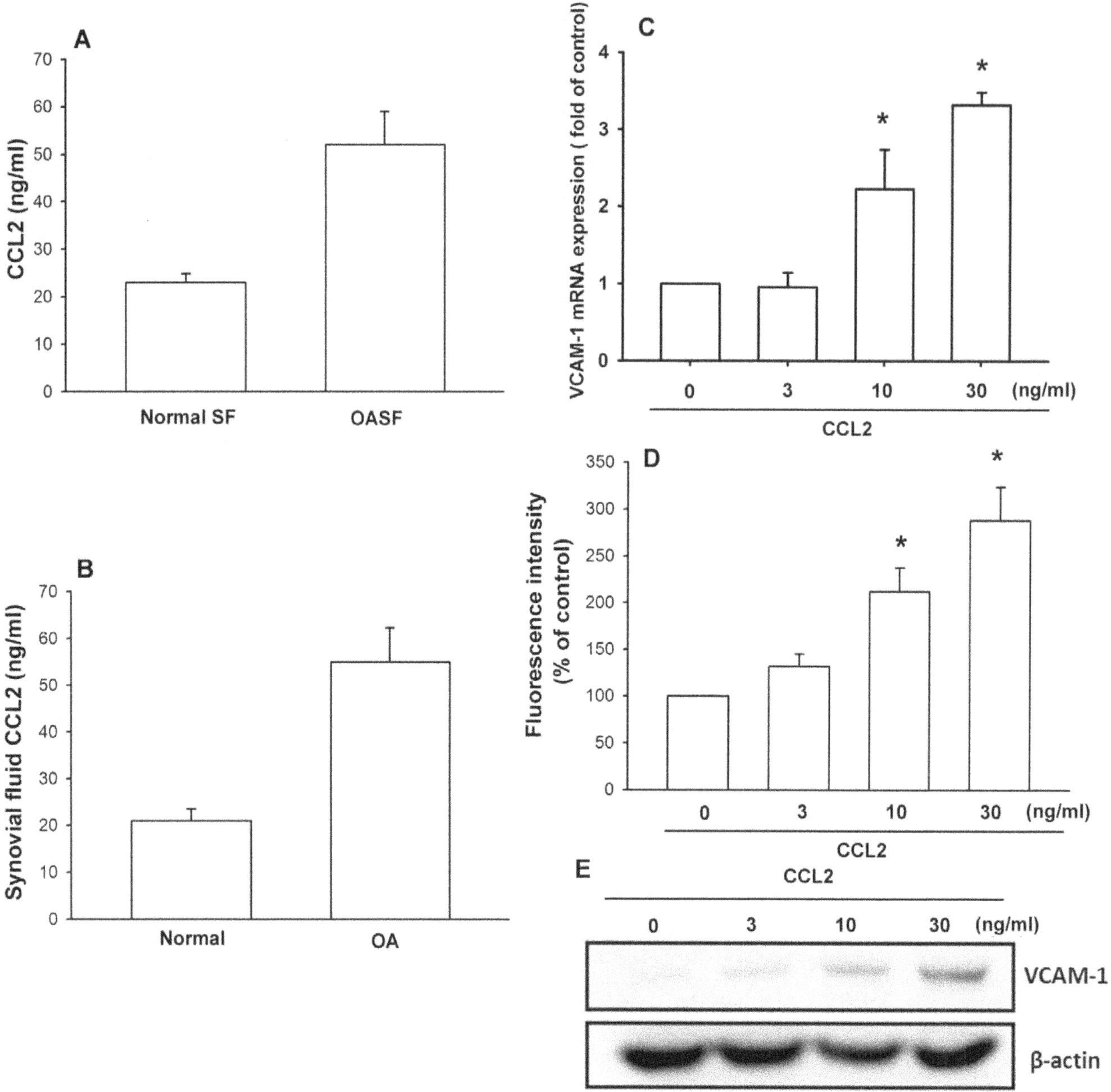

Figure 1. CCL2 increases VCAM-1 expression. (A) Synovial fluid was obtained from normal (n = 12) or osteoarthritis patients (n = 11) and examined with ELISA for the expression of CCL2. (B) Human synovial fibroblasts were cultured for 48 h, and media were collected to measure CCL2 (n = 6). OASFs were incubated with various concentrations of CCL2 for 24 h. The mRNA (C), cell surface (D), and protein expression (E) of VCAM-1 was examined by qPCR, flow cytometry, and Western blotting (n = 4–6). Results are expressed as the mean ± S.E. *: $p<0.05$ as compared with basal level. #: $p<0.05$ as compared with CCL2-treated group.

or transfected them with PKCδ and c-Jun siRNA. Both the pretreatment and transfection significantly inhibited the amount of monocytes adhesion (Fig. 6D&F). On the basis of these results, it appears that CCL2 promoted adhesion of monocytes to OASFs through CCR2, PKCδ, p38MAPK, and AP-1 pathway.

Discussion

OA is a heterogeneous group of conditions associated with defective integrity of articular cartilage as well as related changes in the underlying bone. The chronic inflammatory process is mediated through a complex cytokine network. The factors responsible for initiating the degradation and loss of articular tissues are not completely understood. Although the pathogenesis of the disease remains elusive, up-regulation of adhesion molecules on the surface of the synovial lining may play a key role in recruitment and infiltration of monocytes sites of inflammation in OA [34]. Here we further characterized VCAM-1 as a target protein for the CCL2 signaling pathway that regulates the cell adhesion. We also showed that potentiation of VCAM-1 by CCL2 requires activation of the CCR2, PKCδ, p38MAPK, and AP-1 signaling pathway and promotes monocytes adhesion to OASFs.

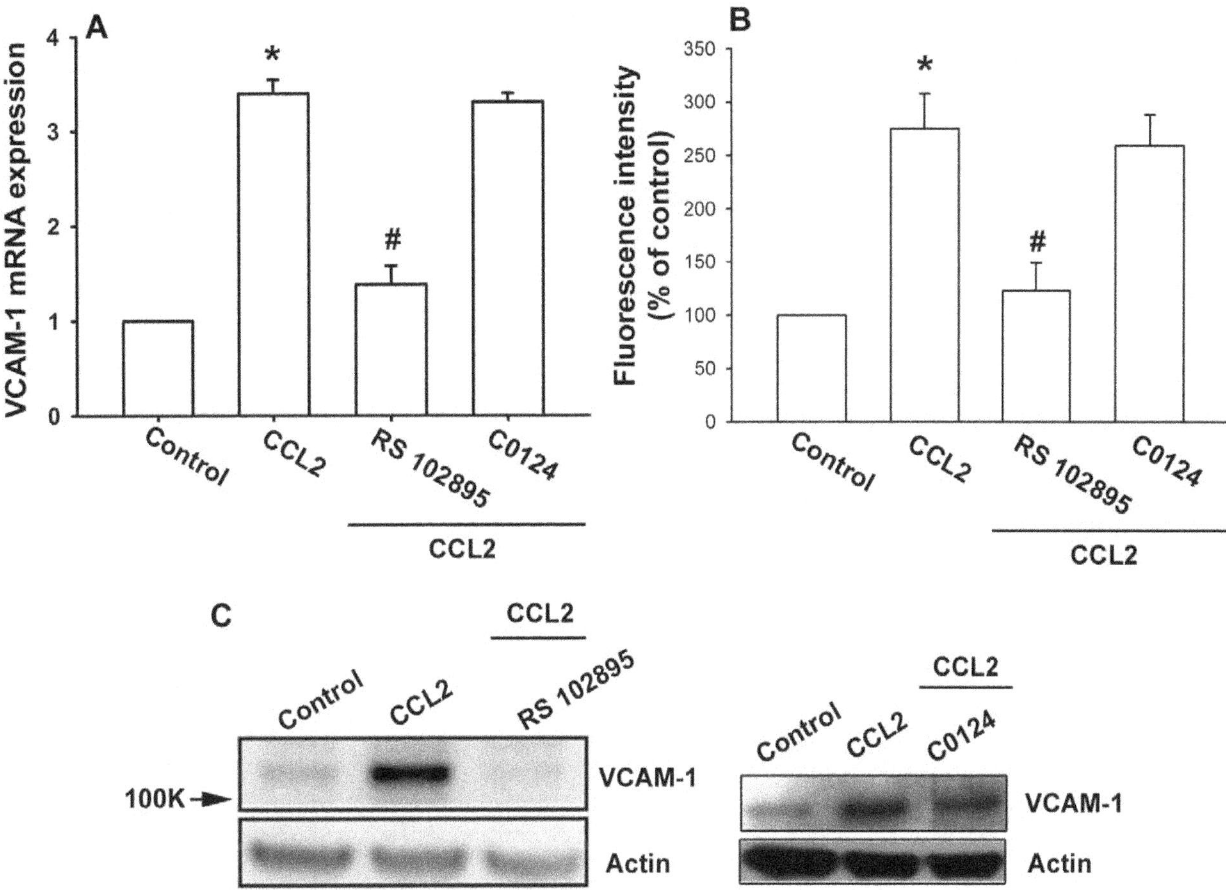

Figure 2. CCL2 increases VCAM-1 expression through CCR2 receptor. OASFs were pretreated for 30 min with RS102895 (400 nM) or C0214 (400 nM) followed by stimulation with CCL2 (30 ng/ml) for 24 h, and VCAM-1 expression was examined by qPCR (A; β-actin was used as internal control), flow cytometry (B), and Western blotting (C) (n = 5–6). Results are expressed as the mean ± S.E. *: $p<0.05$ as compared with basal level. #: $p<0.05$ as compared with CCL2-treated group.

The CC-chemokine is regulated on activation of normal T-cell expression, and secreted CCL2 mediates its biological activities through activation of G protein–coupled receptors, CCR2 or CCR4 [25,26]. It have been reported that CCL2 affects cell migration through binding to cell surface CCR2 or CCR4 receptor [25,26]. In this study, we found that pretreatment of cells with CCR2 inhibitor but not CCR4 inhibitor blocked CCL2-increased VCAM-1 expression. In addition, CCR2 inhibitor also reduced CCL2-induced monocytes adhesion. The results indicated that expression of CCL2/CCR2 axis was associated with VCAM-1 expression and cell adhesion in OASFs.

Several isoforms of PKC have been characterized at the molecular level and have been found to mediate the progress of OA [35]. We demonstrated that the PKC inhibitor GF109203X antagonized the CCL2-mediated potentiation of VCAM-1 expression, suggesting that PKC activation is an obligatory event in CCL2-induced VCAM-1 expression in these cells. In addition, rottlerin also inhibited CCL2-induced VCAM-1 expression. However, previous report indicated that rottlerin is not a specific PKCδ inhibitor but inhibits may other targets [36]. Therefore, we used PKCδ siRNA to confirm PKCδ function in OASFs. We found that PKCδ siRNA inhibited the enhancement of VCAM-1 expression. Incubation of synovial fibroblasts with CCL2 also increased PKCδ phosphorylation. On the other hand, RS102895 blocked the CCL2-induced PKCδ phosphorylation. These data suggest that the CCR2 receptor and PKCδ pathways are required for CCL2-induced VCAM-1 expression.

p38MAPK has been shown to play an important role in VCAM-1 expression in human synovial fibroblasts [37]. In this study, we used a specific p38MAPK inhibitor SB203580 (10 μM) to examine the role of p38MAPK in CCL2-mediated VCAM-1 expression. SB203580 inhibited p38MAPK at a very low dosage (600 nM) but did not affect ERK or JNK activity at a very high dosage (100 μM). Although there is scant evidence that SB303580 blocks other signaling molecules, we still can not rule out the off-target effect of this chemical inhibitor. In this study, we also used a p38MAPK mutant to confirm the role of p38MAPK in CCL2-mediated VCAM-1 expression. However, siRNA can provide a more specific effect in blocking p38MAPK activation.

There are several binding sites for a number of transcription factors including NF-κB, Sp-1, and AP-1 in the 5′ region of the VCAM-1 gene [38]. Recent studies of the VCAM-1 promoter have demonstrated that VCAM-1 induction by several transcription factors occurs in a highly stimulus-specific or cell-specific manner [30,39]. The results of our current study show that AP-1 activation contributes to CCL2-induced VCAM-1 expression in synovial fibroblasts. Pretreatment of cells with an AP-1 inhibitors curcumin or tanshinone IIA reduced CCL2-increased VCAM-1 expression. Therefore, the AP-1 binding site is likely to be the most important site for CCL2-induced VCAM-1 production. The AP-1

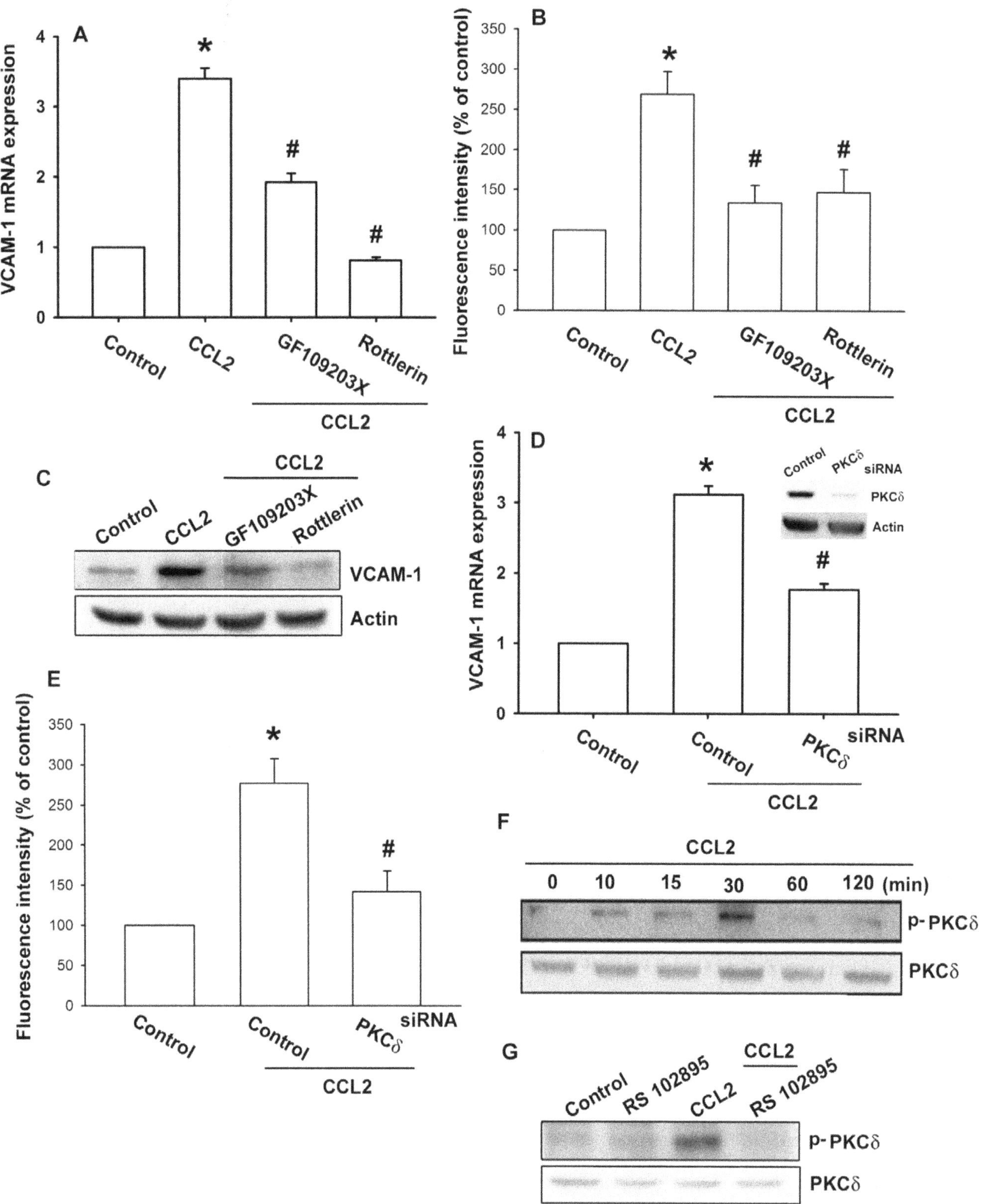

Figure 3. PKCδ is involved in CCL2-induced VCAM-1 expression in synovial fibroblasts. OASFs were pretreated for 30 min with GF109203X (3 μM) or rottlerin (10 μM) followed by stimulation with CCL2 (30 ng/ml) for 24 h, and VCAM-1 expression was examined by qPCR (A), flow cytometry (B), and Western blotting (C) (n = 4–6). OASFs were transfected with PKCδ siRNA for 24 h followed by stimulation with CCL2 for 24 h, and VCAM-1 expression was examined by qPCR (D) and flow cytometry (E). OASFs were incubated with CCL2 for indicated time intervals (n = 4) (F) or pretreated with RS102895 for 30 min before incubation with CCL2 for 30 min (n = 4) (G), and PKCδ phosphorylation was determined by Western blotting (n = 4). Results are expressed as the mean ± S.E. *: $p<0.05$ as compared with basal level. #: $p<0.05$ as compared with CCL2-treated group.

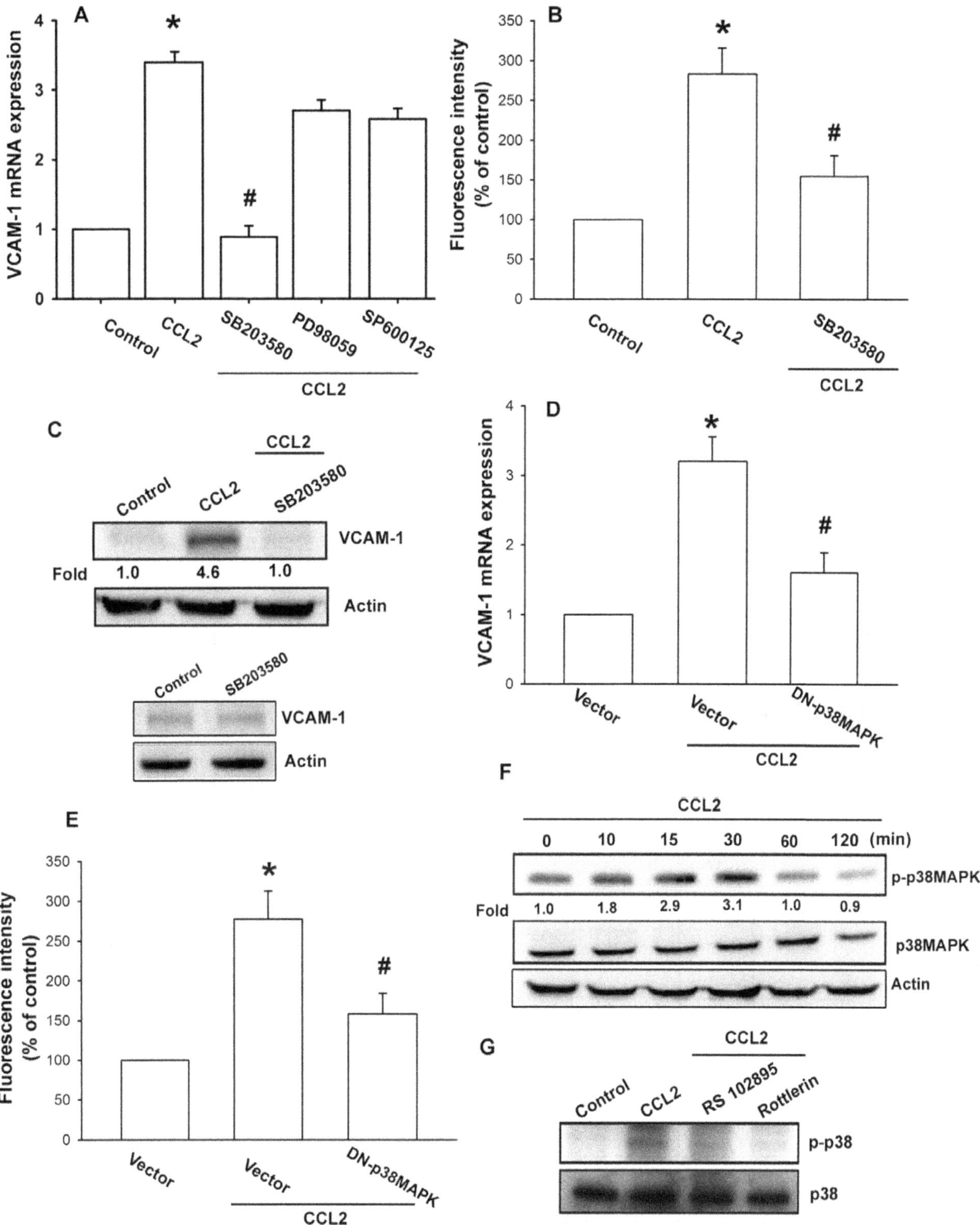

Figure 4. p38MAPK is involved in CCL2-induced VCAM-1 expression in synovial fibroblasts. (A) OASFs were pretreated for 30 min with SB203580 (10 μM), PD98059 (30 μM), or SP600125 (10 μM) followed by stimulation with CCL2 (30 ng/ml) for 24 h, and VCAM-1 expression was examined by qPCR (n = 5). OASFs were pretreated for 30 min with SB203580 followed by stimulation with CCL2 for 24 h, and VCAM-1 expression was examined by flow cytometry (B) and Western blotting (C) (n = 5). OASFs were transfected with p38MAPK mutant for 24 h followed by stimulation with CCL2 for 24 h, and VCAM-1 expression was examined by qPCR (D) and flow cytometry (E) (n = 4). OASFs were incubated with CCL2 for indicated time intervals (F) or pretreated with RS102895 or rottlerin for 30 min before incubation with CCL2 for 30 min (G), and p38 phosphorylation was determined by Western blotting (n = 5). Results are expressed as the mean ± S.E. *: $p<0.05$ as compared with basal level. #: $p<0.05$ as compared with CCL2-treated group.

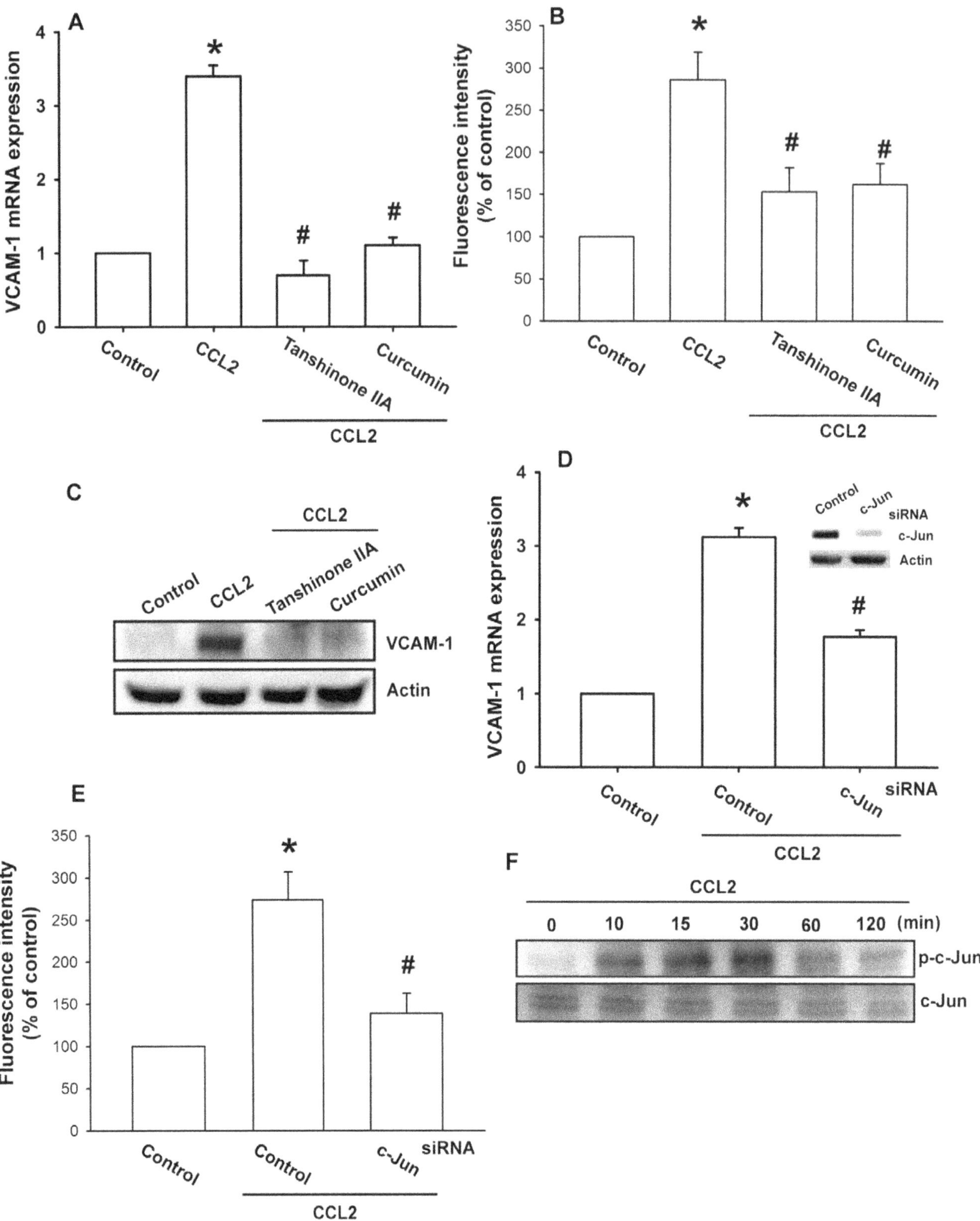

Figure 5. AP-1 is involved in the potentiation of VCAM-1 expression by CCL2. OASFs were pretreated for 30 min with curcumin (3 μM) or tanshinone IIA (5 μM) followed by stimulation with CCL2 (30 ng/ml) for 24 h, and VCAM-1 expression was examined by qPCR (A), flow cytometry (B), and Western blotting (C) (n = 4–6). OASFs were transfected with c-Jun siRNA for 24 h followed by stimulation with CCL2 for 24 h, and VCAM-1 expression was examined by qPCR (D) and flow cytometry (E) (n = 4). (F) OASFs were incubated with CCL2 for indicated time intervals and c-Jun phosphorylation was determined by Western blotting (n = 5). Results are expressed as the mean ± S.E. *: $p<0.05$ as compared with basal level. #: $p<0.05$ as compared with CCL2-treated group.

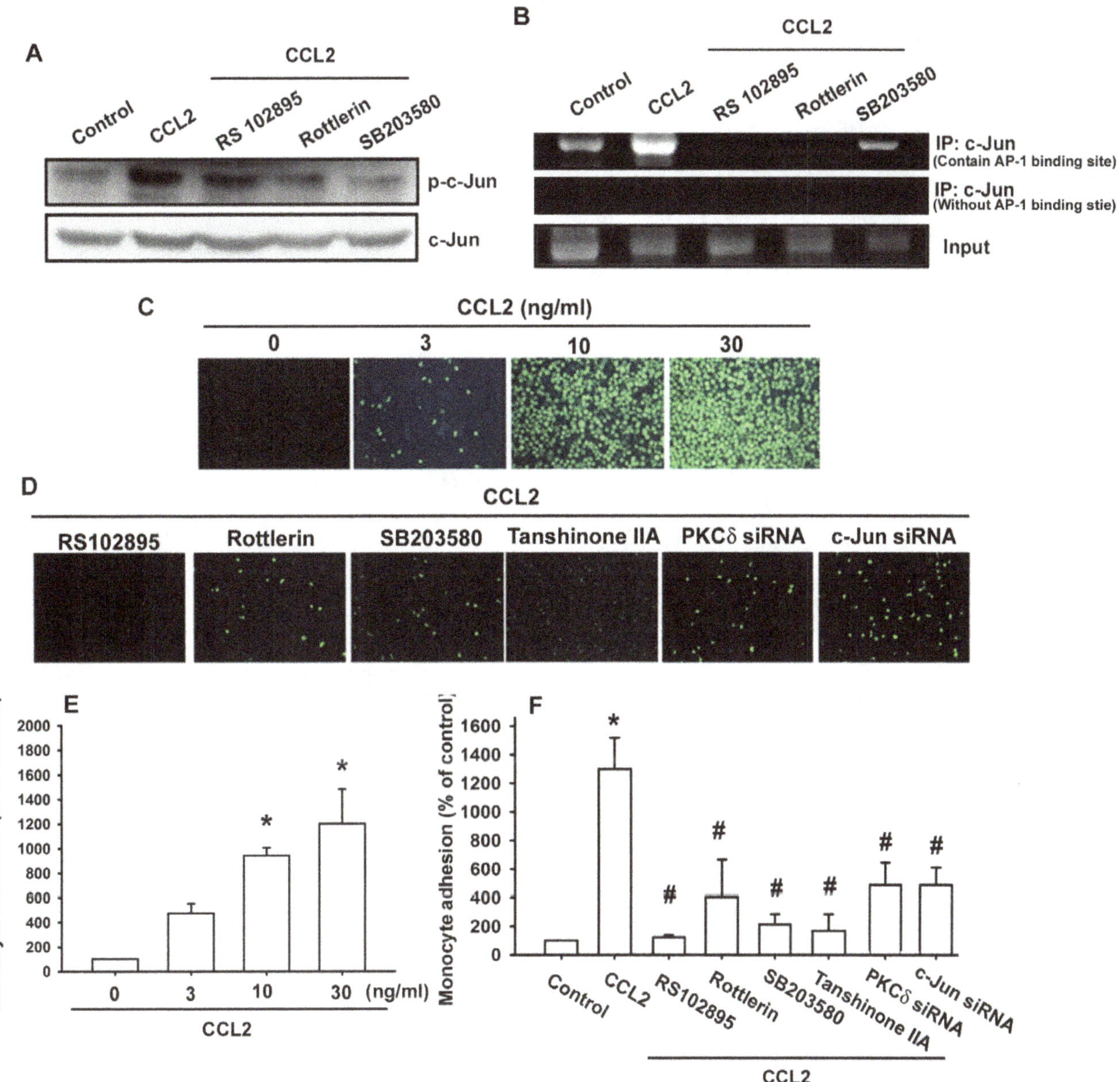

Figure 6. CCL2 induces AP-1 activation and monocytes adhesion through CCR2, PKCδ, and p38 pathway. (A) OASFs were pretreated with RS102895, rottlerin, or SB203580 for 30 min then stimulated with CCL2 for 30 min, and p-c-Jun expression was determined by Western blotting (n = 5). (B) OASFs were pretreated with RS102895, rottlerin, or SB203580 for 30 min then stimulated with CCL2 for 120 min, the chromatin immunoprecipitation assay was then performed (n = 5). OASFs were incubated with various concentrations of CCL2 for 24 h (C&E) or pretreated with RS102895, rottlerin, SB203580, and tanshinone IIA for 30 min or transfected with PKCδ and c-Jun siRNA followed by stimulation with CCL2 for 24 h (D&F) (n = 6). THP-1 cells labeled with BCECF-AM were added to OASFs for 6 h, and then the THP-1 cells adherence was measured by fluorescence microscopy. Results are expressed as the mean ± S.E. *: $p<0.05$ as compared with basal level. #: $p<0.05$ as compared with CCL2-treated group.

sequence binds to members of the Jun and Fos families of transcription factors. These nuclear proteins interact with the AP-1 site as Jun homodimers or Jun-Fos heterodimers formed by protein dimerization through their leucine zipper motifs [40]. The results of our study show that CCL2 induced c-Jun phosphorylation. In addition, c-Jun siRNA abolished CCL2-induced VCAM-1 expression in OASFs. Therefore, c-Jun activation mediates CCL2-increased VCAM-1 expression. Furthermore, CCL2 increased the binding of c-Jun to the AP-1 element within the VCAM-1 promoter, as shown by a chromatin immunoprecipitation assay. Binding of c-Jun to the AP-1 element was attenuated by RS102895, rottlerin, and SB203580. These results indicate that the CCL2 may act through the CCR2, PKCδ, p38MAPK, and AP-1 pathway to induce VCAM-1 production in human OASFs.

In conclusion, we have explored the signaling pathway involved in CCL2 induced VCAM-1 expression in human synovial fibroblasts. CCL2 increases VCAM-1 production by binding to CCR2 receptor, and activating PKCδ and p38 which in turn enhances binding of AP-1, resulting in the transactivation of VCAM-1 expression. The CCL2-mediated CCR2, PKCδ, p38MAPK, and AP-1 pathway promotes monocytes adhesion to human OASFs. These findings may provide a better understanding of the mechanisms of OA pathogenesis.

Acknowledgments

We thank Dr. J. Han for providing the p38MAPK mutant.

Author Contributions

Conceived and designed the experiments: MCC CHT. Performed the experiments: YML CJH YYL. Analyzed the data: YML CJH YYL. Contributed reagents/materials/analysis tools: YML CJH YYL. Wrote the paper: YML MCC CHT.

References

1. Mor A, Abramson SB, Pillinger MH (2005) The fibroblast-like synovial cell in rheumatoid arthritis: a key player in inflammation and joint destruction. Clin Immunol 115: 118–128.
2. Shen PC, Wu CL, Jou IM, Lee CH, Juan HY, et al. (2011) T helper cells promote disease progression of osteoarthritis by inducing macrophage inflammatory protein-1gamma. Osteoarthritis and cartilage/OARS, Osteoarthritis Research Society 19: 728–736.
3. Choy EH, Panayi GS (2001) Cytokine pathways and joint inflammation in rheumatoid arthritis. The New England journal of medicine 344: 907–916.
4. Sakkas LI, Platsoucas CD (2007) The role of T cells in the pathogenesis of osteoarthritis. Arthritis and rheumatism 56: 409–424.
5. Sucosky P, Balachandran K, Elhammali A, Jo H, Yoganathan AP (2009) Altered shear stress stimulates upregulation of endothelial VCAM-1 and ICAM-1 in a BMP-4- and TGF-beta1-dependent pathway. Arterioscler Thromb Vasc Biol 29: 254–260.
6. Qureshi MH, Cook-Mills J, Doherty DE, Garvy BA (2003) TNF-alpha-dependent ICAM-1- and VCAM-1-mediated inflammatory responses are delayed in neonatal mice infected with Pneumocystis carinii. J Immunol 171: 4700–4707.
7. Schett G, Kiechl S, Bonora E, Zwerina J, Mayr A, et al. (2009) Vascular cell adhesion molecule 1 as a predictor of severe osteoarthritis of the hip and knee joints. Arthritis Rheum 60: 2381–2389.
8. Kalichman L, Pantsulaia I, Kobyliansky E (2011) Association between vascular cell adhesion molecule 1 and radiographic hand osteoarthritis. Clin Exp Rheumatol 29: 544–546.
9. Karatay S, Kiziltunc A, Yildirim K, Karanfil RC, Senel K (2004) Effects of different hyaluronic acid products on synovial fluid levels of intercellular adhesion molecule-1 and vascular cell adhesion molecule-1 in knee osteoarthritis. Ann Clin Lab Sci 34: 330–335.
10. Szekanecz Z, Kim J, Koch AE (2003) Chemokines and chemokine receptors in rheumatoid arthritis. Seminars in immunology 15: 15–21.
11. Maghazachi AA, al-Aoukaty A, Schall TJ (1994) C-C chemokines induce the chemotaxis of NK and IL-2-activated NK cells. Role for G proteins. Journal of immunology 153: 4969–4977.
12. Koch AE, Kunkel SL, Harlow LA, Johnson B, Evanoff HL, et al. (1992) Enhanced production of monocyte chemoattractant protein-1 in rheumatoid arthritis. The Journal of clinical investigation 90: 772–779.
13. Levinger I, Levinger P, Trenerry MK, Feller JA, Bartlett JR, et al. (2011) Increased inflammatory cytokine expression in the vastus lateralis of patients with knee osteoarthritis. Arthritis and rheumatism 63: 1343–1348.
14. Akahoshi T, Wada C, Endo H, Hirota K, Hosaka S, et al. (1993) Expression of monocyte chemotactic and activating factor in rheumatoid arthritis. Regulation of its production in synovial cells by interleukin-1 and tumor necrosis factor. Arthritis and rheumatism 36: 762–771.
15. Gong JH, Ratkay LG, Waterfield JD, Clark-Lewis I (1997) An antagonist of monocyte chemoattractant protein 1 (MCP-1) inhibits arthritis in the MRL-lpr mouse model. The Journal of experimental medicine 186: 131–137.
16. Eisinger K, Bauer S, Schaffler A, Walter R, Neumann E, et al. (2012) Chemerin induces CCL2 and TLR4 in synovial fibroblasts of patients with rheumatoid arthritis and osteoarthritis. Experimental and molecular pathology 92: 90–96.
17. Juarranz Y, Gutierrez-Canas I, Santiago B, Carrion M, Pablos JL, et al. (2008) Differential expression of vasoactive intestinal peptide and its functional receptors in human osteoarthritic and rheumatoid synovial fibroblasts. Arthritis and rheumatism 58: 1086–1095.
18. Tang CH, Chiu YC, Tan TW, Yang RS, Fu WM (2007) Adiponectin enhances IL-6 production in human synovial fibroblast via an AdipoR1 receptor, AMPK, p38, and NF-kappa B pathway. Journal of immunology 179: 5483–5492.
19. Tang CH, Hsu CJ, Fong YC (2010) The CCL5/CCR5 axis promotes interleukin-6 production in human synovial fibroblasts. Arthritis and rheumatism 62: 3615–3624.
20. Hsieh MT, Hsieh CL, Lin LW, Wu CR, Huang GS (2003) Differential gene expression of scopolamine-treated rat hippocampus-application of cDNA microarray technology. Life sciences 73: 1007–1016.
21. Wang YC, Lee PJ, Shih CM, Chen HY, Lee CC, et al. (2003) Damage formation and repair efficiency in the p53 gene of cell lines and blood lymphocytes assayed by multiplex long quantitative polymerase chain reaction. Analytical biochemistry 319: 206–215.
22. Huang HC, Shi GY, Jiang SJ, Shi CS, Wu CM, et al. (2003) Thrombomodulin-mediated cell adhesion: involvement of its lectin-like domain. The Journal of biological chemistry 278: 46750–46759.
23. Tseng CP, Huang CL, Huang CH, Cheng JC, Stern A, et al. (2003) Disabled-2 small interfering RNA modulates cellular adhesive function and MAPK activity during megakaryocytic differentiation of K562 cells. FEBS letters 541: 21–27.
24. Lin WN, Luo SF, Lin CC, Hsiao LD, Yang CM (2009) Differential involvement of PKC-dependent MAPKs activation in lipopolysaccharide-induced AP-1 expression in human tracheal smooth muscle cells. Cell Signal 21: 1385–1395.
25. Aragay AM, Mellado M, Frade JM, Martin AM, Jimenez-Sainz MC, et al. (1998) Monocyte chemoattractant protein-1-induced CCR2B receptor desensitization mediated by the G protein-coupled receptor kinase 2. Proceedings of the National Academy of Sciences of the United States of America 95: 2985–2990.
26. Zhang T, Somasundaram R, Berencsi K, Caputo L, Gimotty P, et al. (2006) Migration of cytotoxic T lymphocytes toward melanoma cells in three-dimensional organotypic culture is dependent on CCL2 and CCR4. European journal of immunology 36: 457–467.
27. Chiu YC, Fong YC, Lai CH, Hung CH, Hsu HC, et al. (2008) Thrombin-induced IL-6 production in human synovial fibroblasts is mediated by PAR1, phospholipase C, protein kinase C alpha, c-Src, NF-kappa B and p300 pathway. Mol Immunol 45: 1587–1599.
28. Hsieh HL, Sun CC, Wang TS, Yang CM (2008) PKC-delta/c-Src-mediated EGF receptor transactivation regulates thrombin-induced COX-2 expression and PGE(2) production in rat vascular smooth muscle cells. Biochimica et biophysica acta 1783: 1563–1575.
29. Basu A, Adkins B, Basu C (2008) Down-regulation of caspase-2 by rottlerin via protein kinase C-delta-independent pathway. Cancer Res 68: 2795–2802.
30. Lin WN, Luo SF, Lin CC, Hsiao LD, Yang CM (2009) Differential involvement of PKC-dependent MAPKs activation in lipopolysaccharide-induced AP-1 expression in human tracheal smooth muscle cells. Cellular signalling 21: 1385–1395.
31. Cai K, Qi D, Hou X, Wang O, Chen J, et al. (2011) MCP-1 upregulates amylin expression in murine pancreatic beta cells through ERK/JNK-AP1 and NF-kappaB related signaling pathways independent of CCR2. PloS one 6: e19559.
32. Tang CH, Tsai CC (2012) CCL2 increases MMP-9 expression and cell motility in human chondrosarcoma cells via the Ras/Raf/MEK/ERK/NF-kappaB signaling pathway. Biochemical pharmacology 83: 335–344.
33. Zhou J, Wang KC, Wu W, Subramaniam S, Shyy JY, et al. (2011) MicroRNA-21 targets peroxisome proliferators-activated receptor-alpha in an autoregulatory loop to modulate flow-induced endothelial inflammation. Proceedings of the National Academy of Sciences of the United States of America 108: 10355–10360.
34. Madry H, Luyten FP, Facchini A (2012) Biological aspects of early osteoarthritis. Knee surgery, sports traumatology, arthroscopy : official journal of the ESSKA 20: 407–422.
35. Hamanishi C, Hashima M, Satsuma H, Tanaka S (1996) Protein kinase C activator inhibits progression of osteoarthritis induced in rabbit knee joints. The Journal of laboratory and clinical medicine 127: 540–544.
36. Leitges M, Elis W, Gimborn K, Huber M (2001) Rottlerin-independent attenuation of pervanadate-induced tyrosine phosphorylation events by protein kinase C-delta in hemopoietic cells. Lab Invest 81: 1087–1095.
37. Luo SF, Fang RY, Hsieh HL, Chi PL, Lin CC, et al. (2010) Involvement of MAPKs and NF-kappaB in tumor necrosis factor alpha-induced vascular cell adhesion molecule 1 expression in human rheumatoid arthritis synovial fibroblasts. Arthritis and rheumatism 62: 105–116.
38. Ahmad M, Theofanidis P, Medford RM (1998) Role of activating protein-1 in the regulation of the vascular cell adhesion molecule-1 gene expression by tumor necrosis factor-alpha. The Journal of biological chemistry 273: 4616–4621.
39. Lazzerini G, Del Turco S, Basta G, O'Loghlen A, Zampolli A, et al. (2009) Prominent role of NF-kappaB in the induction of endothelial activation by endogenous nitric oxide inhibition. Nitric oxide : biology and chemistry/official journal of the Nitric Oxide Society 21: 184–191.
40. Wagner EF (2010) Bone development and inflammatory disease is regulated by AP-1 (Fos/Jun). Annals of the rheumatic diseases 69 Suppl 1: i86–88.

Cartilage Regeneration by Chondrogenic Induced Adult Stem Cells in Osteoarthritic Sheep Model

Chinedu C. Ude[1,5], Shamsul B. Sulaiman[1], Ng Min-Hwei[1], Chen Hui-Cheng[2], Johan Ahmad[3], Norhamdan M. Yahaya[3], Aminuddin B. Saim[1,4], Ruszymah B. H. Idrus[1,5]*

1 Tissue Engineering Centre, Universiti Kebangsaan Malaysia Medical Centre, Cheras, Selangor, Malaysia, **2** Department of Clinical Veterinary, Faculty of Veterinary Medicine Universiti Putra Malaysia, Serdang, Selangor, Malaysia, **3** Department of Orthopedic & Traumatology, Universiti Kebangsaan Malaysia Medical Center, Cheras, Selangor, Malaysia, **4** ENT Consultant Clinic, Ampang Putri Specialist Hospital, Ampang, Selangor, Malaysia, **5** Department of Physiology, Faculty of Medicine, Universiti Kebangsaan Malaysia, Kuala Lumpur, Selangor, Malaysia

Abstract

Objectives: In this study, Adipose stem cells (ADSC) and bone marrow stem cells (BMSC), multipotent adult cells with the potentials for cartilage regenerations were induced to chondrogenic lineage and used for cartilage regenerations in surgically induced osteoarthritis in sheep model.

Methods: Osteoarthritis was induced at the right knee of sheep by complete resection of the anterior cruciate ligament and medial meniscus following a 3-weeks exercise regimen. Stem cells from experimental sheep were culture expanded and induced to chondrogenic lineage. Test sheep received a single dose of 2×10^7 autologous PKH26-labelled, chondrogenically induced ADSCs or BMSCs as 5 mls injection, while controls received 5 mls culture medium.

Results: The proliferation rate of ADSCs 34.4±1.6 hr was significantly higher than that of the BMSCs 48.8±5.3 hr (P = 0.008). Chondrogenic induced BMSCs had significantly higher expressions of chondrogenic specific genes (Collagen II, SOX9 and Aggrecan) compared to chondrogenic ADSCs (P = 0.031, 0.010 and 0.013). Grossly, the treated knee joints showed regenerated de novo cartilages within 6 weeks post-treatment. On the International Cartilage Repair Society grade scores, chondrogenically induced ADSCs and BMSCs groups had significantly lower scores than controls (P = 0.0001 and 0.0001). Fluorescence of the tracking dye (PKH26) in the injected cells showed that they had populated the damaged area of cartilage. Histological staining revealed loosely packed matrixes of de novo cartilages and immunostaining demonstrated the presence of cartilage specific proteins, Collagen II and SOX9.

Conclusion: Autologous chondrogenically induced ADSCs and BMSCs could be promising cell sources for cartilage regeneration in osteoarthritis.

Editor: Chi Zhang, University of Texas Southwestern Medical Center, United States of America

Funding: This study was supported by grants from the Malaysian Ministry of Education (UKM-AP-2011-26), (DPP-2013-084) and the grant from the Universiti Kebangsaan Malaysia Medical Center (Tissue Engineering Center Chemical grant: 50-67-01-001). The funders had no role in study design, data collection and analysis, decision to publish, or preparation of the manuscript.

Competing Interests: The authors have declared that no competing interests exist.

* E-mail: ruszyidrus@gmail.com

Introduction

On-going findings indicate that stem cell therapy holds promise as a therapeutic option for many diseases. Among other joint degenerative diseases, the treatment of pathologies in cartilage has posed important unmet challenges to the medical community. Cartilage can be elastic, fibrous or hyaline. The hyaline (articular) cartilage covers the smooth load-bearing tissues lining the ends of long bones within the synovial joints [1]. Articular cartilage functions as a nearly frictionless load-bearing surface in diarthrodial joints, withstanding loads of several times body weight for decades as long as it remains healthy [2]. The unique function and properties of cartilage are provided by their tissue's extracellular matrix which is maintained by a population of cells known as chondrocytes (>5% by volume). Because of its small volume of chondrocytes, as well as aneural, avascular and lack of undifferentiated cells properties, cartilage exhibits little to no intrinsic repair capabilities in response to injury or disease [1] [2]. Osteoarthritis (OA), the most common degenerative joint disease comprises of a heterogeneous group of syndrome that affects all joint tissues; characterized by the degeneration of articular cartilages with loss of matrix, formation of fissures and complete loss of the cartilage surface [3]. Traditional efforts to treat articular cartilage damage include joint lavage, tissue debridement, and microfracture of the subchondral bone; abrasion arthroplasty or the transplantation of autologous or allogeneic osteochondral grafts [3] [4] [5]. Although, some of these procedures have yielded promising clinical results, they are generally not applicable to large degenerative diseases such as osteoarthritis [6].

In recent years, there has been a growing emphasis on the use of undifferentiated progenitor cells for tissue engineering, owing to their ability to expand in culture and to differentiate into multiple cell lineages when cultured under specific growth conditions [7] [8] [9] [10]. Owing to these characteristics, adult stem cells from different tissues have been used in various focal cartilage regenerations [11] [12] [13]. We had earlier shown that a single dose of intraarticular injection of autologous bone marrow stem cells (BMSC) could retard the progressive destruction of cartilage in OA sheep model (8). With the recent plethora of interest to adipose stem cells (ADSC) owing to their abundance and easy harvest, it was included in the present study. Both BMSC and ADSC have shown significant chondrogenic potentials for use in tissue engineering approaches [11] [12]. As the field of cellular transplantation matures, methodologies are needed to longitudinally track and evaluate the functional effect of transplanted cells, thus ascertaining the homing of the injected cells. Among the many tracking agents that can be used is PKH26 dye. This red fluorescence cell tracker was developed by (Horan and Slezak 1989) [14] and can be easily detected by conventional fluorescence microscopy and stably incorporates into the cell membrane, allowing for proliferation assessment [15].

Our main objective is to treat OA with cell based therapy. The specific objectives include: firstly to isolate, culture and differentiate ADSCs and BMSCs into chondrocytes. Secondly, to compare the effectiveness of chondrogenically induced ADSCs and BMSCs in treating surgically induced osteoarthritis in sheep model; thirdly to track the induced cells with PKH26 dye after intraarticular injections.

Material and Methods

Ethics Statement

This study was carried out in strict observation with the recommendation of ACUC international. Ethics approval was granted by Universiti Kebangsaan Malaysia (UKM) Animal Ethics Committee (PP/TEC/RUSZYMAH/25-NOV/342-DEC-2010-JUN-2012) and Universiti Putra Malaysia (UPM) Animal Ethics Committee (RUJ: ACUC 07R6/JULY 07-DEC 09). All surgery was performed under Xylazine and Ketamine anesthesia; and all efforts were made to minimize pain using Tramadol analgesic.

Study Design

Un-castrated male sheep (*Siamese long tail cross*) aged 1–2 years, and weighing 20–25 kg (n = 18) comprising of 6 control, 6 ADSC and 6 BMSC confirmed to be healthy were used. The selections to the groups were done randomly and they were housed in pen with slatted floor at a density of 3 animals per pen. The design was to have arthroscopy evaluation of the right knee joint (week 0) in all groups to rule out any pre-existing chondral lesion before surgical operations at (week 1) leading to OA inductions (week 4–6). Then, the second set of arthroscopy was to reveal any induced lesion. Cells were harvested before and during operations, proliferated, labeled with PKH26 (week 1–3) and induced to chondrogenic lineage (week 4–6) then, intraarticulary injected by week 7. Six weeks afterwards, sheep were euthanized and joint samples examined for cartilage regeneration.

Arthroscopy Evaluations

This procedure was conducted with the aid of an arthroscope (Stryker[R] Endoscopy Santa Clara CA.). Briefly, a lateral parapatelar skin incision was made proximal to the patella, through which the scope was inserted into the stifle joint. With careful navigation, it was guided through the trochlear groove, the medial and lateral condoyle, then to the tibia plateau. This was performed before surgical operations (week 0) on the knee to ascertain any pre-existing chondral lesions. It was subsequently performed after the full induction of OA (week 6) to visualize the extent of degenerative changes and inflammation developed within the various knee regions; before the injection of chondrogenic induced cell treatments.

Osteoarthritis Induction

The surgical protocol was conducted according to our previously optimized method [16]. Sheep were sedated with intravenous (IV) xylazine (0.1 mg/ kg) and induced with IV Ketamine (7 mg/kg). Following intubation sheep were ventilated and maintained on isoflurane (1.5%) in oxygen. Analgesic consisted of IV tramadol 2 mg/kg, intra-operatively and repeated 6–8 hourly post operatively for 2days. Prophylactic antibiotics consisted of amoxicillin 20 mg/kg. A medial parapatelar skin incision was made beginning at a level 2 cm proximal to the patella (P) and extending to the level of the tibial plateau (TP). Subcutaneous tissue was incised, and the lateral fascia was separated from the joint capsule for 1 cm in either direction away from the incision. The joint capsule were incised and the patella was subluxated laterally to expose the trochlear groove, medial and lateral condyles of the distal femur. Anterior cruciate ligament (ACL) removal was performed by first excising its attachment on the medial aspect of the lateral femoral condyle (LFC). The proximal attachment is brought forward and the entire ligament was excised from its tibial attachment. The knee joint was moved in a drawer test to ensure that the entire cruciate ligament had been excised. The medial meniscus was removed by sharp excision. The caudal horn of the meniscus was grasped with a hemostat and its lateral attachment was excised from its tibial attachment. Working from caudal to lateral, then cranial, the meniscus was completely removed. The joint was closed using Vicryl sutures 3.0 and 2.0 (Ethicon Inc. USA) for the knee capsules and muscles respectively and 1.0 for the skins. Meloxicam 0.2 mg/ kg was administered, and repeated once daily for 3 days. Following extubation, sheep was recovered in its pen and monitored daily for inappetence and wound dehiscence until suture removal, 7 days post-operatively.

Sheep Exercise

At the end of three weeks recovery period from surgical injuries, sheep underwent exercise conducted in a confined concrete track of 25 meters long and 1 meter wide, running to and fro twice to complete a 100 meters distance. This lasted for three weeks to increase joint contact stress at the operated knee. After the exercise, they were allowed free movement within a pen of 4×4 m^2.

Harvest of Adipose Tissue

Adipose tissue was harvested from the right infra patella fat pad during the surgical resections at week 1. Briefly, a medial parapatelar skin incision was made beginning at level 2 cm proximal to the patella and extending to the level of tibial plateau. The medial aspect of the vastus medialis and the joint capsule were incised and the patella was luxated laterally to expose the knee fat pad. Ten milliliters of fat pad were harvested and kept at +4°C until further processing.

Harvest of Bone Marrow

After scrubbing the skin area covering the iliac spine and sedation prior to operation, a mini incision was made at the most lateral region. 10 mLs of bone marrow was harvested after, with the aid of a trocar (Cardinal Health Inc. USA) and 50 mls syringe

(Cringe Malaysia) containing heparin 1×10^3 units and was kept at +4°C until further processing.

Isolation of ADSC and BMSC

All samples were processed 6–12 hr after collection. Adipose tissue was minced with a surgical blade (*CE* OEM France Inox) to about 2 mm thick before digestion with an equal volume of 0.6% collagenase II (Gibco USA) in an orbital incubator (Stuart scientific UK) at 37°C, 21 g-force for 2 hr. The digest was filtered with a cell strainer of 100 µm pore (Orange Scientific). The filtrate was then centrifuged (CR3i) to a 4724 g-force for 5 mins at 37°C and the pellet washed with PBS (Sigma USA) twice and basal medium before culture. Bone marrow was isolated and processed using the Ficoll-Paque method (Sigma USA) (16).

Monolayer Cell Culture

Following the isolation of ADSC and BMSC, they were cultured in 6 well plates (Corning Incorporated USA) with Dulbecco's Modified Eagles Medium/F12 (D-MEM/F12)+10% fetal bovine serum medium (Gibco USA), in a Galaxy^R CO_2 incubator (RS Biotech) at humidified atmosphere of 95% O_2, 5% CO_2 and 37°C. After the initial 3 days culture which is necessary for cells to attach; medium was changed every 2 days until the cells were about 90% confluence. They were trypsinized with trypsin-EDTA (Sigma USA), and passaged to T-75 cm^2 flask (Corning Incorporated USA) at a density of 5×10^5 cells for an average of four passages. The viability of the cells was calculated using the trypan blue exclusion procedure and the growth kinetics (population doubling time) was evaluated by dividing the total number of cells at the end of the passage by the initial seeding number. These were recorded at every passage.

Evaluation of Multipotency

Isolated cells from bone marrow and adipose tissue (BMSC and ADSC) were differentiated into the three main cells lineage of mesoderm origin namely: adipocyte, osteocyte and chondrocyte. For the adipogenic inductions, a formula by Buinn Wickham et al [17] was used with modifications. This comprised of Dulbecco's Modified Eagle Media F-10 supplemented with 3% foetal bovine serum, 100 units/mL penicillin, 100 ug/mL streptomycin, 15 mmol/L HEPES buffer solution (pH 7.4), biotin (33 um, Sigma), Calcium Pantothenate (17 um), human recombinant insulin (100 nmol/L), 3-isobutyl-1-methylaxanthine (0.25 mmol/L), and Rosiglitazone (1 umol). Oil red staining was used to evaluate the adipogenic differentiation for lipid deposition. Briefly, the adipogenic cultures were fixed by removing the culture media and gently rinsing the flask with 10 ml sterile DPBS. Then 10 ml, 10% formalin was added and incubated for 30–60 mins at room temperature. The working stock solution of Oil Red O was prepared and the staining was done according to the protocols. After this, sample was washed with tap water and viewed on phase contrast microscope. Lipid appears red and nuclei appear blue.

The osteogenic induction was done using an optimised formula from our lab that comprised of FD+10% FBS medium containing Hans FD/F12, Antibiotic- antimycotic, Glutamax, Vitamin C, Herpes 2.4 mg/ml, and 10% foetal bovine solution (FBS). Other components include dexamethasone, β-glycerophoshate and ascorbic acid-2- phosphate. Medium was changed every three days and the induction period lasted for 21 days. Calcium deposition in the osteogenic differentiated cells was evaluated using Alizarin Red Staining. Alizarin Red was done by fixing the cultures with cold ethanol for 1 hour and rinsed. Fixed cultures were incubated with Alizarin red for I hour, then with boric acid buffer before counterstaining with haematoxylin. The whole stain was evaluated using bright field microscopy (Olympus-CK40).

Chondrogenic induction was done for both BMSCs and ADSCs using an optimised formula from our lab as explained in the section below. Evaluation of chondrogenesis was done using Toluidine blue staining (Gainland UK) to detect the proteoglycans formation and matrix accumulations. Briefly, sections were deparaffinised and dehydrated in distilled water; stained in Toluidine blue working solution for 2–3 minutes before washing in distilled water. Stained sections were dehydrated through (95 and 100) % alcohol; cleared with xylene before mount using DPX fluid (Gibco USA) for microscopic examination to detect extracellular matrix and proteoglycans formation. Cytoplasm stains blue, nuclear materials stain dark blue and cartilage ECM/mast cells stain purple.

PKH26 Staining

Cells were stained following an optimized protocol in our earlier study [18]. Briefly, 2×10^7cells were trypsinized and counted via trypan blue (Gibco USA) exclusion using haemocytometer (Neubauer Improved-Germany) for total cell number and viability before staining. ADSCs were stained with 2 µmol and BMSCs with 8 µmol of PKH26 dye in 15 ml polypropylene tubes. Cells were monitored with light microscope (Olympus-CK40) and live imaging fluorescence microscope (Nikon-Eclipse Ti). After sacrifice, the visible regenerated areas on the treated knee joints were analyzed for the presence of the tissue-engineered chondrocytes with the Confocal Microscope (NIKON -AIR).

Chondrogenic Induction

The chondrogenic medium was prepared following our optimized formula [19], by the addition of Dulbecco's Modified Eagles Medium/F12 (D-MEM/F12) (Gibco USA) 93.5%, Fetal bovine serum and Glutamax (Gibco USA) 1%, Antibiotic antimycotic (Gibco USA) 1%, Vitamin C (Sigma USA) 1%, Insulin transferring selenium (Gibco USA) 1%, IGF-1 (Invitrogen Inc.) 50 ng/ml, Ascorbic acid-2-phosphate (Sigma USA) 50 ug/ml, L- Proline (Sigma USA) 40 ng/ml, Dexamethasone (Invitrogen Inc.) 100 nM and Tissue growth factor-beta 3 (TGF-β3) (Invitrogen Inc.) 10 ng/ml. Immediately after PKH26 staining, cells were cultured in the prepared chondrogenic medium. Medium was changed every 3–4 days and the induction period lasted for three weeks.

Quantitative RT-PCR Assay

Total ribonucleic acid (RNA) from the samples of BMSC and ADSC at early P0 cultures (1week post isolation) and after induction to chondrocytes (6 weeks post isolation), was extracted by dissolution in trizol reagent (Gibco BRL, USA). Complementary DNA was synthesized using the iscript (BIO-RAD) and analyzed for gene expression using the iQ SYBR^R green super mix (BIO-RAD) on MyiQ single colour Real Time polymerase chain reaction (RT-PCR) detection system (BIO-RAD). Primers (Bio-basic Canada.) were used to determine transcript levels in triplicate for a housekeeping gene glyceraldehydes-3-phosphate dehydrogenase (GAPDH) (F: 5^I –ctggtgctgagtacgtggtg–3^I, R: 5^I –cgtcagcagaaggtgcagag–3^I) and four different genes of interest namely: Collagen type II (Col II) (F: 5^I –cctcaagaaggctctgctca–3^I, R: 5^I –atgtcaatgatggggagacg–3^I), Aggrecan Core Protein (Agg) (F: 5^I –taggtggcgaggaagacatc–3^I, R: 5^I –aaacgtgaaaggctcctcag–3^I), SRY (sex determining region y)-box 9 (SOX9 genes) (F: 5^I –tgaatctcctggacccctc–3^I, R: 5^I –cttgtcctcctcgctctcct–3^I) and collagen type I (Col I) (F: 5^I –cggctcctgctcctcttagcg–3^I, R: 5^I –ctgtacgcaggtgactggtg–3^I). Data was analyzed by calculating the

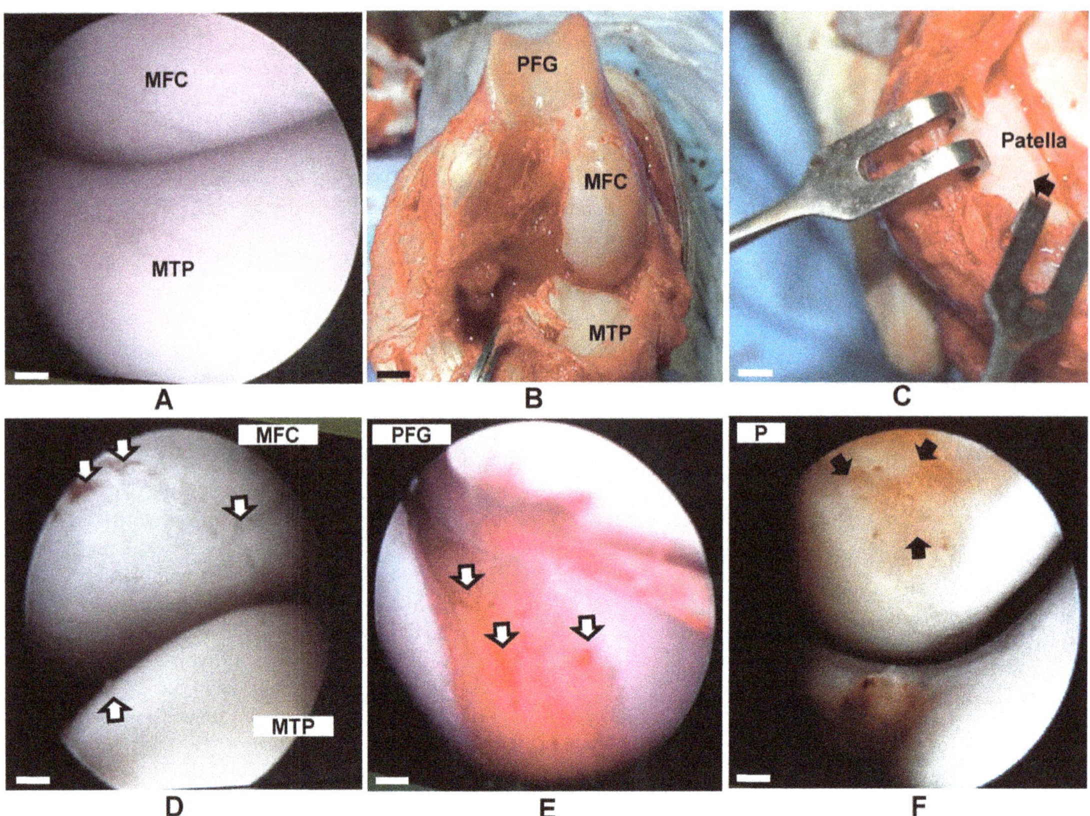

Figure 1. The arthroscopic and arthrotomy representation of the right knee joints before and after surgical inductions. (**a**) The arthroscopic representation of the right knee joints before the surgical operations revealed no chondral lesion on medial femoral condyle (MFC) and medial tibial plateau (MTP). (**b**) The arthrotomy photo during the surgical operations revealed no previous lesions at Patella femoral groove (PFG), medial femoral condyle (MFC), medial tibial plateau (MTP). (**c**) The arthrotomy photo of patella (P) before OA induction revealed no chondral degenerations (black arrow). (**d**) The arthroscopic images after OA inductions at MFC and MTP showed slight indentations and moderate focal lesions (white arrows). (**e**) Arthroscopic images after OA inductions at the PFG revealed severe and prominent chondral erosion (white arrows). (**f**) The arthroscopic images after OA inductions at P, which is the opposite contact of PFG, depicted degenerations of cartilage caused by the frictional contacts. Arthroscopy scale =0.5 cm, Arthrotomy =1.5 cm.

fold differences in gene expressions of the differentiated cells compared to undifferentiated cells after they were normalized to their own GAPDH value.

Intraarticular Injections of Induced BMSCs and ADSCs

On the 7th weeks (1 week after OA inductions), intraarticular injections were done according to our previously optimized method [16]. Briefly the cells were trypsinized, washed with PBS (Gibco USA) and culture medium, resuspended in culture medium at a density of 4×10^6cells/ml in a 5 ml cell injection. Sheep was anesthetized with intravenous (IV) xylazine (0.1 mg/kg) and Ketamine (7 mg/kg); then placed on lateral recumbence. Using the para ligamentous technique, an18-guage needle (Cringe Malaysia) was inserted posterior to the medial edge of the patellar ligament, through the triangle formed by the epicondyle of the femur, the tibia plateau and the notch at their junction. Cell suspension was injected into the operated knee of the BMSC and ADSC samples after aspiration of synovial fluid, while the controls received an equal volume of culture medium. The joint was repeatedly flexed and extended for the dispersal of the injected cells.

International Cartilage Repair Society (ICRS) Evaluation

At the end of six weeks post intraarticular injection, sheep were euthanized. The ICRS scale of OA assessment was used to evaluate the degenerations and cartilage repairs in both the control and test sheep. It has five score grades namely: Grade 0 – Normal; Grade 1 - Soft indentation superficial fissures and cracks; Grade 2 - Lesions extending down to <50% of cartilage depth; Grade 3 - Cartilage defects extending down >50% of cartilage depth to calcified layer; Grade 4 - Severely abnormal, extending down through the subchondral bone. The articular cartilage lesion was graded by two independent blinded orthopaedic scorers.

Haematoxylin and Eosin

Sections of 10 um thickness were stained with Haematoxylin and Eosin to assess cell morphology. Samples from the visible regenerated portions of the patella femoral groove (PFG) on both the treated samples and the degenerated part on the control sheep were deparaffinized with xylene and dehydrated with ethyl alcohol (Essen-Haus Sdn. Bhd). They were stained with Hematoxylin Harris (DAKO, Glostrup Denmark) and counter stained with Eosin (DAKO, Glostrup Denmark). Slides were viewed by the light microscope after dehydration with alcohol and xylene (VWR International LTD).

Safranin O Stain

Slides of 10 um thickness from the patella (P) on both the treated samples and the degenerated part of P on the control sheep were stained with Weigert's iron haematoxylin (Sigma USA)

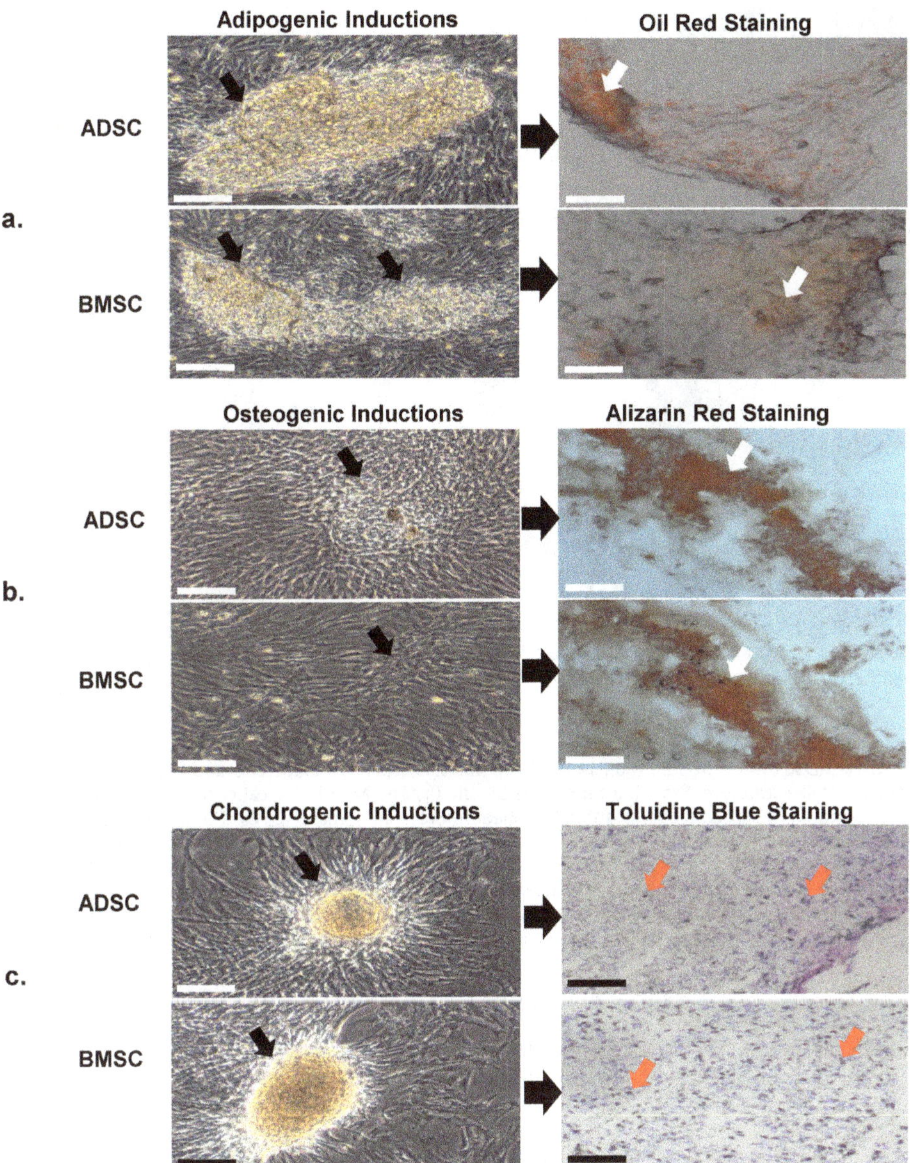

Figure 2. Multipotency evaluations of ADSCs and BMSCs. (**a**) Inverted phase contrast images of the Adipogenic inductions of ADSCs and BMSCs. The image depicted the collection of fat droplets in clusters (black arrows) from day 4 of the inductions process. The oil red staining showed that lipids formed on both induced cell samples, picked up red stain (white arrow) showing their positivity to adipogenic lineage. Scale = 70 µm. (**b**) Inverted phase contrast images of the osteogenic inductions of ADSCs and BMSCs. The picture revealed similar clustered mineralization on both cell samples from day 4 of the inductions process. The evaluation of the induced ADSCs and BMSCs with alizarin red staining demonstrated some mineralization activities (white arrow) showing their commitment to osteogenic lineage. Scale = 70 µm. (**c**) Inverted phase contrast images of the chondrogenic inductions of ADSCs and BMSCs. The picture revealed similar aggregation of the cells in condensations seen in early chondrogenesis from day 4 of the inductions process. The evaluation of the induced ADSCs and BMSCs with toluidine blue staining demonstrated that the condensed matrixes picked up the blue stain (red arrows), showing their positivity to chondrogenic lineage. Scale = 70 µm.

working stock solution. They were further stained with fast green solution (Dako, Denmark), and counter stained with Safranin O solution (Stain pur), before mount using DPX fluid (Gibco USA) for microscopic examination to detect proteoglycan accumulations.

Immunohistochemistry

Sections of 10 um from the regenerated portions of PFG and a subsequent 10 um section of healthy cartilage from the unoperated PFG were pretreated with Tris-buffered saline (TBS) (Sigma, Inc) for one minute. Antibodies were retrieved using pH 9 buffer (DAKO, USA) in boiling water for 20–40 min at 95°C. Antibody binding was blocked by incubation in 10% normal goat serum (Gibco, USA) at 37°C for 30 min. Rabbit anti-sheep Col II, SOX9 and Col I polyclonal antibodies (iDNA Biotechnology Malaysia) were applied as primary antibody at 4°C for 14–18 hr. Sections were incubated with the secondary antibody, sheep anti-rabbit immunoglobin tagged with green fluorescence (iDNA Biotechnology Malaysia) for 1–2 hr and counter stained with 4, 6-diamino-2-phenylindole (DAPI) (Sigma, Inc.). Col II, SOX9 and Col I were detected using confocal microscopy. The native articular cartilage served as the positive control for Col II and

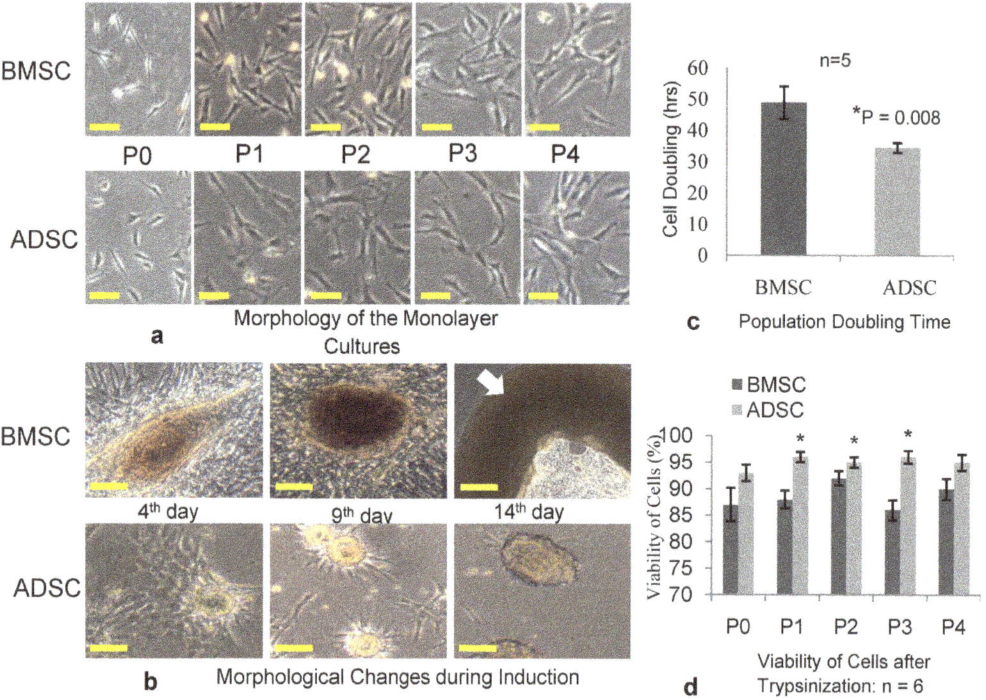

Figure 3. Monolayer analysis of BMSCs and ADSCs. (**a**) The morphological images of the BMSCs and ADSCs from P0 to P4. BMSC looked more spindle upon isolation and early attachment, while ADSCs were broader (P0-P1). Both cell samples attain the same size and shape as the passage progressed from P2–P4 showing more mesenchymal-like structure. Scale bar represents 35 μm. (**b**) The Morphological changes of the cells during chondrogenic differentiation. BMSCs formed the aggregates of cartilage in a film-like sheet, more readily than ADSCs. The aggregates and sheet clumped together (white arrow) to form a firm cartilage structure by 3rd week. ADSCs split its formed aggregates and dispersed on the medium. Scale represents 35 μm. (**c**) The Population doubling time (PDT) of the cell samples during culture. ADSCs were 34.4±1.6 hrs, while that of BMSCs were 48.8±5.3 hrs. ADSCs had a significantly higher growth rate compared to the BMSCs with P value of 0.008. (**d**) The viability of cells after trypsinization, at the end of each passage. From P0–P4, BMSCs had mean viabilities of (87, 88, 92, 86, and 90); while ADSCs had (93, 96, 95, 96, and 95) respectively. ADSCs had higher viabilities at each passage compare to BMSCs but were significantly higher at P1, P2 and P3; $P<0.05$.

SOX9, while the fibrous cartilage served as the positive control for Col I. The regenerated cartilage sections without primary antibody served as negative control for all.

Statistical Analysis

Data were presented as mean ± standard error of mean (SEM) of sample size. The parametric means which compare the means of two samples or treatments in a normal distribution were analyzed using paired student's t-tests. In the gene analysis, we effectively used each sample as its own control hence the correct rejection of a null hypothesis can become much more likely. The ICRS were done using the Mann Whitney U-test for non-parametric mean. Uncertainties were presented within 95% confidence intervals and all statistical analysis was performed using the version 17.0 of the SPSS software.

Results

Arthroscopy and Arthrotomy

The arthroscopy examination conducted on the right knee joints (Fig. 1a) before the surgical operations revealed that the target regions medial femoral condyle (MFC) and medial tibial plateau (MTP were free of chondral lesions.The arthrotomy photos taken during the surgical resections (Fig. 1b & c) still revealed that the Patella femoral groove (PFG), medial femoral condyle (MFC), medial tibial plateau (MTP), and patella (P) had no chondral degenerations. Then after OA inductions (Fig. 1d, e & f), the arthroscopic images showed degenerative and inflammatory changes within the various regions of the knee examined. The MFC and MTP showed moderate focal lesions to slight indentations. The lesions at the patella femoral groove (PFG) were severe and prominent. It was not only seen on the groove, but also at the opposite side patella (P), depicting a degeneration of cartilage caused by the frictional contacts between the two surfaces owing to ACL resection.

Evaluation of Multipotency

Both cell samples from ADSCs and BMSCs demonstrated their capacities for adipogenic differentiations. From the third day of induction, lipid droplets were noticed within the cells and as the induction progressed, the formed droplets clumped together in clusters of shiny oily appearances, though more in ADSCs culture (Fig. 2a). At the end of the induction period, Oil red staining was used to confirm the lipid depositions as seen in early adipogenesis.

Osteogenic differentiation caused both cells to form stratified-like cluster of cells from the fifth day. These clusters, which are typical characters of early mineralization and calcium deposition seen in osteoblasts differentiation multiplied in number throughout the flask from day twelve (Fig. 2b). ADSCs seem to have more of the cluster formations. Alizarin Red stain was used to confirm the presence of calcium deposition and both cells picked up the dye.

On chondrogenic evaluations, both cells showed signs of cell aggregation and matrix deposition from day three, though more prominent in BMSCs culture. As the induction progressed, the

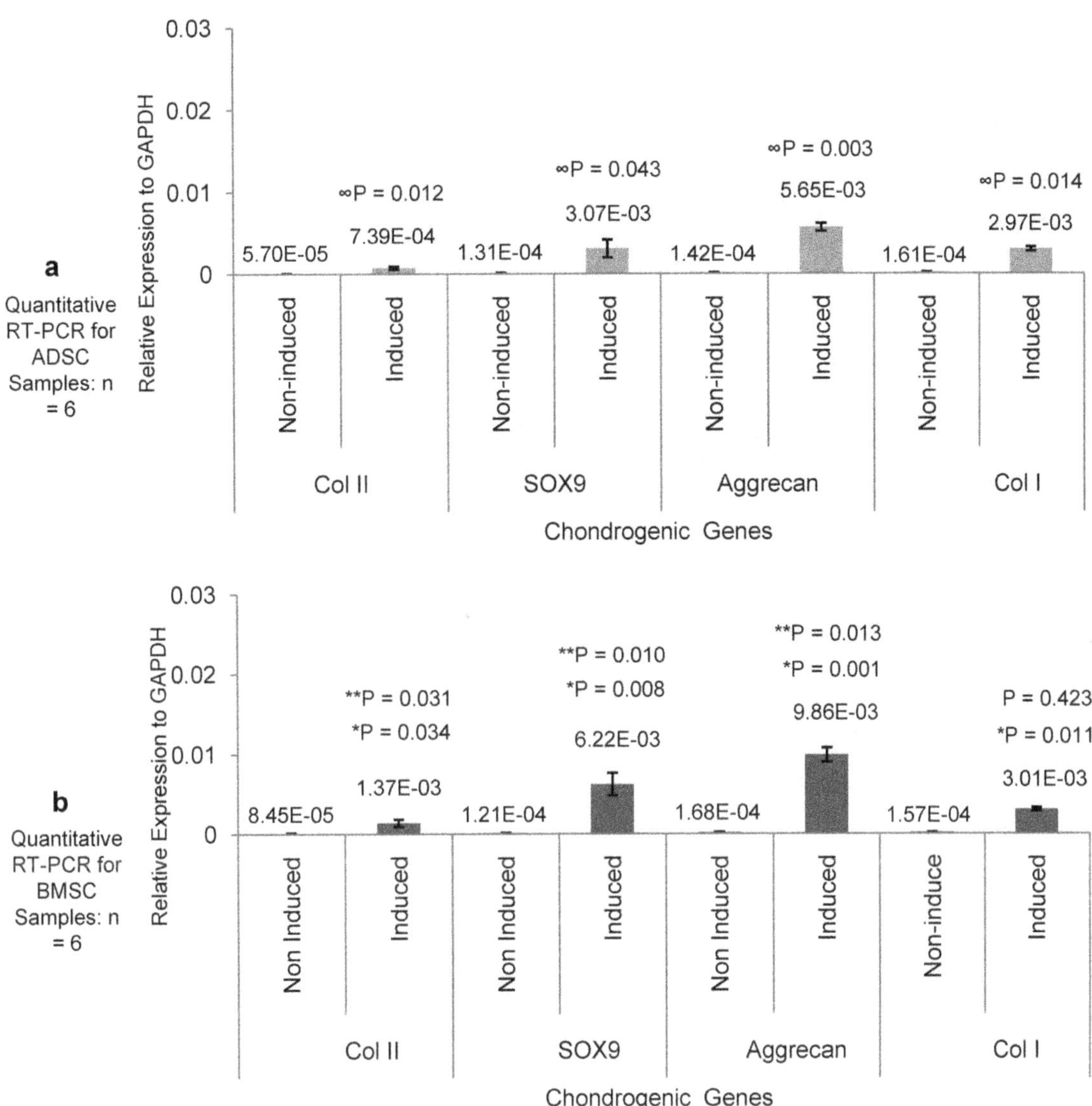

Figure 4. Gene expression analysis of ADSCs and BMSCs. (**a**) Comparison of the gene expressions of chondrogenically induced ADSCs to the uninduced. After 21 days of induction, the induced samples had significantly higher expressions of Col II, SOX9, Aggrecan and Col I genes in fold increases of (12.96, 23.44, 44.36 and 18.44) respectively compare to the uninduced (week 1 post-isolation) cells, with P values (∞) respectively (P< 0.05). (**b**) Comparison of the gene expressions of chondrogenically induced BMSCs to the uninduced. After 21 days of induction, the induced samples had significantly higher expressions of Col II, SOX9, Aggrecan and Col I genes in fold increases of (16.21, 51.40, 120.33 and 19.17) respectively compare to the uninduced (week 1 post-isolation) cells, with P values (*) respectively (P<0.05). Comparing the Induced ADSCs and Induced BMSCs, BMSCs had significantly higher expressions of Col II, Aggrecan and SOX9 genes in fold increases of (1.85, 2.03 and 5.31) respectively with P values (**) (p<0.05). There was no significance difference on Col I expression.

aggregation of cells turned into pockets of nodules with cell sheets folding them (Fig. 2c). This is typical of condensation seen in early chondrogenesis. Toluidine blue stain confirmed the extracellular matrix and proteoglycans formation on both cells.

Monolayer Cultures

After the isolation and culture of stem cells from the same volume of tissues (each 10 mLs of adipose or bone marrow), ADSCs showed more adhesion to the flask and proliferation by the second day. At the fourth day, the attached ADSCs were replicating faster compared to BMSCs. ADSCs were the first to reach confluence at passage zero (P0) in 6 well plates. At P0 and P1, BMSCs look more spindles and smaller in shape than ADSCs. As the passage increased from P2 to P4, both cells get even and looked alike with no differences in shapes and sizes Fig. 3a. Subsequently, the cells morphology during chondrogenesis revealed that BMSCs formed aggregates and matrixes of proteoglycans more readily than ADSCs. As the induction progressed, BMSCs aggregate-matrixes and the cell sheets clumped together to become a firm cartilage structure by the 3rd week of induction. ADSCs on the other hand, did formed aggregates of chondrogenic matrix and proteoglycans but with minimal sheet. From the third day of induction, the formed aggregates split and dispersed on the medium Fig. 3b.

Growth Kinetics and Viability

After the initial P0 cultures, cells were seeded at low density of 5000 cell/cm^2 in 75 cm^2 culture flask. It was observed that ADSCs

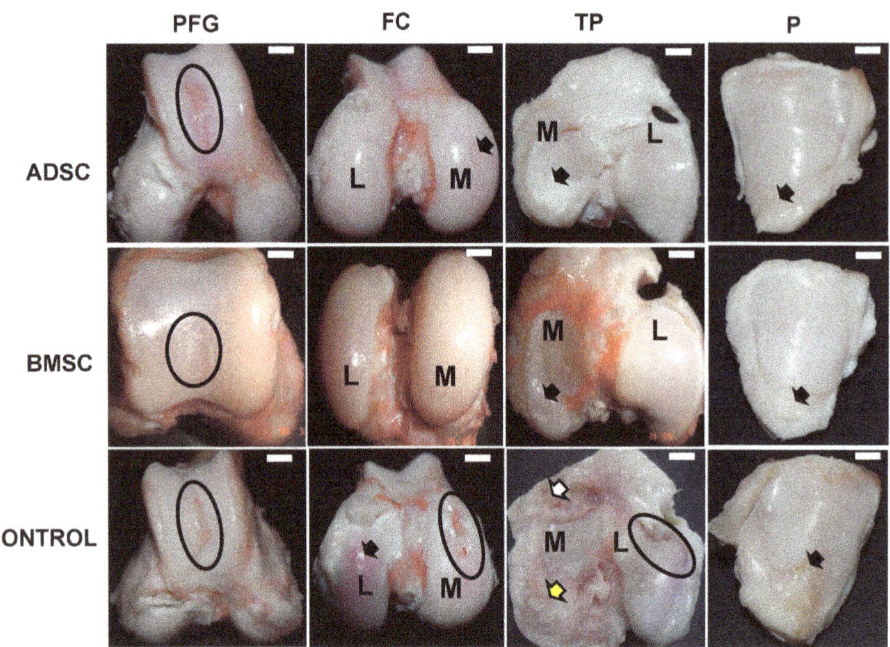

a. Gross Images of Knee representing six regions of the stifle joint at 6 weeks post cell injections: n = 6

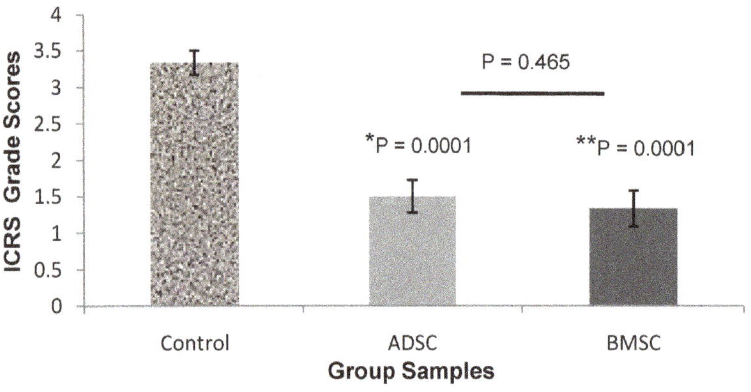

b. ICRS Score Grading: n = 6 each

Figure 5. The gross evaluations of the right knee joint samples. (**a**) The gross images of knee representing the six regions. Patella femoral groove (PFG), medial femoral condyle (MFC), lateral femoral condyle (LFC), medial tibia plateau (MTP), lateral tibia plateau (LTP) and patella (P) were used as reference points. The treated knees showed regenerations. At PFG, the regenerated cartilages had unique morphological appearances different from the native (black ring); the control still retained severe cartilage degeneration (black ring). At MFC, the ADSCs still retain a slight focal defect (black arrow); BMSCs had no sign of defect, while the control retained severe cartilage degeneration (black ring). At LFC, there were no lesions on the treated knees, but the control had reduced cartilage thickness (black arrow). At MTP, both treated samples revealed structural appearances of a crescent regenerating meniscus-like cartilage (black arrow), but none at the control. There is no evidence of meniscus regeneration on the medial tibia plateau (yellow arrow). There is also a remnant of resected spur bone formed at the anterior region of the medial tibia plateau (white arrow), which is a supportive mechanism seen in severe OA. At the LTP, there were no conspicuous lesions at the treated samples but the control retained a severe degeneration (black ring). At P, the control presented worse degeneration compared to either of the ADSCs or BMSCs (black arrows). (M = medial, and L = lateral). Scale represents 1.5 cm. (**b**) Combined gross and histological ICRS grading of the right knee joints. The control sheep scored a mean grade of 3.33±0.2, while the test groups ADSCs and BMSCs scored 1.5±0.2 and 1.3±0.3 respectively. Both treated sheep samples had significantly higher grades (*) and (**) respectively compared to the control $P<0.05$. BMSCs treated sheep had better grade score than ADSCs, but was not significant $P=0.465$.

attained confluence faster than BMSCs from P1 to P4. The proliferation rate of ADSCs was 34.4±1.6 hrs and that of the BMSCs was 48.8±5.3 hrs; thus ADSCs had significantly higher growth rate compared to BMSC $p<0.05$ Fig. 3c. At every trypsinization, BMSCs detached faster than ADSCs using equal volumes of 0.25 M concentration of trypsin EDTA. The viability of cells after trypsinization showed that ADSCs had higher viability at all the passages compared to BMSCs. At the 95% confidence limit, ADSCs viabilities were significantly higher at P1, P2 and P3, Fig. 3d.

Chondrogenic Induction and Gene Expressions

After the normalization with their GAPDH, the expressions of the specific genes for chondrocytes on the induced samples of

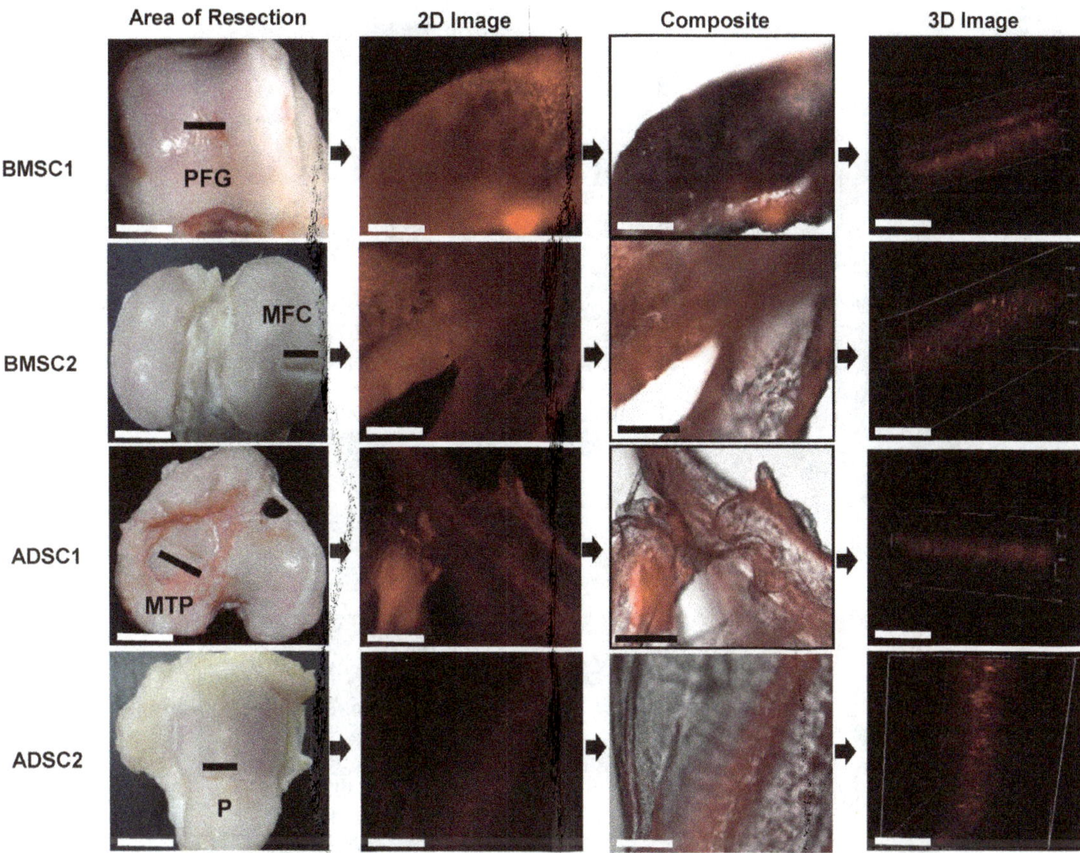

Figure 6. Fluorescence evaluations of PKH26 dye on the resected regenerated cartilages. Samples were taken from PFG and MFC of the BMSCs samples; then from MTP and P of the ADSCs samples. PKH26 fluorescence was shown in 2D, the composite images and 3D images. The composite and 3D confocal images revealed the integration and arrangements of the labeled chondrogenically induced cells. The fluorescence of the dye proved the participation of the injected cells in the cartilage regeneration. Scale: gross images = 1.5 cm and microscopic images = 35 μm.

BMSCs and ADSCs were higher compared to the uninduced samples. Chondrogenically induced ADSCs had 12.96, 23.44, 44.36 and 18.44 folds increases of Col II, SOX9, Aggrecan core protein and Col I genes respectively Fig. 4a, while the chondrogenically induced BMSCs had 16.21, 51.40, 120.33 and 19.17 fold increases respectively which were significant at 95% confidence limit, Fig. 4b. Compared to ADSCs, BMSCs had significantly higher expressions (1.85, 2.03 and 5.31) of Col II, Aggrecan and SOX9 genes respectively but not on Col I ($p<0.05$).

Gross Evaluations

The treated joints had varying degrees of regenerated cartilages. The regenerations at patella-femoral groove (PFG) were more prominent and had a distinct morphological appearance. They were different in appearance compare to the native cartilage and were not present on controls Fig. 5a. The medial femoral condyles (MFC) of the treated sheep had decreased cartilage degenerations and possible cartilage regeneration. They were better that the control samples which showed deep cartilage degeneration. There were no much differences from samples at the lateral femoral condyle (LFC), except for the controls that revealed swollen reduced cartilage thickness which will likely deteriorate with time Fig. 5a. At the medial tibia plateau (MTP), the treated samples had visible signs of cartilage regeneration and most prominently, the formation of a crescent structure-like meniscus in attempt to replace the resected meniscus. The control samples had no signs of meniscus regeneration; instead there was a remnant of spur bone formed at the anterior region of the medial tibia plateau (white arrow), which is a supportive formation seen in severe OA development. There were reduced signs of cartilage degeneration at the lateral tibia plateau (LTP) for the treated sheep samples, but deep cartilage defects on the control samples Fig. 5a. The patella (P) showed reduced cartilage degeneration on the treated samples, while the controls revealed remarkable deep cartilage defects Fig. 5a. Generally, the treated sheep had varying degrees of regenerations, but the control sheep had little evidence of cartilage regeneration and the area of degeneration were prominent in all the regions. On the ICRS grade scale, the control sheep scored a mean grade of 3.3 ± 0.2, while the test groups ADSCs and BMSCs scored 1.5 ± 0.2 and 1.3 ± 0.3 respectively Fig. 5b. Using the 95% confidence interval estimation, both treated knee were highly significant compared to the control with P values of 0.0001 and 0.0001 respectively. BMSCs treated sheep had better scores of ICRS than ADSCs but was not significant $P=0.465$.

Fluorescence of PKH26 Dye

The monolayer pictures of the labeled cells showed the cytoplasm stained with PKH26. Fluorescence microscopic analysis of the resected portions of neo-cartilages from the treated right knee joints revealed red fluorescence of PKH26 on the various regions with visible regenerations Fig. 6. These include: PFG, MFC, MTP and P. The composite images from these regions

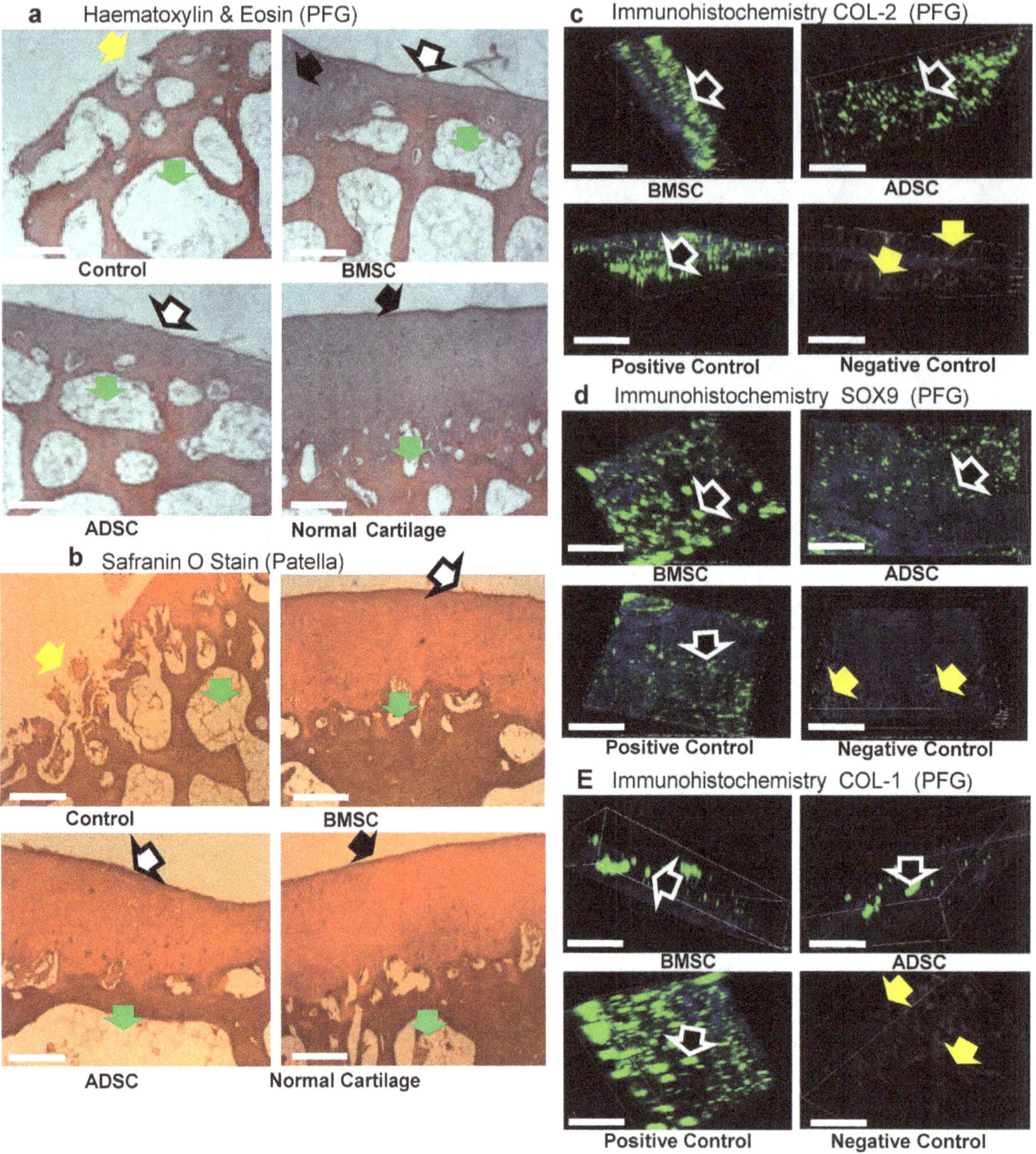

Figure 7. Histological and immunohistochemical evaluations of the right knee joints. (**a**) Haematoxylin and Eosin stain of the right knee joint PFG samples. Yellow arrow points at the exposed area of cartilage, leading to subchondral bone (green arrow) of the control knee joints. Treated samples (BMSCs and ADSCs) reflected regenerated engineered cartilages (white arrows) covering the subchondral bone, though not smoothly packed like the native cartilage (black arrow). Scale represents 70 μm. (**b**) Safranin O stains of the right knee joint (patella) samples. The regenerated cartilage on both treated knee (BMSCs and ADSCs) stained positive (white arrow). They were homogenous to the histochemical properties of accumulated proteoglycans revealed via Safranin O, but not smooth as the native cartilage (black arrow). Yellow arrow points at the degenerated area of cartilage on the control; green arrow, the subchondral bone. Scale represents 70 μm. (**c**) Immunohistochemistry images of the right knee joint (PFG) samples. Collagen type II protein staining for both treated samples (BMSCs and ADSCs) demonstrated positive staining within the ground tissues and were visible throughout the matrixes, evidenced by the green fluorescence tagged with the secondary antibody (black arrow). The native articular cartilage served as positive control (black arrow). The absence of green fluorescence on the ground tissue of the engineered cartilages without the primary antibody (yellow arrow) served as the negative control. Scale represents 35 μm. (**d**) Immunohistochemistry images of the right knee joint (PFG) samples. SOX9 staining for BMSCs and ADSCs demonstrated positivity within the ground tissues and were visible throughout the matrixes by the green fluorescence tagged with the secondary antibody (black arrow). The native articular cartilage served as positive control (black arrow), while the absence of green fluorescence on the ground tissue of the engineered cartilages without the primary antibody (yellow arrow) served as the negative control. Scale represents 35 μm. (**e**) Immunohistochemistry images of the right knee joint (PFG) samples. Collagen type I staining for BMSCs and ADSCs demonstrated diminished positivity within the ground tissues. This occurred mainly as scattered clusters of the green fluorescence tagged with the secondary antibody (black arrow). The fibrous cartilage served as positive control (black arrow), while the absence of green fluorescence on the ground tissue of the engineered cartilages without the primary antibody (yellow arrow) served as the negative control. Scale represents 35 μm. **Note**: The authors wish to state that a superimposed histological image of Safranin O and PKH26 dye or the immuno signals with PKH26 dye would have made better proves of the presence of the injected cells, but owing to technical challenges with these processes and the dye stability, it was not accomplished.

which comprised a phase contrast and the fluorescence image depicted the possible interactions of the labelled cells with the native cartilage. With the confocal microscope, three-dimensional (3-D) layered arrangements of integration of the neo cartilages with the native could be appreciated. The fluorescence confirmed that the injected cells were on the articular surfaces of the treated joints.

Histological Evaluation

The tissue-engineered cartilages from the visible regenerated portions of the PFG on both treated sheep samples showed slight signs of lacunae and cartilage isolated cells on haematoxylin and eosin staining. Though the regenerated cartilages exhibited the stain of well distributed cartilage cells within the basophilic ground substances, they were not smoothly packed like the native cartilage. The controls showed reduced cartilage layer and exposure of the subchondral bone Fig. 7a. The regenerated cartilage from the P on both treated samples stained positive with Safranin O. They were avascular and homogenous in accordance to the accumulated proteoglycans revealed in Safranin O staining. There was no difference in the stains of ADSCs compared to the BMSCs, but the control samples showed deep cartilage defects Fig. 7b. On immunohistochemistry analysis, both treated knee samples from the regenerated portions of PFG demonstrated expressions for Col II (the major oligomeric protein in hyaline cartilage), SOX9 (the main transcription factor for cartilage) and Col 1(a marker of fibrous cartilage) proteins within the ground tissues. Both Col II and SOX9 antigens can be highly visualized throughout the matrix of the engineered cartilages by the green fluorescence of the secondary antibody Fig. 7c and 7d; while the expression of negative marker Col I was scanty present within the ground tissue Fig. 7e.

Discussions

Cell based therapeutic approaches in tissue engineering and regenerative medicine has highlighted the need for the utilization of the abundant, undifferentiated progenitor cells in various tissues [2]. This study compared adult stem cells from adipose tissue (ADSCs) and bone marrow (BMSCs) that were cultured under the same chondrogenic conditions and duration. Both cell samples exhibited multipotency abilities at least, to the three main cell types of mesoderm origin evaluated, adipocyte, osteocyte and chondrocyte. This was in agreement with some of the earlier reports in pluripotency of adult stem cells from various tissues [1] [2] [11] [17] [20]. Our observation that ADSCs has more cells attached than BMSCs from the second day of culture was a further indication as suggested earlier that, ADSCs had relatively abundance cells available as compared to BMSCs [20] [21] [22] [23]. It had also been reported that ADSCs achieved higher passage number compared to BMSCs before senescence [24] [25] [26]. The trypsinization experience suggested that ADSCs may have secreted more extracellular matrixes for adhesion and needed more time to dissolve after the application of trypsin EDTA. This extra cellular matrix might also have protected their contacts with trypsin EDTA thus, gave them higher viability after trypsinization. This is a new observation from this study and needed more experiments for confirmation as it was consistent in all the passages and with different concentrations of trypsin EDTA (data not shown).

Using the same chondrogenic formula which was necessary for a fair comparison of gene expression and cartilage regeneration from both cells, BMSCs had higher expressions on all the four genes compared to ADSCs. Col II which is the most abundant hyaline cartilage oligomeric matrix protein; SOX9, a major transcription factor; aggrecan, the predominant proteoglycan and Col I, a negative marker to hyaline cartilage [20], [27] were highly expressed by the BMSCs. This was reflected on the nature of cartilages formed and the regeneration that followed on the treated sheep. BMSCs induced better than ADSCs using our induction medium, even though they also had higher expression of the fibrotic marker. Immunohistochemistry showed a high presence of SOX9 transcription protein, Col II together with a diminished presence of Col I protein on both treated knee samples. The presence of Col II throughout the matrix of both samples was as a result of the in vivo three-dimensional interactions of the cells. This confirmed the phenotype of maturing hyaline-like cartilages in contrast with the in vitro gene expressions. The diminished expression of Col I was also due to the same course. Previously in our work, we had shown that cartilage induction in two-dimensional monolayer culture flask expressed less Col II and more Col I with cells retaining fibroblastic morphology. These expressions were changed towards typical Col II and polygonal morphology of hyaline-like chondrocytes, when the cells were implanted in vivo under the skin of nude mice [28].

It was reported that ADSCs have reduced or absent transforming growth factor β (TGF- β) receptor ALK-5 [29], and cell surface marker vascular cell adhesion molecule 1 (CD106) [20] thus, under standard chondrogenic differentiation conditions, typically utilizing TGF- β and dexamethasone, BMSCs have an enhanced potential for chondrogenesis compared to ADSCs [24] [30]. However, other reports suggested that ADSCs had been shown to be more efficiently induced towards chondrogenic lineage by a high dose of bone morphogenetic protein-6 (BMP-6) than by TGF-β or other cocktails [20] [29]. Kim and Im reported that higher concentration of growth factors, specifically fivefold of TGF-β and IGF for ADSCs is required to overcome the chondrogenic differences with BMSCs [21] [31] [32].

The arthroscopic and arthrotomy images of the joint before OA inductions showed that they were free of degenerations. Trauma to the ACL, meniscus and isolated cartilage lesions have been reported to be responsible for osteoarthritis of the joint with time [33]. Our combination of resections and exercise regimen caused severe multifocal cartilage degenerations typical of OA. The chondrogenically induced injected cells elicited varying degrees of regenerations on the test samples compared to the controls as represented by the ICRS grading. This reflected decreased cartilage degenerations and increased regenerations on the treated animal compared to controls. In addition, the regeneration of the meniscus seen in the treated animals only is also a remarkable feature in this study, being that naturally, meniscus is less likely to regenerate. Among the many surgical methods to regenerate cartilage [11] [12] [13] [34] [35] [36] microfracture has been the most favorable [33]. Clinical studies of autologous chondrocytes transplantation generally have reported significant improvements in function [2]. However these techniques retain a high probability of fibrous tissue formation, periosteum flap hypertrophy, cell apoptosis, cartilage degeneration, incomplete hyaline cartilage generation and donor site morbidity [26]. These issues have encouraged studies with injectable chondrogenically induced ADSCs and BMSCs in cartilage regenerations. Our results gave hope for the first time, a prospective clinical regeneration of cartilage that does not involve surgical implantations, autologous chondrocytes, invasiveness and related complications in 6 weeks; only a single dose injection of the appropriate number of induced chondrocyte is required to regenerate full chondral degradations.

The histological evaluation of the engineered cartilage with haematoxylin and eosin at PFG, showed the histoarchitectural characteristics of well distributed chondrocytes within the basophilic ground substances. The arrangement of the condensing cartilage could be seen just as earlier reports [20]. The test samples also stained positive for safranin O at P, but presented rough outer periphery compared to the native cartilage.

In our earlier study, it was found that both uninduced BMSC and chondrogenic induced BMSC could retard the progression of OA, though the chondrogenically induced cells indicated better results [8] [16]. There have been varied reports on probable paracrine effects of the pluripotent stem cells to illicit regenerations [37] [38]. Efforts to clarify the authenticity of our claims from possible regenerations done by migrating cells or secretory vesicles necessitated the labeling of both cell samples to ascertain their homing. PKH26 dye was detected on the resected portions of regenerated cartilages in all 4 regions of the right knee joints. This consolidated our previous and the present claim; and proved that the injected chondrogenically induced cells participated in the regeneration of the osteoarthritic lesions within 6 weeks.

Limitations: Considering that sheep matures at about 18months and osteoarthritis is a disease of the elderly, the first limitation to this study was the age of some of the experimental animals. Due to the difficulty in procuring the desired older samples, these teenage sheep were used in our study. Secondly, it was our view to evaluate the dedifferentiating (negative) markers of hyaline cartilage (Collagen I and Collagen X) in order to ascertain the extent of maturity and stability of the engineered cartilages. Collagen I was evaluated, but due to the unavailability of sheep Collagen X primer and antibody at the time of this study, we were unable to verify the hypertrophic status of these engineered cartilages. The last limitation to this study is the inability to circumscribe the injected cells to the lesion site only, to ensure better regeneration. This, if accomplished in the future, will help to save the precious cells only to the desired location.

Conclusions

In this study ADSCs had better cell proliferations, but BMSCs had better chondrogenic inductions and gene expressions. There was no difference of ICRS score between ADSCs and BMSCs treatment. The presence of the tracking dye PKH26 at the resected portions of the neo-cartilages confirmed the participation of our injected cell in the osteoarthritic regeneration, hence both autologous chondrogenically induced ADSCs and BMSCs could be promising cell sources for cartilage regeneration in osteoarthritis.

Acknowledgments

The authors wish to acknowledge the Ministry of Higher Education of Malaysia and the staffs of Tissue Engineering Center Universiti Kebangsaan Malaysia Medical Center.

Author Contributions

Conceived and designed the experiments: CCU SBS NMH CHC JA NMY ABS. Performed the experiments: CCU SBS NMH CHC JA NMY ABS RBHI. Analyzed the data: CCU SBS NMH CHC JA NMY ABS RBHI. Contributed reagents/materials/analysis tools: CCU SBS NMH CHC JA NMY ABS RBHI. Wrote the paper: CCU SBS NMH CHC JA NMY ABS RBHI. Obtaining of funding: ABS RBHI.

References

1. Bradely TE, Diekman OD, Gimbe JM, Guilak F (2010) Isolation of adipose-derived stem cells and their induction to a chondrogenic phenotype. Nature Protocols 5 (7): 1294–1311.
2. Guilak F, Bradely TE, Diekman OD, Montos FT, Gimbe JM (2010) Multipotent adult stem cells from adipose tissue for musculoskeletal tissue engineering. Clin Orthop Relat Res 468: 2530–2540.
3. Murphy CL, Sambanis A (2001) Effect of oxygen tension and alignate encapsulation on restoration of the differentiated phenotype of passaged chondrocyte. Tissue Eng 7: 791–803.
4. Aichroth PM, Patel DV, Moyes ST (1991) A prospective review of arthroscopic debridement for degenerative joint disease of the knee. Int. Orthop 15: 351–355.
5. Aubin PP, Cheah HK, Davis AM, Gross AE (2007) Long-term followup of fresh femoral osteochondral allografs for posttraumatic knee defect. Clin. Orthop. Relat. Res (Suppl 391): S318–S327.
6. Tew SR, Kwan AP, Hann A, Thomson BM, Archer CW (2000) The reactions of articular cartilage to experimental wounding: role of apoptosis. Arthritis Rheum 43: 251–225.
7. Crisan M, Yap S, Casteilla L, Chen CW, Corselli M, Park TS, et al (2008) A perivascular origin for mesenchymal stem cells in multiple human organs. Cell Stem Cell 3:301–313.
8. Al Faqeh H, NorHamdan BMY, Chen HC, Aminuddin BS, Ruszymah BHI (2012) The potential of intra-articular injection of chondrogenic-induced bone marrow stem cells to retard the progression of osteoarthritis in a sheep model. Experimental Gerontology 47: 458–464.
9. Chen K, Man C, Zhang B, Hu J, Zhu S-S (2013) Effect of in vitro chondrogenic differentiation of autologous mesenchymal stem cells on cartilage and subchondral cancellous bone repair in osteoarthritis of temporomandibular joint. International Journal of Oral and Maxillofacial Surgery 42 (2): 240–248.
10. Mifune Y, Matsumoto T, Takayama K, Ota S, Li H, et al (2013) The effect of platelet – rich plasma on the regenerative therapy of muscle derived stem cells for articular repair. Osteoarthritis and Cartilage 21 (1): 175–185.
11. Murphy JM, David JF, Hunziker EB, Barry FP (2003) Stem Cell Therapy in a Caprine Model of Osteoarthritis. Arthritis and Rheumatism. 48(12): 3464–3477.
12. Dragoo JL, Carlson G, Mccormick F, Khan-Farooqi H, Min Z, et al (2007) Healing Full-Thickness Cartilage Defects using Adipose-Derived Stem Cells. Tissue Engineering, 13: 7.
13. Centeno CJ, Busse D, Kisiday J, Keohan C, Freeman M, et al (2008) Increased Knee Cartilage Volume in Degenerative Joint Disease using Percutaneously Implanted, Autologous Mesenchymal Stem Cells. Pain Physician 11: 343–353.
14. Horan PK and Slezak SE (1989) Stable Cell Membrane Labeling; Nature 340: 67–168.
15. Sigma. Staining optimization for PKH Dyes (1993) Research 53: 2360.
16. Alfaqeh H, Norhamdan MY, Chua KH, Chen HC, Aminuddin BS, et al (2008) Cell Therapy for Osteoarthritis in Sheep Model, gross and histological assessment. The Medical Journal of Malaysia. 63(Supp A): 37.
17. Wickham MQ, Erickson GR, Gimble JM, Vail TP, Guilak F (2003) Multipotent Stromal Cells Derived From the Infrapatellar Fat Pad of the Knee. Clinical Orthopaedics & Related Research: July 2003 - Volume 412 - Issue - pp 196–212 doi: 10.1097/01.blo.0000072467.53786.ca.
18. Ude CC, Shamsul BS, Ng MH, Chen HC, Aminuddin BS (2012) Bone marrow and adipose stem cells can be tracked with PKH26 until post staining passage 6 *invitro and invivo*. Tissue and Cell. doi: 10.1016/j.tice.
19. Alfaqeh HH, Chua KH, Aminuddin BS, Ruszymah BHI (2011) Growth medium with low medium and transforming growth factor beta 3 promotes better chondrogenesis of bone marrow-derived stem cells in vitro and invivo. Saudi Med. J. 32 (6): 640–641.
20. Brian OD, Christopher RR, Donald PL, Arnold IC, Guilak F (2010) Chondrogenesis of adult stem cells from adipose tissue and bone marrow: Induction by growth factors and cartilage-derived matrix. Tissue Engineering: part A. Vol.16.
21. Aust L, Devlin B, Foster SJ, Halvorsen YD, Hicok K, et al. (2004) Yield of human adipose-derived adult stem cells from liposuction aspirates. Cytotherapy 6:7.
22. Oedayrajsingh-Varma MJ, VanHam SM, Knippenberg M, Helder Mn, Klein-Nulend J, et al. (2006) Adipose tissue-derived mesenchymal stem cell yield and growth characteristics are affected by the tissue-harvesting procedure. Cytotherapy. 8:166–177.
23. Im GI, Shin YW, Lee KB (2005) Do adipose tissue-derived mesenchymal stem cells have the same osteogenic and chondrogenic potential as bone marrow-derived cells? Osteoarthritis Cartilage/OARS, Osteoarthritis Res Soc. 13: 845.
24. Rider DA, Dombrowski C, Sawyer AA, Ng GH, Leong D, et al. (2008) Autocrine fibroblast growth factor 2 increases the multipotentiality of human adipose-derived mesenchymal stem cells. Stem Cells (Dayton), 26: 1598.
25. Izadpanah R, Trygg C, Patel B, Kriedt C, Dufour J, et al. (2006) Biologic properties of mesenchymal stem cells derived from bone marrow and adipose tissue. J Cell Biochem. 99: 1285.
26. Puetzer JL, Petitte JN, Loboa EG (2010) Tissue Engineering Part B: Reviews. 16(4): 435–444.
27. Mehlhorn AT, Niemeyer P, Kaiser S, Finkenzeller G, Stark GB, et al. (2006) Differential expression pattern of extracellular matrix molecules during chondrogenesis of mesenchymal stem cells from bone marrow and adipose tissue. Tissue Eng. 12: 2853.
28. Munirah S, Aminuddin BS, Samsudin OC, Chua KH, Fuzina NH (2005) The re-expression of Collagen II, Aggrecan and SOX9 in tissue engineered hman

articular cartilage. Tissue Engineering and Regenerative Medicine 2(4): 347–355.

29. Hennig T, Lorenz H, Thiel A, Goetzke K, Dickhut A (2007) Reduced chondrogenic potential of adipose tissue derived stromal cells correlates with an altered TGF beta receptor and BMP profile and is overcome by BMP-6. J Cell Physiol, 211: 682.
30. Adila AH, Ruszymah BHI, Aminuddin BS, Somasumdaram S, Chuaa KH (2012) Characterization of human adipose-derived stem cells and expression of chondrogenic genes during induction of cartilage differentiation. Clinics, 67(2): 99–106.
31. Kim HJ, and Im GI (2009) Chondrogenic differentiation of adipose tissue-derived mesenchymal stem cells: greater doses of growth factor are necessary. J Orthop Res. 27: 612.
32. Sha'ban M, Samsudin OC, NorHamdan MY, Aminuddin BS, Ruszymah BHI (2012) Sox-9 transient transfection enhances chondrogenic osteoarthritic in vitro: Preliminary Analysis. Tissue Engineering and Regenerative Medicine. 8(1) 32–41.
33. Hunziker EB (2002) Articular cartilage repair: basic science and clinical progress. A review of the current status and prospects. Osteoarthritis and Cartilage. 10:432–463.
34. Saw KY, Adam A, Shahrin M, Tay YG, Kunaseegaran R, et al (2010) Articular Cartilage Regeneration with Autologous Peripheral Blood Progenitor Cells and Hyaluronic Acid after Arthroscopic Subchondral Drilling: A Report of 5 Cases with Histology. J. Arthro 11: 054 Doi: 10. 1016/.
35. Maumus M, Guérit D, Toupet K, Jorgensen C, Noël D (2011) Mesenchymal Stem Cell-Based Therapies in Regenerative Medicine: Applications in Rheumatology. Stem Cell Res. Ther. 2 (2): 14.
36. Pak J (2011) Regeneration of Human Bones in Hip Osteonecrosis and Human Cartilage in Knee Osteoarthritis with Autologous Adipose Tissue-Derived Stem Cells: A Case Series. Pak Journal of Medical Case Reports, 5:296.
37. Gnecchi M, Zhang Z, Aiguo N, Dzau VJ (2008) Paracrine Mechanisms in Adult Stem Cell Signaling and Therapy. Circ Res. 103:1204–1219.
38. Ratajczak MZ, Kucia M, Jadczyk T, Greco NJ, Wojakowski W (2012) Pivotal role of paracrine effects in stem cell therapies in regenerative medicine: can we translate stem cell-secreted paracrine factors and micro vesicles into better therapeutic strategies? Leukemia. 26, 1166–1173.

Disease Progression and Phasic Changes in Gene Expression in a Mouse Model of Osteoarthritis

Richard F. Loeser[1]*, Amy L. Olex[2], Margaret A. McNulty[3], Cathy S. Carlson[3], Michael Callahan[4], Cristin Ferguson[4], Jacquelyn S. Fetrow[2,5]

1 Department of Internal Medicine, Section of Molecular Medicine, Wake Forest University School of Medicine, Winston-Salem, North Carolina, United States of America, **2** Department of Computer Science, Wake Forest University, Winston-Salem, North Carolina, United States of America, **3** Department of Veterinary Population Medicine, College of Veterinary Medicine, University of Minnesota, St. Paul, Minneapolis, United States of America, **4** Department of Orthopedic Surgery, Wake Forest University School of Medicine, Winston-Salem, North Carolina, United States of America, **5** Department of Physics, Wake Forest University, Winston-Salem, North Carolina, United States of America

Abstract

Osteoarthritis (OA) is the most common form of arthritis and has multiple risk factors including joint injury. The purpose of this study was to characterize the histologic development of OA in a mouse model where OA is induced by destabilization of the medial meniscus (DMM model) and to identify genes regulated during different stages of the disease, using RNA isolated from the joint "organ" and analyzed using microarrays. Histologic changes seen in OA, including articular cartilage lesions and osteophytes, were present in the medial tibial plateaus of the DMM knees beginning at the earliest (2 week) time point and became progressively more severe by 16 weeks. 427 probe sets (371 genes) from the microarrays passed consistency and significance filters. There was an initial up-regulation at 2 and 4 weeks of genes involved in morphogenesis, differentiation, and development, including growth factor and matrix genes, as well as transcription factors including Atf2, Creb3l1, and Erg. Most genes were off or down-regulated at 8 weeks with the most highly down-regulated genes involved in cell division and the cytoskeleton. Gene expression increased at 16 weeks, in particular extracellular matrix genes including Prelp, Col3a1 and fibromodulin. Immunostaining revealed the presence of these three proteins in cartilage and soft tissues including ligaments as well as in the fibrocartilage covering osteophytes. The results support a phasic development of OA with early matrix remodeling and transcriptional activity followed by a more quiescent period that is not maintained. This implies that the response to an OA intervention will depend on the timing of the intervention. The quiescent period at 8 weeks may be due to the maturation of the osteophytes which are thought to temporarily stabilize the joint.

Editor: Francois Rannou, Cochin Hospital (AP-HP), and the University Paris Descarte, France

Funding: Supported by an Innovative Research Award from the Arthritis Foundation, The Wake Forest University Translational Science Institute, NIH Musculoskeletal Training Grant (T32 AR050938) and NIH Orthopaedics and Skeletal Biology Training Grant (T32 AR052272). The funders had no role in study design, data collection and analysis, decision to publish, or preparation of the manuscript.

Competing Interests: The authors have declared that no competing interests exist.

* E-mail: rloeser@wakehealth.edu

Introduction

Osteoarthritis (OA) affects over 27 million people in the United States and is similarly prevalent across the globe, making it the most common cause of chronic disability in adults [1,2]. There are a number of well established risk factors for OA that include age, obesity, prior joint injury, genetics, joint anatomy, and occupational history related to joint use [3]. Current treatments for OA are limited and no treatment has been conclusively shown to alter disease progression. A better understanding of the biological factors which drive disease progression, particularly early-stage disease, is needed in order to develop more targeted therapies to stop or slow progression.

Studies of human OA are limited by its multifactorial nature, the lack of tissue that can be obtained at various stages of the disease and difficulties in defining disease onset. Basic mechanistic studies often are performed with tissue obtained at the time of joint replacement, which represents end-stage disease. These studies have focused largely on changes present in the articular cartilage; however, OA is a condition that affects the joint as an organ including not only the cartilage but also subchondral bone, synovium, ligaments and, in the knee, the meniscus (reviewed in [4]).

Various animal models of OA have been developed in order to study the disease process under more controlled conditions where disease onset and stages of progression can be better defined and evaluated. A commonly used model in mice is the destabilized medial meniscus (DMM) model where OA is surgically induced by transection of the medial meniscotibial ligament. In this model, OA results from altered joint biomechanics and the pathologic changes of cartilage destruction, subchondral bone thickening, and osteophyte formation are similar to the changes seen in human OA [5]. We recently used this model to compare the changes in OA severity and gene expression in young and older adult mice at a single time point of 8 weeks after DMM surgery [6]. The severity of OA changes in the joint of the older adult mice (12 months old at the time of surgery) was about twice that of the younger adult mice (12 weeks old at surgery) and significant differences were noted in the genes that were up and down-regulated at that time point.

The present study was designed as a time-course experiment to evaluate changes in gene expression during the development of OA and to compare these changes to the histologic progression of the disease. The recently reported comparison of gene expression at the 8 week time point in young adult and older adult mice [6] was a sub-study of the present work, but because of the lack of sufficient numbers of older animals the time course study only includes the young adult mice. Similar to the previous report, the histological assessment and the gene microarray analysis were designed in a manner which considered OA as a disease of the joint as an organ and, thus, were not limited to a single tissue within the joint. The general hypothesis was that different stages of the disease process would be characterized by unique gene expression signatures. Knowledge of the biological processes regulated by these genes could provide new information about the OA disease process. The results demonstrated progressive histological changes of OA beginning within two weeks of DMM surgery and progressing over the 16 week time course. These were accompanied by phasic changes in gene expression, with the peak number of up-regulated genes found at 4 weeks after induction of OA, a significant decline in expression at 8 weeks, and an increase again at 16 weeks with different clusters of genes being more prominent at each time point.

Materials and Methods

Animals and surgical induction of OA

Male C57BL/6 mice (n = 129) were purchased from Charles River Inc. and were 12 weeks of age at the time of DMM surgery or sham surgery performed as a control. Animal use was carried out in strict accordance with the recommendations in the Guide for the Care and Use of Laboratory Animals of the National Institutes of Health. The protocol was approved by the Wake Forest School of Medicine Animal Care and Use Committee (protocol #A09-622). All surgery was performed under isoflurane anesthesia, and all efforts were made to minimize suffering. Butorphanol (2.5mg/kg) was administered in the event of pain.

Details of animal housing and induction of OA have been recently published [6]. Mice were operated on in waves and at the time of surgery were randomly assigned to a surgical group and termination time point so that the date when the surgery was performed would not influence the results. For the present study, a group of 9 mice was used for collection of RNA at time 0 (before surgery) when the animals were 12 weeks old. For the other time points, 6 DMM and 6 sham controls were sacrificed at 2, 4, 8, and 16 weeks after surgery for histological analysis and 9 DMM and 9 sham controls were sacrificed at each time point for RNA isolation. As noted above, the histological sections and RNA used for the 8 week time point were from the same samples as those previously reported [6] but here were reanalyzed as part of the time course study.

Histological analysis

Hind limbs from both the operated side and the contralateral side of each animal were dissected and processed for histological analysis. The details of fixation, processing, and sectioning, as well as the histological analysis, were as recently published [6,7]. In brief, hematoxylin and eosin and safranin-O mid-coronal sections of each stifle joint were obtained and representative sections from each joint graded by an evaluator (MAM) blinded to group assignment. The evaluation included the Articular Cartilage Structure (ACS) score (0–12), Safranin-O (Saf-O) staining score (0–12), articular cartilage thickness and area,% chondrocyte cell death, subchondral bone area and thickness, and osteophyte total area. Because the most severe changes were consistently found on the tibial side of the joints, the analysis was focused on the tibial plateaus. Synovitis is only apparent in severe disease in this model and given the lack of sufficient numbers of severe samples there was no attempt to score synovial changes.

Immunohistochemistry was performed on sections from 3 DMM and 4 sham control mice at the 16-week time point in order to examine tissue distribution of type III collagen, fibromodulin and proline-arginine-rich end leucine-rich repeat protein (Prelp). Antigen retrieval and blocking steps were as recently described [6]. Primary antibodies were acquired from Abcam Inc (Cambridge, MA) and included rabbit polyclonal antibodies to Collagen III (ab7778), Prelp (ab103868), and fibromodulin (ab81443). Secondary antibodies and detection were as described [6]. Immunostained sections were graded for cell and matrix staining using a scale of no immunopositivity (−) to marked immunopositivity (++++).

RNA preparation and microarray analysis

Knee joint tissue from the medial joint compartment was obtained from the time 0 group and the operated hind limbs from the other time points and processed for RNA isolation as described [6]. The tissue included tibial plateau and femoral condyle articular cartilage, subchondral bone with any osteophytes, meniscus, and the joint capsule with synovium. The tissue was treated with RNAlater® (Invitrogen) prior to freezing and storage at −80°C. RNA was extracted by homogenization using the Precellys 24 tissue homogenizer (Bertin Technologies purchased from MO BIO) as described [6] and the amount and quality of the RNA was determined using an Agilent 2100 Bioanalyzer.

RNA was pooled prior to microarray analysis such that 3 randomly selected samples from each surgical group and time point were pooled to create a each biological replicate. Because 9 mice were used for each experimental group, a total of three biological replicates per group were analyzed using the Affymetrix Mouse Genome 430 2.0 oligonucleotide arrays as described [6]. One replicate pool, which was from week two DMM mice, did not meet the RNA integrity level needed for microarray analysis; thus, this pool was not analyzed further, leaving two pools for the week two DMM mice.

Normalization and processing of microarray data

Microarrays were imaged and the resulting data normalized using systematic variation normalization (SVN) as previously described [6,8]. Reported data included the $\log_2$ of the signal intensity and the Affymetrix detection p-value for each probe set. Because some genes had more than one probe set, we provide results for both numbers of genes and probe sets when the numbers differed. The complete dataset has been provided to the Gene Expression Omnibus (GEO) repository (accession number GSE41342). Relative gene expression in the samples collected from the sham-operated control animals was calculated to identify those genes that changed as the animals aged over the 16 week time course independent of DMM-induced OA. For this analysis, sham gene expression was calculated as the signal log ratio (SLR) of the average time 0 intensity (baseline un-operated controls) to each sham replicate pool for each time point. The average of the time 0 intensity was used to ensure a consistent baseline, and each biological replicate of the sham arrays was analyzed individually to allow biological consistency to be measured in the analysis. The SLR is the $\log_2$ of the fold change and so an SLR of 0.5 = 1.4-fold. After SLR calculations, each probe set had 12 associated SLR values (3 for each time point—2, 4, 8 and 16 weeks), which together are referred to as the "sham time course".

Relative gene expression changes for the DMM time course were calculated to identify those genes that changed over time due to the DMM-induced changes in the joints. For this analysis, the sham results were used as a time-matched control (sham 2 weeks used as control for DMM 2 weeks etc.). Sham replicate signal intensities for each time point were averaged to ensure a consistent baseline for each replicate. DMM gene expression was then calculated as the time-matched signal log ratio of the average sham intensity to each DMM replicate for each time point, where each DMM replicate was analyzed individually. After SLR calculations, each probe set had 11 associated SLR values (2 for the 2 week time point, and 3 each for 4, 8 and 16 weeks), which are referred to as the "DMM time course".

Filtering and clustering of microarray data

Relative gene expression for the sham time course and DMM time course was filtered for differentially expressed genes with consistent expression changes over time as previously described [9] with a few alterations. Briefly, both data sets were filtered in a step-wise fashion as illustrated in **Figure 1**. Replicate time courses were filtered individually in the first two steps to identify those transcripts that were significantly detected on the chip over background (detection p-value $<=0.06$ for all time points and control), and for those that were differentially expressed in at least one time point (SLR ≥ 0.5 or ≤ -0.5 which converts to ≥ 1.4-fold and ≤ -1.4-fold). These data sets were intersected to identify those probe sets that passed the first two filtering steps independently in all replicates. Finally, transcripts were filtered for consistency of expression pattern (Pearson's correlation; PCC) and magnitude (Euclidean distance; ED) over time. An all-by-all comparison was done for each replicate time course profile resulting in 3 PCC and 3 ED scores for each probe set. Requiring all 6 scores to pass selected criteria was found to be too strict (data not shown). Therefore, only 2 of the 3 PCC and ED scores were required to pass selected cutoffs: PCC $>=0.70$ (a standard statistical threshold for positive correlation) and ED $<=0.60$ or $<=0.81$ for the DMM and sham time courses, respectively (the median ED score for each data set). Additionally, due to the missing 2-week DMM data for one of the replicates, all PCC and ED comparisons with this time course were done using only the 4-, 8- and 16-week time points. Probe sets passing all filtering criteria were considered to have been consistently and significantly expressed.

Filtered DMM time course gene expression data were clustered using the updated consensus clustering option provided by version 3 of SC^{2}ATmd [10]—sham time course data was not clustered in this work. The option to perform consensus clustering using a threshold to identify genes that cluster together less than 100% of the time was added to SC^{2}ATmd's functionality since its original release. This was implemented by converting the consensus matrix to an adjacency matrix and then using MATLAB's depth first search algorithm to identify consensus clusters. A figure of merit (FOM) analysis was run to determine the optimal number of clusters present in each replicate data set and to identify which clustering algorithm formed the most homogeneous clusters with respect to Euclidean distance [9,11]. As determined by the FOM analysis, consensus clustering was run using 10 starting clusters with k-means as the clustering algorithm and Euclidean distance as the distance metric. Each replicate data set was clustered 10 times, and a consensus over all 30 runs was calculated. Performing more than 10 iterations on each replicate did not significantly improve cluster homogeneity (data not shown). Probe sets clustering together 83% of the time were identified as a consensus cluster. Increasing or decreasing this threshold resulted in small clusters with many singletons or large clusters that were uninformative, respectively; thus, the 83% threshold was chosen as an acceptable balance between these two extremes

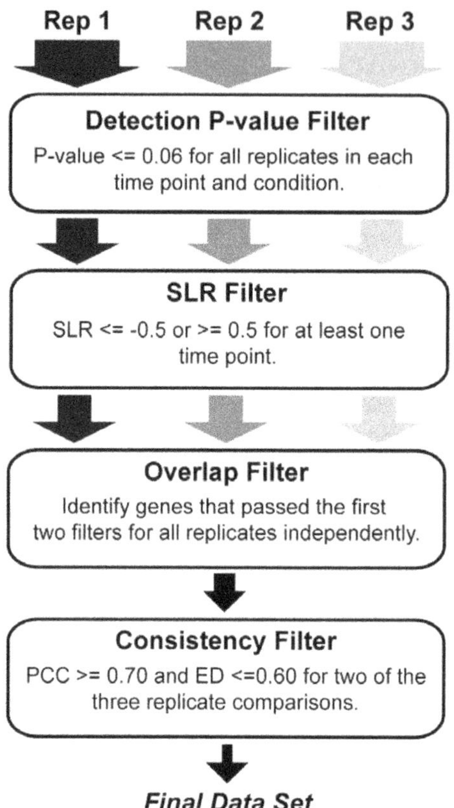

Figure 1. Flow chart of filtering process. After data normalization, SLR values were calculated as described in the methods, and replicate pools were randomly paired to obtain 3 complete time courses—referred to as Rep 1, Rep 2 and Rep 3. The first 2 filtering steps were done for each replicate independently, and identified probe sets that were significantly detected on the chip (detection p-value filter; all p-values $<=0.06$) as well as significantly differentially expressed (SLR filter; SLR was $<=-0.5$ or $>=0.5$ for any one time point). The overlap filter intersected all three filtered lists to identify the set of probe sets that passed the first 2 filtering steps independently in all replicates. Finally, probe sets were filtered for consistency in pattern (PCC score) and magnitude (ED score) of expression over time across all replicate time courses (consistency filter), where 2 of the 3 PCC scores had to be $>=0.70$, and 2 of the 3 ED scores had to be $<=0.60$. Those probe sets passing all filtering criteria were considered consistently and significantly differentially expressed across the time course in all 3 biological replicates, and were used for further analysis. Results of this process on each of the data sets described in the text can be found in Tables S1 and S2.

Annotation analysis

Annotation enrichment analysis was performed using the Database for Annotation, Visualization, Integration and Discovery (DAVID) [12,13]. The Functional Annotation Clustering tool provided by DAVID was run using the Affymetrix Mouse 430 2.0 chip as background, with all other options left at their default settings. Annotations of clusters were considered significant if the Enrichment Score was greater than or equal to 1.3 (equivalent to a p-value $<=0.05$).

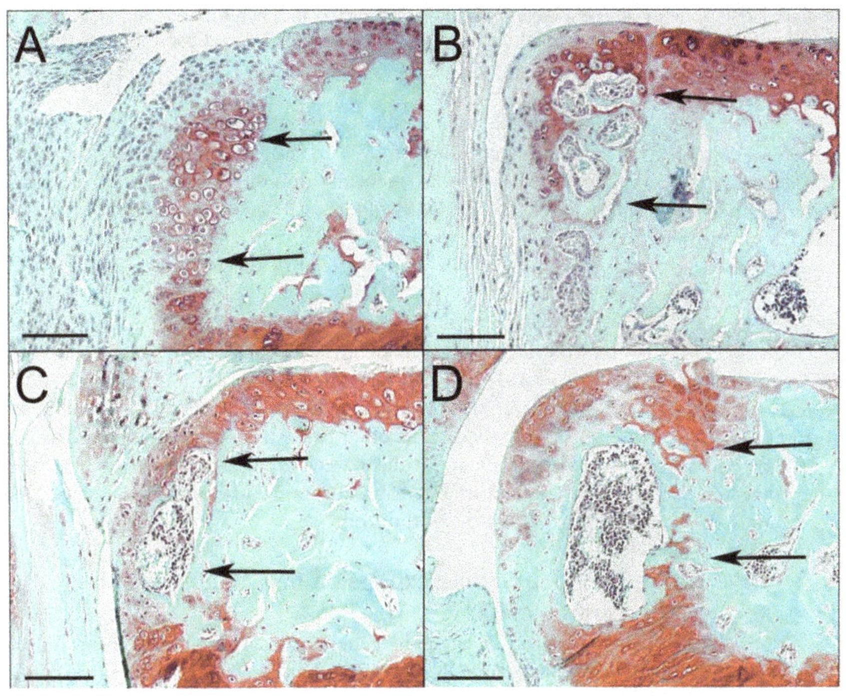

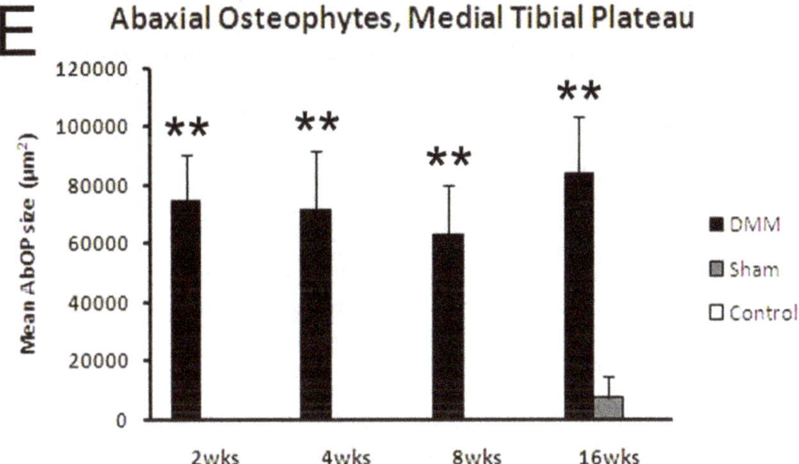

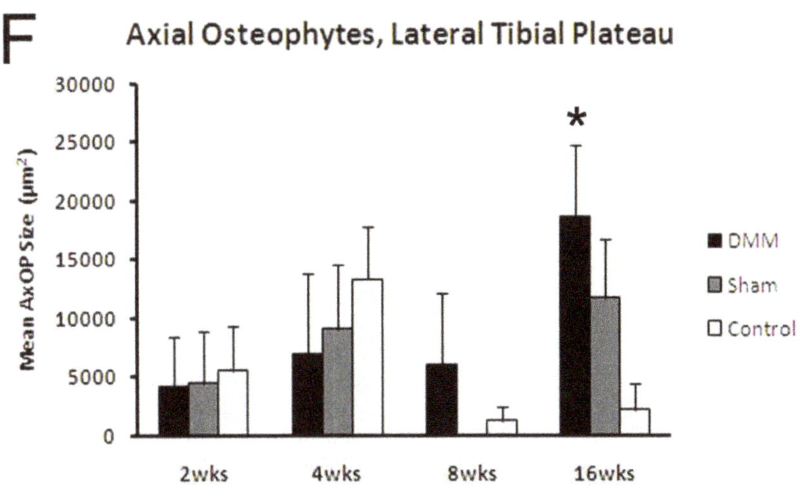

Figure 2. Histology results demonstrating osteophyte formation over the time course. Sections from DMM joints obtained 2 weeks (A), 4 weeks (B), 8 weeks (C), and 16 weeks (D) after DMM surgery were stained with safranin-O. Bar = 100 μm. Arrows point to the original medial abaxial joint margin and abaxial osteophytes that formed at this site. These start as chondrophytes at 2 weeks (A) and progressively mature.

Histomorphometric measures included the size of the abaxial osteophytes on the medial plateau (E) and axial osteophytes on the lateral plateau (F) for the DMM, sham, and contralateral control groups as indicated. **p<0.0001 vs sham and control; *p = 0.02 vs sham and control by ANOVA.

Real-time PCR

Real-time PCR was performed using samples of RNA from the same pools used for the microarrays as previously described [6] using the SYBR®Green-based method with optimized primer sets obtained in the RT2 qPCR Primer Assays (SABiosciences/Qiagen) and with TATA box-binding protein (TBP) used to normalize relative expression.

Statistical analysis

Analysis of the microarray data is presented above. The histological data and the real time PCR data were found to be normally distributed. Histological data from both the lateral and medial tibial plateaus was evaluated using ANOVAs (intra-animal comparisons) and repeated measures analyses (inter-animal comparisons) using SPSS version 17.0 (IBM Corp, Somers, NY). The real time PCR results at each individual time point for sham controls and DMM animals were analyzed using t tests with StatView 5.0 software (SAS, Cary, NC).

Results

Histologic progression of joint tissue changes induced by DMM surgery

The sham operated joints and the contralateral control (non-operated joints from sham and DMM animals) demonstrated minimal to no pathological changes over the 16 week time course. Among the earliest changes observed in the DMM joints at 2 weeks after surgery were abaxial osteophytes in the medial tibial plateau. Osteophytes were primarily cartilaginous at 2 weeks, were ossified at 4 weeks, and were composed of trabecular bone that contained marrow spaces occupied by hematopoietic tissue at 8 and 16 weeks (**Figure 2A, B, C, D**). Interestingly, the cross-sectional area of the osteophytes did not change significantly from 2–16 weeks (**Figure 2E**). Much smaller and more variable axial osteophytes were noted on the lateral tibial plateaus but, unlike the medial abaxial osteophytes, their size was not significantly different among the three groups until 16 weeks after surgery, when they were significantly larger in the DMM relative to the sham and contralateral control joints (**Figure 2F**).

There were mild articular cartilage lesions noted at 2 weeks in the medial tibial plateaus of the DMM joints, resulting in an increase in the articular cartilage structure score and an increase in the Saf-O scores relative to sham and contralateral control joints at this time point (**Figure 3**). The articular cartilage structure scores increased progressively over the 16 weeks in the DMM joints while the Saf-O scores remained more stable over time. At 16 weeks, there was a mild increase in the articular cartilage structure score at the lateral tibial plateau in the DMM joints but the mean score was less than half of that seen in the medial tibial plateau (**Figure 3G**). No significant differences were seen among the groups or time points for Saf-O scores in the lateral tibial plateaus (data not shown). In addition, there were no significant differences in articular cartilage thickness over the course of the study in any of the groups (data not shown).

Chondrocyte death in the medial tibial plateau articular cartilage was significantly increased at 4 weeks in the DMM and sham joints relative to the non-operated controls, and increased further in the DMM joints at 8 and 16 weeks (**Figure 4A**). Dead chondrocytes also were apparent in the lateral tibial plateaus at week 16 but the area occupied by dead chondrocytes was less than half that in the medial tibial plateau, nor was there a difference in this parameter among the surgical groups at any time point (**Figure 4B**). We have recently published evidence for chondrocyte death in the DMM model at 8 weeks after surgery including findings of positive TUNEL staining consistent with apoptosis [14]; thus, the mechanism of cell death was not pursued in the present study.

The subchondral bone was thicker in the medial tibial plateau than the lateral tibial plateau in all three groups and at all time points (**Table 1**). At all time points, the subchondral bone thickness and area were larger in the medial tibial plateau of the DMM group than in the other two groups, although this difference was only significant at the 4-week time point. In all groups, there was a gradual increase in subchondral bone thickness and area over the 16 weeks of the study.

Changes in gene expression over time in the sham control joints

To detect changes in gene expression occurring over the 16 week time period of the study that could be due to aging of the animals, we analyzed the gene expression results in the sham joints relative to the time 0 baseline. Filtering of the data revealed 347 genes (406 probe sets) significantly and consistently regulated over time in the sham joints. A complete list of these genes is provided in File S1. The 2-week time point had the largest number of up-regulated genes and this was followed by a progressive decrease in expression of the majority of genes over the 16 week time course (**Figure 5A and 5B**). The set of 347 genes was analyzed by DAVID's Functional Annotation Clustering tool [12], which identified 36 groups of significantly over-represented annotations with enrichment scores ≥1.3 (File S1). Most of the annotations were related to signal peptide, extracellular matrix, development, differentiation and morphogenesis, consistent with a maturation process occurring over the 16 week time course.

A small subset of 25 genes remained up-regulated over the time course (File S1). Functional Annotation Clustering was performed on this subset of genes, and only one group of significantly over-represented annotations was identified. This group of terms included plasma membrane, glycoprotein, immune response, and cell surface linked signal transduction terms.

Gene expression in DMM joints relative to sham controls

The time course results for changes in expression in the DMM joints relative to time-matched sham joints revealed 371 genes (427 probe sets) that were significantly and consistently regulated over the three biological replicates (File S2). Examination of a heat map of these genes as well as the SLR distributions (**Figure 6A and 6B**) reveals a phasic pattern. The majority of genes were up-regulated at 2 and 4 weeks followed by reduced expression or down-regulation at 8 weeks and then some increase in expression at 16 weeks although not to the level of weeks 2 and 4.

These results were much different from the time course results noted in the sham joints, consistent with changes in gene expression due to induction of OA by the DMM surgery. An overlap analysis revealed 94 genes (97 probe sets) that were in common in the DMM/sham and sham/baseline control datasets (**Figure 7A** and File S3). Many of these were extracellular matrix genes including Prelp, fibromodulin, several collagens (Types IV, V, XII, XVI, and XXII), and biglycan. A heat map revealed that

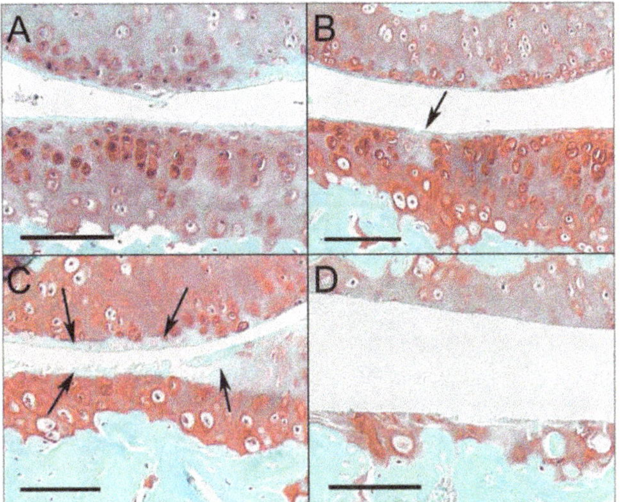

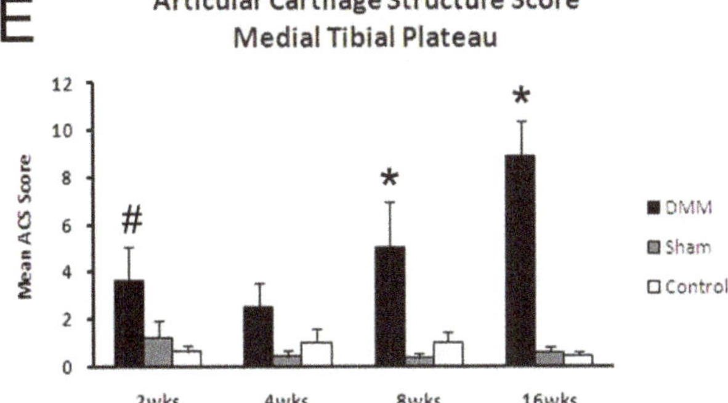

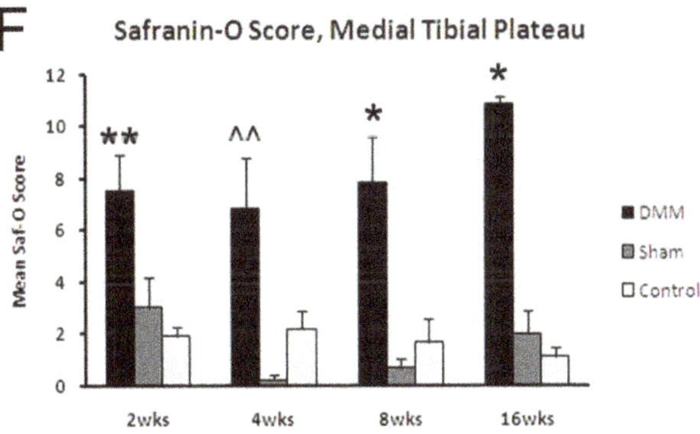

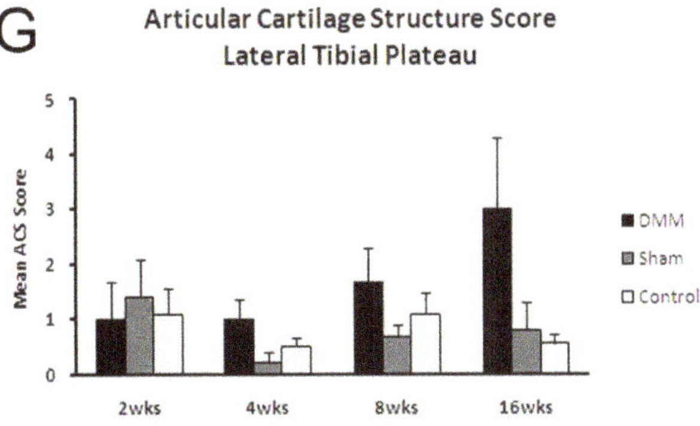

Figure 3. Histology results demonstrating articular cartilage lesions over the time course. Sections from DMM joints obtained 2 weeks (A), 4 weeks (B), 8 weeks (C), and 16 weeks (D) after DMM surgery were stained with safranin-O. Bar = 100 μm. Arrows indicate an early cartilage lesion in the medial tibial plateau at 4 weeks (B) and a more severe lesion at 8 weeks (C) on the medial tibial plateau (lower tissue in image) and the femoral condyle (upper tissue in image). Note advanced articular cartilage loss at 16 weeks. Articular cartilage structure scores (E) and safranin-O scores (F) for the medial tibial plateaus and articular cartilage structure scores for the lateral tibial plateau (G) are shown for the DMM, sham, and contralateral control groups as indicated. *$p<0.05$ vs sham and control; ^^$p=0.01$ vs sham; **$p<0.01$ vs control; #$p<0.05$ vs control by ANOVA.

almost all of these genes displayed very different expression profiles. Most were down-regulated over time in the sham controls but up-regulated in the DMM joints, particularly at 2 and 4 weeks (**Figure 7B**). Of the 94 genes in common between the DMM and sham joints, almost all were up-regulated in the DMM joint, with the exception of three: H2afz (predicted gene 6722///H2A histone family, member Z), Alms1(Alstrom syndrome 1), and Adhfe1(iron-containing alcohol dehydrogenase), which were down-regulated in the DMM joints. These genes do not have any known role in joint development or in OA.

The 94 genes in common between DMM/sham and sham/baseline were analyzed by DAVID. This returned 10 significant annotation groups (File S3) that included terms such as extracellular matrix, cell adhesion, collagen, skeletal development, EGF-like domains, fibronectin, leucine rich repeats, and endoplasmic reticulum.

Consensus clustering of the genes regulated during the development of OA in the DMM joints

Consensus clustering of genes with altered expression after DMM surgery identified 27 clusters with 2 or more probe sets and 38 genes (39 probe sets) that were classified as outliers (singletons). The complete list of the genes found in each cluster and the DAVID analysis for the clusters are found in File S2. Heat maps of the largest 16 clusters are shown in **Figure 8** and reveal striking differences in the temporal patterns of gene expression over the 16 week time course. The significant annotations for these clusters from DAVID analysis are shown in **Table 2**.

Only clusters 5, 7, 10 and 12 exhibited significant down-regulation at specific time points. Cluster 5 contained genes down-regulated at week 4; cluster 10, genes down-regulated at weeks 4 and 8; and clusters 7 and 12, genes down-regulated at week 8. Cluster 5 genes were not associated with any significantly over-represented annotations, but this cluster of 27 genes (32 probe sets) included Cytl1 (cytokine-like 1), which has been shown to be expressed during chondrogenesis and to promote chondrocyte differentiation through stimulation of Sox9 transcriptional activity [15]. Cluster 10, also down-regulated at week 4, with continuing down-regulation in week 8, contained 11 genes. No functions were significantly over-represented in this cluster and none of these genes were associated with osteoarthritis in the literature. Cluster 10 contained a phosphatase, several kinases and four genes whose function involves nucleotide binding. Clusters 7 and 12, both down-regulated at week 8, consisted of 19 and 11 genes (21 and 11 probe sets), respectively. Significantly over-represented annotations identified by DAVID in cluster 7 included mitotic cell cycle, cell cycle process, cell division, and cytoskeleton. S100b, which had been used in the past as a marker for chondrogenesis [16] was in this cluster. Over-represented annotations in cluster 12 all involved carbohydrate metabolism.

Significant up-regulation of gene expression at 16 weeks was seen in clusters 15 and 16, both of which also exhibited high up-regulation at week 4. Cluster 15 consisted of 7 probe sets covering three genes; Prelp, Col3a1 (collagen, type III, alpha 1), and Fmod (fibromodulin). Prelp and fibromodulin were also present in the

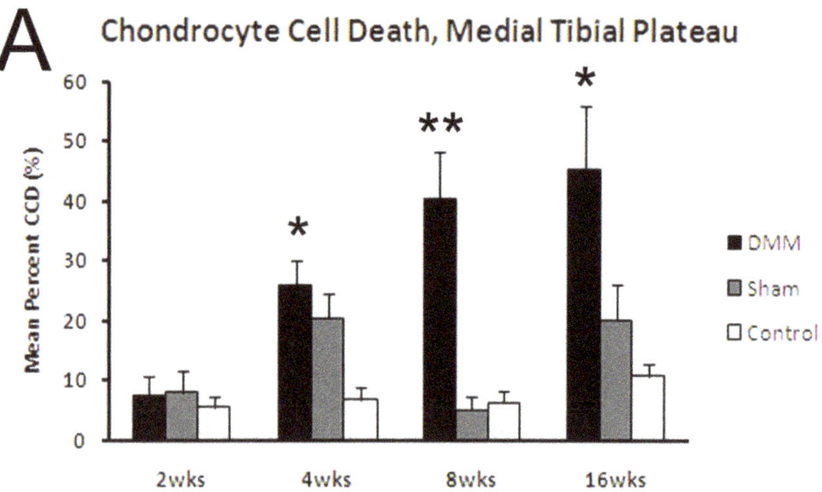

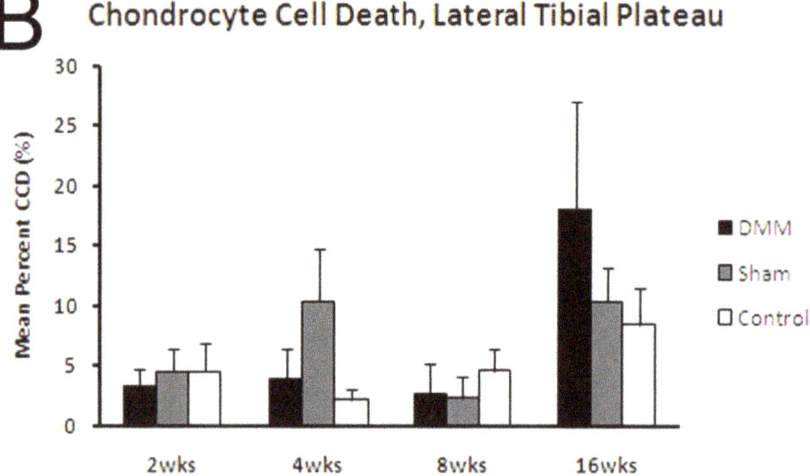

Figure 4. Histologic analysis of chondrocyte death over the time course. Dead chondrocytes were counted on H&E sections from the medial tibial plateau (A) and lateral tibial plateau (B) from DMM, sham, and contralateral control joints at the various time points after surgery. *$p<0.05$ vs sham and control joints; **$p<0.001$ vs sham and control joints by ANOVA.

DMM/sham-Sham/baseline overlap gene list reported above, where they were found to be highly down-regulated at 16 weeks in the sham joints; however, these genes were highly up-regulated in the DMM joints. Cluster 16 was comprised of four probe sets, representing 3 genes: Col14a1 (collagen, type XIV, alpha 1), Bgn (biglycan), and Fbln7 (fibulin 7), all associated with the extracellular matrix. Col14a1 was identified in a microarray analysis of human tissue [17]; while Bgn was previously associated with chondrogenesis and extracellular matrix turnover in osteoarthritis [18].

Genes in clusters 3 and 11 displayed temporal profiles of up-regulation only at 4 weeks, with little significant change in expression from control at any other time point. Cluster 3 contained 45 genes (48 probe sets), with significant annotations that included regulation of transcription, DNA binding, regulation of RNA metabolic process, zinc ion binding, and transcription. Potential genes of interest were NFκB activating protein, Atf2 and Erg. Cluster 11 was composed of 11 genes, which exhibited no significantly over-represented functions. One of the genes in this cluster was Asb13, an ankyrin repeat and SOCS box-containing protein.

Clusters 1, 2, 4, 9, and 14 contained genes that exhibit strong up-regulation at 4 weeks, with less up-regulation at 2 weeks. Cluster 1 contained 48 genes (54 probe sets) representing genes whose significant annotations include embryonic organ morphogenesis, positive regulation of cell differentiation and developmental process. This cluster included several genes thought to be involved in joint biology and/or OA including syndecan 4, Bmp-1, and Timp-2. Cluster 2 contained 39 genes (52 probe sets) for genes also up-regulated at 2 and 4 weeks. The cluster included over-represented annotations for collagen, signal peptide, extracellular region, extracellular matrix, cell adhesion and glycosaminoglycan binding. Genes of potential interest in this cluster included collagen genes such as Col5a1 and Col16a1, growth factor-related genes such as Igf1 and Egfr, MMP-14, and biglycan. (Note, biglycan is represented by three probe sets on this mouse chip, two of which are found in cluster 16 and 1 in cluster 2). Clusters 4, 9, and 14 contained 33, 16 and 8 genes (33, 18, and 8 probe sets), respectively. DAVID did not identify any function annotations over-represented any of these clusters. Cluster 4 genes included two glutathione peroxidases, Gpx7 and Gpx8, perhaps suggesting some redox-related event.

Table 1. Histomorphometric measures of subchondral bone area and thickness in DMM and sham control joints.

	Time	Treatment Group	Medial Tibial Plateau	ANOVA	Lateral Tibial Plateau	ANOVA
SCB Area	2 week	DMM	85777 (±12232)	NS	42703 (±5768)	NS
SCB Area	2 week	Sham	66140 (±8668)	NS	46342 (±6410)	NS
SCB Area	2 week	Control	70557 (±5895)	NS	48279 (±4694)	NS
SCB Area	4 week	DMM	116943 (±18235)	p = 0.011	67074 (±5367)	NS
SCB Area	4 week	Sham	71067 (±11028)	p = 0.011	57426 (±8690)	NS
SCB Area	4 week	Control	71758 (±5284)	p = 0.011	55541 (±5293)	NS
SCB Area	8 week	DMM	147622 (±13141)	NS	50446 (±8643)	NS
SCB Area	8 week	Sham	122046 (±19956)	NS	68432 (±11352)	NS
SCB Area	8 week	Control	103391 (±9112)	NS	62735 (±5925)	NS
SCB Area	16 week	DMM	144786 (±21706)	NS	75524 (±16120)	NS
SCB Area	16 week	Sham	124481 (±23749)	NS	62240 (±10563)	NS
SCB Area	16 week	Control	116784 (±15843)	NS	66090 (±7798)	NS
SCB Thickness	2 week	DMM	74.1 (±9.4)	NS	40.5 (±4.6)	NS
SCB Thickness	2 week	Sham	58.7 (±6.2)	NS	45.7 (±5.7)	NS
SCB Thickness	2 week	Control	63.3 (±5.3)	NS	45.5 (±4.1)	NS
SCB Thickness	4 week	DMM	99.2 (±13.4)	p = 0.011	56.3 (±4.0)	NS
SCB Thickness	4 week	Sham	64.2 (±9.8)	p = 0.011	51.9 (±7.8)	NS
SCB Thickness	4 week	Control	63.5 (±4.3)	p = 0.011	49.8 (±4.1)	NS
SCB Thickness	8 week	DMM	120.8 (±9.9)	NS	48.4 (±5.1)	NS
SCB Thickness	8 week	Sham	99.4 (±11.3)	NS	69.0 (±11.7)	NS
SCB Thickness	8 week	Control	90.8 (±7.2)	NS	57.0 (±4.7)	NS
SCB Thickness	16 week	DMM	111.9 (±20.4)	NS	66.2 (±9.8)	NS
SCB Thickness	16 week	Sham	106.8 (±15.7)	NS	60.1 (±7.9)	NS
SCB Thickness	16 week	Control	101.2 (±12.6)	NS	60.1 (±6.2)	NS

Subchondral bone (SCB) area (μm^2) and thickness (μm) were measured as detailed in the Materials and Methods. The p values are the ANOVA values between the treatment groups within each time point and the significance noted was between the DMM vs sham and contralateral controls. For each group and each time point sections from an n of 6 animals were measured.

Clusters 6, 8, and 13 also displayed the most up-regulation at week 4, but to a lesser extent than clusters 1, 2, 4, 9, and 14. Cluster 6 included 23 genes (24 probe sets) whose DAVID-identified over-represented annotations included signal peptide, glycoprotein, cell adhesion, serine/threonine kinase signaling pathway, skeletal system development and growth factor activity. Genes of particular interest included TGFβ2 and TGFβ3, latent TGFβ binding protein and Ddr2. Cluster 8 contained 19 genes for which the significant gene annotations included cell adhesion and contained COMP and Mmp13 which are thought to be important markers of the OA process. Cluster 13 included 9 genes for which there were no significantly over-represented functions. One of these, Enpp3, a pyrophosphatase, has been previously associated with osteoarthritis [19].

Overall, the analysis of gene clusters based on the metrics of both shape and magnitude of the time profile provided insight into the temporal process of osteoarthritis development. Only a few genes were down-regulated as part of this process, and those were down-regulated mainly at 4 and/or 8 weeks. Many more genes were up-regulated and most of the up-regulated genes displayed up-regulation at 4 weeks, with lesser up-regulation at 2 and 16 weeks. The phasic process was clearly visualized in these clusters, with the gene expression at 8 weeks being significantly different from gene expression at the other time points. This difference was consistent across all replicates.

Tissue distribution of type III collagen, fibromodulin, and Prelp

Based on the results of the consensus clustering, we choose to immunostain for type III collagen, fibromodulin, and Prelp, in order to determine which tissues might be providing the signals noted by gene expression at week 16. A total of 3 DMM and 4 sham control mice were studied and representative images are shown in **Figure 9** The tissue distribution of immunopositivity was similar between the two surgical groups; however, certain tissue types (e.g. fibrocartilage) were more prevalent in the DMM mice. Type III collagen immunopositivity was present in a pericellular distribution in articular cartilage and the meniscus and was located more diffusely in ligaments, the joint capsule, and the synovium as well as in the fibrocartilage located over osteophytes (**Table 3**). It was also present in the vascular endothelium. Fibromodulin immunopositivity was present in low numbers of articular chondrocytes, minimally in meniscus, and variably in synovium. Immunopositivity was more intense and involved more chondrocytes in fibrocartilage, notably over osteophytes, than in articular cartilage. Some bone marrow cells, including megakaryocytes also were positive. Immunopositivity for Prelp was present in ligaments (particularly at the site of ligamentous attachments to bone), periosteum, and fibrous connective tissue. Most chondrocytes were negative; however the

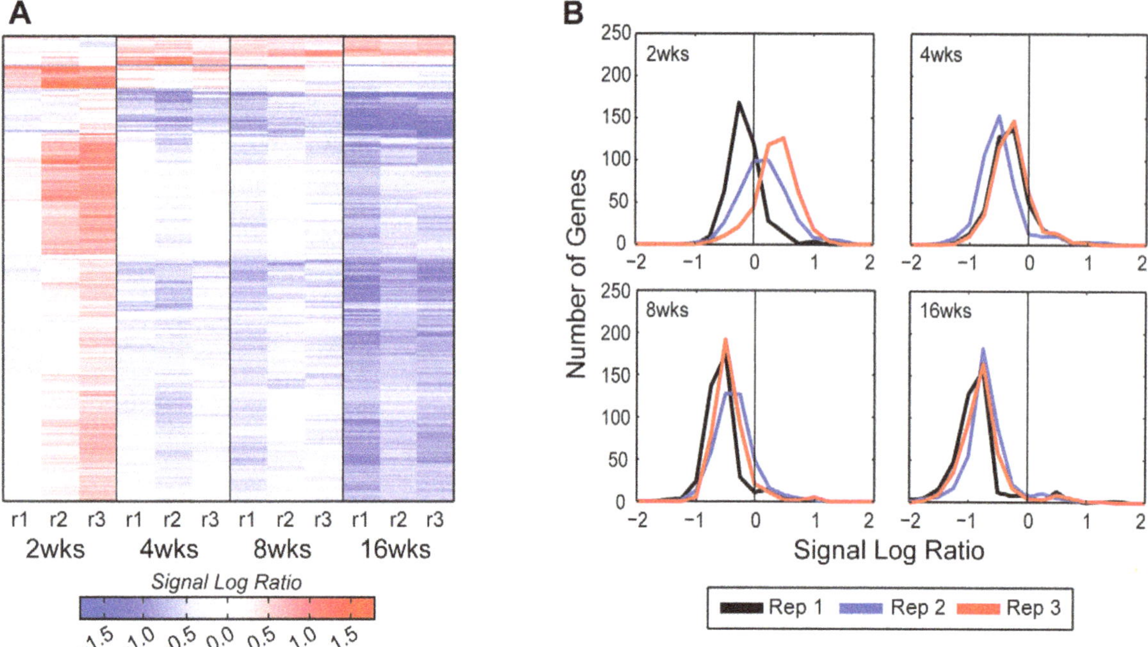

Figure 5. Global view of the differentially expressed genes in the sham time course. A) A heat map illustrates that the majority of differentially expressed genes (406 probe sets for 347 genes), in the sham time course are down-regulated, with few being up-regulated over time. Heat map rows represent genes, and columns represent replicates of each time points. Red indicates up-regulation, blue down-regulation and white indicates no change in gene expression from the respective control (see Methods). B) Gene expression distributions of the sham time course exhibit a uni-modal distribution throughout the experiment; however, the distributions center becomes shifted toward the negative side of zero at 4 weeks, indicating a global down-regulation of these genes over time due to aging. An SLR of zero is marked by a vertical line on the graph, and replicate time courses are colored as follows: replicate 1 = black, replicate 2 = blue, replicate 3 = red.

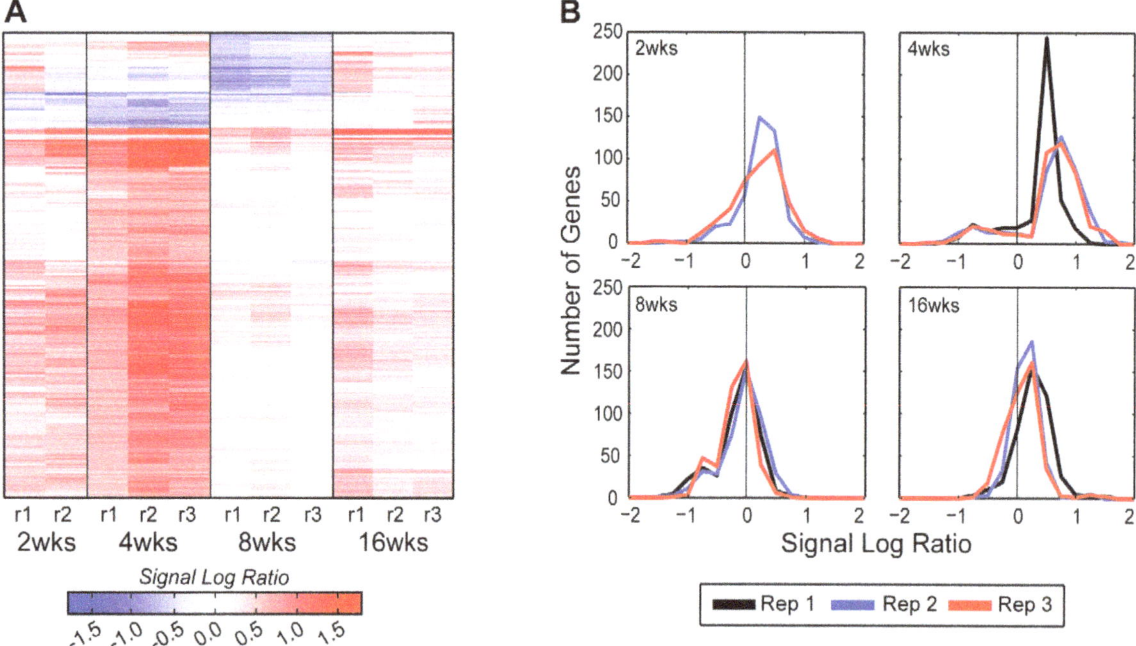

Figure 6. Global view of the differentially expressed genes in the DMM time course. A) The heat map illustrates that the majority of differentially expressed genes (427 probe sets for 371 genes) were up-regulated throughout the DMM time course, except for a small group of genes, which were down-regulated 4 and 8 weeks after surgery (see Figure 5A legend for heat map formatting details). B) The DMM time course exhibits a bi-modal distribution at 4 and 8 weeks after surgery, with the majority of genes being up-regulated at 4 weeks and not different from control at 8 weeks (see Figure 5B legend for formatting details).

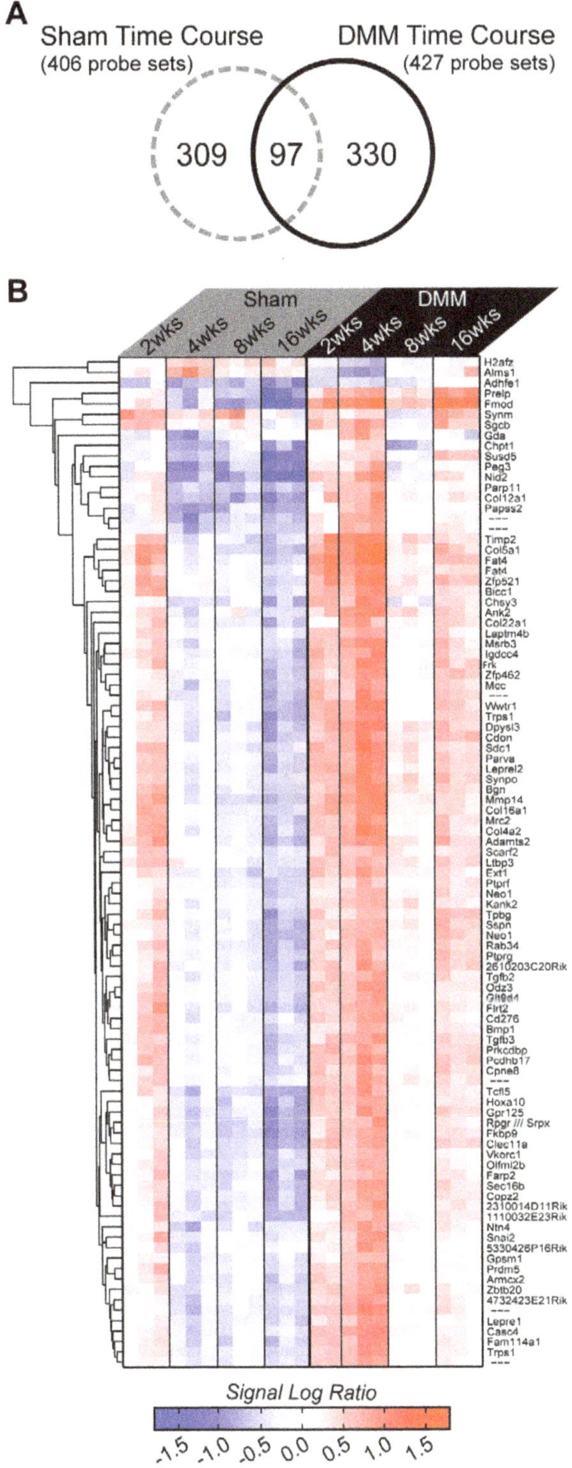

Figure 7. The group of genes differentially expressed in both sham and DMM data sets. Intersection of the 406 differentially expressed sham time course probe sets and the 427 DMM time course probe sets revealed 97 probe sets (94 genes) found in both data sets. A) A Venn diagram illustrates the number of probe sets in each data set as well as the overlap, and indicates that the majority of genes with OA induced expression changes are not altered in sham joints. B) A heat map of gene expression changes for the 97 intersecting probe sets was created using hierarchical agglomerative clustering and Euclidean distance, with sham expression on the left and DMM expression on the right. The heat map is formatted as in Figures 5A and 6A with the addition of the hierarchical dendrogram on the left and the gene names on the right.

matrix of degenerative cartilage and fibrocartilage was strongly immunopositive.

Real-time PCR results for selected genes

We selected a set of 16 genes to evaluate using RT-PCR based on genes tested in our previous study [6] where we had compared RT-PCR results at the 8 week time point in young and older adult mice. The average fold change in the DMM relative to sham controls for this gene set was highest at 4 weeks and lowest at 8 weeks (**Table 4**) which was consistent with the overall pattern of the 371 genes found to be significantly regulated in DMM vs sham joints on the microarrays (**Figure 6**). Genes with significant upregulation at 4 weeks included aggrecan, asporin, Ccl21, Cxcr7, Dkk3, Htra1, Igf-1, periostin, and Sfrp2. Looking across the time course, none of the genes examined were significantly up- or down-regulated in DMM relative to sham joints at all 4 time points; however, Ccl21, Cxcr7, Igf-1, and Sfrp2 were up-regulated at 3 of 4 time points. The two Wnt pathway regulators that were examined, Dkk3 and Sfrp2, were both significantly up-regulated at the early time points as was Col3a1. Unlike Dkk3 and Sfrp2, Col3a1 was also highly expressed at 16 weeks, consistent with the microarray results. Although type X collagen has been used as a marker of chondrocyte hypertrophy, which is thought to contribute to the development of OA, we actually observed a decrease in its expression at two weeks and no significant increase at the later time points. MMP-13 was increased at 2, 4, and 16 weeks in DMM relative to joints, as was noted on the microarrays, but due to variability among the 3 pools it did not reach statistical significance.

Discussion

Both the histologic and gene expression analysis support a phasic process for the development of OA in this model. The early phases at 2 and 4 weeks after DMM surgery were the most active in terms of gene expression at a time when the earliest cartilage lesions in the medial tibial plateau were very mild but abaxial chondrophytes had already formed. The chondrophytes matured to osteophytes as the articular cartilage lesions became more severe but, interestingly, this was accompanied by a significant decline in overall gene expression at the 8 week time point. In addition to the differences in overall gene expression, the findings from cluster analysis showed that each time point studied had a unique gene signature that also supports a phasic process.

Perhaps most striking was the decline in gene expression at 8 weeks after surgery. There was a significant down-regulation of genes regulating cell proliferation while matrix remodeling genes that were up-regulated at 2 and 4 weeks were mostly off, suggesting that a quiescent phase had been reached. However, at 16 weeks this pattern had changed and was accompanied by significant cartilage loss in the medial tibial plateau while cartilage damage and chondrocyte death was beginning to be evident in the lateral tibial plateau along with the appearance of lateral axial osteophytes. Because RNA for the gene arrays was only isolated from the medial side of the joint, the changes in gene expression observed at 16 weeks were not due to the disease progressing laterally but rather reflect more advanced disease medially. The lack of time points between 4 and 8 weeks and 8 and 16 weeks prevents any conclusions about the length of the quiescent phase.

The significant expression of Prelp, Col3a1, and fibromodulin at 16 weeks suggests that a matrix repair or a "wound healing response" was active. At 16 weeks, the articular cartilage from the DMM group had severe lesions in the medial tibial plateau with some loss of cartilage. This suggested that the signal at 16 weeks

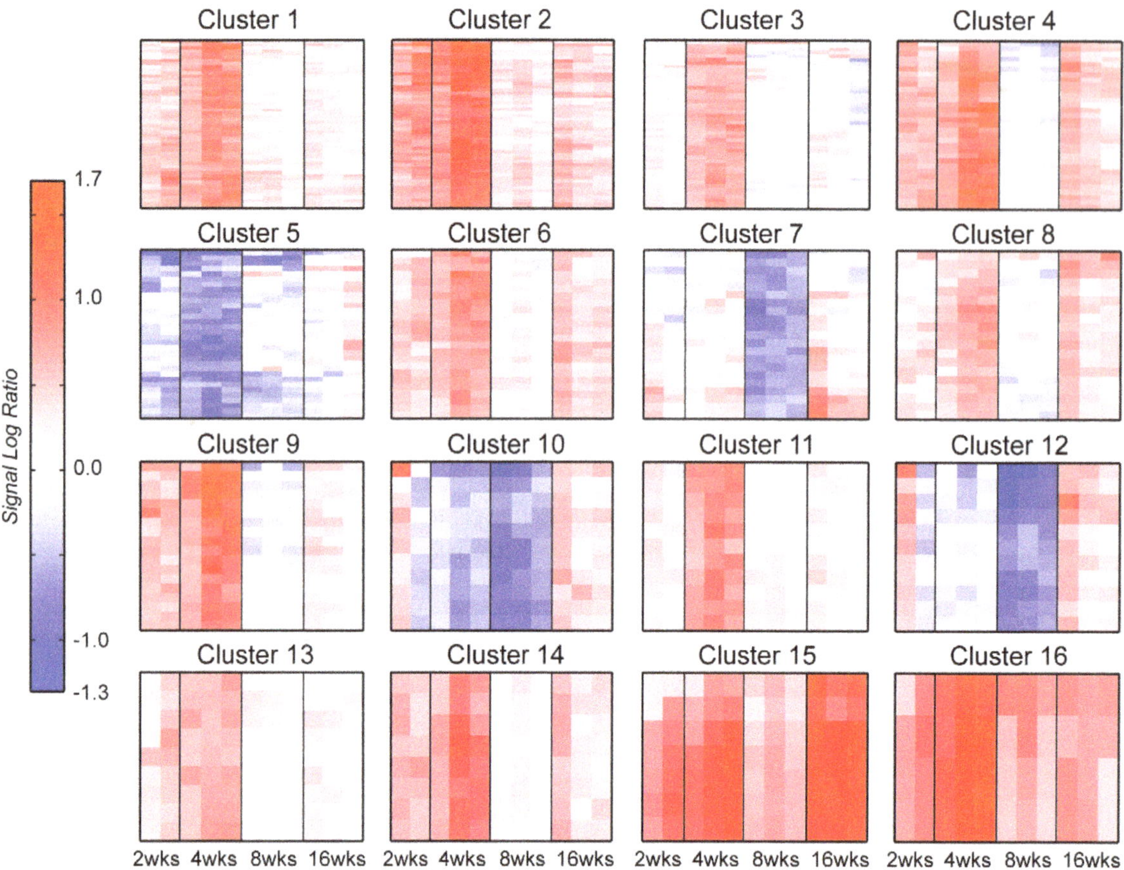

Figure 8. Heat maps of the largest 16 consensus clusters in the DMM time course. Rows represent genes and columns are time point replicates in the following order: 2 weeks rep2, rep3; 4-, 8- and 16 weeks rep1, rep2, rep3. Red indicates up-regulation, blue down-regulation and white indicates no change in expression from the sham time-matched control. All heat maps in this figure are colored on the same scale for easy comparison with maximum up-regulation at 1.7 SLR and maximum down-regulation at −1.3 SLR. A variety of expression patterns are present with most including significant up-regulation at 4 weeks. Only four clusters contain down-regulated genes (clusters 5, 7, 10 and 12), and cluster 15 is the only one with significant up-regulation 16 weeks after surgery.

for these genes may have come from either early changes on the femoral side, since some femoral tissue was included for RNA extraction, or more likely, from other joint structures such as the meniscus, synovium, ligaments and subchondral bone. Immunostaining revealed that ligaments and the fibrocartilage found over osteophytes were common locations for all three proteins. These results are consistent with previous studies that examined the location and function of these proteins. Prelp is thought to play a role in matrix organization through interactions with collagen, as does the small leucine-rich proteoglycan fibromodulin [20,21]. Deletion of fibromodulin in mice leads to OA, possibly via weakened ligaments and tendons [22]. However, a recent study that revealed a role for complement activation in OA demonstrated increased levels of fibromodulin in OA synovial fluid and found that fibromodulin could promote the activation of complement [23]. Overexpression of Prelp has been shown to disrupt normal collagen fiber formation in skin [24] and, in contrast to fibromodulin, it is an inhibitor of complement activation [25]. Thus, too little or too much fibromodulin and Prelp could contribute to OA.

Increased expression of type III collagen has been previously noted in human OA cartilage [26,27] and it has been found in normal cartilage in fibrils containing type II collagen [28]. We noted a pericellular location for type III collagen in articular cartilage and the meniscus. It is not known what role type III collagen could have in the OA joint. In the set of 371 genes that were differentially expressed in DMM vs sham joints, we observed increased expression, at one or more time points, in a large number of collagen genes that are likely part of an attempted repair response. These included the alpha 1 chain of types III, V, XII, XIV, XVI, and XXII collagen and the alpha 2 chain of type IV collagen, along with the collagen processing genes, procollagen c-endopeptidase enhancer protein and procollagen-lysine, 2-oxoglutarate 5-dioxygenase 1.

The phasic changes in gene expression noted in the DMM knees were not the result of aging of the animals over the 16 week time course. Changes in gene expression were noted when we compared the 12 week old animals at baseline (un-operated) and the sham controls over the 16 week time course but these differed significantly from the changes in gene expression noted in the DMM relative to sham joints. This was seen in the overlap analysis where the changes over time in expression in the DMM joints were most often in the opposite direction to changes over time in the sham joints. This was most evident for Prelp and fibromodulin which were significantly down-regulated at week 16 in the sham controls but increased in the DMM joints. Interestingly, immunopositivity for both of these proteins was notably stronger and more extensive in fibrocartilage over osteophytes than in

Table 2. Significant DAVID annotations for the top 16 Gene Clusters.

Cluster	Significant DAVID Annotations
1	Embryonic organ morphogenesis, inner ear morphogenesis, embryonic organ development, positive regulation of cell differentiation, positive regulation of developmental process, regulation of cell proliferation
2	Collagen, signal peptide, disulfide bond, glycoprotein, extracellular region, extracellular matrix, cell adhesion, glycosaminoglycan binding
3	Regulation of transcription, DNA binding, regulation of RNA metabolic process, Zinc finger C2H2-like, transition metal ion binding
4	None significant
5	None significant
6	Signal, signal peptide, glycoprotein, glycosylation site:N-linked, disulfide bond, cell adhesion, phosphorus, metabolic process, transmembrane receptor protein serine/threonine kinase signaling pathway, skeletal system development/morphogenesis, enzyme linked receptor protein signaling pathway, protein amino acid phosphorylation, growth factor, growth factor activity, regulation of cell proliferation
7	Mitotic cell cycle, cell cycle phase/process, nuclear/cell division, organelle fission, cytoskeletal protein binding, intracellular non-membrane-bounded organelle,
8	Cell adhesion, biological adhesion
9	None significant
10	None significant
11	None significant
12	Carbohydrate metabolism, glucose/hexose/monosaccharide metabolic process
13	None significant
14	None significant
15	Extracellular matrix, secreted, disulfide bond, signal peptide, glycoprotein
16	Extracellular matrix, secreted, disulfide bond, signal peptide, glycosylation site:N-linked, glycoprotein

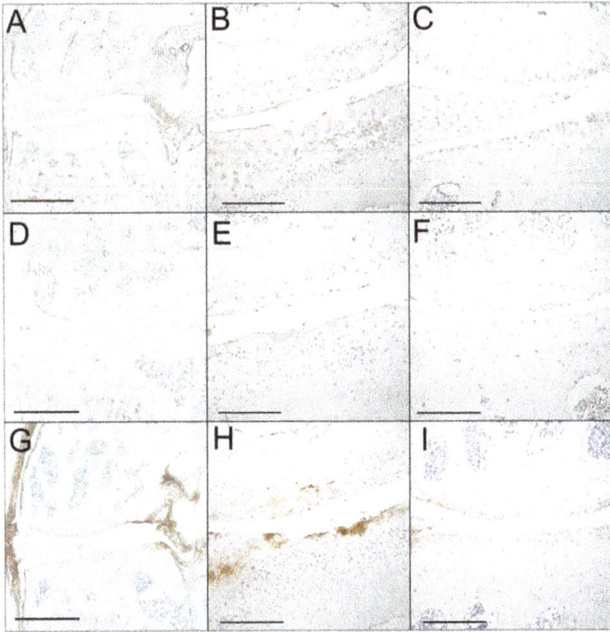

Figure 9. Immunolocalization of type III collagen, fibromodulin, and Prelp. Sections from mice in the 16 week-old sham and DMM groups were immunostained as detailed in the Methods using antibodies to type III collagen (A,B,C), fibromodulin (D,E,F) and Prelp (G,H,I). A, D, and G are 4x views of sham control joints to demonstrate overall tissue distribution. B, E, and H are 20x views of DMM joints and C, F, and I are 20x views of sham control joints. Bar =1 mm for 4X, 200um for 20X.

articular or meniscal cartilage. In addition, immunopositivity for Prelp was increased in degenerative cartilage matrix compared with normal cartilage. In the sham time course analysis, most genes exhibited an up-regulation of expression at 2 weeks followed by a progressive decline out to 16 weeks, compared to time zero. Many of these genes were involved in morphogenesis and development, suggesting the animals were more actively growing at the start of the study and then growth likely slowed. Importantly, the progressive increase in subchondral bone area and thickness were the only histologic measures that changed with time in all groups (control, sham and DMM).

We have recently reported a comparison of the 8 week time point results included in the present study with results from the same time point in animals that were 12 months-old at the time of DMM surgery [6]. The histologic OA severity in the older mice was about twice that of the younger mice and significantly more genes were up-regulated in the older mice. The 8 week comparisons suggest that the older mice develop OA more rapidly after DMM surgery than the younger mice, a result which could have contributed to the differences in gene expression at 8 weeks. A major difference between the young and older mice was in the expression of muscle related genes which were up-regulated in the older mice and either down-regulated or unchanged in the younger mice. Consistent with greater importance of the muscle-related genes in the older mice, we did not find significant annotations for muscle in the time course study using young mice. It would be of interest to do a time course study in the 12 month-old mice to determine if a phasic progression is also found. We did compare the DMM vs sham gene expression from the 8 week time point in the 12 month old mice to the other time points in the younger mice and found the most genes in common at 16 weeks (158 genes) suggesting more rapid progression in the older mice (data not shown).

Table 3. Immunostaining results for Prelp, Type III collagen, and Fibromodulin.

Tissue	Prelp	Type III collagen	Fibromodulin
Ligaments	+++/++++	+	+/−
Periosteum	+++	+	+/−
Fibrous connective tissue	++	+	−
Articular cartilage chondrocytes	−	−	+/−
Articular cartilage matrix	+/−	++ (mainly pericellular matrix)	−
Meniscus chondrocytes	+/−	+	+/−
Meniscus matrix	+/−−	++ (mainly pericellular matrix)	+
Bone	−	−	−
Bone marrow	−	−	++
Growth plate chondrocytes	+/−	−	−
Growth plate matrix	+/−	+/−	+
Fibrocartilage	++	++ (mainly pericellular matrix of chondrocytes)	++
Skeletal muscle	−	+ (perimysium only)	+/−
Synovium	−	+++	+/++
Degenerate/fibrillated cartilage	++/+++	++	++
Vascular endothelium	−	++++ (also vessel wall)	−

Prelp = proline-arginine-rich end leucine-rich repeat protein. Sections from 3 DMM and 4 sham control animals at 16 weeks after surgery were graded on a scale from no immunopositivity (−) to marked immunopositivity (++++). The results presented are the consensus grades from all animals evaluated. The degenerate/fibrillated cartilage was only present in the DMM animals.

A phasic progression of OA was suggested by a previous study in humans where radiographic progression was related to changes in serial measures of serum COMP, as an OA biomarker [29]. Interestingly, we found that COMP, along with MMP-13, clustered with genes that were up-regulated during times of increased activity at 2, 4, and 16 weeks and were down-regulated at 8 weeks when activity was lowest. One potential explanation for a phasic process would be the maturation of osteophytes which have been proposed to stabilize the joint mechanics [30]. Our observation that chondrophytes had already formed by 2 weeks after surgery to destabilize the meniscus is consistent with the hypothesis that joint destabilization stimulates their formation.

Table 4. Real time PCR results for selected genes showing fold change in DMM joints relative to sham controls.

Time point	2 weeks		4 weeks		8 weeks		16 weeks	
Gene name	**fold change**	**p value**	**fold change**	**p value**	**fold change**	**p value**	**fold change**	**p value**
Adamts5	0.37	NS	0.26	NS	0.86	NS	0.96	NS
Aggrecan	2.53	NS	5.90	0.006	1.06	NS	2.00	NS
Asporin	1.45	NS	2.50	0.04	1.60	0.05	2.00	NS
Ccl21	1.48	NS	2.41	0.001	2.27	0.003	1.57	0.05
Ccr7	0.48	0.006	1.00	NS	1.83	0.05	1.00	NS
Cxcr7	2.43	NS	2.77	0.03	1.51	0.02	2.99	0.03
Col3	2.24	0.05	4.28	NS	1.93	NS	3.34	0.004
Col10	0.48	0.02	0.25	NS	1.75	NS	1.17	NS
Dkk 3	4.27	0.01	2.50	0.02	1.77	NS	2.50	NS
Htra1	1.39	NS	4.09	0.01	1.81	0.008	3.00	NS
Igf-1	1.88	NS	3.50	0.0004	3.00	0.002	3.00	0.008
IL33	1.50	NS	1.50	NS	1.61	0.05	1.88	NS
Mmp3	3.68	0.03	10.57	NS	2.32	0.007	2.22	NS
Mmp13	1.48	NS	2.00	NS	1.08	NS	1.46	NS
Periostin	4.48	NS	3.38	0.009	1.44	NS	1.75	NS
Sfrp2	2.92	0.01	2.81	0.002	1.56	0.01	1.29	NS
Average fold change	2.07		3.11		1.71		2.01	

Increased expression of Bmp-1, TGFβ2 and TGFβ3 at the early time points is also consistent with their presumed role in stimulating osteophyte formation [31]. The stabilization, however, appeared to be transient because cartilage loss was marked at 16 weeks and gene expression was increased relative to 8 weeks.

There are important limitations to the present study. Because RNA was not isolated from individual tissues it is not possible to determine which specific tissue (cartilage, bone, meniscus, ligament, synovium) contributed to the changes in gene expression. Also, if a gene is expressed in a single tissue, pooling of tissues will reduce the signal to a lower level than what would have been observed in the individual tissue. That is the likely explanation for the overall lower levels of gene expression observed in the present study when compared to work using a single tissue. Based on the immunostaining for type III collagen, fibromodulin, and Prelp, as well as immunostaining for IL-33, periostin, and CCL21 reported in our previous study [6], it appears that multiple joint tissues can be responsible for changes in gene expression consistent with the joint operating as an organ rather than as individual tissues. Therapeutic interventions for OA which target key processes occurring in multiple joint tissues rather than a single tissue should be more effective than those targeting a single tissue. Another limitation is that the DMM model may or may not reflect human OA disease pathogenesis. Certainly the histologic features in cartilage and bone are similar, but in human OA there may be more disease activity in the synovium than in the DMM model. Finally, we studied gene expression, and not protein production, and these do not always correlate. Immunohistochemical studies to assess changes at the protein level are not sensitive enough to detect differences noted at the level of gene expression, unless either the differences in expression are marked, or the protein being examined is only detected in diseased tissue and not in normal tissue.

Further studies will be needed to determine the importance of these findings for human OA. An important implication of the results is that the degree of response to an intervention given during a phasic process will depend on the timing of the intervention. Pre-clinical studies using animal models most often start the intervention at the same time or just after the start of the OA process while in human trials participants are likely to be at various stages of the disease process when the intervention is initiated. Finding markers of various disease stages in OA could be used to direct targeted therapy to the proper phase of the disease when the target is most active.

Supporting Information

Table S1 Filtering results for the sham time course.

Table S2 Filtering results for the DMM time course.

File S1 Excel file of 406 Sham filtered probe sets and DAVID results. Results are presented as signal log ratio (SLR) which is the $\log_2$ of the fold change and so an SLR of 0.5 = 1.4-fold. A positive number would be up-regulation and negative number down-regulation.

File S2 Excel file of 427 DMM filtered probe sets and DAVID results. Results are presented as signal log ratio as described for supplemental file 1.

File S3 Excel file of 97 common probe sets and DAVID results.

Acknowledgments

We thank Mary Zhao for technical assistance and the microarray core facility of the Comprehensive Cancer Center of Wake Forest University for performing the microarrays. We also thank Paula Overn in the Comparative Pathology Shared Resource of the Masonic Cancer Center, University of Minnesota, for developing the immunostaining protocols and preparing the immunohistochemistry sections.

Author Contributions

Conceived and designed the experiments: RFL ALO MAM CSC MC CF JSF. Performed the experiments: RFL ALO MAM CSC MC. Analyzed the data: RFL ALO MAM CSC JSF. Contributed reagents/materials/analysis tools: ALO JSF. Wrote the paper: RFL ALO MAM CSC MC CF JSF.

References

1. Lawrence RC, Felson DT, Helmick CG, Arnold LM, Choi H, et al. (2008) Estimates of the prevalence of arthritis and other rheumatic conditions in the United States: Part II. Arthritis Rheum 58: 26–35.
2. (2010) Prevalence of doctor-diagnosed arthritis and arthritis-attributable activity limitation --- United States, 2007–2009. MMWR Morb Mortal Wkly Rep 59: 1261–1265.
3. Blagojevic M, Jinks C, Jeffery A, Jordan KP (2010) Risk factors for onset of osteoarthritis of the knee in older adults: a systematic review and meta-analysis. Osteoarthritis Cartilage 18: 24–33.
4. Loeser RF, Goldring SR, Scanzello CR, Goldring MB (2012) Osteoarthritis: A disease of the joint as an organ. Arthritis Rheum 64: 1697–1707.
5. Glasson SS, Blanchet TJ, Morris EA (2007) The surgical destabilization of the medial meniscus (DMM) model of osteoarthritis in the 129/SvEv mouse. Osteoarthritis Cartilage 15: 1061–1069.
6. Loeser RF, Olex A, McNulty MA, Carlson CS, Callahan M, et al. (2012) Microarray analysis reveals age-related differences in gene expression during the development of osteoarthritis in mice. Arthritis Rheum 64: 705–717.
7. McNulty MA, Loeser RF, Davey C, Callahan MF, Ferguson CM, Carlson CS (2011) A comprehensive histological assessment of osteoarthritis lesions in mice. Cartilage 2: 354–363.
8. Chou JW, Paules RS, Bushel PR (2005) Systematic variation normalization in microarray data to get gene expression comparison unbiased. J Bioinform Comput Biol 3: 225–241.
9. Olex AL, Hiltbold EM, Leng X, Fetrow JS (2010) Dynamics of dendritic cell maturation are identified through a novel filtering strategy applied to biological time-course microarray replicates. BMC Immunol 11: 41.
10. Olex AL, Fetrow JS (2011) SC(2)ATmd: a tool for integration of the figure of merit with cluster analysis for gene expression data. Bioinformatics 27: 1330–1331.
11. Yeung KY, Haynor DR, Ruzzo WL (2001) Validating clustering for gene expression data. Bioinformatics 17: 309–318.
12. Huang DW, Sherman BT, Lempicki RA (2009) Systematic and integrative analysis of large gene lists using DAVID bioinformatics resources. Nat Protoc 4: 44–57.
13. Huang DW, Sherman BT, Lempicki RA (2009) Bioinformatics enrichment tools: paths toward the comprehensive functional analysis of large gene lists. Nucleic Acids Res 37: 1–13.
14. McNulty MA, Loeser RF, Davey C, Callahan MF, Ferguson CM, et al. (2012) Histopathology of naturally occurring and surgically induced osteoarthritis in mice. Osteoarthritis Cartilage 20: 949–956.
15. Kim JS, Ryoo ZY, Chun JS (2007) Cytokine-like 1 (Cytl1) regulates the chondrogenesis of mesenchymal cells. J Biol Chem 282: 29359–29367.
16. Wolff DA, Stevenson S, Goldberg VM (1992) S-100 protein immunostaining identifies cells expressing a chondrocytic phenotype during articular cartilage repair. J Orthop Res 10: 49–57.
17. Karlsson C, Dehne T, Lindahl A, Brittberg M, Pruss A, et al. (2010) Genome-wide expression profiling reveals new candidate genes associated with osteoarthritis. Osteoarthritis Cartilage 18: 581–592.
18. Embree MC, Kilts TM, Ono M, Inkson CA, Syed-Picard F, et al. (2010) Biglycan and fibromodulin have essential roles in regulating chondrogenesis and extracellular matrix turnover in temporomandibular joint osteoarthritis. Am J Pathol 176: 812–826.

19. Johnson K, Hashimoto S, Lotz M, Pritzker K, Goding J, et al. (2001) Up-regulated expression of the phosphodiesterase nucleotide pyrophosphatase family member PC-1 is a marker and pathogenic factor for knee meniscal cartilage matrix calcification. Arthritis Rheum 44: 1071–1081.
20. Bengtsson E, Neame PJ, Heinegard D, Sommarin Y (1995) The primary structure of a basic leucine-rich repeat protein, PRELP, found in connective tissues. J Biol Chem 270: 25639–25644.
21. Neame PJ, Tapp H, Azizan A (1999) Noncollagenous, nonproteoglycan macromolecules of cartilage. Cell Mol Life Sci 55: 1327–1340.
22. Jepsen KJ, Wu F, Peragallo JH, Paul J, Roberts L, et al. (2002) A syndrome of joint laxity and impaired tendon integrity in lumican- and fibromodulin-deficient mice. J Biol Chem 277: 35532–35540.
23. Wang Q, Rozelle AL, Lepus CM, Scanzello CR, Song JJ, et al. (2011) Identification of a central role for complement in osteoarthritis. Nat Med 17: 1674–1679.
24. Grover J, Lee ER, Mounkes LC, Stewart CL, Roughley PJ (2007) The consequence of PRELP overexpression on skin. Matrix Biol 26: 140–143.
25. Happonen KE, Furst CM, Saxne T, Heinegard D, Blom AM (2012) PRELP protein inhibits the formation of the complement membrane attack complex. J Biol Chem 287: 8092–8100.
26. Aigner T, Bertling W, Stoss H, Weseloh G, von der Mark K (1993) Independent expression of fibril-forming collagens I, II, and III in chondrocytes of human osteoarthritic cartilage. J Clin Invest 91: 829–837.
27. Fukui N, Ikeda Y, Ohnuki T, Tanaka N, Hikita A, et al. (2008) Regional differences in chondrocyte metabolism in osteoarthritis: A detailed analysis by laser capture microdissection. Arthritis Rheum 58: 154–163.
28. Young RD, Lawrence PA, Duance VC, Aigner T, Monaghan P (2000) Immunolocalization of collagen types II and III in single fibrils of human articular cartilage. J Histochem Cytochem 48: 423–432.
29. Sharif M, Kirwan JR, Elson CJ, Granell R, Clarke S (2004) Suggestion of nonlinear or phasic progression of knee osteoarthritis based on measurements of serum cartilage oligomeric matrix protein levels over five years. Arthritis Rheum 50: 2479–2488.
30. Pottenger LA, Phillips FM, Draganich LF (1990) The effect of marginal osteophytes on reduction of varus-valgus instability in osteoarthritic knees. Arthritis Rheum 33: 853–858.
31. Scharstuhl A, Glansbeek HL, Van Beuningen HM, Vitters EL, Van Der Kraan PM, et al. (2002) Inhibition of endogenous tgf-Beta during experimental osteoarthritis prevents osteophyte formation and impairs cartilage repair. J Immunol 169: 507–514.

16

Positive Selection on the Osteoarthritis-Risk and Decreased-Height Associated Variants at the *GDF5* Gene in East Asians

Dong-Dong Wu[1], Gui-Mei Li[2], Wei Jin[2], Yan Li[1], Ya-Ping Zhang[1,2*]

1 State Key Laboratory of Genetic Resources and Evolution, Kunming Institute of Zoology, Chinese Academy of Sciences, Kunming, China, **2** Laboratory for Conservation and Utilization of Bio-resource, Yunnan University, Kunming, China

Abstract

GDF5 is a member of the bone morphogenetic protein (BMP) gene family, and plays an important role in the development of the skeletal system. Variants of the gene are associated with osteoarthritis and height in some human populations. Here, we resequenced the gene in individuals from four geographically separated human populations, and found that the evolution of the promoter region deviated from neutral expectations, with the sequence evolution driven by positive selection in the East Asian population, especially the haplotypes carrying the derived alleles of 5′ UTR SNPs rs143384 and rs143383. The derived alleles of rs143384 and rs143383, which are associated with a risk of osteoarthritis and decreased height, have high frequencies in non-Africans and show strong extended haplotype homozygosity and high population differentiation in East Asian. It is concluded that positive selection has driven the rapid evolution of the two osteoarthritis osteoarthritis-risk and decreased height associated variants of the human *GDF5* gene, and supports the suggestion that the reduction in body size during the terminal Pleistocene and Holocene period might have been an adaptive process influenced by genetic factors.

Editor: Thomas Mailund, Aarhus University, Denmark

Funding: This work was supported by grants from the National Natural Science Foundation of China (31061160189). The funders had no role in study design, data collection and analysis, decision to publish, or preparation of the manuscript.

Competing Interests: The authors have declared that no competing interests exist.

* E-mail: zhangyp@mail.kiz.ac.cn

These authors contributed equally to this work.

Introduction

Humans are characterized by many unique traits, such as cognitive ability, language speaking, special skeletal anatomy, and susceptibility to diseases, which distinguish us from our closest relative, the chimpanzee (reviewed in [1]). In addition, modern humans exhibit substantial phenotypic variation, e.g., susceptibility to diseases, metabolism, skin pigmentation, eye and hair color, body mass, height, and craniofacial differences shaped by the skeletal system. Many studies have examined the genetic bases of the evolutionary patterns of these phenotypes and have identified the role of positive selection on genes in processes such as brain development in the human lineage and skin pigmentation among modern human populations (reviewed in [2,3]). Similarly, in our previous studies we had concluded that positive selection in human skeletal genes had driven population differentiation in non-African populations [4], and identified a few skeletal genes that were subjected to this natural selection [5,6]. To better understand the evolutionary forces acting upon skeletal genes, and associated traits, here we studied another critical skeletal gene, *GDF5*, in modern human populations.

GDF5 (growth differentiation factor 5) is a member of the bone morphogenetic protein (BMP) gene family and the TGF-beta superfamily and plays an essential role in the skeletal development. GDF5 is expressed in the primordial cartilage of appendicular skeleton, with little expression in the axial skeleton such as vertebrae and ribs [7], and is required for the normal formation of bones and joints in the limbs, skull, and axial skeleton [8]. Several kinds of skeletal disorders (e.g., acromesomelic dysplasia, Hunter-Thompson Type [9]; brachydactyly, type C [10]; chondrodysplasia, Grebe type [11]; fibular hypoplasia and complex brachydactyly [12]) are caused by mutations in the *GDF5* gene. The allele A of the SNP rs143383 in the 5′ promoter region of the *GDF5* gene was found to be associated with an increased risk of osteoarthritis, and shows decreased transcriptional activity of *GDF5* in chondrogenic cells [13–15]. In addition, this allele is associated with decreased height, which may be due to the lower expression of *GDF5* that could lead to a reduction in limb bone growth [16].

The functional importance of *GDF5* in skeletal development raises the possibility that this gene may contribute to the evolution of the human skeletal system. Evidence indicates that the human skeletal system has evolved rapidly since the advent of agriculture [17] suggesting that the selective pressures on skeletal genes changed during this process. Indeed, skeletal genes do demonstrate high population differentiation among different human populations, which was driven by positive selection [4]. The genetic basis, however, of the evolution of human skeletal system largely remains undocumented. Here we studied the population variation of the human *GDF5* gene by sequencing alleles from 142 individuals from four geographically separated populations from Africa,

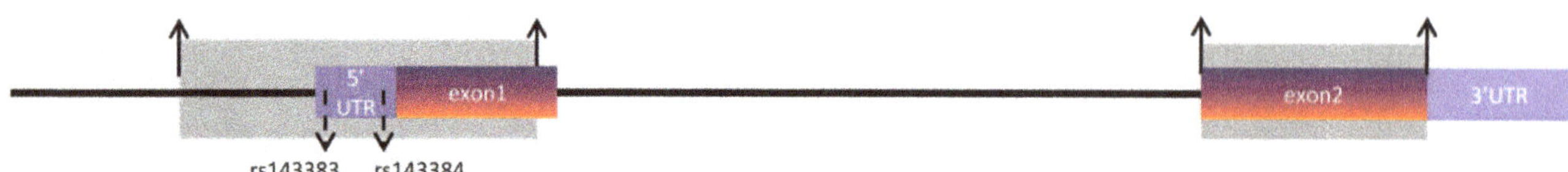

Figure 1. Structure of the human *GDF5* gene structure. The human *GDF5* gene is composed of two exons. The two regions sequenced in this study are denoted by the two rectangles.

Europe, East Asia and South Asia. Positive selection was identified as operating on the 5′ UTR region of the gene in the East Asian population, with the target of selection being the derived alleles of the SNPs rs143384 and rs143383.

Results

Of the 284 chromosomes sequenced, 13 mutations were identified in the 1359 bp exon 1 region, which includes 5′ UTR and some coding sequences of *GDF5* (Fig. 1). To better study the sequence variation, we used the SNPs to construct haplotypes using the PHASE program [18,19], and identified 16 haplotypes. Table 1 summarizes the population genetics data, including values for the nucleotide diversity, Tajima's D, Fu and Li's D, D*, F and F*, and Fay and Wu's H (see Materials and Methods). Population demographic history is the major confounding factor affecting the detection of positive selection. For example, negative values of Tajima's D can be attributed to population expansion, positive selection, or negative selection [2,20], therefore, we used coalescence simulations, incorporating best-fit demographic parameters for the populations including European, African, and East Asian [21], to better understand the demographic histories of the populations. The results of the simulations indicated it was mostly positive selection rather than demographic effect that generated the variation of *GDF5*, although the factor of demographic effect can not be excluded absolutely. In the East Asian population, Fu and Li's D, and D* demonstrated significantly lower values with a *P*-value lower than 0.05. In the 875 bp sequenced exon 2 region 4 mutations were detected and 6 haplotypes were constructed. For this region the population variation did not deviate from the expectation of neutrality (Table 2). The observations for the exon 2 data support the hypothesis that positive selection, and not demographic history, operated on the 5′ UTR region, as demographic history should influence all parts of the gene similarly, and thus would be expected to produce the same pattern of polymorphisms in both the exons 1 and 2 regions. The difference in the patterns seen in the exon 1 and exon 2 regions thus means that demographic history cannot explain the exon 1 pattern.

Within the 5′ UTR region of the *GDF5* gene there are two SNPs, rs143384 (A/G, derived allele is A) and rs143383 (A/G, derived allele is A), which have high derived allele frequencies in the East Asian population (61.84%, and 60.53%, respectively, Fig. 2A). These two SNPs demonstrate significantly strong linkage disequilibrium ($r^2 = 0.857$). We divided the 5′ UTR haplotypes into those carrying a derived allele and those carrying an ancestral allele of the SNPs. In the East Asian population only one haplotype carried the A-A pattern composed by the two derived SNP alleles and has a frequency of 60.53% (Fig. 2B). The high derived allele frequency was driven mostly by positive selection, to generate high haplotype homogeneity and was not destroyed by recombination. In contrast, the A-A haplotype is not found in our sequenced Africans (Fig. 2B). The World-wide allele frequency distribution also did not find the A-A allele in the sequenced Africans, despite the high derived allele frequencies in non-African populations (Fig. 3).

The derived allele A of SNP rs143384 is contained by two haplotypes, and these haplotypes demonstrate lower nucleotide diversity, lower Tajima's D, and significant lower Fu and Li's D* and F* ($P<0.05$) relative to haplotypes carrying the ancestral allele G (Table 3). The derived allele of the other SNP, rs143383, is contained by only one haplotype, which has a frequency of 60.53%. Haplotypes carrying the derived alleles also diverge from the others in the phylogenetic network (Fig. 4). In the Africans, there are no derived alleles at these two SNPs (Fig. 2, and Fig. 3), which indicates that these two SNPs were generated mostly after the "out of African" event. We also calculated the allele age of the derived alleles using the formula $t=[-2p/(1-p)]\ln p$, which considered that allele evolved under a model of neutral evolution [22,23], where p is the allele frequency and t is age, measured in units of 2*N (effective population size) generations. With a generation time of 20–25 years and N = 10000, the ages of the derived alleles of SNPs rs143384 and rs143383 are 311,552~389,440, 307,950~384,937 years, respectively. These results suggest that the derived alleles could not reach the high

Table 1. Population statistics summary of exon1 region.

Exon1 region (1359 bp, 12 SNPs)	Nucleotide Diversity	Tajima's D	Fu and Li's D	Fu and Li's F	Fu and Li's D*	Fu and Li's F*	Fay and Wu's H
African ($N^a = 66$)	6.209E-04	−0.451	0.052	−0.129	0.067	−0.115	0.703
European (N = 72)	7.954E-04	0.652	−0.207	0.077	−0.189	0.089	−0.176
East Asian (N = 76)	9.897E-04	−0.446	**−2.693**	−2.292	**−2.583**	−2.205	−0.217
South Asian (N = 70)	1.097E-03	0.470	0.230	0.365	0.239	0.370	0.865
Whole populations (N = 284)	1.052E-03	−0.604	−1.531	−1.422	−1.507	−1.404	0.761

The bolds are values significantly lower than 0 with P-value<0.05 by simulating human demographic history incorporating human best-fit model.
[a]is the number of chromosomes.

Table 2. Population statistics summary of exon 2 region.

Exon2 region (875 bp, 4 SNPs)	Nucleotide Diversity	Tajima's D	Fu and Li's D	Fu and Li's F	Fu and Li's D*	Fu and Li's F*	Fay and Wu's H
African (N = 66)	1.082E-03	0.976	−0.508	−0.059	−0.486	−0.042	0.386
European (N = 72)	5.665E-04	0.331	−1.011	−0.708	−0.991	−0.688	−0.333
East Asian (N = 76)	9.360E-04	0.639	−0.540	−0.204	−0.521	−0.188	−0.069
South Asian (N = 70)	9.488E-04	1.653	0.713	1.163	0.715	1.163	0.298
Whole populations (N = 284)	9.115E-04	0.409	−1.816	−1.273	−1.804	−1.263	0.132

observed frequencies (61.84%, 60.53%) under neutral evolution after the event of "out of Africa", which only occurred about 100,000 years ago [24]. This suggests that positive selection may have been driving these two derived alleles to high frequencies.

Further evidence for positive selection comes from the high population differentiation of the SNPs rs143384 and rs143383 among human populations. Here, we computed the Fst values of the SNPs based on three human populations using African (YRI), European (CEU), and East Asian (EA) data from HapMap to evaluate population differentiation. Fst values among the three populations at SNPs rs143383 and rs143384 are 0.544 and 0.499, respectively, which are higher than the Fst values of other SNPs in the gene regions of chromosome 20 (99.1%, 98.4% percentile rank) (Fig. 5A). Fst for the two SNPs between European and African are 0.664 and 0.597, for rs143383 and rs143384, respectively, values that are higher than the Fst values of SNPs in gene region of chromosome 20 (99.6%, 99.3% percentile rank) (Fig. 5D). Fst for the two SNPs between East Asian and African are 0.735 and 0.705, for rs143383 and rs143384, respectively, values that are higher than the Fst values of SNPs in the gene regions of

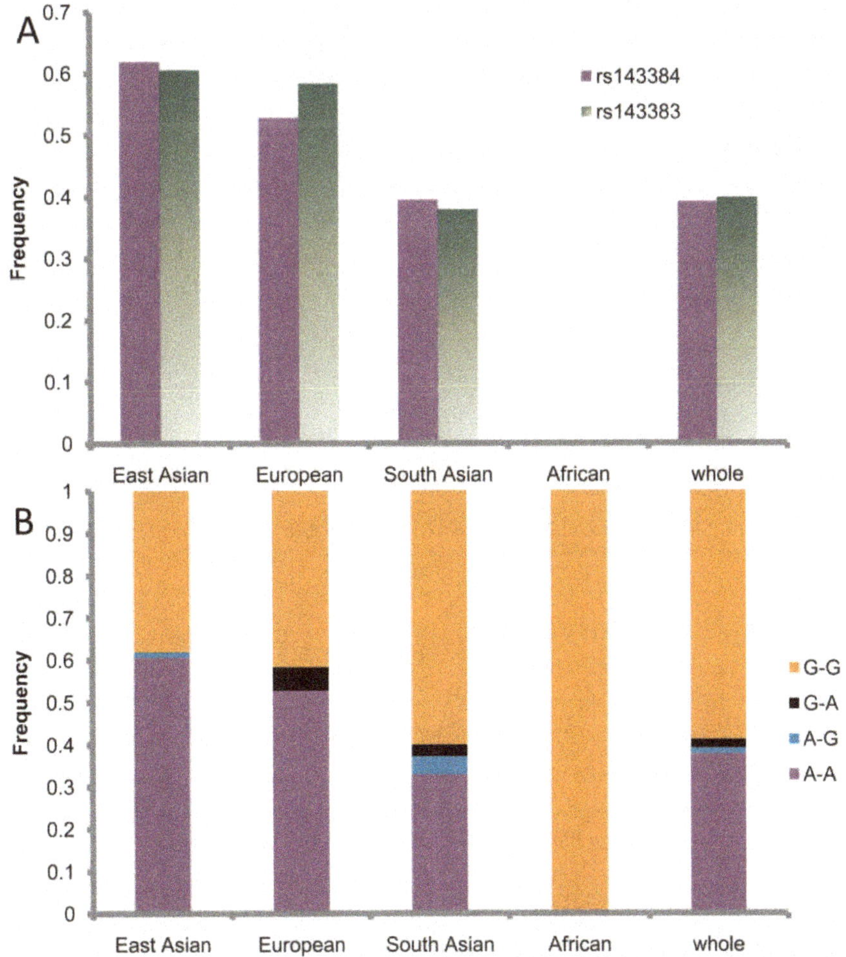

Figure 2. SNP allele frequencies in the *GDF5* gene. (A) Allele frequencies of haplotypes constructed using SNP rs143384 and rs143383 in four separate populations and the whole population. (B) Derived allele frequencies of the two SNPs in the four populations and the whole population.

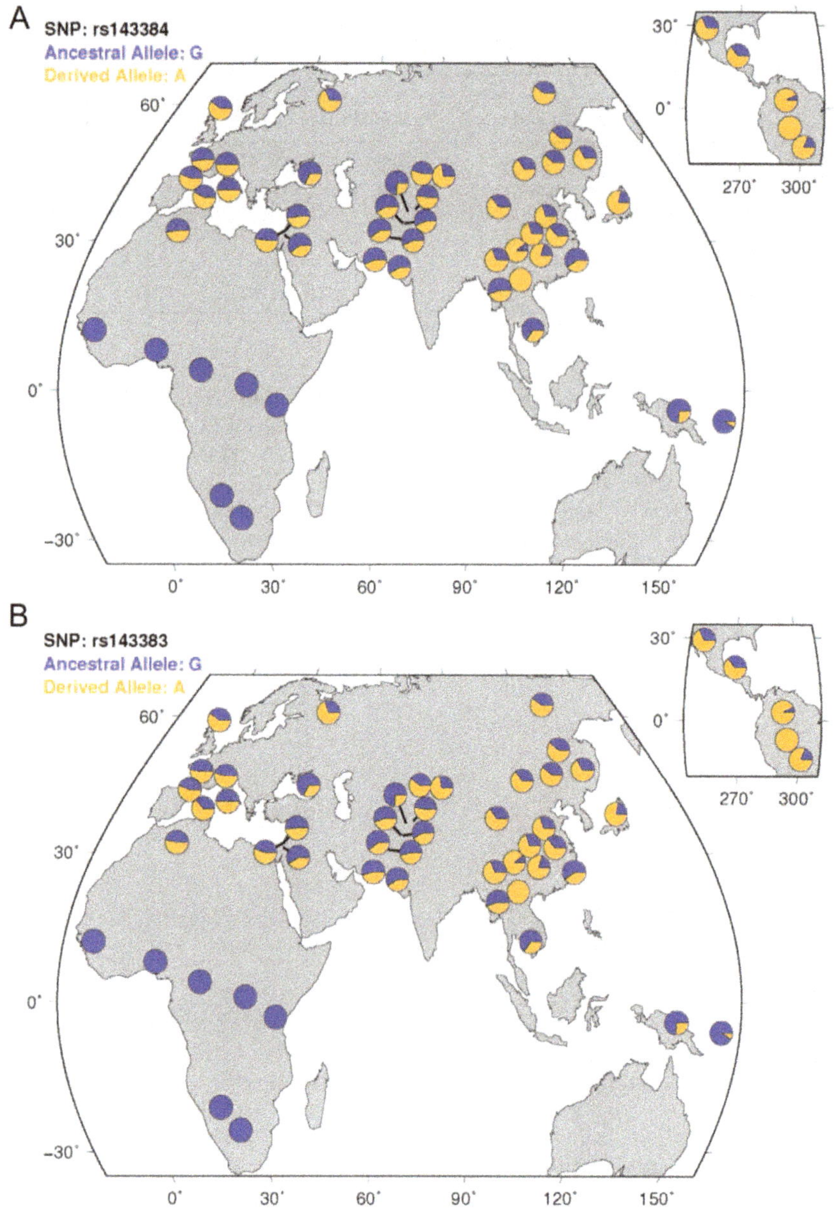

Figure 3. World-wide allele frequency distribution of the two SNPs rs143384 and rs143383. The data were downloaded from http://hgdp.uchicago.edu/.

chromosome 20 (99.5%, 99.3% percentile rank) (Fig. 5C). The Fst values of the two SNPs between East Asian and European, however, are not significantly higher (Fig. 5B). To further refine our analysis we performed a sliding window analysis of Fst values of other SNPs on chromosome 20 using a 50 kb window size and 25 kb step size. The Fst values of the two *GDF5* SNPs between Europeans and Africans are higher than the 95% percentile rank value for 50 kb regions of chromosome 20 (Fig. 5E).

To better understand the evolutionary pattern of *GDF5* in the human population we studied the extended haplotype homozygosity (EHH) of the *GDF5* exon 1 region in four populations, using the entire chromosome 20 phased haplotypes as empirical data. In the East Asian population, the major haplotype at the *GDF5* exon 1 and promoter core region (Fig. 4, haplotype in the ellipse), which contains the derived alleles of SNPs rs143383 and rs143384, reached 10.8986, 4.6377, and 6.7391 at 300 kb, 500 kb and 1000 kb upstream of *GDF5* core region, all of which are higher than the 95% percentile rank values (Fig. 6). These values support the conclusion that positive selection targeted the derived alleles of SNPs rs143383 and rs143384 in the East Asian population (Fig. 6).

We employed an approach described in [25] to roughly estimate the ages of derived alleles of SNPs rs143384 and rs143383, using formula EHH≈Pr (Homozygosity) = e^{-2rg}, namely, $-\ln(\text{EHH})\approx g*2r$, where Pr(Homozygosity) is the probability that two chromosomes are homozygous at recombination distance r from the core, given identity by decent from a common ancestor g generations ago. Here, we used linear regression of $-\ln$ (EHH) and 2r to evaluate the value of g based on the EHH data in East Asian. As in Fig. 7, the age of derived allele of SNP rs143384,

Table 3. Population statistics summary of haplotypes carrying derived allele A and ancestral allele G of SNP rs143384.

rs143384 derived allele A	Allele Frequency	Nucleotide Diversity	Tajima's D	Fu and Li's D	Fu and Li's F	Fu and Li's D*	Fu and Li's F*
African (N = 0)	0	*N.A.*	*N.A.*	*N.A.*	*N.A.*	*N.A.*	*N.A.*
European (N = 38)[a]	52.78%	*N.A.*	*N.A.*	*N.A.*	*N.A.*	*N.A.*	*N.A.*
East Asian (N = 47)	61.84%	9.395E-05	−1.702	−1.752	−2.033	**−2.984**	**−3.026**
South Asian (N = 26)	39.39%	3.736E-04	−0.869	0.973	0.527	0.968	0.518
Whole populations (N = 111)	39.08%	1.302E-04	−1.493	−0.300	−0.811	−0.288	−0.798
rs143384 ancestral allele G	**Allele Frequency**	**Nucleotide Diversity**	**Tajima's D**	**Fu and Li's D**	**Fu and Li's F**	**Fu and Li's D***	**Fu and Li's F***
African (N = 66)	100%	6.209E-04	−0.451	0.052	−0.129	0.067	−0.115
European (N = 34)	47.22%	2.846E-04	−1.075	−0.341	−0.650	−0.302	−0.611
East Asian (N = 29)	38.16%	5.111E-04	−0.824	−2.100	−2.028	−1.958	−1.889
South Asian (N = 44)	60.61%	5.585E-04	−0.408	−0.090	−0.220	−0.064	−0.196
Whole populations (N = 173)	60.92%	5.421E-04	−1.230	−1.179	−1.431	−1.152	−1.407

Bolds are values significantly lower than 0 with P-value<0.05 detected by DnaSP v 5.0 program.
[a]European population contains only one haplotype carrying derived allele of rs143384.

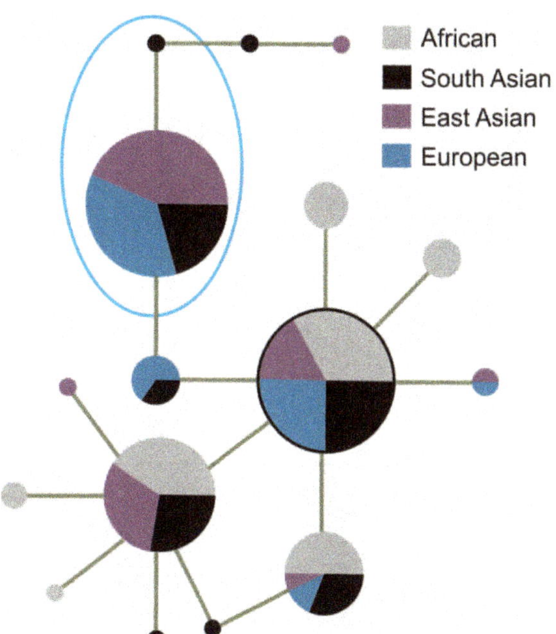

Figure 4. Median-joining phylogenetic network of the 16 haplotypes at at the exon 1 region. Each haplotype is represented by a circle with its area proportional to its frequency. The ancestral haplotype is outlined by a black line. The two haplotypes in the ellipse are the haplotypes that carry the derived allele at SNPs rs143383 and rs143384.

t = g*25 = 499.2*25 = 12,480 years, and the age of derived allele of SNP 143383, t = g*25 = 488.1*25 = 12,203 years.

Discussion

Our previous study indicated that positive selection operated on skeletal genes in non-African populations, including Europeans and East Asians [4]. Here, we describe positive selection acting in East Asian populations on a skeletal gene, *GDF5*, which plays a crucial role in the skeletal system. Positive selection probably targeted the derived alleles of SNPs rs143383 and rs143384 in the *GDF5* gene. The advantage of the derived alleles of these two SNPs is not clear. Strong evidence indicates that the derived allele of SNP rs143383 is associated with an increased risk of osteoarthritis, which is associated with decreased transcriptional activity of the *GDF5* gene in chondrogenic cells [13–16]. Lower expression of *GDF5* should lead to a reduction in limb bone growth and, as expected, the derived allele of rs143383 is associated with decreased height [16]. The two SNPs demonstrate significantly strong linkage disequilibrium, with the frequencies of the A-A and G-G haplotypes being 37.68% and 58.80%, respectively. The function of rs143383 on the expression of *GDF5* is influenced by the state of the rs143384 SNP [26]. Positive selection has driven the frequency of the derived alleles of these two SNPs to very high levels, leading to the associated decrease in height and increased risk of osteoarthritis (Fig. 8).

There is a decline in average human body mass, both in size and stature, began in the Late Pleistocene and early Holocene (~12,000 years BP) [27,28]. During this period, humans transited from lifestyle of close-contact ambush hunting of large mammals to the foraging and collecting of small animals. With the advent of agriculture, humans could produce food rather than needing to foraging for food [27,28]. Technological improvements decreased

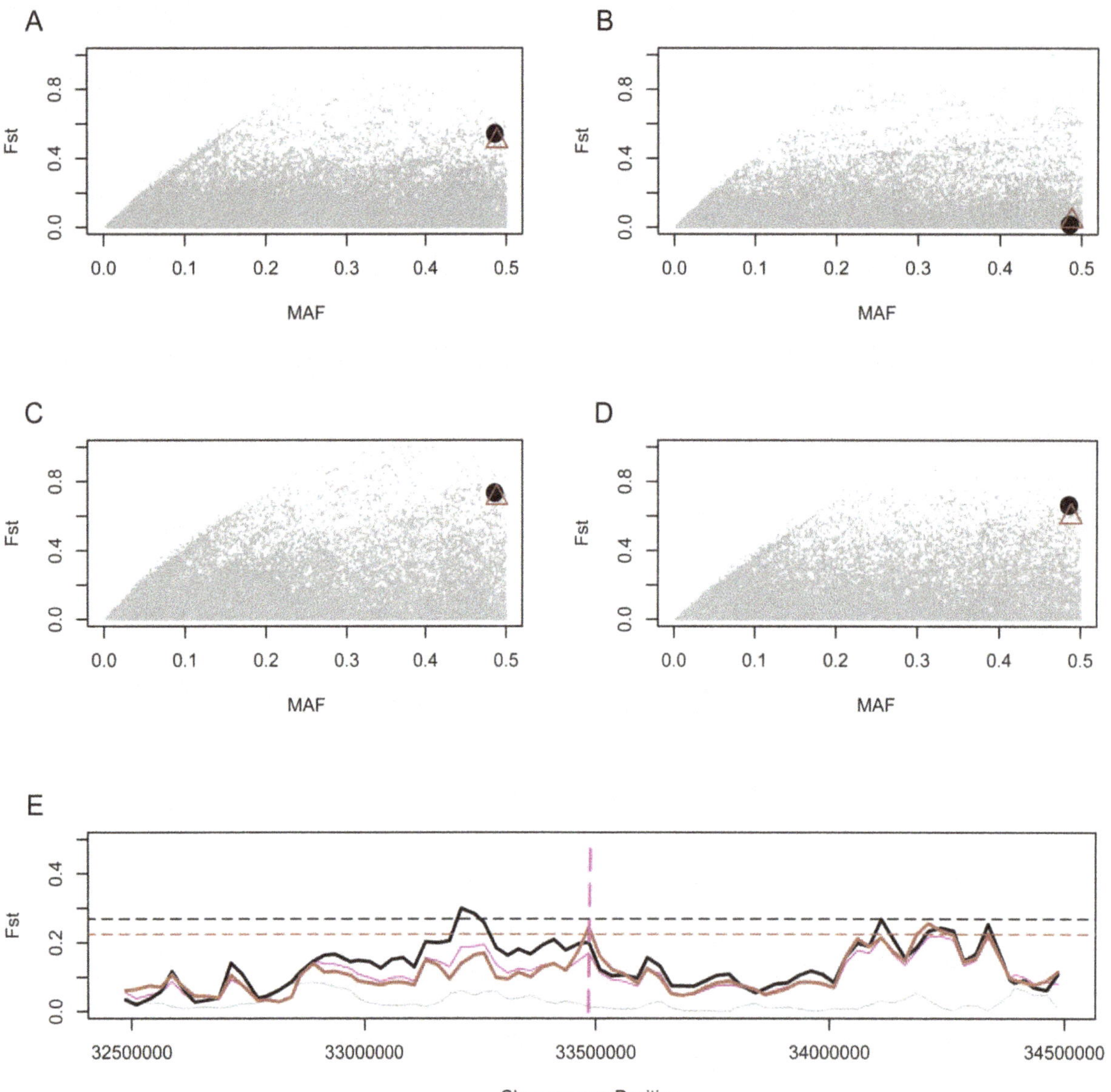

Figure 5. Fst distribution of SNPs across chromosome 20 gene regions. (A): Fst among the three populations vs minor allele frequencies (MAF). Big green dot and triangle represent SNPs rs143383 and rs143384. (B) Fst between East Asians and Europeans vs minor allele frequencies (MAF). (C) Fst between East Asians and Africans vs minor allele frequencies (MAF). (D) Fst between Africans and Europeans vs minor allele frequencies (MAF). (E) Sliding window analysis of Fst. Purple, black, brown and gray lines represent Fst among the three populations, Fst between East Asians and Africans, Fst between Africans and Europeans, Fst between East Asians and Europeans, respectively. The vertical line represents the position of *GDF5* gene. Black and brown horizontal lines represent the 95% percentile rank values of Fst values between East Asians and Africans and Fst between Africans and Europeans, respectively.

the selective advantage of having a larger body, which is metabolically expensive to maintain. Nutritional inadequacies and the spread of infectious disease during the Holocene may also help explain the reductions in human body size [27,28]. Changes associated with food production appeared to be developmental rather than genetic, however, the reduction in body size may also be due to genetic factors [27].

The ages of the derived alleles of SNPs rs143383 and rs143384 are ~12,000 years supporting the hypothesis that the Late Pleistocene–Early Holocene decline in human body size results from a genetic factor that was driven by positive selection. Humans with smaller body size might have some advantages, and thus elevated probability of survival, due to the poor socio-economic conditions under nutritional stress [29,30]. The decline in body size continued through the Neolithic, after which it was reversed in Europeans [27]. It had been concluded that when humans migrated to Europe they increased their body mass and height to facilitate their adaptation to this cold climatic area [31].

A question raised by our analysis is how can variants associated with diseases be positively selection for a fitness advantage? There are two main reasons to resolve this paradox. First, some characters that were adaptively evolved in the past may become maladaptive in a changing environment [3]. For *GDF5*, the derived alleles might have been positively selection for their advantage in the past, such as lower height, which would have increased survival in an environment with a lack of food. That

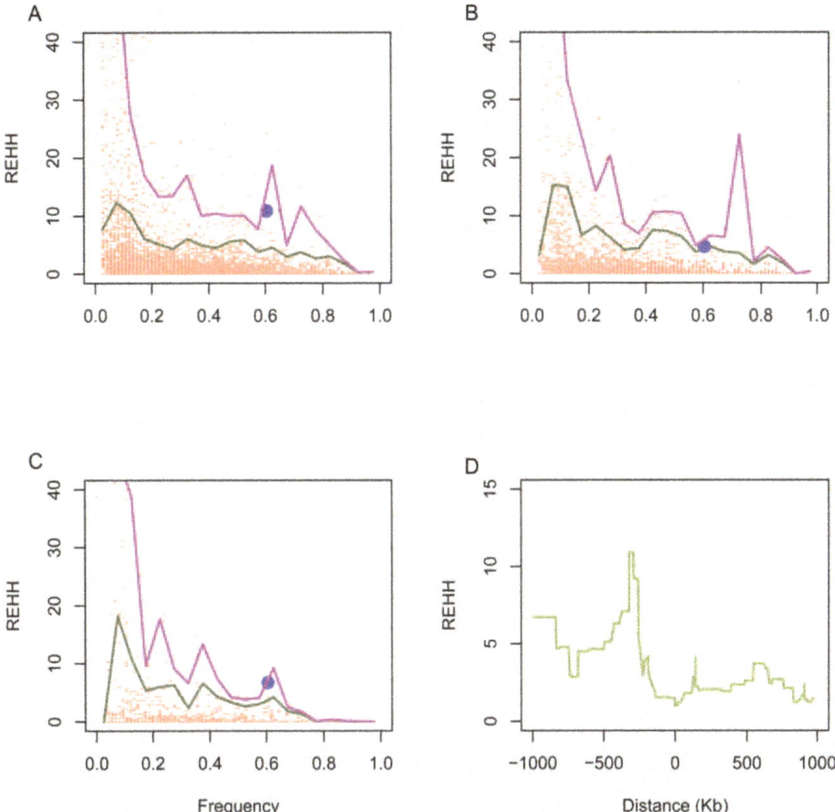

Figure 6. REHH of the core haplotypes on chromosome 20 and *GDF5*. REHH distributions at (A) 300 kb, (B) 500 kb, and (C) 1000 kb upstream and downstream of the core haplotypes. The two lines represent the 99% and 95% percentile rank values. Big dots are the major haplotype at the *GDF5* gene. (D) REHH of the major core haplotype at the *GDF5* gene at varying physical distances (kb).

advantage, however, may no longer be necessary. This would be similar to the example of the seven-repeat (7R) allele of the human dopamine receptor D4 (*DRD4*) gene. The 7R allele is associated with attention-deficit hyperactivity disorder (ADHD), however, people carrying this allele may have had an advantage in moving from one place to another during the colonization of world, and thus was driven to high frequency by positive selection [32,33]. A second reason is gene pleiotropy. Pleiotropy means that a mutation that is advantageous in one instance can be unfavorable in another [3]. Osteoarthritis is probably a byproduct of the rapid evolution of human skeletal system. Furthermore, osteoarthritis is a disease associated with ageing, and is rare in individuals below the age of 45 years [14]. This means that the disease of osteoarthritis contributes very little to the fitness of the patient, as it only affects them after reproducing.

Materials and Methods

Sequencing of *GDF5* alleles in modern humans

GDF5 gene sequences from a total of 142 unrelated human individuals, including 33 Africans, 36 Europeans, 38 East Asians and 35 South Asians, were chosen randomly from the Human Genome Diversity Cell Line Panel [34], were amplified by PCR and sequenced for two regions that include the two exons of the *GDF5* gene (Fig. 1). DNA sequencing was performed on an ABI 3730 automated DNA sequencer. Primer and PCR condition are available on request. Sequences were analyzed by DNAStar software. *GDF5* allele sequences of all individuals were submitted to GenBank under accession numbers GU831600–GU831883.

Population variation analysis based on the re-sequenced data

SNPs detected in the resequenced *GDF5* alleles were used to construct haplotypes using the program PHASE [18,19]. Median-joining network for the inference of haplotype genealogy was constructed by Network 4.5.1.0 [35]. The derived allele of each SNP was determined by comparing with the chimpanzee and orangutan sequences from UCSC genome database (http://genome.ucsc.edu/). Nucleotide diversity, which is the mean pairwise sequence difference, was calculated by the program DnaSP 5.0 [36]. A series population genetics parameters, Tajima's D [37], Fu and Li's D, F, D*, and F* [38,39], and Fay and Wu's H [40], were used to measure deviation from neutrality in each population. Demographic history and natural selection can both generate similar patterns of population variation. For example, negative values of Tajima's D, Fu and Li's D, F, D*, F* can be due to either positive selection or population expansion. Accordingly, coalescent simulations were constructed that incorporate the best-fit demographic parameters, as described in [21], to calculate the significance of the deviation from neutrality.

EHH analysis

Data on the genotypes of SNPs of chromosome 20 for the individuals that we resequenced for *GDF5* were downloaded from the Harvard HGDP-CEPH Genotypes for Population Genetics Analyses FLAT FILES SUPPLEMENT 10 from http://www.cephb.fr/en/hgdp/. We merged the SNPs data at *GDF5* to the genotyped data for chromosome 20 and constructed haplotypes

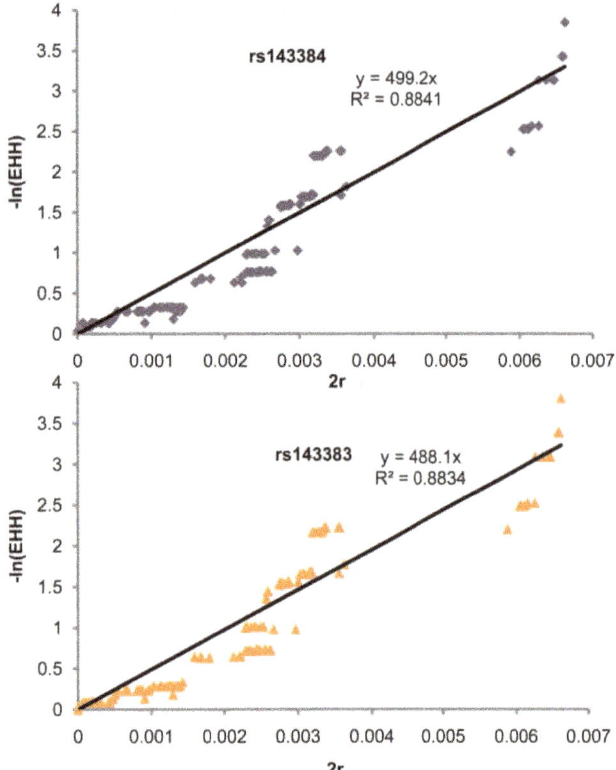

Figure 7. Evaluation of the ages of the derived alleles of SNPs rs143383 and rs143384 by linear regression of −ln(EHH) and 2r.

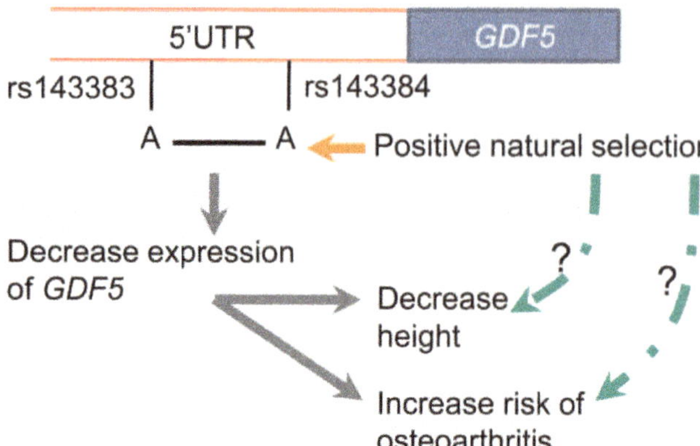

Figure 8. Positive natural selection operated upon the derived alleles of SNPs rs143384 and rs143383.

for each chromosome using the fastPHASE program [41]. Positively selected alleles or haplotypes will quickly become accumulate, and tend to have strong extended haplotype homozygosity with surrounding loci as recombination would not have time to disrupt it [42]. Here, the extended haplotype homozygosity (EHH) and REHH (relative EHH) for each haplotype at 300 kb, 500 kb, and 1000 kb upstream and downstream of the core region were calculated by the Sweep program (http://www.broadinstitute.org/mpg/sweep/). In addition, the world-wide allele frequency distribution of the two GDF5 SNPs rs143384 and rs143383 was downloaded from the hgdp selection browser (http://hgdp.uchicago.edu/cgi-bin/gbrowse/HGDP/).

Population differentiation analysis

Population differentiation of the SNPs on chromosome 22 was described in Wu and Zhang [43], which employed method from Weir BS and Cockerham [44,45], and HapMap Phase II (release 24, NCBI36) [46] for the three populations: African (YRI panel including 60 Yoruban individuals from Ibadan), European (CEU panel including 60 individuals of Utah residents with ancestry from northern and western Europe) and East Asian (EA panels including 45 Han Chinese (HCB) and 45 Japanese from Tokyo (JPT)). A sliding window analysis was performed with a window size of 50 kb and a step size of 25 kb.

Acknowledgments

We thank Prof. David Irwin for improving the writing of the manuscript.

Author Contributions

Conceived and designed the experiments: DDW GML WJ YPZ. Performed the experiments: GML WJ. Analyzed the data: DDW YL. Contributed reagents/materials/analysis tools: DDW YL GML WJ. Wrote the paper: DDW YPZ.

References

1. Varki A, Altheide TK (2005) Comparing the human and chimpanzee genomes: searching for needles in a haystack. Genome Res 15: 1746–1758.
2. Sabeti PC, Schaffner SF, Fry B, Lohmueller J, Varilly P, et al. (2006) Positive natural selection in the human lineage. Science 312: 1614–1620.
3. Wu DD, Zhang YP (2008) Positive Darwinian selection in human population: A review. Chinese Science Bulletin 53: 1457–1467.
4. Wu DD, Zhang YP (2010) Positive selection drives population differentiation in the skeletal genes in modern humans. Hum Mol Genet 19: 2341–2346.
5. He F, Wu DD, Kong QP, Zhang YP (2008) Intriguing balancing selection on the intron 5 region of LMBR1 in humanpopulation. PloS one 3: 2948.
6. Wu DD, Jin W, Hao XD, Tang NLS, Zhang YP Evidence for Positive Selection on the Osteogenin (BMP3) Gene in Human Populations. PloS one 5: e10959.
7. Chang SC, Hoang B, Thomas JT, Vukicevic S, Luyten FP, et al. (1994) Cartilage-derived morphogenetic proteins. New members of the transforming growth factor-beta superfamily predominantly expressed in long bones during human embryonic development. J Biol Chem 269: 28227–28234.
8. Settle SH, Rountree RB, Sinha A, Thacker A, Higgins K, et al. (2003) Multiple joint and skeletal patterning defects caused by single and double mutations in the mouse Gdf6 and Gdf5 genes. Dev Biol 254: 116–130.
9. Thomas JT, Lin K, Nandedkar M, Camargo M, Cervenka J, et al. (1996) A human chondrodysplasia due to a mutation in a TGF-β superfamily member. Nat Genet 12: 315–317.
10. Yang W, Cao L, Liu W, Jiang L, Sun M, et al. (2008) Novel point mutations in GDF5 associated with two distinct limb malformations in Chinese: brachydactyly type C and proximal symphalangism. J Hum Genet 53: 368–374.
11. Thomas JT, Kilpatrick MW, Lin K, Erlacher L, Lembessis P, et al. (1997) Disruption of human limb morphogenesis by a dominant negative mutation in CDMP1. Nat Genet 17: 58–64.
12. Faiyaz-Ul-Haque M, Ahmad W, Zaidi SHE, Haque S, Teebi AS, et al. (2002) Mutation in the cartilage-derived morphogenetic protein-1 (CDMP1) gene in a kindred affected with fibular hypoplasia and complex brachydactyly (DuPan syndrome). Clin Genet 61: 454–458.
13. Miyamoto Y, Mabuchi A, Shi D, Kubo T, Takatori Y, et al. (2007) A functional polymorphism in the 5′ UTR of GDF5 is associated with susceptibility to osteoarthritis. Nat Genet 39: 529–533.
14. Southam L, Rodriguez-Lopez J, Wilkins JM, Pombo-Suarez M, Snelling S, et al. (2007) An SNP in the 5′-UTR of GDF5 is associated with osteoarthritis susceptibility in Europeans and with in vivo differences in allelic expression in articular cartilage. Hum Mol Genet 16: 2226–2232.
15. Chapman K, Takahashi A, Meulenbelt I, Watson C, Rodriguez-Lopez J, et al. (2008) A meta-analysis of European and Asian cohorts reveals a global role of a functional SNP in the 5′UTR of GDF5 with osteoarthritis susceptibility. Hum Mol Genet 17: 1497.

16. Sanna S, Jackson AU, Nagaraja R, Willer CJ, Chen WM, et al. (2008) Common variants in the GDF5-UQCC region are associated with variation in human height. Nat Genet 40: 198–203.
17. Larsen CS (1995) Biological changes in human populations with agriculture. Ann Rev Anthropol 24: 185–213.
18. Stephens M, Donnelly P (2003) A comparison of bayesian methods for haplotype reconstruction from population genotype data. Am J Hum Genet 73: 1162–1169.
19. Stephens M, Smith NJ, Donnelly P (2001) A new statistical method for haplotype reconstruction from population data. Am J Hum Genet 68: 978–989.
20. Bamshad M, Wooding SP (2003) Signatures of natural selection in the human genome. Nat Rev Genet 4: 99–111.
21. Schaffner SF, Foo C, Gabriel S, Reich D, Daly MJ, et al. (2005) Calibrating a coalescent simulation of human genome sequence variation. Genome Res 15: 1576–1583.
22. Slatkin M, Rannala B (2000) Estimating allele age. Annu Rev Genomics Hum Genet 1: 361–385.
23. Kimura M, Ohta T (1973) The age of a neutral mutant persisting in a finite population. Genetics 75: 199–212.
24. Nei M (1995) Genetic support for the out-of-Africa theory of human evolution. Proc Natl Acad Sci USA 92: 6720–6722.
25. Voight BF, Kudaravalli S, Wen X, Pritchard JK (2006) A map of recent positive selection in the human genome. PLoS Biol 4: e72.
26. Egli RJ, Southam L, Wilkins JM, Lorenzen I, Pombo-Suarez M, et al. (2009) Functional analysis of the osteoarthritis susceptibility-associated GDF5 regulatory polymorphism. Arthritis & Rheumatism 60: 2055–2064.
27. Ruff C (2002) Variation in human body size and shape. Annu Rev Anthropol 31: 211–232.
28. Hawks J (2011) Selection for smaller brains in Holocene human evolution. arXiv:11025604v1.
29. Frisancho AR, Sanchez J, Pallardel D, Yanez L (1973) Adaptive significance of small body size under poor socio-economic conditions in southern Peru. Am J Phys Anthrop 39: 255–261.
30. Stini WA (1975) Adaptive strategies of human populations under nutritional stress. Physiological and Morphological Adaptation and Evolution: The Hague, Netherlands: Mouton. pp. 387–408.
31. Leppaeluoto J, Hassi J (1991) Human physiological adaptations to the arctic climate. Arctic 44: 139–145.
32. Ding Y-C, Chi H-C, Grady DL, Morishima A, Kidd JR, et al. (2002) Evidence of positive selection acting at the human dopamine receptor D4 gene locus. Proc Natl Acad Sci USA 99: 309–314.
33. Harpending H, Cochran G (2002) In our genes. Proc Natl Acad Sci USA 99: 10–12.
34. Cann HM, De Toma C, Cazes L, Legrand MF, Morel V, et al. (2002) A human genome diversity cell line panel. Science 296: 261–262.
35. Bandelt HJ, Forster P, Rohl A (1999) Median-joining networks for inferring intraspecific phylogenies. Mol Biol Evol 16: 37–48.
36. Librado P, Rozas J (2009) DnaSP v5: a software for comprehensive analysis of DNA polymorphism data. Bioinformatics 25: 1451–1452.
37. Tajima F (1989) Statistical method for testing the neutral mutation hypothesis by DNA polymorphism. Genetics 123: 585–595.
38. Fu YX (1997) Statistical tests of neutrality of mutations against population growth, hitchhiking and background selection. Genetics 14: 915–925.
39. Fu YX, Li WH (1993) Statistical tests of neutrality of mutations. Genetics 133: 693–709.
40. Fay JC, Wu CI (2000) Hitchhiking under positive Darwinian selection. Genetics 155: 1405–1413.
41. Scheet P, Stephens M (2006) A fast and flexible statistical model for large-scale population genotype data: applications to inferring missing genotypes and haplotypic phase. Am J Hum Genet 78: 629–644.
42. Sabeti PC, Reich DE, Higgins JM, Levine HZP, Richter DJ, et al. (2002) Detecting recent positive selection in the human genome from haplotype structure. Nature 419: 832–837.
43. Wu DD, Zhang YP (2011) Different level of population differentiation among human genes. BMC Evol Biol 11: 16.
44. Weir BS, Cockerham CC (1984) Estimating F-statistics for the analysis of population structure. Evolution 38: 1358–1370.
45. Akey JM, Zhang G, Zhang K, Jin L, Shriver MD (2002) Interrogating a high-density SNP map for signatures of natural selection. Genome Res 12: 1805–1814.
46. The International HapMap Consortium (2007) A second generation human haplotype map of over 3.1 million SNPs. Nature 449: 851–861.

17

Functional Annotation of Rheumatoid Arthritis and Osteoarthritis Associated Genes by Integrative Genome-Wide Gene Expression Profiling Analysis

Zhan-Chun Li[1], Jie Xiao[2], Jin-Liang Peng[3], Jian-Wei Chen[1], Tao Ma[1], Guang-Qi Cheng[1], Yu-Qi Dong[1], Wei-li Wang[1], Zu-De Liu[1]*

1 Department of Orthopaedic Surgery, Ren Ji Hospital, School of Medicine, Shanghai Jiao Tong University, Shanghai, P. R. China, **2** Department of Anesthesiology, Ren Ji Hospital, School of Medicine, Shanghai Jiao Tong University, Shanghai, P. R. China, **3** School of Biomedical Engineering/MED-X Research Institute, Shanghai Jiao Tong University, Shanghai, P. R. China

Abstract

Background: Rheumatoid arthritis (RA) and osteoarthritis (OA) are two major types of joint diseases that share multiple common symptoms. However, their pathological mechanism remains largely unknown. The aim of our study is to identify RA and OA related-genes and gain an insight into the underlying genetic basis of these diseases.

Methods: We collected 11 whole genome-wide expression profiling datasets from RA and OA cohorts and performed a meta-analysis to comprehensively investigate their expression signatures. This method can avoid some pitfalls of single dataset analyses.

Results and Conclusion: We found that several biological pathways (*i.e.*, the immunity, inflammation and apoptosis related pathways) are commonly involved in the development of both RA and OA. Whereas several other pathways (*i.e.*, vasopressin-related pathway, regulation of autophagy, endocytosis, calcium transport and endoplasmic reticulum stress related pathways) present significant difference between RA and OA. This study provides novel insights into the molecular mechanisms underlying this disease, thereby aiding the diagnosis and treatment of the disease.

Editor: Ted S. Acott, Casey Eye Institute, United States of America

Funding: This study was supported by Shanghai Natural Science Foundation, China (No. 13ZR1424900) and Medical-Engineering Joint Fund of Shanghai Jiao Tong University (No. YG2011MS41). The funders had no role in study design, data collection and analysis, decision to publish, or preparation of the manuscript.

Competing Interests: The authors have declared that no competing interests exist.

* E-mail: zudeliu001@163.com

Introduction

Rheumatoid arthritis (RA) is a common chronic systemic autoimmune disease that mainly affects the flexible joints. It is characterized by the inflammation of articular synovial. The lasting recurrent inflammation of synovial can lead to the deformation and destruction of cartilage and bones, which could result in disability of the patients [1,2]. RA mainly occurs in the 30~70 years old people and is more frequent in females than males. More than 1% of the world's population may be affected by RA [3,4]. This disease brings great physiological and psychological burden to patients. However, the biological causes for RA remain largely unknown. Although infectious agents including viruses, bacteria and fungi have long been suspected, none has been comprehensively proved [5,6]. Previous researches have also investigated the potential associations between RA and environmental factors, such as smoking, vitamin D deficiency, etc [7,8]. It is now generally believed that the pathogenesis of RA is closely related to genetic factors. Certain genes such as the human leukocyte antigen (HLA). HLA-DR4 and DW4 antigen, were identified in more than 90% of the patients. These pathological factors are referred to as the RA-shared epitope [3,9].

Osteoarthritis (OA) is another main type of chronic disease that affects the joints. The major pathological feature of OA is the degradation of articular cartilage and subchondral bone, and this may lead to the rigidity deformity and dysfunction of the joints [10]. The incidence of this disease in more than 50 years old people is as high as 80%. Etiological factors of OA include the mechanical injury, overweight, impairment of peripheral nerves, etc [11]. Osteoarthritis is different from rheumatoid arthritis in that there are extra-articular manifestations for rheumatoid arthritis. In addition, these diseases have different pathological manifestations for the synovial. RA is characterized by synovial cell hypertrophy and hyperplasia, infiltration of lymphocytes and inflammatory cells, whereas OA has fewer leukocytic infiltrates [12,13].

Recently, large efforts have been made to screen the genetic factors involved in RA and OA by high-throughput methods [14,15]. Several key genes and diagnostic markers have been identified for these diseases. However, the integrative analysis of multiple factors that contribute to the development of RA and OA appears to be a challenging task, and the underlying pathogenesis of RA and OA remain far from being understood. In this study, we compiled several whole-genome gene expression profiling datasets from RA and OA. Then we used a meta-analysis method to identify the aberrantly expressed genes. The subsequent functional annotation of these genes was performed based on gene ontology (GO) and Kyoto Encyclopedia of Genes and Genomes (KEGG) analysis [16,17]. We demonstrated that several biological pathways are highly enriched in both RA and OA associated genes, such as chemokine signaling pathway, regulation of autophagy, focal adhesion, etc. Whereas other pathways, including regulation of autophagy, endocytosis, calcium transport and endoplasmic reticulum stress related pathways, are differentially influenced in the RA and OA respectively. This analysis provides a novel insight into the pathophysiological processes involved in these diseases. In addition, it would help to prioritize putative targets for further experimental studies and develop novel therapeutic strategies in preventing the RA and OA.

Materials and Methods

Sample Collection

We first queried the PubMed and related literatures to collect the expression profiling datasets from RA, OA and the corresponding normal control (NT) tissues. The following key words and their combinations were used: "rheumatoid arthritis, osteoarthritis, gene expression, microarray". We only retained the original experimental works that analyzed the gene expression profiling between RA, OA and NT samples, respectively. Non-human studies, review articles and integrated analysis of expression profiles were excluded (**Figure 1**). At last, a total of 15 expression profiling datasets from 11 studies were collected (**Table 1**).

Data Preprocessing

In this study, a global normalization method to minimize the data inconsistency and heterogeneity was used. We used the *Z-score* transformation approach to calculate the expression intensities for each probe of the gene expression profiles [18]. *Z-scores* were calculated according to the following formula:

$$Z-score=\frac{x_i-\bar{x}}{\delta}.$$

where x_i represents raw intensity data for each gene; $\bar{x}$ represents average gene intensity within a single experiment and δ represents standard deviation (SD) of all of the measured intensities.

Statistical Analysis

To give an overview of the global shifts of gene expression between pathological and normal tissues, we first calculated the pairwise Euclidean distances for samples from RA, OA and NTs according to the following the formula:

$$D=\sqrt{\sum_{i=1}^{n}(x_{i1}-x_{i2})^2}.$$

The significance analysis of microarray (SAM) algorithm was then used to identify the differentially expressed genes between pathological and control samples. The SAM procedure first calculate the "relative difference" score for each gene based on a modified *t-test* method, then a subsequent permutation analysis was

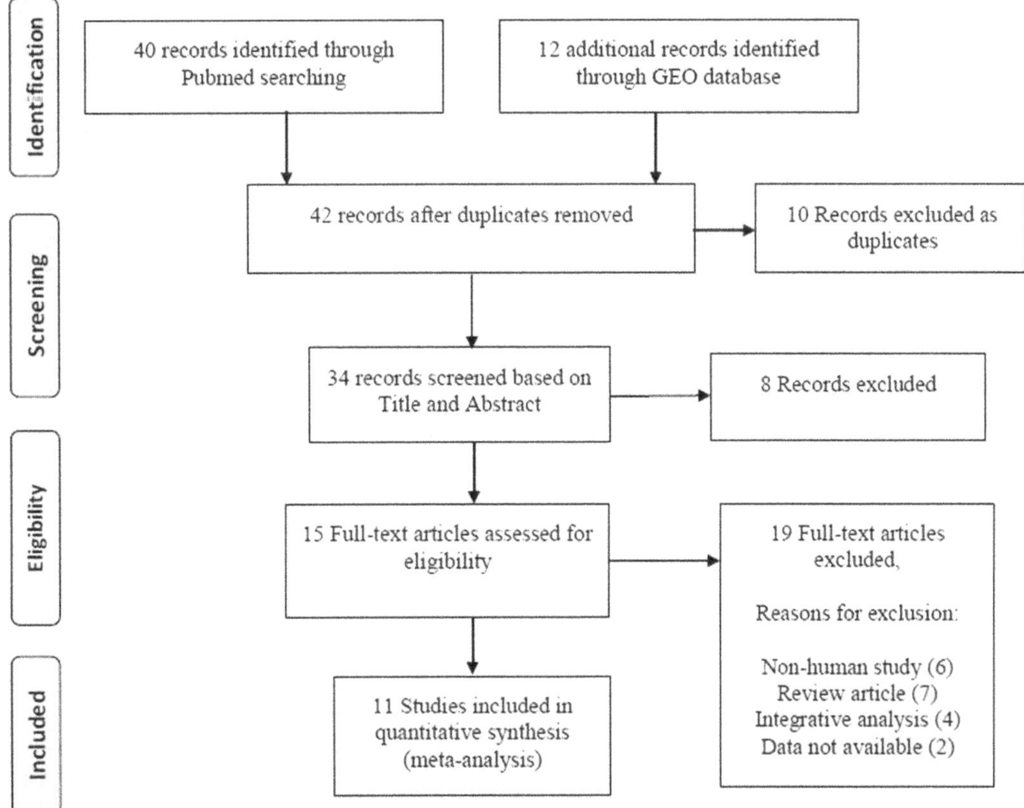

Figure 1. Flowchart of the selected process of microarray datasets for the meta-analysis.

Table 1. Characteristics of analyzed datasets.

GEO Acc	PMID	Publish date	tissue type	Platforms	Number of samples
GSE1919	20858714	4-Nov-04	synovial	Affymetrix HGU95A	5 OA
					5 NC
					5 RA
GSE2053	20858714	10-Dec-04	synovial	HUMAN UNIGENE SetI Part 1	4 NC
					4 RA
GSE3698	16508983	6-Jun-06	synovial	Human Unigene3.1 cDNA Array 37.5K v1.0	18 RA
					19 OA
GSE7669	21474483	30-Aug-07	synovial	Affymetrix HGU95 2.0	6 RA
					6 OA
GSE9027	17665400	13-Sep-07	synovial		28 RA
GSE12021	18721452	2-Sep-08	synovial	Affymetrix HGU133A HGU133B Array	20 OA
					22 RA
					13 NC
GSE17755	21496236	21-Aug-10	peripheral blood	Hitachisoft AceGene Human Oligo Chip 30K 1 Chip Version	112 RA
					8 NC
					45 NC
GSE27390	21679443	31-May-11	bone marrow	Affymetrix HGU133 Plus 2.0	9 RA
					11 OA
GSE29746	22021863	25-Oct-11	synovial	Whole Human Genome Microarray 4x44K G4112F	9 RA
					11 OA
GSE36700	17469140	27-Mar-12	synovial	Affymetrix HGU133 Plus 2.0	6 OA
					7 RA
GSE39340		22-Oct-12	synovial	Illumina HumanHT-12 V4.0 expression beadchip	10 RA
					7 OA

A total of 11 expression profiles comparing RA, OA and NTs samples were collected in this study. Their GEO accession number, PubMed ID, publish date, tissue type, expression platform and number of samples were listed.

used to compute false discovery rate (*FDR*) [19]. To get the best balance between the number of significant calls and the lowest *FDR* for the dataset tested, we used *FDR* <0.05 and |log fold change| >1 as the criteria for significant difference.

Functional Annotation

In order to examine the biological significance of the differentially expressed genes, we performed GO and KEGG enrichment analysis to investigate their functional and pathway implications. The online based software GeneCoDis3 was used to perform this analysis [20]. The differentially expressed genes and all the expressed genes were submitted as the gene list and background list, respectively. The 5% cut-off of the FDR was used.

Results

Short Overview of the Studies Included

In recent years, many studies have used microarray technology to analyzed the whole genome expression proofing in samples of RA and OA. In this study, a total of 11 expression profiling datasets were collected, which include 383 samples. The characteristics of all these datasets included in this analysis were listed as **Table 1**. Among the 11 datasets, nine studies focused on synovial tissues and two studies focused on peripheral blood and bone marrow-derived mononuclear cells, respectively. More than half (six) of these studies focused on the differentially expressed genes between RA and OA samples, whereas four studies focused on the expression profiling of RA or OA and the corresponding NT samples, and one study only provided the expression profiling from RA samples.

Global Changes in Gene Expression in RA and OA Samples

Normalization is an important issue for comparison of microarray datasets. The heterogeneity of different datasets may lead to difficulties for comparing the results directly. The improperly normalized data used in microarray comparisons may run a high risk of skewing comparison results and reduces the credibility of individual gene change measurements. Towards this end, a global transformation of *z-score* was used to normalize all the expression profiling data retrieved for RA and OA. After filtering the normalized data, a total of 14,047 genes were detected in more than 60% of the samples. By using the assembled expression compendium, we investigated the global shifts of gene expression between RA, OA and NTs samples respectively. The average Euclidean distance was calculated to measure expression divergence between individual samples. As indicated in **Figure 2**, the expression divergence between OA and corresponding NT samples is significantly larger than that between RA and NT samples (Mann-Whitney U test, *P-value* <1e-6). We found that expression divergence between pathological samples and NTs is significantly larger than the distance between pathological samples of RA and OA samples (Mann-Whitney U test, *P-value*: 2.37e-57 and 1.12e-83 respectively,). This indicates that the similarities of expression signatures between RA and OA and several pathogenesis in common may contribute to the development of these diseases.

Identification of Differentially Expressed Genes from RA *vs.* NT Samples

To obtain the genetic markers involved in the development and progression of RA and OA, the SAM method was used to identify the differentially expressed genes between pathological and control samples. At last, a total of 201 genes were found to be differentially expressed between RA and NT samples with the threshold of *FDR* <0.05 and minimal two-fold changes of expression. Among those differentially expressed genes, 35 genes were up-regulated and 166 genes were down-regulated in RA samples compared with the NT samples, respectively. The full list of these genes was provided in **Table S1**. The top 10 up-regulated and down-regulated genes for RA *vs.* NT were listed in **Table 2**, which include the *DCTN1, GABRR3, SOX18, ALPK2, UCP2, GGTL3, GNGT2, ABHD11, ETV3, NPCDR1*, etc. The gene with the most significant expression difference between RA and OA is Dynactin subunit 1 (*DCTN1*), which presents a ~1437.67 fold higher expression in RA samples. *DCTN1*, encoding the largest subunit of dynactin, is involved in a diverse array of cellular functions, including the centripetal movement of lysosomes and endosomes, spindle formation, chromosome movement, nuclear positioning, and axonogenesis. Conversely, the gene with the most significant expression divergence and higher expression in RA samples (151.59 fold) is *NPCDR1*. Some of the deregulated genes have been previously reported to be closely related to the development of RA.

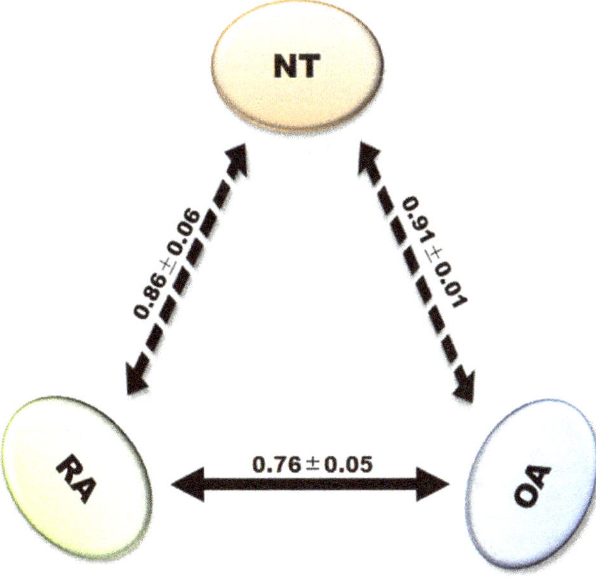

Figure 2. Average expression distances between RA, OA and NT samples. The average distances and the standard errors were labeled in the figure. The distance between pathological samples (RA or OA) and NTs is significantly larger than the distance between RA and OA samples.

For example, the single nucleotide polymorphism within the *UCP2* gene was identified to associate with many chronic inflammatory diseases including RA and systemic lupus erythematosus (SLE) [21]. Activated *PIAS1* gene was identified to repress the transcription of inflammatory genes [22], repression of *PIAS1* related pathways have some effects for the treatment of inflammatory disorders such as RA and atherosclerosis [23].

Identification of Differentially Expressed Genes from OA *vs.* NT Samples

With the same analytic procedure described above, we identified 244 genes to be differentially expressed in OA samples comparing with NT samples, which include 45 up-regulated and 199 down-regulated genes. The full gene list and the top deregulated gene list for OA *vs.* NT samples were listed in **Table S2** and **Table 3**, respectively. Specifically, the top deregulated genes for OA *vs.* NT samples include the *DPM2, MUS81, VAMP2, ZBTB33, NUP62, RHBDD1, PDZD7, PLEKHG4, ABCG1, TCEA3*, etc. Several of these genes have been identified to be involved in the development RA or OA samples, including *COL2* [24], *Gal-9* [25,26], *MUS81* [27] and *ABCG1* [28].

Functional Annotation of Differentially Expressed Genes

To gain insights into the biological roles of these differentially expressed genes from RA and OA *vs.* NT samples, we performed a GO categories enrichment analysis. GO category provides a descriptive framework of functional annotation and classification for gene sets analysis. GO categories are organized into three groups: biological process, molecular function and cellular component. In our work, only biological process and molecular function categories were considered. The functional enrichment work was performed by a web-based software, GeneCoDis3. With the *FDR* <0.05, we found GO terms for molecular functions significantly enriched in protein binding (GO:0005515), metal ion binding and DNA binding (GO:0003677), while for biological processes, the enriched GO terms were regulation of transcription (GO:0006355), embryonic limb morphogenesis (GO:0030326) and otic vesicle development (GO:0071599) (**Figure 3**).

To further evaluate the biological significance for the differentially expressed genes, we also performed the KEGG pathway enrichment analysis. The top enriched biological pathways associated with RA and OA include chemokine signaling pathway, glycosaminoglycan biosynthesis-chondroitin sulfate, SNARE interactions in vesicular transport, endocytosis, autophagy, etc. (**Table 4**). The chemokine pathway, for example, has long been suspected to involve in the development of RA. The chemokines are a family of small cytokines or signaling proteins secreted by cells, which function is to control cells of the immune system during processes of immune surveillance. Many chemokines could participates in the inflammatory response and attracts immune cells to the site of inflammation [29]. The genes involved in chemokines signaling pathway was identified to be altered in both RA *vs.* NT and OA *vs.* NT. The *CXCL2*, for example, also known as *GRO2*, is implicated in the recruitment of neutrophils from the circulation system to the sites of inflammation [30], it is constitutively expressed in resting OA cells, which supports the idea that some circumstances OA can be considered inflammatory disease [31].

As for apoptosis, genes involved in the regulation of cell survival and anti-apoptosis and autophagy related pathways are significantly affected, such as the mitogen-activated protein kinases (MAPK) pathways. MAPK comprises a family of serine/threonine protein kinases that implicated in the regulation of key cellular processes including cell survival, proliferation, differentiation and

Table 2. Summary of differentially expressed genes between RA *vs.* NT samples.

Gene Symbol	Description	Score (D)	Fold Change	Status
DCTN1	dynactin 1	3.46	1437.67	down-regulated
GABRR3	gamma-aminobutyric acid (GABA) A receptor, rho 3	3.23	130.1	down-regulated
SOX18	SRY (sex determining region Y)-box 18	4.32	70.33	down-regulated
ALPK2	alpha-kinase 2	3.96	64.95	down-regulated
UCP2	uncoupling protein 2	3.85	52.75	down-regulated
MITD1	microtubule interacting and transport, domain containing 1	3.15	46.12	down-regulated
SMEK1	SMEK homolog 1, suppressor of mek1	3.64	35.59	down-regulated
BANF1	barrier to autointegration factor 1	3.46	33.62	down-regulated
PIAS1	protein inhibitor of activated STAT, 1	3.25	33.18	down-regulated
GFOD2	glucose-fructose oxidoreductase domain containing 2	3.38	30.77	down-regulated
TSPAN1	tetraspanin 1	−3.13	−48.9	up-regulated
HSPB2	heat shock 27kDa protein 2	−4.52	−50.67	up-regulated
NEK6	NIMA-related kinase 6	−10.5	−56.03	up-regulated
COL2	collagen, type II, alpha 1	−3.62	−62.02	up-regulated
LGALS9	lectin, galactoside-binding, soluble, 9	−4.85	−64.47	up-regulated
GGTL3	gamma-glutamyltransferase 7	−3.23	−79.05	up-regulated
GNGT2	guanine nucleotide binding protein (G protein), gamma transducing activity polypeptide 2	−9.81	−89.35	up-regulated
ABHD11	abhydrolase domain containing 11	−4.03	−95.86	up-regulated
ETV3	ets variant 3	−3.66	−106.96	up-regulated
NPCDR1	nasopharyngeal carcinoma, down-regulated 1	−4.79	−151.59	up-regulated

The symbol name, description, D score and the expression fold change were provided.

Table 3. Summary of differentially expressed genes between OA *vs.* NT samples.

Gene Symbol	Description	Score (D)	Fold Change	Status
DPM2	dolichyl-phosphate mannosyltransferase polypeptide 2	4.18	697.61	down-regulated
MUS81	MUS81 structure-specific endonuclease	4.3	236.6	down-regulated
VAMP2	vesicle-associated membrane protein 2	6.38	220.45	down-regulated
ZBTB33	zinc finger and BTB domain containing 33	3.67	25366	down-regulated
NUP62	nucleoporin 62kDa	3.24	157.76	down-regulated
LOXL3	lysyl oxidase-like 3	4.84	111.57	down-regulated
LIMK2	LIM domain kinase 2	3.88	76.61	down-regulated
ZNF593	zinc finger protein 593	3.73	65.5	down-regulated
MRPS5	mitochondrial ribosomal protein S5	4.24	54.33	down-regulated
SMYD2	SET and MYND domain containing 2	3.62	31.41	down-regulated
MAN2	alpha Mannosidase II	−4.51	−87.45	up-regulated
SDCCAG1	NEMF nuclear export mediator factor	−6.12	−97.84	up-regulated
IGSF8	immunoglobulin superfamily, member 8	−6.9	−100.79	up-regulated
PBX1	pre-B-cell leukemia homeobox 1	−5.22	−133.75	up-regulated
KIAA1128	CCSER2 coiled-coil serine-rich protein 2	−6.9	−195.25	up-regulated
RHBDD1	rhomboid domain containing 1	−6.18	−231.9	up-regulated
PDZD7	PDZ domain containing 7	−4.48	−286	up-regulated
PLEKHG4	pleckstrin homology domain containing, family G (with RhoGef domain) member 4	−8.78	−337.12	up-regulated
ABCG1	ATP-binding cassette, sub-family G (WHITE), member 1	−3.87	−441.27	up-regulated
TCEA3	transcription elongation factor A (SII), 3	−8.37	−1241.14	up-regulated

The symbol name, description, D score and the expression fold change were provided.

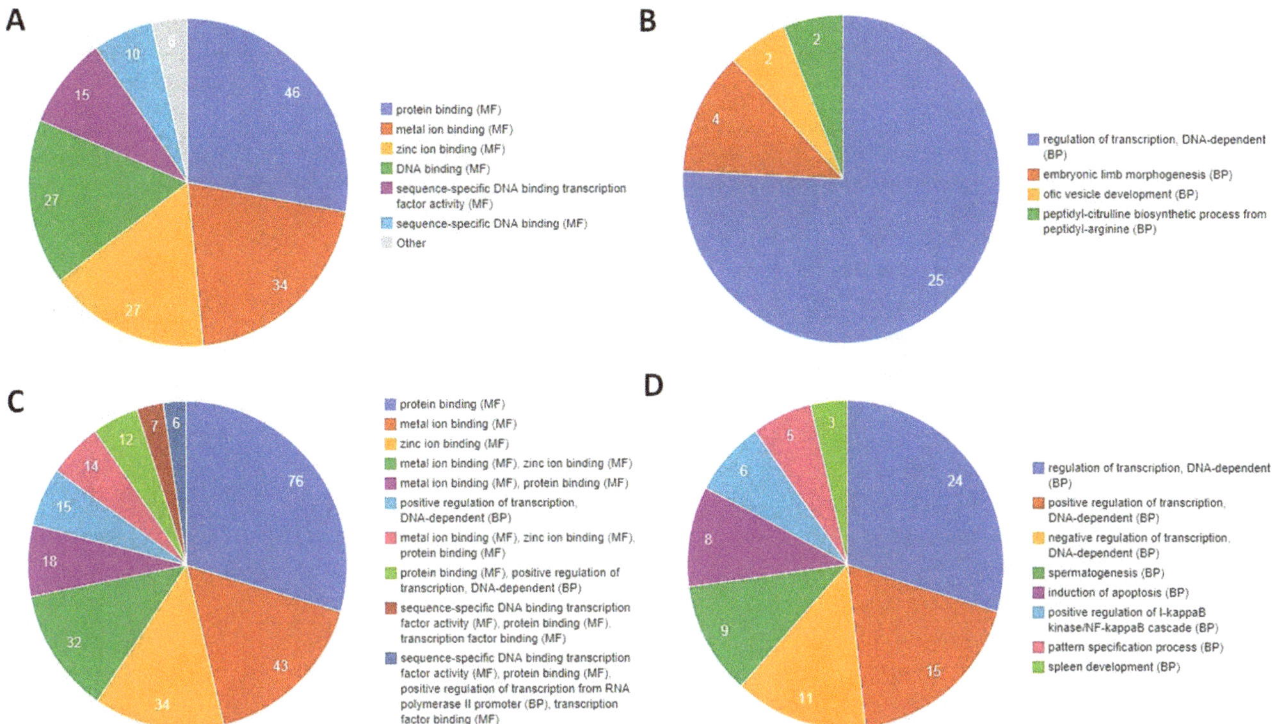

Figure 3. Enriched GO terms of differentially expressed genes between RA and OA *vs.* NT samples. (A) molecular functions for differentially expressed genes of RA *vs.* NT samples; (B) biological process for differentially expressed genes of RA *vs.* NT samples; (C) molecular functions for differentially expressed genes of OA *vs.* NT samples; (D) biological process for differentially expressed genes of OA *vs.* NT samples.

apoptosis as well as cellular stress and inflammatory responses. The respective genes in MAPK pathway showed altered expression levels in RA and OA patients of this study. Involvement of MAPK in the regulation of the synthesis of inflammation mediators and the development of RA have been widely identified [32]. Inhibitors targeting MAPK related pathways have been developed and the preclinical data indicated that they exhibit anti-inflammatory activities. This makes them the potential targets of anti-inflammatory therapy for these diseases [33].

Focal adhesion kinase (FAK) is another pathway that known to play a key role in cell proliferation and migration. Members of this family, which include FAK and PYK2 and their associated signaling intermediates, have been implicated in cell adhesion, migration and osteoclast differentiation [34]. GRB2 is one of the interaction factors of FAK that facilitate intracellular signaling [35]. This gene was found to be up-regulated in both of the diseases, and this may be responsible for the activation of the FAK family signaling and results in the adhesion and migration of the pathological cells.

Discussion

Rheumatoid arthritis and osteoarthritis are the most commonly observed types of arthritis. However, the underlying causes of RA and OA remain largely unknown. Understanding the pathogenesis could have important implications for drug development and treatment for these diseases. Genetic researches on RA and OA have pursued throughout the last years. For example, the whole genome expression profiling studies by using microarrays. Gene expression profiling studies are capable of identifying differences in transcription of thousands of genes on a genome-wide scale. This technique may investigate the pathophysiology of complex genetic tracts and the altered molecular pathways. The first genome wide comparisons of gene expression of RA and OA was performed by Ungethuem *et al.* in 2006. To date, a total of 11 microarray mRNA profiling studies comparing RA and OA with control tissue have been published. Combination and comparison of these studies may have the potential to substantiate and filter the results of each single study and may provide further insights into the pathogenesis of these diseases. However, the heterogeneity of the datasets may run a risk of skewing comparison results and reduces the credibility of gene expression change measurements. To this end, we collected those published expression profiling datasets and used a global normalization method to calculate the expression level for each gene. This algorithm used in this study could reduce heterogeneity of different datasets and make them comparable. Then we performed a systemic meta-analysis based on re-analysis of primary data sets to retrieve RA and OA associated genes. Followed functional implication analysis was performed to investigate their physiological impact in development of these diseases. To our knowledge, no other systematic meta-analysis of gene profiling has been performed to investigate the differences and similarities between RA and OA. The present study suggests several promising genes and may provide a clue to the role of these genes played in the development of these diseases.

Based on our results, it is evident that inflammation as well as apoptotic processes are key elements in the development and progression of RA since several inflammation- and apoptosis-associated genes were identified. For example, the *Gal-9*. *Gal-9* is a kind of immunity associated gene that plays a role in inflammatory responses. This gene has previously been proved to be a ligand of T cell Ig and mucin domain (*Tim-3*). It was reported that *Tim-3* expression is higher in patients with inflammatory disorders such as RA compared to controls [36]. In this case, up-regulation of

Table 4. KEGG pathway enrichment of genes differentially expressed RA and OA *vs.* NT samples.

Sample type	KEGG pathway	Number of genes	Entrez gene ID	*P-value*
OA vs. NT	Chemokine signaling pathway	5	2920 2869 409 9844 2309	0.0168
OA vs. NT	Endocrine and other factor-regulated calcium reabsorption	5	56302 6546 490 793 8766	0.0179
OA vs. NT	Glycosaminoglycan biosynthesis - chondroitin sulfate	3	55501 64132 10090	0.0286
OA vs. NT	SNARE interactions in vesicular transport	3	6844 53407 113189	0.0462
OA vs. NT	NF-KAPPA B signaling	5	27040 29760 8915 10015 2637	0.0439
OA vs. NT	PPAR signaling pathway	3	1376 364 10999	0.0726
OA vs. NT	Protein processing in endoplasmic reticulum	4	50613 9695 3300 4217	0.0726
OA vs. NT	Phagosome	3	53407 23673 30835	0.0726
OA vs. NT	Pathogenic Escherichia coli infection	3	9181 999 10092	0.0726
OA vs. NT	MAPK signaling pathway	3	999 9844 6197	0.0726
OA vs. NT	Focal adhesion	3	6844 3783 3912	0.0974
OA vs. NT	Oxidative phosphorylation	4	9997 4519 28487 4512	0.0981
OA vs. NT	Endocytosis	3	2869 23096 409	0.0996
RA vs. NT	Vasopressin-regulated water reabsorption	3	6844 51164 1639	0.0175
RA vs. NT	Glyoxylate and dicarboxylate metabolism	3	4190 48 847	0.0275
RA vs. NT	Chemokine signaling pathway	3	2885 2793 2829	0.0493
RA vs. NT	Regulation of autophagy	3	25989 5562 9474	0.0339
RA vs. NT	NF-KAPPA B signaling	4	29760 8915 8091 9020	0.0339
RA vs. NT	SNARE interactions in vesicular transport	3	6844 9527 9482	0.0339
RA vs. NT	Oxidative phosphorylation	5	4508 9997 4519 28487 4512	0.0421
RA vs. NT	Citrate cycle (TCA cycle)	3	4190 48 945406	0.0421
RA vs. NT	mTOR signaling pathway	3	25989 5562 1978	0.0421
RA vs. NT	Adherens junction	3	81 6615 7414	0.0781
RA vs. NT	Wnt signaling pathway	4	56998 6093 9475 51176	0.0781
RA vs. NT	MAPK signaling pathway	4	9448 4773 7151 4217	0.0793
RA vs. NT	Pathogenic Escherichia coli infection	3	9181 999 4690	0.0793
RA vs. NT	Focal adhesion	3	81 2885 3912	0.0841
RA vs. NT	Bacterial invasion of epithelial cells	3	10163 999 9844	0.0841

The number of differentially expressed genes in a specific pathway, enriched gene ID and adjusted *P-values* calculated by fisher's exact test were included.

Gal-9 may enhance the *Tim-3-Tim-3L* interactions in synovial and improve the symptoms of inflammation.

In addition, we found that the NF-κB signaling pathway may play significant role in these diseases. NF-κB is a key transcription factor that regulates a variety of genes involved in immune response, cell differentiation and proliferation. Incorrect activation of NF-κB was suggested to associate with cancer, inflammatory and autoimmune diseases, septic shock and viral infection [37]. It has previously indicated that Interleukin-1 beta (*IL-1β*) gene was induced in the RA patient-derived synovial fibroblast cell line MH7A by cigarette smoke condensate [38]. NF-κB binding sites were found in the promoter region of *IL-1β* gene. Therefore, this indicated that aberrant expression of the genes relevant of NF-κB signaling pathway may play a pathological role in the development of RA and OA.

Abnormalities in the mitochondria have been a topic of interests into the study of arthritis. It has been reported that mutation frequency of mtDNA is significantly higher in the inflamed synovial compared with normal synovial. This high mutation frequency is caused by the inflammatory mediators of TNFα and interferon γ (IFNγ) and eventually results in the changes of microenvironment and function of mitochondria [39]. Here, we reported that expressions of certain genes related to the function of mitochondria were altered in RA patients. Notably, the relevant genes, which include the *ATP6, SCO2, CYTB, DN1, COX1, ANT1,* are mainly function in oxidative phosphorylation, whereas dysfunction in oxidative phosphorylation related genes is closely related to the systemic juvenile idiopathic arthritis and endemic osteoarthritis [40,41]. This largely indicates that both RA and OA can be classified as mitochondrial disorder.

Although RA and OA samples share many similarities of their respective gene expression profiles and a number of pathways show comparable variance in both of these diseases, thus reflecting basic common pathomechanism of these joint diseases. However, RA and OA samples can be clearly differentiated regarding gene expression variances in other pathways. In OA, the pathways affected by expression variances include calcium ion transport, PPAR signaling pathway, protein processing in endoplasmic reticulum (ER), phagosome and endocytosis related pathways, etc. Calcium is the essential structural component of the skeletal system. Adequate calcium intake is the basis of osteoblast growth. Observation of the dysregulated expression of calcium related gene may partially explain why calcium pyrophosphate dihydrates accumulate in synovial of OA patients [42,43]. Endocytosis and autophagy are the major pathways for materials to be transported into the lysosomes in cells. The former is responsible for uptake of extracellular constituents and the latter for degradation of cytoplasmic constituents. Several common factors and pathways that regulate the endocytosis and autophagy has been identified [44]. Since there is a high correlation between autophagy activation and the severity of experimental osteoarthritis [45], we may speculate the causal relationship between the deregulation of endocytosis related genes and the development of OA.

ER stress refers to as the enhanced expression of normal or folding-defective proteins and the accumulation of unfolded protein in ER by stimuli. This process has been shown to participate in many disease, including diabetes, inflammation, and neurodegenerative disorders [46]. It was also indicated that ER stress may contribute to chondrocyte apoptosis along with OA progression, which was closely associated with an enhanced apoptotic response and a reduced protective response by cells [47]. Therefore, molecules that regulate the ER stress response would be candidate targets for treatment of this disease.

In contrast to OA, RA-specific pathways are involved in vasopressin-regulated water reabsorption, adherens junction, etc. As a proinflammatory hormone, vasopressin can stimulate the cell proliferation in chondrocytes that derived from patients with RA [48]. Adherens junctions are protein complexes that occur at cell-cell junctions in epithelial tissues to create ephemeral connections with counterparts from adjacent cells. The inflamed synovial tissue undergoes remodeling during the course of RA, the synovial lining becomes hyperplastic and forms a condensed tissue [49]. Genes related to the adherens junctions pathway is speculated to involve in this process and their abnormal expression may enhance the development of RA. Identification of interferon signaling and bacterial invasion related pathways suggests that some of the cases are indeed caused by microbial infection. In addition, other canonical pathways that involved in the RA development, such as the Wnt signaling and mTOR signaling pathways, were also identified in this analysis [50,51]. These affected pathways and the respective genes reported here may provide the basis for further analyses of the pathogenesis and the differences between RA and OA on a cellular and molecular level.

In conclusion, by collecting the whole genome expression data sets from different platforms, multiple biological markers were identified for RA and OA. This work is important to characterize the specific roles of those genes involved in the pathogenesis of RA and OA. Functional analysis of these genes may provide additional insights into the complex process of these diseases. In addition, this analysis may help to improve the diagnosis and treatment of these diseases.

Supporting Information

Table S1 Full lists of the differentially expressed genes between RA *vs.* NT samples. The symbol name, D score and the expression fold change were provided.

Table S2 Full lists of the differentially expressed genes between OA *vs.* NT samples. The symbol name, D score and the expression fold change were provided.

Acknowledgments

We thank the two anonymous reviewers for their valuable suggestions.

Author Contributions

Conceived and designed the experiments: ZCL ZDL. Performed the experiments: ZCL JX JP JC TM GC YD WW. Analyzed the data: ZCL JX. Contributed reagents/materials/analysis tools: JX JP. Wrote the paper: ZDL.

References

1. Huber LC, Distler O, Tarner I, Gay RE, Gay S, et al. (2006) Synovial fibroblasts: key players in rheumatoid arthritis. Rheumatology (Oxford) 45: 669–675.
2. Bartok B, Firestein GS (2010) Fibroblast-like synoviocytes: key effector cells in rheumatoid arthritis. Immunol Rev 233: 233–255.
3. Scott DL, Wolfe F, Huizinga TW (2010) Rheumatoid arthritis. Lancet 376: 1094–1108.
4. Firestein GS (2003) Evolving concepts of rheumatoid arthritis. Nature 423: 356–361.
5. Alvarez-Lafuente R, Fernandez-Gutierrez B, de Miguel S, Jover JA, Rollin R, et al. (2005) Potential relationship between herpes viruses and rheumatoid arthritis: analysis with quantitative real time polymerase chain reaction. Ann Rheum Dis 64: 1357–1359.
6. Balandraud N, Roudier J, Roudier C (2004) Epstein-Barr virus and rheumatoid arthritis. Autoimmun Rev 3: 362–367.
7. Albano SA, Santana-Sahagun E, Weisman MH (2001) Cigarette smoking and rheumatoid arthritis. Semin Arthritis Rheum 31: 146–159.
8. Wen H, Baker JF (2011) Vitamin D, immunoregulation, and rheumatoid arthritis. J Clin Rheumatol 17: 102–107.
9. Plenge RM, Seielstad M, Padyukov L, Lee AT, Remmers EF, et al. (2007) TRAF1-C5 as a risk locus for rheumatoid arthritis–a genomewide study. N Engl J Med 357: 1199–1209.
10. Kingsbury SR, Conaghan PG (2012) Current osteoarthritis treatment, prescribing influences and barriers to implementation in primary care. Prim Health Care Res Dev 13: 373–381.
11. Brandt KD, Dieppe P, Radin E (2009) Etiopathogenesis of osteoarthritis. Med Clin North Am 93: 1–24, xv.
12. Baecklund E, Iliadou A, Askling J, Ekbom A, Backlin C, et al. (2006) Association of chronic inflammation, not its treatment, with increased lymphoma risk in rheumatoid arthritis. Arthritis Rheum 54: 692–701.
13. Franklin J, Lunt M, Bunn D, Symmons D, Silman A (2006) Incidence of lymphoma in a large primary care derived cohort of cases of inflammatory polyarthritis. Ann Rheum Dis 65: 617–622.
14. Heruth DP, Gibson M, Grigoryev DN, Zhang LQ, Ye SQ (2012) RNA-seq analysis of synovial fibroblasts brings new insights into rheumatoid arthritis. Cell Biosci 2: 43.
15. Zhang R, Fang H, Chen Y, Shen J, Lu H, et al. (2012) Gene expression analyses of subchondral bone in early experimental osteoarthritis by microarray. PLoS One 7: e32356.
16. Ashburner M, Ball CA, Blake JA, Botstein D, Butler H, et al. (2000) Gene ontology: tool for the unification of biology. The Gene Ontology Consortium. Nature Genetics 25: 25–29.
17. Kanehisa M, Araki M, Goto S, Hattori M, Hirakawa M, et al. (2008) KEGG for linking genomes to life and the environment. Nucleic Acids Res 36: D480–484.
18. Cheadle C, Vawter MP, Freed WJ, Becker KG (2003) Analysis of microarray data using Z score transformation. J Mol Diagn 5: 73–81.
19. Tusher VG, Tibshirani R, Chu G (2001) Significance analysis of microarrays applied to the ionizing radiation response. Proc Natl Acad Sci U S A 98: 5116–5121.
20. Tabas-Madrid D, Nogales-Cadenas R, Pascual-Montano A (2012) GeneCodis3: a non-redundant and modular enrichment analysis tool for functional genomics. Nucleic Acids Res 40: W478–483.
21. Yu X, Wieczorek S, Franke A, Yin H, Pierer M, et al. (2009) Association of UCP2-866 G/A polymorphism with chronic inflammatory diseases. Genes Immun 10: 601–605.
22. Liu B, Shuai K (2008) Targeting the PIAS1 SUMO ligase pathway to control inflammation. Trends Pharmacol Sci 29: 505–509.
23. Sikora KA, Fall N, Thornton S, Grom AA (2012) The limited role of interferon-gamma in systemic juvenile idiopathic arthritis cannot be explained by cellular hyporesponsiveness. Arthritis Rheum 64: 3799–3808.
24. Fraser A, Fearon U, Billinghurst RC, Ionescu M, Reece R, et al. (2003) Turnover of type II collagen and aggrecan in cartilage matrix at the onset of inflammatory arthritis in humans: relationship to mediators of systemic and local inflammation. Arthritis Rheum 48: 3085–3095.
25. Seki M, Sakata KM, Oomizu S, Arikawa T, Sakata A, et al. (2007) Beneficial effect of galectin 9 on rheumatoid arthritis by induction of apoptosis of synovial fibroblasts. Arthritis Rheum 56: 3968–3976.
26. Lee J, Park EJ, Noh JW, Hwang JW, Bae EK, et al. (2012) Underexpression of TIM-3 and blunted galectin-9-induced apoptosis of CD4+ T cells in rheumatoid arthritis. Inflammation 35: 633–637.

27. Daouti S, Latario B, Nagulapalli S, Buxton F, Uziel-Fusi S, et al. (2005) Development of comprehensive functional genomic screens to identify novel mediators of osteoarthritis. Osteoarthritis Cartilage 13: 508–518.
28. Collins-Racie LA, Yang Z, Arai M, Li N, Majumdar MK, et al. (2009) Global analysis of nuclear receptor expression and dysregulation in human osteoarthritic articular cartilage: reduced LXR signaling contributes to catabolic metabolism typical of osteoarthritis. Osteoarthritis Cartilage 17: 832–842.
29. Reedquist KA, Tak PP (2012) Signal transduction pathways in chronic inflammatory autoimmune disease: small GTPases. Open Rheumatol J 6: 259–272.
30. De Filippo K, Dudeck A, Hasenberg M, Nye E, van Rooijen N, et al. (2013) Mast cell and macrophage chemokines CXCL1/CXCL2 control the early stage of neutrophil recruitment during tissue inflammation. Blood.
31. Scaife S, Brown R, Kellie S, Filer A, Martin S, et al. (2004) Detection of differentially expressed genes in synovial fibroblasts by restriction fragment differential display. Rheumatology (Oxford) 43: 1346–1352.
32. Thalhamer T, McGrath MA, Harnett MM (2008) MAPKs and their relevance to arthritis and inflammation. Rheumatology (Oxford) 47: 409–414.
33. Kaminska B (2005) MAPK signalling pathways as molecular targets for anti-inflammatory therapy–from molecular mechanisms to therapeutic benefits. Biochim Biophys Acta 1754: 253–262.
34. Shahrara S, Castro-Rueda HP, Haines GK, Koch AE (2007) Differential expression of the FAK family kinases in rheumatoid arthritis and osteoarthritis synovial tissues. Arthritis Res Ther 9: R112.
35. Schlaepfer DD, Broome MA, Hunter T (1997) Fibronectin-stimulated signaling from a focal adhesion kinase-c-Src complex: involvement of the Grb2, p130cas, and Nck adaptor proteins. Mol Cell Biol 17: 1702–1713.
36. Lee J, Oh JM, Hwang JW, Ahn JK, Bae EK, et al. (2011) Expression of human TIM-3 and its correlation with disease activity in rheumatoid arthritis. Scand J Rheumatol 40: 334–340.
37. Gilmore TD (1999) The Rel/NF-kappaB signal transduction pathway: introduction. Oncogene 18: 6842–6844.
38. Adachi M, Okamoto S, Chujyo S, Arakawa T, Yokoyama M, et al. (2013) Cigarette Smoke Condensate Extracts Induce IL-1-Beta Production from Rheumatoid Arthritis Patient-Derived Synoviocytes, but Not Osteoarthritis Patient-Derived Synoviocytes, Through Aryl Hydrocarbon Receptor-Dependent NF-Kappa-B Activation and Novel NF-Kappa-B Sites. J Interferon Cytokine Res 33: 297–307.
39. Harty LC, Biniecka M, O'Sullivan J, Fox E, Mulhall K, et al. (2012) Mitochondrial mutagenesis correlates with the local inflammatory environment in arthritis. Ann Rheum Dis 71: 582–588.
40. Ishikawa S, Mima T, Aoki C, Yoshio-Hoshino N, Adachi Y, et al. (2009) Abnormal expression of the genes involved in cytokine networks and mitochondrial function in systemic juvenile idiopathic arthritis identified by DNA microarray analysis. Ann Rheum Dis 68: 264–272.
41. Li C, Wang W, Guo X, Zhang F, Ma W, et al. (2012) Pathways related to mitochondrial dysfunction in cartilage of endemic osteoarthritis patients in China. Sci China Life Sci 55: 1057–1063.
42. Kumarasinghe DD, Sullivan T, Kuliwaba JS, Fazzalari NL, Atkins GJ (2012) Evidence for the dysregulated expression of TWIST1, TGFbeta1 and SMAD3 in differentiating osteoblasts from primary hip osteoarthritis patients. Osteoarthritis Cartilage 20: 1357–1366.
43. Robier C, Neubauer M, Fritz K, Lippitz P, Stettin M, et al. (2013) The detection of calcium pyrophosphate crystals in sequential synovial fluid examinations of patients with osteoarthritis: once positive, always positive. Clin Rheumatol 32: 671–672.
44. Lamb CA, Dooley HC, Tooze SA (2013) Endocytosis and autophagy: Shared machinery for degradation. Bioessays 35: 34–45.
45. Carames B, Hasegawa A, Taniguchi N, Miyaki S, Blanco FJ, et al. (2012) Autophagy activation by rapamycin reduces severity of experimental osteoarthritis. Ann Rheum Dis 71: 575–581.
46. Yoshida H (2007) ER stress and diseases. FEBS J 274: 630–658.
47. Takada K, Hirose J, Senba K, Yamabe S, Oike Y, et al. (2011) Enhanced apoptotic and reduced protective response in chondrocytes following endoplasmic reticulum stress in osteoarthritic cartilage. Int J Exp Pathol 92: 232–242.
48. Petersson M, Bucht E, Granberg B, Stark A (2006) Effects of arginine-vasopressin and parathyroid hormone-related protein (1–34) on cell proliferation and production of YKL-40 in cultured chondrocytes from patients with rheumatoid arthritis and osteoarthritis. Osteoarthritis Cartilage 14: 652–659.
49. Kiener HP, Lee DM, Agarwal SK, Brenner MB (2006) Cadherin-11 induces rheumatoid arthritis fibroblast-like synoviocytes to form lining layers in vitro. Am J Pathol 168: 1486–1499.
50. Kudryavtseva E, Forde TS, Pucker AD, Adarichev VA (2012) Wnt signaling genes of murine chromosome 15 are involved in sex-affected pathways of inflammatory arthritis. Arthritis Rheum 64: 1057–1068.
51. Laragione T, Gulko PS (2010) mTOR regulates the invasive properties of synovial fibroblasts in rheumatoid arthritis. Mol Med 16: 352–358.

Moxibustion Treatment for Knee Osteoarthritis: A Multi-Centre, Non-Blinded, Randomised Controlled Trial on the Effectiveness and Safety of the Moxibustion Treatment versus Usual Care in Knee Osteoarthritis Patients

Tae-Hun Kim[1,2]⁹, Kun Hyung Kim[1,3]⁹, Jung Won Kang[4], MinHee Lee[1], Kyung-Won Kang[1], Jung Eun Kim[1], Joo-Hee Kim[1], Seunghoon Lee[1], Mi-Suk Shin[1], So-Young Jung[1], Ae-Ran Kim[1], Hyo-Ju Park[1], Hee-Jung Jung[1], Ho Sueb Song[5], Hyeong Jun Kim[6], Jin-Bong Choi[7], Kwon Eui Hong[8], Sun-Mi Choi[1]*

1 Korea Institute of Oriental Medicine, Dae-Jeon, South Korea, **2** College of Korean medicine, Gachon University, Seongnam, South Korea, **3** Department of Acupuncture & Moxibustion, Korean medicine hospital, Pusan National University, Yangsan, South Korea, **4** Department of Acupuncture & Moxibustion, College of Korean Medicine, Kyung-Hee University, Seoul, South Korea, **5** Kyungwon University Incheon Gill Oriental Medical Hospital, Incheon, South Korea, **6** Semyung University Jecheon Oriental Medical Hospital, Jecheon, South Korea, **7** Dongshin University Gwangju Oriental Hospital, Gwangju, South Korea, **8** Department of Acupuncture and Moxibustion, Daejeon University, Daejeon, South Korea

Abstract

Introduction: This study tested the effectiveness of moxibustion on pain and function in chronic knee osteoarthritis (KOA) and evaluated safety.

Methods: A multi-centre, non-blinded, parallel-group, randomised controlled trial compared moxibustion with usual care (UC) in KOA. 212 South Korean patients aged 40–70 were recruited from 2011–12, stratified by mild (Kellgren/Lawrence scale grades 0/1) and moderate-severe KOA (grades 2/3/4), and randomly allocated to moxibustion or UC for four weeks. Moxibustion involved burning mugwort devices over acupuncture and Ashi points in affected knee(s). UC was allowed. Korean Western Ontario and McMaster Universities Questionnaire (K-WOMAC), Short Form 36 Health Survey (SF-36v2), Beck Depression Inventory (BDI), physical performance test, pain numeric rating scale (NRS) and adverse events were evaluated at 5 and 13 weeks. K-WOMAC global score at 5 weeks was the primary outcome.

Results: 102 patients (73 mild, 29 moderate-severe) were allocated to moxibustion, 110 (77 mild, 33 moderate severe) to UC. K-WOMAC global score (moxibustion 25.42+/−SD 19.26, UC 33.60+/−17.91, p<0.01, effect size =0.0477), NRS (moxibustion 44.77+/−22.73, UC 56.23+/−17.71, p<0.01, effect size =0.0073) and timed-stand test (moxibustion 24.79+/−9.76, UC 25.24+/−8.84, p=0.0486, effect size =0.0021) were improved by moxibustion at 5 weeks. The primary outcome improved for mild but not moderate-severe KOA. At 13 weeks, moxibustion significantly improved the K-WOMAC global score and NRS. Moxibustion improved SF-36 physical component summary (p=0.0299), bodily pain (p=0.0003), physical functioning (p=0.0025) and social functioning (p=0.0418) at 5 weeks, with no difference in mental component summary at 5 and 13 weeks. BDI showed no difference (p=0.34) at 5 weeks. After 1158 moxibustion treatments, 121 adverse events included first (n=6) and second degree (n=113) burns, pruritus and fatigue (n=2).

Conclusions: Moxibustion may improve pain, function and quality of life in KOA patients, but adverse events are common. Limitations included no sham control or blinding.

Trial Registration: Clinical Research Information Service (CRIS) KCT0000130

Editor: D. William Cameron, University of Ottawa, Canada

Funding: This study was supported by the "Development of Acupuncture, Moxibustion and Meridian Standard Health Technology" project of the Korea Institute of Oriental Medicine (K12010). The funders had no role in study design, data collection and analysis, decision to publish, or preparation of the manuscript.

Competing Interests: The authors have declared that no competing interests exist.

* Email: smchoi@kiom.re.kr

⁹ These authors contributed equally to this work.

Introduction

Knee osteoarthritis (KOA) is a common disease which is related to the chronic degenerative changes of knee joint structures [1]. The prevalence of KOA is expected to increase in future because of rising life expectancy [1] and increasing obesity population [2]. Pharmacological treatments are usually recommended for the relief of pain but severe adverse effects related to drug therapy are suggested to be a significant limitation for use [3]. In this point, to discover and to test effectiveness and safety of non-pharmacological interventions is necessary for the vulnerable patients who need long term treatment for KOA.

Moxibustion is a representative non-drug intervention in East Asian traditional medicine. Generally, moxibustion is a method of direct or indirect acupuncture-point stimulation using burned dried mugwort. Although moxibustion is not well known in European countries, it may have been used there in the distant past; several soot marks were found on the body of Ötzi the 'Tyrolean Ice Man', half of which were coincident with classic acupuncture points [4].

Moxibustion has been used in clinical practice for conditions such as rheumatic diseases, digestive dysfunction (e.g. dyspepsia, diarrhoea and constipation), and gyneco-obstetric problems (i.e., hot flush and breech presentation of foetus, etc.); however, conclusive evidence on its effectiveness in treating these conditions has yet to be established because few rigorous, full-scale randomised controlled trials have been performed. Moxibustion seems to be effective in the treatment of KOA, but there is currently no rigorous evidence supporting this conclusion [5]. In addition, information on the safety of invasive procedures using burned moxibustion cones is needed.

The primary objective of this study was to test the effect of moxibustion on the pain and function of chronic KOA patients in a pragmatic way. Additionally, the severity and frequency of adverse events (AEs) related to moxibustion treatment were evaluated.

Methods

This was a multi-centre, randomised controlled, parallel-group, open clinical trial conducted in South Korea. The study protocol was published previously [6]. Participants aged 40 to 70 years with idiopathic osteoarthritis of the knee were recruited through advertisement using local newspapers between June 30, 2011, and January 19, 2012. Idiopathic KOA was diagnosed according to the clinical guidelines of the American College of Rheumatology: the participants should have pain at one or both knees with a daily average of over 40 points on the 0-to-100 numeric rating scale (NRS) and meet at least 3 of the following 6 conditions: age of 50 to 70 years, stiffness within 30 minutes of waking in the morning, crepitus, bony tenderness, bony enlargement or no palpable warmth [7]. Participants with positive rheumatoid factor (RF) in blood chemistry or a history of rheumatoid arthritis, cancer, traumatic injury or significant deformity of the knee, knee-replacement surgery, knee arthroscopy within the last 2 years, steroid injection within the last 3 months or viscosupplement injection and joint-fluid injection within the last 6 months were excluded. Four local research hospitals, namely Oriental Hospital of Daejeon University (Korea Institute of Oriental Medicine), Kyungwon University Incheon Gill Oriental Medical Hospital, Dongshin University Gwangju Oriental Hospital and Semyung University Jecheon Oriental Medicine Hospital, participated in this trial. The protocol for this trial, supporting CONSORT checklist and STRICTA checklist are available as supporting information; see Checklist S1, Checklist S2 and Protocol S1.

Random sequences for allocation were generated with a computer software package (SAS Version 9.1.3, SAS institute. Inc., Cary, NC) by an independent statistician. To avoid casual baseline imbalances in KOA severity, stratification was performed by separate randomisation of each stratum according to the Kellgren/Lawrence scale: both knee x-rays of anterior-posterior and lateral view was obtained from all the patients before allocation. Radiologist read x-rays and graded patient's status based on the Kellgren/Lawrence scale. Participants with grades 0 and 1 were considered as one stratum, and those with grades 2, 3 and 4 were considered as the other stratum. Block size for the randomization was 4 with an allocation ratio of 1: 1. Opaque, sealed envelopes containing serial numbers with a stratification code were used for allocation concealment, and the participants were assigned at the second visit by opening the envelopes in a sequential manner. To reduce the selection bias, the outcome was assessed by individuals who had not participated in the moxibustion treatment. Outcome assessors were intended to be blinded in the study protocol, but outcome assessors were not blinded to the treatment actually, because they became to know about the patients' allocation result from the different visit frequencies in moxibustion group and usual care group as the study went on.

Ethics statement

The institutional review boards of each participating research centre including Oriental Hospital of Daejeon University, Kyungwon University Incheon Gill Oriental Medical Hospital, Dongshin University Gwangju Oriental Hospital and Semyung University Jecheon Oriental Medicine Hospital reviewed and approved the study protocol before the enrolment of the first patient (2011. 7. 19.). Participants were informed about the moxibustion therapy including moxibustion devices, stimulating methods, intensity and frequency of treatment and possible adverse events. After that, written informed consent was obtained from each participant.

Interventions

Moxibustion was used for experimental intervention, and a usual care group was used as the comparator. In the moxibustion group, moxibustion therapy on the affected knee(s) was offered at six standard acupuncture points (ST36, ST35, ST34, SP9, Ex-LE04 and SP10), plus up to two points of 'Ashi' unilaterally, if needed, three times per week for four weeks. Points were chosen according to the traditional Korean medicine (TKM) literature and to the consensus of four TKM doctors with clinical and research experience. Ashi meant tender points which were not included in classic acupuncture points [8] and were often selected as treatment points of moxibustion for KOA [9,10]. For patients with pain in both knees, treatments were provided bilaterally. A total of three moxibustion cones were applied indirectly to each point per treatment session. Each burned moxibustion cone was held in place for approximately 5 to 10 minutes and was removed when a patient could no longer tolerate the stimulation. Smokeless, paper devices which had a cylindric shape with a diameter of 1.9 cm and a length of 2.1 cm were used to hold the mugwort for the indirect treatments which means that there is no direct contact between moxibustion and skin (Manina moxibustion, Haitnim Bosung Inc., South Korea). All moxibustions were attached to the skin by adhesive placed on the base of each paper device. Moxibustion was delivered by board-certified KM doctors or postgraduate TKM doctors who had at least 2 years of clinical experience following the standard 6 years of education in KM. To enhance TKM doctor's adherence to the study protocol, all treatment providers were encouraged to attend one-day education program on the moxibustion method. All patients received an educational leaflet containing basic information about KOA such as definition, pathology, current treatment options including drug therapy, supplements and hyaluronic acid or steroid injection and recommendations on the principles of self-exercise, good postures and rules for daily activities avoiding exaggerating symptoms. In addition, participants were instructed in exercises to stretch hamstrings and calf muscles and strengthen muscles related to the function of knee joints by research TKM doctors. The frequency and intensity were not prescribed equally but participants were encouraged to increase them along with the physical fitness.

Each component of usual care was based on previous evidence of benefits in the management of KOA [11]. Co-interventions allowed to both groups in all study periods included surgery, conventional medication, physical therapy, acupuncture, herbal medicine, over-the-counter drugs and other active treatments.

Before allocation, all participants were asked to rate their expectations on a 0-to-9 (higher expectation) numeric scale. The question was as follows: "To what degree do you expect moxibustion to relieve your symptoms?".

Outcomes

The primary outcome was measured by the Korean Western Ontario and McMaster Universities Questionnaire (K-WOMAC) global score [12]. This was a Korean-translated validated version of WOMAC which was widely used for the evaluation of knee pain and function related to osteoarthritis [13]. It consisted of 24 questions about knee pain, stiffness and physical function. Individual questions were summed up in three domains each and global score was calculated as well through summing up of these three subscales which ranges 0 to 100 (the worst) [6]. The Short-Form 36 Health Survey (SF-36v2) was assessed for quality of life evaluation [14]. The Beck Depression Inventory (BDI) was used to measure the severity of depression [15]. Physical performance affected by disability related to KOA was evaluated [16,17]. Three functional tests were assessed for each participant: the timed-stand test, standing-balance test and six-minute walk test [18]. The 7-day average score on the pain-numeric rating scale from 0 (least pain) to 100 (most pain) was assessed. All the outcomes were assessed up to 13 weeks after first visit principally. We used validated Korean-translated tools for all outcome assessment except physical performance test. In our study, unit of analysis were individual patients not affected knees. Patients with pain in one knee and in both knees were included without discrimination. Outcomes for knee pain and function were observed in the knee with more severe symptoms. Blood chemistry including C-reactive protein and erythrocyte sedimentation rate at 5 weeks and cost-effectiveness at 5 and 13 weeks were assessed as secondary outcomes. These results will be published elsewhere in future.

To evaluate safety, we assessed the occurrence of adverse events (AEs) related to moxibustion during the trial. Local and systemic AEs were assessed in every visit. If unexpected responses related to moxibustion occurred, the type, severity and frequency were reported. The severity of each AE was graded 1 (mild) to 3 (severe) according to Spilker's AE classification [19,20]. Burn wounds were diagnosed as first to third degree [21]. All outcomes were assessed by separate outcome assessors who did not participate in moxibustion treatment. AEs related to usual care treatments were not assessed in this study.

Because there were no field-specific standards for data deposition available for moxibustion study, data related to the study results could not be publicly assessed.

Statistical analysis

The study sample size was calculated from the unpublished internal data of our pilot-study which was conducted with 40 KOA patients at Korea Institute of Oriental Medicine in 2010. In the pilot-study, only patients with grades over 2 on the Kellgren/Lawrence scale were included at first but we extended inclusion criteria during the study due to a low participation rate. We adopted revised inclusion criteria in this multi-centre trial. The mean difference and pooled standard deviation of the K-WOMAC global score between the moxibustion and usual care groups was estimated to be 15.4 and 6.65, respectively. With a two-sided 5% significance level, 80% power and 20% dropout rate, a total of 212 participants needed to be recruited.

To compare key baseline characteristics between the two groups, the Chi-squared test or Fisher's exact test for categorical data and the t-test or the Wilcoxon rank-sums test for continuous data were conducted after the Kolmogorov–Smirnov test for normality. Age and body mass index which might affect the severity of KOA symptom were not controlled in both groups for all analysis. Most outcomes (i.e., K-WOMAC, pain NRS, BDI, Physical Function Test and SF-36v2) were analysed using analysis of covariance (ANCOVA), with baseline scores and individual research centres as covariates. However, because KOA patients with different disease severity were allocated equally in 2 groups through stratified randomization method based on the Kellgren/Lawrence scale, KOA grade of each participant was not used as covariates. Eta-squared (η^2) was calculated as an effect-size estimate in the ANCOVA statistic model [22]. The T-scores of each domain for the SF-36v2 assessment were calculated using Health Outcomes Scoring software 4.5 (QualityMetric Incorporated, Lincoln, RI). All statistical analyses were conducted on an intention-to-treat basis at a 95% significance level. The last observation carried forward (LOCF) method was used to input missing data. All statistical analyses were conducted using SAS statistical software. There was no Data Monitoring Committee in this study.

Results

A total of 251 participants were recruited, and 212 KOA patients met the inclusion criteria. Incheon, Gwangju and Jecheon hospitals recruited 60 participants each, and Daejeon centre recruited 32 participants. Of these, 102 patients (73 for mild and 29 for moderate to severe KOA) were placed in the moxibustion group and 110 (77 for mild and 33 for moderate to severe KOA) were placed in the usual care group. During the study, 5 participants in the moxibustion group and 9 participants in control group dropped out (figure 1). Five participants in the moxibustion group and eight in the control group were dropped out due to withdrawal of consent. Other reasons for the dropout in control group were admission to other hospital due to other diseases and incomplete participation during the clinical trial.

Median duration of knee pain was 4 years [2 to 6 years] in the moxibustion group and 3 years [1 to 6 years] (interquartile ranges) in the usual care group. According to the Kellgren/Lawrence scale, most participants had mild-to-moderate KOA. Many patients had previously tried physical therapy, acupuncture treatment and glucosamine administration for KOA. Including age and body mass index, all baseline characteristics did not show significant different between groups. In addition, there was no significant difference between the groups in terms of their expectations of the effectiveness of moxibustion (Table 1).

K-WOMAC

The global K-WOMAC score (primary outcome) showed significant differences between the 2 groups at 5 weeks (25.42 (SD 19.26) in the moxibustion group and 33.60 (17.91) in the usual care group; $p<0.01$) and 13 weeks (26.70 (18.82) in the moxibustion group and 34.69 (18.67) in the control group; p<

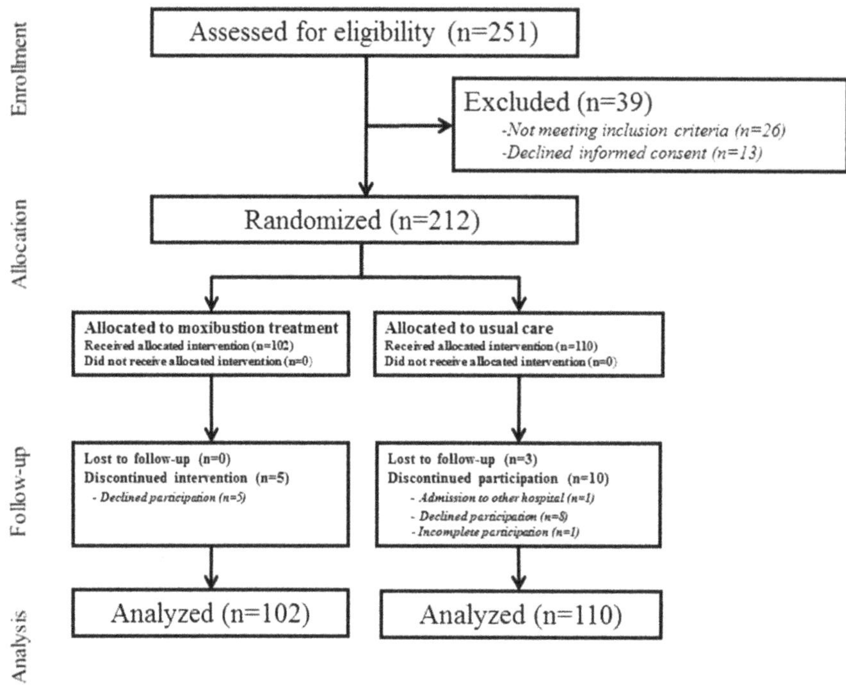

Figure 1. Study flow chart.

Table 1. Demographic Data in the moxibustion and usual care Groups.

Characteristics	Moxibustion group (n = 102)	Usual care group (n = 110)	p-value
Age, year (median [25% to 75% IQR])*	56 [52 to 62]	57 [51 to 62]	0.74
Sex M/F, No.†	17/85	16/94	0.67
Duration of knee pain, year (median [25% to 75% IQR])*	4 [2,6]	3 [1,6]	0.28
Body mass index, Kg/m^2 (mean, standard deviation)‡	24.77, 2.63	24.09, 2.94	0.08
Kellgren/Lawrence scale§			0.3579
Grade 0	24	36	
Grade 1	49	41	
Grade 2	25	29	
Grade 3	4	3	
Grade 4	0	1	
Past experience of surgery for knee osteoarthritis (yes/no)§	2/100	0/110	0.23
Past experience of anti-arthritic medication for knee osteoarthritis (yes/no)†	28/73	37/71	0.31
Past experience of physical therapy for knee osteoarthritis (yes/no)†	53/49	60/50	0.71
Past experience of acupuncture treatment for knee osteoarthritis (yes/no)†	34/67	41/68	0.55
Past experience of intra-articular injection treatment for knee osteoarthritis (yes/no)†	23/78	29/80	0.52
Past experience of glucosamine administration for knee osteoarthritis (yes/no)†	33/68	36/74	0.99
Assessment of expectation on the effectiveness of moxibustion (median [25% to 75% IQR])*	7 [6 to 9]	7 [5 to 8]	0.33

*The Wilcoxon rank sum test was used for statistical analysis.
†The Chi-squared test was used for statistical analysis.
‡The t-test was used for statistical analysis.
§Fisher's exact test was used for statistical analysis. IQR: interquartile range.

Table 2. Primary and secondary outcomes at each visit.

	Moxibustion group (n = 102, mean, SD)			Usual care group (n = 110, mean, SD)			P-value		Effect size (η^2)***	
	Baseline	5 weeks	13 weeks	Baseline	5 weeks	13 weeks	5 weeks	13 weeks	5 weeks	13 weeks
K-WOMAC (mean, SD)*										
Global score (total)	34.16, 16.80	25.42, 19.26	26.70, 18.82	34.15, 18.01	33.60, 17.91	34.69, 18.67	<0.01	<0.01	0.0477	0.0518
*Mild severity (Grade 0 and 1) ***	*32.19, 16.88*	*22.14, 17.74*	*23.53, 16.64*	*30.75, 17.37*	*30.95, 17.58*	*32.08, 18.10*	*<0.01*	*<0.01*		
*Moderate to severe severity (Grade 2,3 and 4) ***	*39.10, 15.81*	*33.69, 20.72*	*34.66, 21.76*	*43.03, 17.25*	*41.06, 17.32*	*41.42, 18.62*	*0.2554*	*0.3021*		
Pain score	6.93, 3.48	5.07, 3.75	5.18, 3.83	7.21, 3.8	7.14, 3.94	7.32, 3,98	<0.01	<0.01	0.0532	0.0595
Stiffness score	2.87, 1.6	2.26, 1.67	2.51, 1.68	3.12, 1.82	2.95, 1.75	3.2, 1.78	0.0043	0.0061	0.0226	0.0267
Function score	24.35, 12.91	18.09, 14.46	19.01, 13.89	23.83, 13.29	23.51, 12.94	24.17, 13.68	<0.01	0.0001	0.0391	0.0412
Pain-NRS (mean, SD)*	57.02, 14.3	44.77, 22.73	40.53, 26.63	57.63, 12.93	56.23, 17.71	54.26, 19.61	<0.01	<0.01	0.0073	0.0075
BDI (mean, SD)*	9.85, 7.11	8.94, 7.15	8.75, 6.95	9.8, 7.2	9.63, 7.13	9.03, 6.44	0.34	0.64	0.0023	0.0005
Physical performance test (mean, SD)*										
Timed-stand test (sec)	27.34, 19.16	24.79, 19.77	22.85, 9.76	26.03, 8.83	25.24, 8.84	25.76, 9.09	0.0486	0.0006	0.0021	0.0307
Standing balance test	3.56, 0.79	3.59, 0.71	3.70, 0.58	3.64, 0.67	3.67, 0.59	3.64, 0.69	0.52	0.26	0.0012	0.0048
Six minute walk test (m/ 6 min)	493.8, 95.1	486.1, 81.3	489.2, 79.3	480.1, 78.2	481.8, 80.4	479.0, 78.0	0.51	0.68	0.0008	0.0004

*ANCOVA was used for the statistical analysis of changes from baseline between two groups on each outcome at 5 weeks and 13 weeks (covariate: baseline value and participating research centre).
**Grades were evaluated by Kellgren/Lawrence scale.
***Eta-squared ($\eta 2$) was calculated as an effect-size estimate in the ANCOVA statistic model. K-WOMAC: Korean version of Western Ontario and McMaster Universities Questionnaire; NRS: numeric rating scale; BDI: Beck Depression Inventory.

0.01). According to Cohen's benchmark for effect size [22], a small-to-medium effect size was observed at 5 weeks (0.0477) and 13 weeks (0.0518, Table 1).

All subcategories of K-WOMAC showed significant improvement following moxibustion treatment at 5 weeks and 13 weeks. The pain score showed a comparatively large effect size at 5 weeks (0.0532) and 13 weeks (0.0595, Table 2).

Pain NRS

Moxibustion treatment improved the average pain NRS significantly compared with usual care at 5 weeks (44.77 (SD 22.73) with moxibustion and 56.23 (17.71) with usual care, $p< 0.01$) and 13 weeks (40.53 (26.63) with moxibustion and 54.26 (19.61) with usual care, $p<0.01$, Table 2); however, comparatively small effect sizes were observed at 5 weeks (0.0073) and 13 weeks (0.0075).

Physical performance test

Moxibustion significantly improved knee function for standing and sitting in a chair (as evaluated by the timed-stand test) compared to usual care at 5 weeks (24.79 (9.76) in the moxibustion group and 25.24 (8.84) in the usual care group; $p = 0.0486$) and 13 weeks (22.85 (9.76) in the moxibustion group and 25.76 (9.09) in the usual care group; $p = 0.0006$). No significant improvement was observed in the standing-balance test ($p = 0.52$ at 5 weeks and $p = 0.26$ at 13 weeks) or six-minute walk test ($p = 0.51$ at 5 weeks and $p = 0.68$ at 13 weeks). All results of the three physical performance tests showed relatively small effect sizes at 5 weeks (0.0021 in the timed-stand test, 0.0012 in the standing-balance test and 0.0008 in six-minute walk test) and 13 weeks (0.0307, 0.0048 and 0.0004 respectively).

BDI

BDI scores improved in the moxibustion group after treatment, but there was no significant difference between the 2 groups at 5 weeks (8.94 (7.15) with moxibustion and 9.63 (7.13) with usual care; $p = 0.34$) and 13 weeks (8.75 (6.95) and 9.03 (6.44); $p = 0.64$). Only small effect sizes were observed in BDI at 5 weeks (0.0023) and 13 weeks (0.0005).

SF-36

The physical component summary (PCS) showed significant improvement following moxibustion treatment at 5 weeks ($p = 0.0299$) and at 13 weeks ($p = 0.0023$), but there was no significant difference between groups in mental component summary (MCS) at 5 weeks ($p = 0.2124$) and 13 weeks ($p = 0.3129$). Bodily pain (BP) showed significant improvement following moxibustion both at 5 weeks ($p = 0.0003$) and 13 weeks ($p = 0.005$). Physical functioning (PF) and social functioning (SF) also showed better results at 5 weeks ($p = 0.0025$ in PF and $p = 0.0418$ in SF), but there was no significant difference between the 2 groups in other domains. Small effects sizes were observed in PCS (0.0147 at 5 weeks and 0.0307 at 13 weeks) and in MCS (0.0034 at 5 weeks and 0.0031 at 13 weeks). Among 8 domains of SF-36, only BP showed small to moderate effect sizes at 5 weeks (0.0437) and 13 weeks (0.0410) and others showed only small effect sizes (Table 3).

Adverse events

One hundred and two participants in the experimental group were subjected to moxibustion for a total of 1,158 treatments, with 121 AEs related to the treatment (10.45%). Among these 102 participants, 48 patients experienced AEs at least once during the

Table 3. The short-form 36 health survey (SF-36v2) results at each visit.

	Moxibustion group (n = 102, mean, SD)			Usual care group (n = 110, mean, SD)			P-value		Effect size (η^2)*	
	Baseline	5 weeks	13 weeks	Baseline	5 weeks	13 weeks	5 weeks	13 weeks	5 weeks	13 weeks
Physical Component Summary (PCS)	42.39, 6.81	44.32, 6.5	44.43, 6.39	41.19, 6.92	41.89, 7.25	41.31, 7.33	0.0299	0.0023	0.0147	0.0307
Mental Component Summary (MCS)	49.24, 10.13	50.71, 9.77	48.80, 9.45	49.96, 10.19	49.69, 10.59	50.23, 10.48	0.2124	0.3129	0.0034	0.0031
Physical Functioning (PF)	39.98, 8.00	42.04, 7.64	40.79, 7.90	40.51, 7.34	39.74, 7.86	39.62, 7.45	0.0025	0.1214	0.0269	0.0087
Role-Physical (RP)	44.96, 9.88	45.55, 10.12	45.49, 9.74	45.11, 8.92	46.19, 9.12	44.42, 9.47	0.5640	0.2893	0.0010	0.0042
Bodily pain (BP)	45.48, 7.87	49.16, 8.10	48.68, 7.63	43.07, 7.68	44.18, 8.53	43.80, 9.04	0.0003	0.0005	0.0437	0.0410
General Health (GH)	43.23, 8.13	44.39, 9.12	44.19, 8.56	42.13, 8.99	42.70, 7.97	43.72, 8.61	0.3110	0.7561	0.0029	0.0003
Vitality (VT)	48.35, 10.46	50.12, 10.29	50.41, 10.82	46.55, 9.72	47.39, 10.63	48.30, 10.97	0.1725	0.4290	0.0054	0.0021
Social Functioning (SF)	48.79, 9.43	50.85, 8.18	49.23, 8.61	49.50, 7.91	49.05, 9.22	48.77, 8.35	0.0418	0.4487	0.0121	0.0020
Role-Emotional (RE)	44.63, 11.78	45.55, 11.86	42.92, 12.02	45.75, 10.96	45.47, 11.66	44.84, 11.65	0.6133	0.3688	0.0007	0.0027
Mental Health (MH)	47.56, 10.07	49.66, 10.02	48.12, 9.66	48.28, 11.01	47.99, 10.79	48.82, 11.03	0.0865	0.6976	0.0083	0.0005

ANCOVA was used for the statistical analysis of changes from baseline between two groups on each outcome at 5 weeks and 13 weeks (covariate: baseline value and participating research centre).
*Eta-squared (η2) was calculated as an effect-size estimate in the ANCOVA statistic model.

treatment periods, and 7 participants experienced AEs more than 5 times. First degree burn wounds occurred 6 times, and second degree burns occurred 113 times. Systemic AEs, including pruritus and fatigue, were seen in 2 participants. When AEs were graded according to the Spilker's AE classification, mild AEs occurred 99 times and moderate AEs occurred 21 times. There was only one severe AE.

Discussion

A total of 212 patients with mild-to-moderate KOA participated in this trial. Dropout rate in the moxibustion group was about 4.9% and that in control group was 11.8%. From the results of this study, 4 weeks of moxibustion treatment improved the global score and sub-scores (pain, stiffness and function) by K-WOMAC and decreased the pain NRS significantly compared with the usual care control at 5 and 13 weeks. However, BDI did not show significant difference between groups at 5 and 13 weeks. Among all domains of SF-36, PCS and BP at both 5 and 13 weeks and PF at 5 week showed significant improvement with moxibustion treatment compared to the control group. Physical performance for sitting and standing from a chair was significantly improved in the moxibustion group than in the usual care group but there were no significant improvements in standing balance and six minute walk test. Approximately 47% of participants experienced at least one AE (mostly burn wounds); the majority of the AEs were second-degree burns.

Recent systematic reviews suggested that moxibustion might be effective in the treatment of KOA, but the supporting evidence was not conclusive because of limitations including methodological flaws, comparatively small sample sizes, inappropriate outcome assessments and poor reporting of adverse events in the previous clinical trials on moxibustion [5,23]. In this study, we adopted a rigorous clinical trial design to reduce possible bias. Sequence generation and allocation concealment were conducted appropriately. Although blinding of participants was impossible, separate outcome assessors participated in the outcome assessment to reduce performance bias. To ensure a considerable degree of external validity, 4 local research centres in different regions of South Korea participated in this study. The appropriate sample size was calculated from the results of a previous pilot study: 212 participants constituted a larger sample size than was used in previous moxibustion trials [5]. Apart from simple evaluation of pain intensity and participants' ratings of improvement used in previous studies, we assessed various core outcome domains, including physical (physical performance test) and emotional (BDI) functioning, a disease-specific outcome such as K-WOMAC and quality of life (SF-36) to report the results more completely [24]. In addition to these quantitive outcomes, we also conducted a qualitative research for assessing KOA patients' experiences of moxibustion in the perspective of mixed-methods approach whose results were published elsewhere [25]. These various outcomes can suggest evidence useful to understand the effect of moxibustion treatment in the multidimensional aspects. Previous studies using moxibustion reported comparatively low incidence rates of AEs [26] and reported only minor AEs [5]; however, from the explicit AE assessment of this study, as conducted according to the pre-defined reporting criteria, we found that AEs occurred frequently and that moxibustion could induce moderate-to-severe AEs. These factors contribute to the validity of the results and are a major strong point of this study.

This study has several weak points as well. First, sham moxibustion was not used for this study. Several types of sham moxibustion devices have been invented [27,28] and some have been used in the clinical trials [29,30]. However, these types of sham devices cannot apply to those who have experience of moxibustion because they have thick membrane between moxibustion and human skin which blocks heat and chemical discharge from the moxibustion so participants cannot feel appropriate moxibustion stimulation [27,28]. In addition, current studies with sham moxibustion might have potential bias in blinding the patients: a clinical trial did not suggest any blinding test results at all [29] and another trial showed incomplete blinding successfulness where sensitivity was high in verum moxibustion group but low in sham group[30]. We found that appropriate sham device which was completely inactive physiologically but seemed similar to verum moxibustion, was not available currently. In this sense, we adopted usual care as comparison intervention. Second, moxibustion is used in clinical practice with wide heterogeneity in the original materials, stimulating methods, frequency, duration, selection of points, etc [5]. The original purpose of this study was to evaluate the benefit and harm of moxibustion treatment itself, so we used manufactured moxibustion of standardised quality. In this sense, the moxibustion used in this trial is not fully representative and is only one typical intervention among various moxibustions. Third, moxibustion is currently used only in Asia (not in European countries), and the participants' expectations were high in this study. Non-specific effects of moxibustion may have an important role in symptom management, as is the case for other non-drug interventions such as acupuncture. Thus, the study results must be interpreted in a limited context. Fourth, outcome assessors were not blinded which might introduce detection bias in this study. To reduce bias, separate independent researchers, who did not conduct treatments, participated in the outcome assessments but this could not ensure low risk of bias in the outcome assessment procedure. Fifth, we allowed any types of co-interventions to both groups during the study periods. We expected that the pattern of usage of treatments for KOA would not be changed easily during the comparatively short period if past usage of usual care components in the baseline stage were similar in two groups. However, it could not be an appropriate explanation on the potential bias that free access to various treatment options might not introduce considerable imbalance of additional treatments between the groups. Finally, AEs related to usual care treatments were not evaluated appropriately in this study. We tried to assess the AEs related to moxibustion rigorously but we did not pay enough attention to the usage of usual care interventions and related AEs which might overestimate the frequency of AEs in the moxibustion group.

One thing we need to declare is that we eased the inclusion criteria because a low participation rate was observed in the pilot study when only patients with grades over 2 on the Kellgren/Lawrence scale were recruited. We adopted the clinical criteria of the American College of Rheumatology as the diagnostic criteria for KOA [7], so we included KOA patients regardless of the severity as evaluated via X-ray. Instead, stratified randomisation was conducted to avoid baseline imbalances in KOA severity. As a result, significant improvement of the K-WOMAC global scale in the moxibustion group was observed in the mild-KOA group but not in the moderate-to-severe-KOA group. This result may have originated from the unequal number of participants with mild ($n = 146$) versus moderate-to-severe KOA ($n = 62$).

Interestingly, the effect sizes of K-WOMAC pain subscale and SF-36 bodily pain component were similar each other but the effect size of pain-NRS was smaller than those of K-WOMAC pain. The pain-NRS is a valid and easy tool for evaluating pain intensity related to KOA [31] but it also has been criticized for its simplicity which prohibits understanding complexity of patient's pain experience [32]. KOA is a chronic condition and many factors are associated with pain experience of the patients with KOA. In this sense, we assume that K-WOMAC pain subscale and SF-36 bodily pain might reflect more closely to the patient's change of pain-related experience than pain-NRS did and it might introduce huge difference in the effect sizes among the evaluation tools.

In future studies, it may be necessary to recruit only patients with moderate-to-severe KOA to evaluate whether moxibustion is effective only in mild cases. To evaluate the specific effect of moxibustion, standardization of original material and practice procedure for moxibustion is necessary and a proper control intervention including sham moxibustion should be developed and used in clinical trials, although such a control would be difficult to devise. Factors contributing to the effect of moxibustion, including selection of acupuncture points and moxibustion devices, intensity, frequency and duration of treatment and the moxibustion method (i.e., direct or indirect application), should be divided and tested in a separate study to evaluate the individual effects. Finally, the long-term outcome of this treatment must be evaluated.

Supporting Information

Checklist S1 A CONSORT checklist.

Checklist S2 A STRICTA checklist.

Protocol S1 Published protocol of this study.

Author Contributions

Conceived and designed the experiments: THK KHK. Performed the experiments: THK KHK JWK MHL KWK JEK SHL MSS SYJ ARK HJP HJJ HSS JHK JBC HJK KEH SMC. Analyzed the data: MHL. Wrote the paper: THK. Study monitoring: HJJ.

References

1. Felson DT, Lawrence RC, Dieppe PA, Hirsch R, Helmick CG, et al. (2000) Osteoarthritis: new insights. Part 1: the disease and its risk factors. Ann Intern Med 133: 635–646.
2. Niu J, Zhang YQ, Torner J, Nevitt M, Lewis CE, et al. (2009) Is obesity a risk factor for progressive radiographic knee osteoarthritis? Arthritis Rheum 61: 329–335.
3. Silverstein FE, Faich G, Goldstein JL, Simon LS, Pincus T, et al. (2000) Gastrointestinal toxicity with celecoxib vs nonsteroidal anti-inflammatory drugs for osteoarthritis and rheumatoid arthritis: the CLASS study: A randomized controlled trial. Celecoxib Long-term Arthritis Safety Study. JAMA 284: 1247–1255.
4. Dorfer L, Moser M, Spindler K, Bahr F, Egarter-Vigl E, et al. (1998) 5200-year-old acupuncture in central Europe? Science 282: 242–243.
5. Choi TY, Choi J, Kim KH, Lee MS (2012) Moxibustion for the treatment of osteoarthritis: a systematic review and meta-analysis. Rheumatol Int 32: 2969–2978.
6. Lee S, Kim KH, Kim TH, Kim JE, Kim JH, et al. (2013) Moxibustion for treating knee osteoarthritis: study protocol of a multicentre randomised controlled trial. BMC Complement Altern Med 13: 59.
7. (2000) Recommendations for the medical management of osteoarthritis of the hip and knee: 2000 update. American College of Rheumatology Subcommittee on Osteoarthritis Guidelines. Arthritis Rheum 43: 1905–1915.
8. Zhao JS (2010) [Research and identification of the concept and terminology of "tender-point"and "Ashi-point"]. Zhen Ci Yan Jiu 35: 388–390.
9. Li ZD, Cao LH, Wang SC (2009) [Effect of moxibustion in treating knee joint osteoarthritis and its relation with contents of hyaluronic acid in serum and synovial fluid]. Zhongguo Zhong Xi Yi Jie He Za Zhi 29: 883–885.
10. Ren XM, Cao JJ, Shen XY, Wang LZ, Zhao L, et al. (2011) [Knee osteoarthritis treated with moxibustion: a randomized controlled trial]. Zhongguo Zhen Jiu 31: 1057–1061.
11. Conaghan PG, Dickson J, Grant RL (2008) Care and management of osteoarthritis in adults: summary of NICE guidance. BMJ 336: 502–503.
12. Bellamy N, Buchanan WW, Goldsmith CH, Campbell J, Stitt LW (1988) Validation study of WOMAC: a health status instrument for measuring clinically important patient relevant outcomes to antirheumatic drug therapy in patients with osteoarthritis of the hip or knee. J Rheumatol 15: 1833–1840.
13. Bae SC, Lee HS, Yun HR, Kim TH, Yoo DH, et al. (2001) Cross-cultural adaptation and validation of Korean Western Ontario and McMaster Universities (WOMAC) and Lequesne osteoarthritis indices for clinical research. Osteoarthritis Cartilage 9: 746–750.
14. Maruish ME, Turner-Bowker DM (2009) A guide to the development of certified modes of Short Form survey administraion. Lincoln: QualityMetric Incorported.
15. Beck AT, Ward CH, Mendelson M, Mock J, Erbaugh J (1961) An inventory for measuring depression. Arch Gen Psychiatry 4: 561–571.
16. Guralnik JM, Simonsick EM, Ferrucci L, Glynn RJ, Berkman LF, et al. (1994) A short physical performance battery assessing lower extremity function: association with self-reported disability and prediction of mortality and nursing home admission. J Gerontol 49: M85–94.
17. Wang C, Schmid CH, Hibberd PL, Kalish R, Roubenoff R, et al. (2008) Tai Chi for treating knee osteoarthritis: designing a long-term follow up randomized controlled trial. BMC Musculoskelet Disord 9: 108.
18. Mark DH (1994) The predictive capabilities of clinical tests: the 6-minute walk. JAMA 271: 661–662.
19. Raisch DW, Troutman WG, Sather MR, Fudala PJ (2001) Variability in the assessment of adverse events in a multicenter clinical trial. Clin Ther 23: 2011–2020.
20. Spilker B (1991) Guide to Clinical Trials. New York Raven Press. 612–635 p.
21. Wasiak J, Cleland H (2009) Burns (minor thermal). Clin Evid (Online) 2009.
22. Ellis PD (2010) The essential guide to effect sizes. New York: Cambridge University Press.
23. Choi TY, Kim TH, Kang JW, Lee MS, Ernst E (2011) Moxibustion for rheumatic conditions: a systematic review and meta-analysis. Clin Rheumatol 30: 937–945.
24. Turk DC, Dworkin RH, Allen RR, Bellamy N, Brandenburg N, et al. (2003) Core outcome domains for chronic pain clinical trials: IMMPACT recommendations. Pain 106: 337–345.
25. Son HM, Kim DH, Kim E, Jung SY, Kim AR, et al. (2013) A qualitative study of the experiences of patients with knee osteoarthritis undergoing moxibustion. Acupunct Med 31: 39–44.
26. Park JE, Lee SS, Lee MS, Choi SM, Ernst E (2010) Adverse events of moxibustion: a systematic review. Complement Ther Med 18: 215–223.
27. Parj K-e, Han C-h, Kang K-w, Shin M-s, Oh D-s, et al. (2007) A sham moxibustion device and Masking test. Korean Journal of Oriental Medicine 13: 93–100.
28. Zhao B, Wang X, Lin Z, Liu R, Lao L (2006) A novel sham moxibustion device: a randomized, placebo-controlled trial. Complement Ther Med 14: 53–60; discussion 61.
29. Park JE, Sul JU, Kang K, Shin BC, Hong KE, et al. (2011) The effectiveness of moxibustion for the treatment of functional constipation: a randomized, sham-controlled, patient blinded, pilot clinical trial. BMC Complement Altern Med 11: 124.
30. Lee J, Yoon SW (2013) Efficacy and Safety of Moxibustion for Relieving Pain in Patients With Metastatic Cancer: A Pilot, Randomized, Single-Blind, Sham-Controlled Trial. Integr Cancer Ther.
31. Hawker GA, Mian S, Kendzerska T, French M (2011) Measures of adult pain: Visual Analog Scale for Pain (VAS Pain), Numeric Rating Scale for Pain (NRS Pain), McGill Pain Questionnaire (MPQ), Short-Form McGill Pain Questionnaire (SF-MPQ), Chronic Pain Grade Scale (CPGS), Short Form-36 Bodily Pain Scale (SF-36 BPS), and Measure of Intermittent and Constant Osteoarthritis Pain (ICOAP). Arthritis Care Res (Hoboken) 63 Suppl 11: S240–252.
32. de CWAC, Davies HT, Chadury Y (2000) Simple pain rating scales hide complex idiosyncratic meanings. Pain 85: 457–463.

Ultrasound Can Detect Macroscopically Undetectable Changes in Osteoarthritis Reflecting the Superficial Histological and Biochemical Degeneration: Ex Vivo Study of Rabbit and Human Cartilage

Kohei Nishitani[1]*, Masahiko Kobayashi[1], Hiroshi Kuroki[2], Koji Mori[3], Takaaki Shirai[1], Tsuyoshi Satake[1], Shinnichiro Nakamura[1], Ryuzo Arai[1], Yasuaki Nakagawa[1,4], Takashi Nakamura[1,4], Shuichi Matsuda[1]

1 Department of Orthopaedic Surgery, Graduate School of Medicine, Kyoto University, Kyoto, Japan, **2** Department of Physical Therapy, Human Health Sciences, Graduate School of Medicine, Kyoto University, Kyoto, Japan, **3** Department of Applied Medical Engineering Science, Graduate School of Medicine, Yamaguchi University, Ube, Japan, **4** Department of Orthopaedic surgery, National Hospital Organization Kyoto Medical Center, Kyoto, Japan

Abstract

Recognizing subtle cartilage changes in the preclinical stage of osteoarthritis (OA) is essential for early diagnosis. To this end, the ability of the ultrasound signal intensity to detect macroscopically undetectable cartilage change was investigated. In this study, cartilage of rabbit OA model and human OA samples was examined by macroscopic evaluation, ultrasound signal intensity, histology with Mankin scores, and Fourier transform infrared imaging (FTIRI) analysis. Rabbit OA was induced by anterior cruciate ligament transection and evaluated at 1, 2, 4 and 12 weeks. Twenty human samples were harvested during total knee arthroplasty from OA patients who had macroscopically normal human cartilage (ICRS grade 0) on the lateral femoral condyle. In the animal study, there was no macroscopic OA change at 2 weeks, but histology detected degenerative changes at this time point. Ultrasound signal intensity also detected degeneration at 2 weeks. In human samples, all samples were obtained from macroscopically intact site, however nearly normal ($0 \leq$ Mankin score <2), early OA ($2 \leq$ Mankin score <6), and moderate OA ($6 \leq$ Mankin score <10) samples were actually intermixed. Ultrasound signal intensity was significantly different among these 3 stages and was well correlated with Mankin scores ($R = -0.80$) and FTIR parameters related to collagen and proteoglycan content in superficial zone. In conclusion, ultrasound can detect microscopic cartilage deterioration when such changes do not exist macroscopically, reflecting superficial histological and biochemical changes.

Editor: Oreste Gualillo, SERGAS, Santiago University Clinical Hospital, IDIS Research Laboratory 9, NEIRID Lab, Spain

Funding: This study was funded by Grant of Japan Sports Medicine Foundation, Inc. in 2007. This study was also supported by Grants-in-Aid for Scientific Research in Japan (No. 20240057). The funders had no role in study design, data collection and analysis, decision to publish, or preparation of the manuscript.

Competing Interests: The authors have declared that no competing interests exist.

* E-mail: nkohei@kuhp.kyoto-u.ac.jp

Introduction

Osteoarthritis (OA) is a slow progressive degenerative joint disease and is a leading cause of impaired mobility in the elderly [1]. Although it is clear that the early diagnosis of OA is important, there is no established method to detect very early or subtle changes in the OA cartilage. Clinically, plain radiographs are still the gold standard for staging OA. However, in the early stage of OA, little or no changes are apparent in plain radiographs [1]. Magnetic resonance imaging is more powerful tool than plain radiographs for the early diagnosis of OA, however cost and availability still remain significant hurdles [2]. It is useful to develop methods to detect such early changes in the cartilage. Moreover, basic studies detecting subtle changes in the cartilage matrix that accompany the progression of OA are pivotal in improving diagnostic methods.

Quantitative ultrasound is a candidate method for detecting subtle changes in the cartilage [3]. Various unique ultrasound devices have been used to investigate cartilage and the potential of ultrasound to evaluate subtle changes in the cartilage is promising [3,4]. We developed our ultrasound noncontact method to evaluate the cartilage in an animal model. More recently, an ultrasound noncontact arthroscopy probe was used to evaluate knee and elbow cartilage during surgery [5,6,7]. Our recent report shows that the ultrasound signal intensity (US signal intensity) is useful for differentiating normal (ICRS grade 0) from slightly degenerated cartilage (ICRS grade 1) [7]. We believe that this ultrasonic noncontact probe is useful in evaluating subtle changes in the cartilage.

Our hypothesis is that the US signal intensity is sufficiently sensitive to detect the microscopic degeneration of articular cartilage. Therefore, we determined whether ultrasound can detect macroscopically undetectable histological changes in OA by using a rabbit OA model. We also used human macroscopically intact cartilage samples (ICRS grade 0) to clarify the ability of ultrasound to differentiate cartilage that has such intact surface.

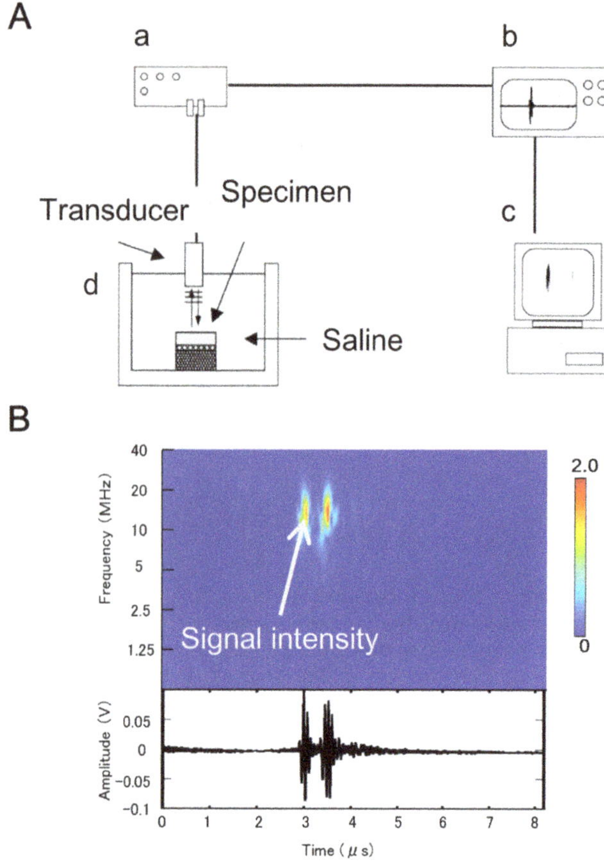

Figure 1. A scheme of the ultrasound measurement system. A) The ultrasound measurement system consists of a transducer, a pulser/receiver (a), a digital oscilloscope (b), and a personal computer (c), and saline bath and probe (d). B) typical A-mode echogram (lower) and its wavelet map (upper) of the cartilage. Each diagram has 2 peaks. The left one is a reflex echo from the surface, and the right one is from the subchondral bone. The wavelet map provides comprehensive information on the transient distribution of the intensity and frequency of an echo wave. US signal intensity is shown by graduation on the wavelet map.

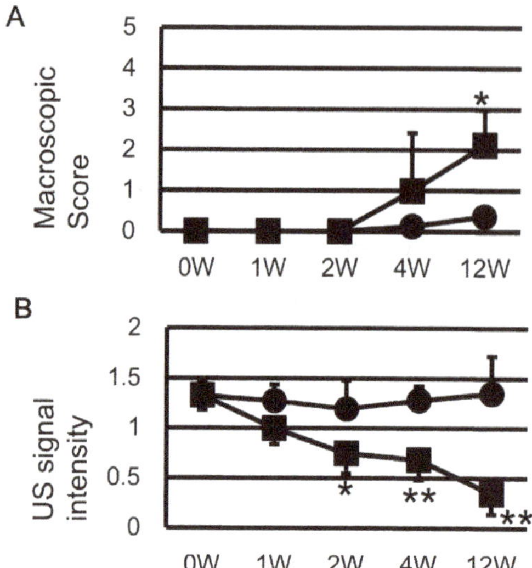

Figure 2. US signal intensity detected the deterioration of rabbit cartilages ahead of the macroscopic change. A) Macroscopic score of sham and ACLT side showed significant difference only at 12 weeks. B) US signal intensity of ACLT side decreased overtime and had significant difference to the sham side as early as 2 weeks. *: $p<0.05$ to sham side. **: $p<0.01$ to sham side.

Materials and Methods

Ethics Statement

All animal studies were conducted in accordance with principles by Kyoto University Committee of Animal Resources, based on International Guiding Principles for Biomedical Research Involving Animals. All procedures for this study were approved by Kyoto University Committee of Animal Resources (Permit Number: Med Kyo 10184). For all human species, ethical approval for this study was granted by the ethics committee of Kyoto University Graduate School and Faculty of Medicine. Written informed consent was provided and obtained from all study participants.

Animal Samples

Eighteen skeletally matured female Japanese white rabbits (weight, 4.0–4.5 kg) were used. Two rabbits (4 knees) were allocated to 0-week control, and 4 were randomly allocated into 4 groups that were examined at 1, 2, 4, or 12 weeks after surgery. They were individually housed at 22°C and 50% humidity with a 14/10-h light/dark cycle and had free access to food and water. For operations, intravenous pentobarbital sodium (25 mg/kg) was used to induce and maintain general anesthesia. An intraarticular injection (3 mL) of 1% lidocaine to each knee was used and a medial parapatellar incision was made to expose both knee joints. Bilateral anterior cruciate ligaments were exposed, and left anterior cruciate ligament transection (ACLT) was carefully performed. The joint capsule and skin incision were closed. The rabbits were allowed full weight-bearing postoperatively. The animals were sacrificed by an intravenous injection of pentobarbital sodium (100 mg/kg) and were macroscopically evaluated by two orthopaedic surgeons. In brief, cartilage changes were graded on a scale from 0 to 5 (0, intact surface normal in appearance; 1, minimal fibrillation; 2, overt fibrillation, distinguished surface irregularity, or cracks; 3, erosion from 0 to 2 mm; 4, erosion from 2 to 5 mm; 5, erosion >5 mm) [8]. The cartilage samples were stored at −20°C before use.

Human Samples

Human articular cartilage samples were obtained from a series of total knee arthroplasties of OA. Patients were diagnosed as OA according to the criteria of the American College of Rheumatology [9]. The KL grading system was used to score knees [10]. The cartilage of the weight-bearing area of the lateral femoral condyle was graded, using the International Cartilage Repair Society (ICRS) grading system by two experienced orthopaedic surgeons [11]. Patients were included in the study only when there was an ICRS grade 0 lesion in the weight-bearing area of the lateral femoral condyle. Eventually, three males and 17 females (mean age, 73.9 years; range, 55–82) (10 patients with KL grade 3 and 10 patients with KL grade 4) were involved in this study. One cylindrical osteochondral plug (diameter, 6 mm) for each patient was harvested from the center of the ICRS grade 0 lesion. The cartilage samples were stored at −20°C before use.

Ultrasound Evaluation

The ultrasonic measurement system with noncontact probe has been described previously and provides a quantitative assessment of tissues properties [5,12,13]. In brief, the transducer is 3 mm in

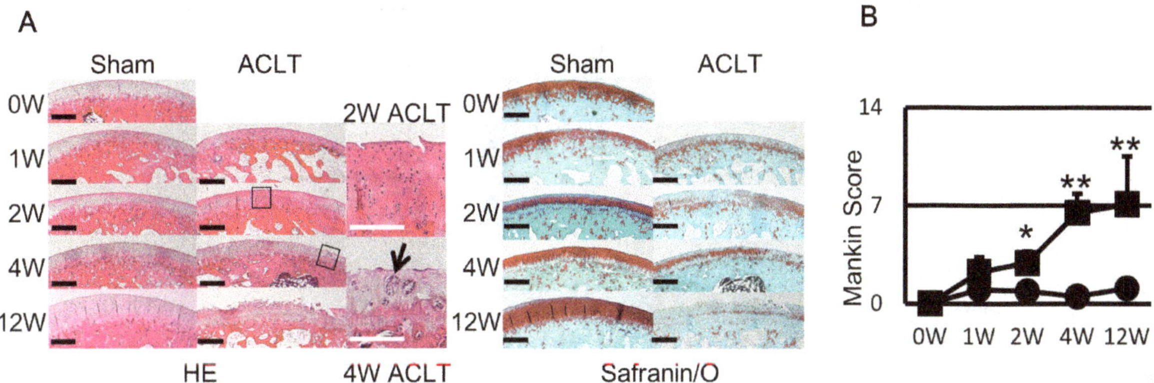

Figure 3. Histological sections and Mankin score of rabbit cartilages also showed OA change at 2 weeks. A) OA change such as fibrillation of the surface and decrease of safranin/O stainingwas detected from 2 weeks and deteriorated overtime. At 12 weeks, most of samples clearly showed OA change with fissures and further decrease of safranin/O staining. In HE, Black boxes of 2W and 4W ACLT side are showed in right column. Black arrow indicates the cloning of chondrocytes. D) Mankin score of ACLT side increased overtime and there was significant difference after 2 weeks, like US signal intensity. Black bar in histology indicates 100 µm and white bar indicates 50 µm. *: p<0.05 to sham side. **: p<0.01 to sham side.

diameter, and the center frequency of the ultrasonic signal is 10 MHz (Figure 1A). While examining cartilage, 2 large-amplitude groups of reflected waves are observed: one is from the cartilage surface and the other is from the subchondral bone (Figure 1B). The maximum magnitude of the wave reflected from the articular cartilage surface on the wavelet map was defined as US signal intensity. Each animal specimen was examined at 3 different sites: at the center, and 5 mm anterior and posterior to the center of the weight-bearing area. Each measurement was performed twice, and data from the 3 points were averaged. Each human specimen was examined at the center of the cylindrical osteochondral plug; each measurement was performed twice, and the average value was used.

Histological Analysis

Samples were fixed in 4% paraformaldehyde. Animal and Human samples were decalcified with 0.25 mol/L ethylenediaminetetraacetic acid in phosphate-buffered saline solution (pH 7.4) and Morse's solution (10% sodium citrate and 22.5% formic acid), respectively. Sagittal sections (6-µm thick) were cut, stained with hematoxylin and eosin (HE) and safranin O/fast green (safranin/O). Histological scoring of the cartilage was performed by two blinded investigators and averaged by using the Mankin scoring system with the following 4 categories: cartilage structure (6 points), cartilage cells (3 points), staining (4 points), and tidemark integrity (2 points); normal and severely degenerated cartilage scoring 0 and 14, respectively [14]. Referring to the classification of Mankin and his colleagues, human specimens were classified into 4 stages based on their Mankin scores: nearly normal ($0 \leq$ Mankin score <2), early OA ($2 \leq$ Mankin score <6), moderate OA ($6 \leq$ Mankin score <10), and late OA ($10 \leq$ Mankin score ≤ 14) [15,16].

FTIRI Evaluation

FTIRI was used to determine the spatial distribution of proteoglycan and collagen. The paraffin sections were mounted on metal plates and deparaffinized. A Fourier transform infrared spectrometer (FT-IR-460 PLUS, JASCO, Tokyo) coupled to a microscope (Intron-IRT-30, JASCO, Tokyo) was used for data acquisition. Spatial pixel size was 20×20 µm. Spectral resolution was set to 4 cm^{-1} wavenumber, and a spectral region of 2000~670 cm^{-1} was collected. An integrated absorbance area of the carbohydrate region (1150–950 cm^{-1}) and that under the amide I peak (1710–1595 cm^{-1}) were defined as the proteoglycan and collagen contents, respectively [17,18]. Two slices were evaluated for each cartilage and the averaged collagen and proteoglycan contents of the superficial zone and whole cartilage were used for quantitative analysis.

Statistical Analysis

All values are means ± standard deviation. Student's *t*-test was used for comparing sham and ACLT sides in the animal study. One-way ANOVA with a post hoc comparison was used to analyze differences among OA stages in the human study. Pearson's linear correlation coefficient was used to determine correlations between the ultrasound and FTIRI parameters. Spearman's correlation coefficient was used to determine correlations between the ultrasound parameter and Mankin scores. Statistical significance was set at $P<0.05$.

Results

Animal Specimens

The sham side of the LFC showed little OA-like changes throughout the experimental period. At 1 or 2 weeks, there was no visible change at the LFC in the ACLT side. At 4 weeks, some rabbits exhibited slight LFC fibrillation in ACLT side. At 12 weeks, most rabbits exhibited fibrillation at the LFC of ACLT side. The macroscopic scores of the LFC were significantly higher only at 12 weeks (Figure 2A).

Ultrasound Evaluation (Figure 2B)

The US signal intensity of the ACLT side decreased with time. At 2 weeks, the US signal intensity of ACLT (0.74±0.20) was significantly lower than that of sham (1.19±0.29). At 4 and 12 weeks, the US signal intensity of the LFC (0.68±0.20 and 0.34±0.21, respectively) decreased further and was significantly lower than sham side (1.28±0.14 and 1.35±0.37, respectively).

Histological Evaluation (Figure 3A)

At one week, both the ACLT and sham sides showed reduced safranin/O staining. At 2 weeks, although the safranin/O staining

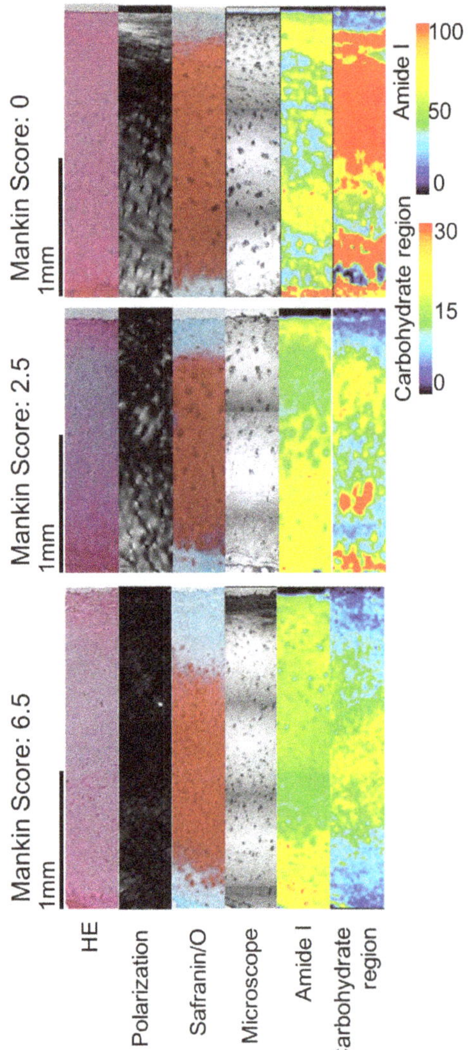

Figure 4. Though gross surface appearance was similar, histology section showed variety of OA stages. Histological section of the representative samples of each stage. HE, poralized microscope of HE, Safranin/O, Microscope for FTIR region of interest, Amide I mapping of FTIR and Carbohydrate region mapping of FTIR are shown. Upper panel is patient 1, middle is patient 2 and lower is patient 7. Black bar indicate 1 mm. Nearly normal cartilage showed a smooth surface, superficial collagen fiber network parallel to the surface, dense Safranin/O staining, Amid I rich area in superficial layer and Carbohydrate region rich areas in whole layer. As cartilage degeneration, these findings disappear or decrease.

of the sham side looked restored, the surfaces of the ACLT group appeared crackled and the safranin/O staining was not restored, and started to show OA-like changes. At 4 weeks, the safranin/O staining of the sham side was completely restored. The ACLT side exhibited fibrillation of the cartilage surface and chondrocyte cloning. At 12 weeks, the sham side appeared normal, whereas the ACLT side exhibited progression of OA-like changes, including fibrillation increase, chondrocyte cloning, and decrease in safranin/O staining. The Mankin scores (Figure 3B) of the ACLT side continuously increased and the Mankin scores of both sides were significantly different at 2, 4 and 12 weeks.

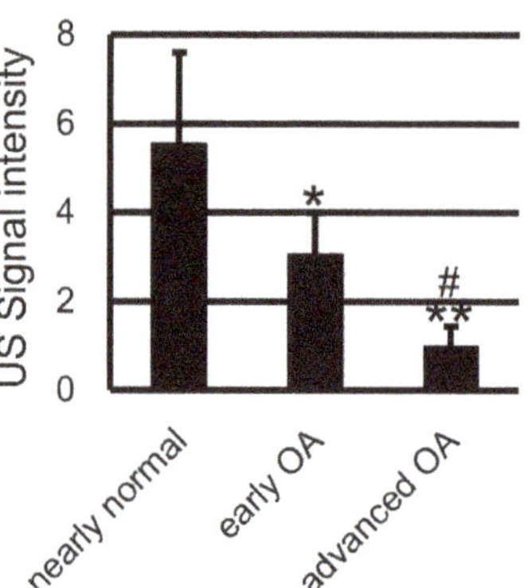

Figure 5. US signal intensity of macroscopically intact human specimens was considerably different among 3 histological stages. US signal intensity of the nearly normal cartilage was significantly higher than that of early OA or moderate OA cartilage. There was also difference between early OA and moderate OA. *: $p<0.05$ to nearly normal stage. **: $p<0.01$ to nearly normal stage. #: $p<0.05$ to early OA stage. ##: $p<0.01$ to early OA stage.

Human Specimens

Two specimens were excluded due to unsuccessful decalcification process of the paraffin sections. Mankin scores ranged widely (0 to 8), although all samples were obtained from ICRS grade 0 sites. The samples were classified into the following stages: nearly normal (3 samples), early OA (12 samples), and moderate OA (3 samples). There were no samples which were classified as late stage.

Histological Evaluation (Figure 4)

Samples in the nearly normal stage had smooth surface, dense safranin/O staining, and columnar chondrocyte arrangements. FTIRI mapping showed Amide I rich area in superficial zone and Carbohydrate region rich area along with Safranin/O staining. In the early OA stage, samples showed slight fibrillation and reduced safranin/O staining and its amide I and carbohydrate region rich area decreased. In the moderate OA stage, fibrillation became obvious and chondrocyte arrangement became random, safranin/O staining decreased, and the amide I or carbohydrate rich area was not seen.

Ultrasound Evaluation (Figure 5)

US signal intensity of the nearly normal stage was significantly higher than early or moderate stage, and US signal intensity of early stage was significantly higher than moderate stage.

Table 1. Correlation of Mankin Score and its subcategories with US signal intensity.

	Correlation with US signal Intensity	
	correlation coefficient	**P value**
Mankin Score	−0.80	<0.001
I. structure	−0.72	0.002
II. cells	−0.67	0.004
III. Safranin/O staining	−0.58	0.01
IV. Tidemark	−0.42	0.06

Table 2. Correlation of Amide I and Carbohydrate region value with US signal intensity.

		Correlation with US signal Intensity	
		correlation coefficient	**P value**
Amide I value	superficial zone	0.82	<0.001
	whole zone	0.06	0.80
Carbohydrate region value	superficial zone	0.74	<0.001
	whole zone	0.61	0.006

Correlation with Ultrasound Parameter

US signal intensity was significantly correlated with Mankin scores and its sub categories, including structure, cells, and safranin/O staining, but not tidemark (Table 1). There was a strong correlation between US signal intensity and the amide I value of the superficial zone. On the other hand, there was no significant correlation between US signal intensity and the amide I values of the whole zone (Table 2). Meanwhile, there was a significant correlation between US signal intensity correlated to carbohydrate region values of both the whole zone and the superficial zone, and correlation with the superficial zone was greater than that of whole zone (Table 2).

Discussion

The US signal intensity was able to detect macroscopically undetectable OA changes in both animal and human samples. In the animal part, there were no macroscopic changes in the ACLT side at 2 weeks; however, the US signal intensity of the ACLT side was already lower than that of the sham side. The histological Mankin scores also showed degenerative changes in the sham side at 2 weeks. Although all the human samples appeared intact, some samples were histologically degenerated. There was a significant difference among the US signal intensity of nearly normal, early OA, and moderate OA samples.

In the animal study, the US signal intensity detected cartilage deterioration when changes could only be identified histologically. OA changes were not macroscopically identified until 4 weeks after ACLT. However, upon histological evaluation, changes in OA, such as tiny crackle on the cartilage or decreased safranin/O staining, were observed at 2 weeks. Thus, ultrasound differentiated changes at this early stage.

In the human samples, although all cartilage samples were obtained from macroscopically intact areas (ICRS grade 0), Mankin scores varied widely. Three moderate OA samples out of 20 were actually diagnosed as normal by a trained orthopaedic surgeon. In clinical situations, orthopaedic surgeons mainly diagnose cartilage changes macroscopically. Thus, evaluating articular cartilage solely based on external findings is unreliable and more objective and distinct decision standards are required. We think US signal intensity with noncontact probe is possible candidate for objective evaluation of cartilage quality.

In human species, the correlation between US signal intensity and the subcategory of Mankin score showed the strongest correlation with structure which was largely from the superficial layer information but no correlation with tidemark which was from the information of deep region. US signal intensity was also strongly correlated with the amide I value of the superficial zone, but not with the whole zone. In terms of the correlation between US signal intensity and carbohydrate region value, correlation of superficial zone was greater than that of whole zone. The correlation of ultrasound reflection to collagen or proteoglycan content is previously reported [19,20,21]. Moreover, we and other groups reported that the reflected ultrasound waves provide superficial information of the cartilage [19,22,23]. The numerical analysis of ultrasonic propagation in articular cartilage from another study of our group suggests that the collagen content from the surface to one wave length (1600[m/s]/10 MHz = 0.16 mm) is correlated with US signal intensity [24]. Since the depth of the superficial zone was ~100 μm, the information of the superficial zone was included in the depth of ultrasonic propagation. The depth of rabbit cartilage was 100–200 μm, which was adequate for our evaluation device. Thus, these correlations with the superficial zone information shows that US signal intensity reflect the cartilage degeneration of superficial zone.

There are some disagreement concerning the use of US signal intensity [25,26], as US signal intensity cannot directly measure any intrinsic physical characteristics. However, we have found a strong correlation between US signal intensity and some clinically important elements of the cartilage. Moreover, the present study revealed that ultrasound can detect macroscopically undetectable change in OA. Our ultimate goal is to improve the diagnostic use of arthroscopic ultrasound systems in order to detect early degeneration in human articular cartilage.

Although the current study demonstrates clinically important findings, it has some limitations. First, the number of animals and human samples is limited. In the human study, only 20 samples were evaluated, which is too small for analyzing subgroups including gender or age. Second, instead of biochemical analysis, FTIRI with univariate-based spectral analysis was used to evaluate cartilage and determine the spatial distribution of materials of interest including collagen and proteoglycan. Amide I and carbohydrate lesion values were used to measure collagen and proteoglycan, respectively, although we did not determine their actual amounts. Nowadays, it is reported that multivalent analysis provides more accurate concentration revealing subtle change [27]. In this study, even with a simple univariate data analysis, we could find the surface change in human OA cartilage. Third, the precise qualitative analysis of the type of collagen was not performed; amide I reflects the total amount of collagen but cannot distinguish its type. Type-II collagen is predominant in articular cartilage, and we obtained a strong correlation between amide I and type-II collagen in OA cartilage in the pretest [28]. Therefore, we believe the data mainly represent changes in type-II collagen, but the data for amide I involves type-I and other minor collagen types. Finally, our current method of ultrasound evaluation could not be performed from the outside of the skin. We believe that our method is less- invasive because of the availability during arthroscopic surgery using non-contact probe, however this methods is not non-invasive. In parallel with the further accumulation of the basic information, we think it important to improve the method so as to evaluate and quantitate the cartilage from the skin surface.

In conclusion, we showed the ability of ultrasound to distinguish microscopic OA change in both animal and human cartilage, especially reflecting the information of the degeneration of superficial zone. We believe that the ultrasound is a potential method for diagnosing early subtle changes in OA at the preclinical stage.

Acknowledgments

The authors thank to Dr. Ko Yasura, Dr. Yukihiro Okamoto and Dr. Mikiko Miura for their technical help and valuable discussion.

Author Contributions

Conceived and designed the experiments: KN MK YN. Performed the experiments: KN T. Shirai T. Satake. Analyzed the data: KN MK HK. Contributed reagents/materials/analysis tools: HK KM SN RA TN SM. Wrote the paper: KN MK.

References

1. Felson DT (2006) Clinical practice. Osteoarthritis of the knee. N Engl J Med 354: 841–848.
2. Van Dyck P, Kenis C, Vanhoenacker FM, Lambrecht V, Wouters K, et al. (2013) Non-invasive imaging of cartilage in early osteoarthritis. Bone Joint J; 95: 738–746.
3. Kiviranta P, Lammentausta E, Toyras J, Kiviranta I, Jurvelin JS (2008) Indentation diagnostics of cartilage degeneration. Osteoarthritis Cartilage 16: 796–804.
4. Hattori K, Ikeuchi K, Morita Y, Takakura Y (2005) Quantitative ultrasonic assessment for detecting microscopic cartilage damage in osteoarthritis. Arthritis Res Ther 7: R38–46.
5. Nishitani K, Nakagawa Y, Gotoh T, Kobayashi M, Nakamura T (2008) Intraoperative acoustic evaluation of living human cartilage of the elbow and knee during mosaicplasty for osteochondritis dissecans of the elbow: an in vivo study. Am J Sports Med 36: 2345–2353.
6. Nishitani K, Shirai T, Kobayashi M, Kuroki H, Azuma Y, et al. (2009) Positive effect of alendronate on subchondral bone healing and subsequent cartilage repair in a rabbit osteochondral defect model. Am J Sports Med 37 Suppl 1: 139S–147S.
7. Kuroki H, Nakagawa Y, Mori K, Kobayashi M, Nakamura S, et al. (2009) Ultrasound properties of articular cartilage immediately after osteochondral grafting surgery: in cases of traumatic cartilage lesions and osteonecrosis. Knee Surg Sports Traumatol Arthrosc 17: 11–18.
8. Wang SX, Laverty S, Dumitriu M, Plaas A, Grynpas MD (2007) The effects of glucosamine hydrochloride on subchondral bone changes in an animal model of osteoarthritis. Arthritis Rheum 56: 1537–1548.
9. Altman R, Asch E, Bloch D, Bole G, Borenstein D, et al. (1986) Development of criteria for the classification and reporting of osteoarthritis. Classification of osteoarthritis of the knee. Diagnostic and Therapeutic Criteria Committee of the American Rheumatism Association. Arthritis Rheum 29: 1039–1049.
10. Kellgren JH, Lawrence JS (1957) Radiological assessment of osteo-arthrosis. Ann Rheum Dis 16: 494–502.
11. Kleemann RU, Krocker D, Cedraro A, Tuischer J, Duda GN (2005) Altered cartilage mechanics and histology in knee osteoarthritis: relation to clinical assessment (ICRS Grade). Osteoarthritis Cartilage 13: 958–963.
12. Mori K (2002) Measurement of the mechanical properties of regenerated articular cartilage using wavelet transformation. Vol. 6, 6 ed. Tokyo: Elsevier 133–142 p.
13. Kuroki H, Nakagawa Y, Mori K, Ohba M, Suzuki T, et al. (2004) Acoustic stiffness and change in plug cartilage over time after autologous osteochondral grafting: correlation between ultrasound signal intensity and histological score in a rabbit model. Arthritis Res Ther 6: R492–504.
14. Mankin HJ, Dorfman H, Lippiello L, Zarins A (1971) Biochemical and metabolic abnormalities in articular cartilage from osteo-arthritic human hips. II. Correlation of morphology with biochemical and metabolic data. J Bone Joint Surg Am 53: 523–537.
15. Ehrlich MG, Houle PA, Vigliani G, Mankin HJ (1978) Correlation between articular cartilage collagenase activity and osteoarthritis. Arthritis Rheum 21: 761–766.
16. Murata M, Trahan C, Hirahashi J, Mankin HJ, Towle CA (2003) Intracellular interleukin-1 receptor antagonist in osteoarthritis chondrocytes. Clin Orthop Relat Res 409: 285–95.
17. Camacho NP, West P, Torzilli PA, Mendelsohn R (2001) FTIR microscopic imaging of collagen and proteoglycan in bovine cartilage. Biopolymers 62: 1–8.
18. Boskey A, Camacho NP (2007) FT-IR imaging of native and tissue-engineered bone and cartilage. Biomaterials 28: 2465–2478.
19. Kuroki H, Nakagawa Y, Mori K, Kobayashi M, Yasura K, et al. (2006) Maturation-dependent change and regional variations in acoustic stiffness of rabbit articular cartilage: an examination of the superficial collagen-rich zone of cartilage. Osteoarthritis Cartilage 14–8: 784–792.
20. Hattori K, Takakura Y, Tanaka Y, Habata T, Kumai T, et al. (2006) Quantitative ultrasound can assess living human cartilage. J Bone Joint Surg Am 88 Suppl 4: 201–212.
21. Saarakkala S, Laasanen MS, Jurvelin JS, Torronen K, Lammi MJ, et al. (2003) Ultrasound indentation of normal and spontaneously degenerated bovine articular cartilage. Osteoarthritis Cartilage 11: 697–705.
22. Hattori K, Uematsu K, Matsumoto T, Ohgushi H (2009) Mechanical effects of surgical procedures on osteochondral grafts elucidated by osmotic loading and real-time ultrasound. Arthritis Res Ther 11: R134.
23. Viren T, Saarakkala S, Kaleva E, Nieminen HJ, Jurvelin JS, et al. (2009) Minimally invasive ultrasound method for intra-articular diagnostics of cartilage degeneration. Ultrasound Med Biol 35: 1546–1554.
24. Mori K, Nakagawa Y, Kuroki H, Ikeuchi K, Nakashima K, et al. (2006) Non-Contact Evaluation for Articular Cartilage Using Ultrasound. JSME International Journal, series A 49: 242–249.
25. Saarakkala S, Jurvelin JS, Zheng YP, Nieminen HJ, Toyras J (2007) Quantitative information from ultrasound evaluation of articular cartilage should be interpreted with care. Arthroscopy 23: 1137–1138.
26. Zheng YP, Huang YP (2008) More intrinsic parameters should be used in assessing degeneration of articular cartilage with quantitative ultrasound. Arthritis Res Ther 10: 125.
27. Kobrina Y, Rieppo L, Saarakkala S, Pulkkinen HJ, Tiitu V, et al. (2013) Cluster analysis of infrared spectra can differentiate intact and repaired articular cartilage. Osteoarthritis Cartilage 21: 462–469.
28. Nishitani K, Kobayashi M, Nakagawa Y, Nakamura T (2011) Detection of early degeneration of osteoarthritis cartilage by evaluating collagen content with Fourier transform infrared imaging and ultrasound. The journal of Japanese Society of Clinical Sports Medicine 19: 258–264 in Japanese.

20

Sphingolipids in Human Synovial Fluid - A Lipidomic Study

Marta Krystyna Kosinska[1], Gerhard Liebisch[2], Guenter Lochnit[3], Jochen Wilhelm[4], Heiko Klein[1], Ulrich Kaesser[5], Gabriele Lasczkowski[6], Markus Rickert[1], Gerd Schmitz[2], Juergen Steinmeyer[1]*

1 Department of Orthopedics, Justus-Liebig-University Giessen, Giessen, Germany, **2** Department of Clinical Chemistry and Laboratory Medicine, University Hospital Regensburg, Regensburg, Germany, **3** Department of Biochemistry, Justus-Liebig-University Giessen, Giessen, Germany, **4** Medical Clinic II/IV, Justus-Liebig-University Giessen, Giessen, Germany, **5** Internistisches Praxiszentrum am Krankenhaus Balserische Stiftung, Giessen, Germany, **6** Institute of Forensic Medicine, Justus-Liebig-University Giessen, Giessen, Germany

Abstract

Articular synovial fluid (SF) is a complex mixture of components that regulate nutrition, communication, shock absorption, and lubrication. Alterations in its composition can be pathogenic. This lipidomic investigation aims to quantify the composition of sphingolipids (sphingomyelins, ceramides, and hexosyl- and dihexosylceramides) and minor glycerophospholipid species, including (lyso)phosphatidic acid, (lyso)phosphatidylglycerol, and bis(monoacylglycero)phosphate species, in the SF of knee joints from unaffected controls and from patients with early (eOA) and late (lOA) stages of osteoarthritis (OA), and rheumatoid arthritis (RA). SF without cells and cellular debris from 9 postmortem donors (control), 18 RA, 17 eOA, and 13 lOA patients were extracted to measure lipid species using electrospray ionization tandem mass spectrometry - directly or coupled with hydrophilic interaction liquid chromatography. We provide a novel, detailed overview of sphingolipid and minor glycerophospholipid species in human SF. A total of 41, 48, and 50 lipid species were significantly increased in eOA, lOA, and RA SF, respectively when compared with normal SF. The level of 21 lipid species differed in eOA SF versus SF from lOA, an observation that can be used to develop biomarkers. Sphingolipids can alter synovial inflammation and the repair responses of damaged joints. Thus, our lipidomic study provides the foundation for studying the biosynthesis and function of lipid species in health and most prevalent joint diseases.

Editor: Paul Proost, University of Leuven, Rega Institute, Belgium

Funding: This work was supported in part by a grant of the DRB foundation and by the "LipidomicNet" project, funded within the Seventh Framework Programme of the European Union (Grant agreement number 202272). The funders had no role in study design, data collection and analysis, decision to publish, or preparation of the manuscript. No additional external funding was received for this study.

Competing Interests: The authors have declared that no competing interests exist.

* E-mail: juergen.steinmeyer@ortho.med.uni-giessen.de

Introduction

Synovial fluid (SF) can be viewed as an ultrafiltrate of plasma that contains locally synthesized factors, such as cytokines; growth factors; and lubricating compounds, such as lubricin, hyaluronic acid, and phospholipids. The chief functions of SF are shock absorption; load bearing; lubrication of articular surfaces, such as those of cartilage, the meniscus, tendons, and ligaments; and nutrition and communication medium of joints.

Altered composition or concentrations of SF components are linked to osteoarthritis (OA) and rheumatoid arthritis (RA) [1–3]. A precise profile of the chemical composition of SF during disease-related alterations will increase our knowledge about the pathogenesis and possible options to treat these joint diseases.

Sphingolipids (SLs) are a class of lipids that include ceramide (Cer) species, sphingomyelins (SMs) and more complex glycosphingolipids. A common constituent of all SLs is the sphingoid base, which is an organic aliphatic amino alcohol sphingosine (SPH) or a structurally similar compound [4]. The metabolic pathways of SLs form complex networks of reactions that involve many enzymes and intermediate metabolites that are needed for the biosynthesis, degradation, and remodeling of individual SLs [4–6].

SLs are structural components of plasma membranes and bioactive molecules that have significant functions in proliferation and growth as well as differentiation, cellular signal transduction, and apoptosis in many mammalian cells for instance fibroblast-like synoviocytes (FLSs) and neural cells [7–11]. The function of SLs depends on their acyl chain length and degree of saturation.

The balance between levels of individual SLs is critical. For instance, sphingosine-1-phosphate (S1P) antagonizes Cer-mediated apoptosis [9]. Exogenous Cer in turn was reported to regulate proliferation in human FLSs from OA and RA patients [7]. Treatment of FLSs with micromolar concentrations of C6-Cer inhibits proliferation through G_o/G_1 arrest, similar to what has been observed after serum starvation [7].

Cardiolipins (CLs) are tetra-acylated glycerophospholipids that are part of the inner mitochondrial membranes in eukaryotic cells. CLs regulate energy production [12,13], whereas free radical oxidation products of CLs are important mediators of mitochondria-dependent apoptosis [14–16]. Altered levels and composition of CLs are linked to diseases, such as diabetes [13], heart failure [13,17], Parkinson disease [18], and a rare cardiomyopathy, known as Barth syndrome [19].

Bis(monoacylglycero)phosphate (BMP) is an acidic phospholipid and an isomer of phosphatidylglycerol (PG). BMPs are formed on the surface of intralysosomal vesicles during the degradation of PGs and CLs and stimulate the enzymatic hydrolysis of membrane-bound SLs. The highest levels of negatively charged BMPs are found in the internal vesicles of lysosomes, and the concentration of BMPs increases as late endosomes convert into lysosomes [20]. BMPs are important for endosomal and lysosomal function, and altered levels of BMP species have been reported in a group of diseases, known as lysosomal storage disorders, in which lysosomal dysfunction leads to the accumulation of secondary metabolites, as observed in Gaucher disease, Fabry disease, mucopolysaccharidosis, Pompe disease, and drug-induced phospholipidosis [20,21].

Phosphatidic acid (PA) is a biosynthetic precursor of lipids, like PGs, CLs, and BMPs. There are two lipids that are chemically similar to PA: lysophosphatidic acid (LPA) and cyclic PA (cPA). LPA has an identical chemical structure to PA, except that it contains a single fatty acid (FA). LPA regulates many physiological and pathophysiological responses and is one of the most active naturally occurring lipids [22]. cPA act as a lipid mediator with several biological activities. Notably, cPA was recently reported to possess some antiinflammatory and chondroprotective activities in a rabbit model of OA [23].

The normal use of articular joints may damage cells found within SF which may be thus an additional source of many components of SF, including intracellular lipids that are not actively secreted into the SF. Chondrocytes, synovial lining cells, leukocytes (predominantly T cells), and cells from the meniscus, tendon, and ligaments are normally found at the borderline of SF or in SF. In addition, SF is an ultrafiltrate of the plasma so that lipids might also derive from the blood.

The levels, composition, and functions of SL, CL, LPA, PA, BMP, PG and lysophosphatidylglycerol (LPG) species in SF are unknown. Thus, we aimed to identify and quantify SL, CL, LPA, PA, LPG, PG, and BMP species. In particular, we wanted to investigate whether these lipid species are related to the health status of synovial joints using SF from normal donors as well as from patients with RA, early (eOA) or with late stages (lOA) of OA.

Materials and Methods

Inclusion and Exclusion Criteria

The SF originated from 9 deceased donors, 18 patients with RA and 30 patients with OA (Table 1). The present study was approved by the Ethical Review Committee of the Faculty of Medicine (Justus-Liebig-University of Giessen, Germany), and all patients provided written informed consent to donor samples for research. The Ethical Review Committee (protocol #62/06) waived the need for consent to be obtained from relatives of deceased donors since a judicial order to perform autopsy existed and, furthermore, to avoid additional emotional drain on relatives.

We used the Outerbridge classification scale (OU) to subcategorise the osteoarthritic changes in the joints as early (eOA) and late (lOA) stages of the disease [24]. For this, the 6 cartilage surfaces of the patella, trochlea and the medial and lateral sides of the femoral condyles and the tibia were macroscopically evaluated and the resulting cumulative OU score was divided by six in order to obtain an average score valid for the entire joint. Early osteoarthritic disease stages were defined as those which showed an average score ≤ 2, while late stages of the disease were defined as those with an OU score >2. Patients with RA were classified as described in the guidelines of the American College of Rheumatology [25]. SF was removed during autopsies of knee healthy donors at the Institute of Forensic Medicine, University of Giessen at the times after death described in Figure 1.

The SF was withdrawn into a syringe either during an arthroscopy (eOA) or during an otherwise necessary knee puncture (RA). In contrast, the SF of patients with late stage disease (lOA) was obtained during a knee prosthetic implantation.

Processing of the Synovial Fluid

The SF was processed as described elsewhere [26]. Briefly, SF was macroscopically evaluated, pressed through a 1.2 micron filter, and then 10% (v/v) inhibitors were added in order to inhibit proteases and phospholipases. This was followed by centrifugation of the SF for 45 min at 16,100×g and RT in order to pellet the cellular debris [26,27]. Finally, the supernatant was frozen at $-86°C$ for further lipid analysis.

Extraction of Sphingolipids and Phospholipids

The cell and cellular debris-free supernatant was extracted in the presence of internal lipid standards (Avanti Polar Lipids, Alabaster, AL, USA) in order to specifically quantify extracellular SMs and Cer species [26,28]. In addition, aliquots of the SF supernatant were extracted with butanol in order to determine hexosylceramide (HexCer) species, dihexosylceramide (Hex_2Cer) species, sphingoid bases, sphingosylphosphorylcholine (SPC) [29], S1P, LPAs, CLs, BMPs, PGs, and PAs [30,31]. In brief, SF was first buffered with 400 µl 30 mM citric acid and 40 mM disodium hydrogen phosphate. Lipids were then extracted with 1-butanol, dried, and redissolved in 50 µl ethanol.

Mass Spectrometric Quantification of Lipid Species

As already described the SM and Cer species were determined using electrospray ionisation mass spectrometry (ESI-MS/MS) [28,32]. In addition, we used MS/MS after liquid chromatographic separation (LC-MS/MS) to determine HexCer species, Hex_2Cer species, sphingoid bases, SPC [29], S1P, LPAs [30], CLs, BMPs, PGs and PAs [31]. Lipid species were annotated as published [33].

Data Analysis

A possible dilution of SF by a joint effusion would result in a clearly reduced concentration of certain lipids as determined by ESI-MS/MS. The liver produces urea which is not synthesized or metabolized in articular joints. Urea diffuses without any restriction across the synovium and can therefore be used to evaluate unknown dilution. The dilution effect was corrected by the method described by Kraus *et al* [26,34]. For this purpose, the concentration of urea was first measured in both SF and serum so that a dilution factor for the SF according to Kraus *et al* [34] could be calculated. Urea was determined using a commercially available kit (BioAssay Systems, Hayward, CA, USA).

Statistical Analysis of the Measured Values Obtained

In our exploratory study, a non-Gaussian distribution of the measured values was assumed so that a non-parametric statistical analysis was carried out. The Kruskal-Wallis test was used to identify statistically significant differences in the levels of lipid species between different cohorts. The false discovery rate was controlled at 5% (Benjamini-Hochberg adjustment).. For the selected species, the Steel-Dwass multiple comparisons was applied to determine statistically significant differences in lipid concentrations between individual cohorts (control, eOA, lOA, RA) while controlling the family-wise error-rate at 5%.

Table 1. Characteristics of synovial fluid donors.

	Postmortem donors. n = 9	Patients with eOA. n = 17	Patients with lOA. n = 13	Patients with RA. n = 18
Age	22 (21–25)	36 (25–49)	70 (67–74)	64 (49–71)
female/male	1/8	6/11	7/6	14/4
BMI	24.8 (20.8–25.2)	24.7 (22.6–26.9)	27.7 (25.8–30.1)	29.5 (24.8–32.8)
CRP	nd	0.5 (0.5–1.0)	1.6 (1.13–1.85)	13.2 (5.3–38.8)
No. of cells/μl SF	nd	nd	nd	6100 (2588–12,925)
DAS28	nd	nd	nd	3.48 (3.32–4.56)

Inclusion criteria: both genders, age 18–85 years inclusive, BMI<40, CRP≤3 mg/L, and all CRP levels for RA. Exclusion criteria: joint infection; severe liver or kidney disease; any surgery within the last 3 months; knee joint surgery within the last 6 months; diabetes mellitus (OA); drug abuse; intraarticular treatment with hyaluronate; or corticosteroid treatment within the last 3 months; HIV infection; tumor/cancer.

We used the statistical software "R" version 2.14.0 to perform the Kruskal-Wallis test, Benjamini-Hochberg adjustment as well as the Steel-Dwass tests. The data obtained are presented as medians with interquartile ranges for the box plots. The values quoted in the text represent the median together with the interquartile range in brackets.

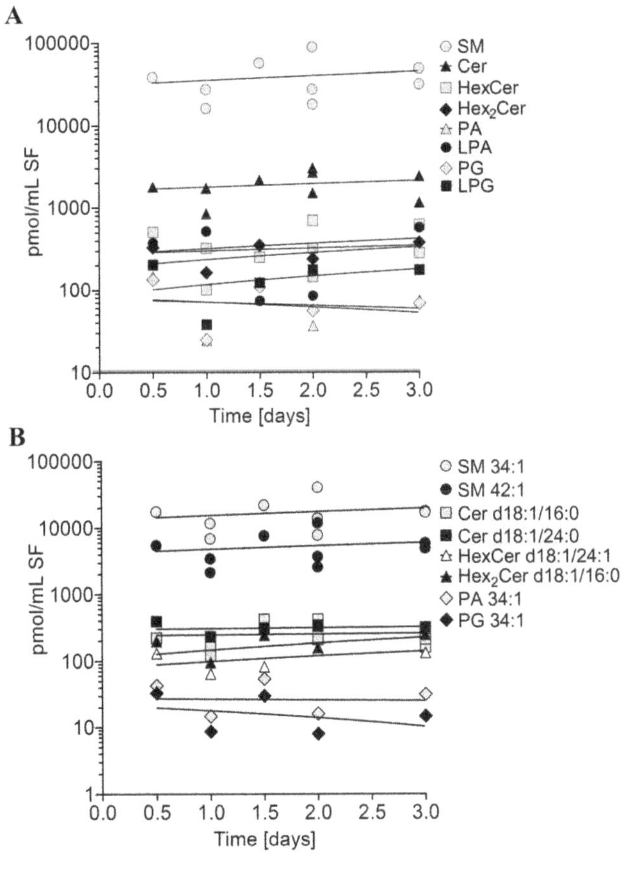

Figure 1. Postmortem stability of lipids extracted from human synovial fluid of healthy knee joints used as controls. Lipids were determined by electrospray ionization tandem mass spectrometry (ESI-MS/MS) or liquid chromatography coupled with tandem mass spectrometry (LC-MS/MS) as outlined in *Material and Methods.* Values are displayed as a scatterplot of the concentration of each lipid class and species by postmortem time. (**A**): Lipid classes, (**B**): Lipid species. SM-sphingomyelin, Cer-ceramide, HexCer-hexosylceramide (most likely glucosylceramide), Hex_2Cer-dihexosylceramide (most likely lactosylceramide), PA-phospatidic acid, LPA-lysophosphatidic acid, PG-phosphatidylglycerol, LPG-lysophosphatidylglycerol.

Results

Sphingomyelin Molecular Species

Using established ESI-MS/MS method the changes in the concentrations of SM species were examined (28). Of the SL classes that we examined, SMs were the most abundant in SF. The concentration of total SMs in control SF was 39 nmol/ml, multiplying 2.4-fold in eOA (92 nmol/ml; $p<0.05$), 4.4-fold in lOA (172 nmol/ml; $p\leq0.001$), and 3.2-fold in RA (126 nmol/ml; $p\leq0.001$). Nineteen SM species, based on the length and saturation of the attached FAs, were identified in human SF as shown in Figure 2. SM 34:1 was the predominant species among SMs, accounting for 38% to 44% of total SMs in all cohorts (Figure 2). In addition, versus control SF, 19 SM species were elevated by 2.4-fold (2.2–2.8-fold; $p<0.05$) in eOA, 4.8fold (4.1–5.4-fold; $p<0.001$) in lOA, and in RA SF 3.5-fold (2.8–4.2-fold; $p\leq0.001$). Notably, all SM species had risen approximately 2-fold in SF from eOA to lOA ($p\leq0.05$, Figure 2).

Ceramide Molecular Species

In order to quantify Cer species, ESI-MS/MS analysis was used. Furthermore, LC-MS/MS method was performed to quantify HexCer and Hex_2Cer species. Within analysed SLs, the second most prominent group of SLs in human SF was Cer species. The concentration of total Cer species was 1.4 nmol/ml in SF from controls, elevated 2-fold in SF from eOA (2.8 nmol/ml; n.s.), 3.9-fold in lOA SF (5.5 nmol/ml; $p\leq0.01$), and 3-fold in SF from RA (4.2 nmol/ml; $p\leq0.001$). Six Cer species were identified; Cer d18:0/24:0 was the predominant species (Figure 3A). As expected, the level of most Cer species was higher in lOA and RA SF, such as Cer d18:1/16:0, Cer d18:1/22:0, Cer d18:1/23:0, and Cer d18:1/24:1. Notably, most Cer species contained saturated FAs, constituting 68.9% to 74.9% of total Cer species in all cohorts (Figure 3A).

Further, the molecular species of HexCer and Hex_2Cer were quantified. Five HexCer species and 5 Hex_2Cer species were detected in human SF (Figure 3B and 4A). The percentage distribution of these species differed slightly between all cohorts, except for Hex_2Cer d18:1/24:0 which was high in eOA, and Hex_2Cer d18:1/24:1, which was low in eOA (Figure 4A). HexCer species and Hex_2Cer species were low in control SF but higher in the SF of all other cohorts. In comparison with control SF, the concentrations of HexCer species increased by 3.9-fold (3.4–4.2-fold; $p\leq0.001$) in eOA, 5.8-fold (4.8–6.1-fold; $p\leq0.01$) in lOA,

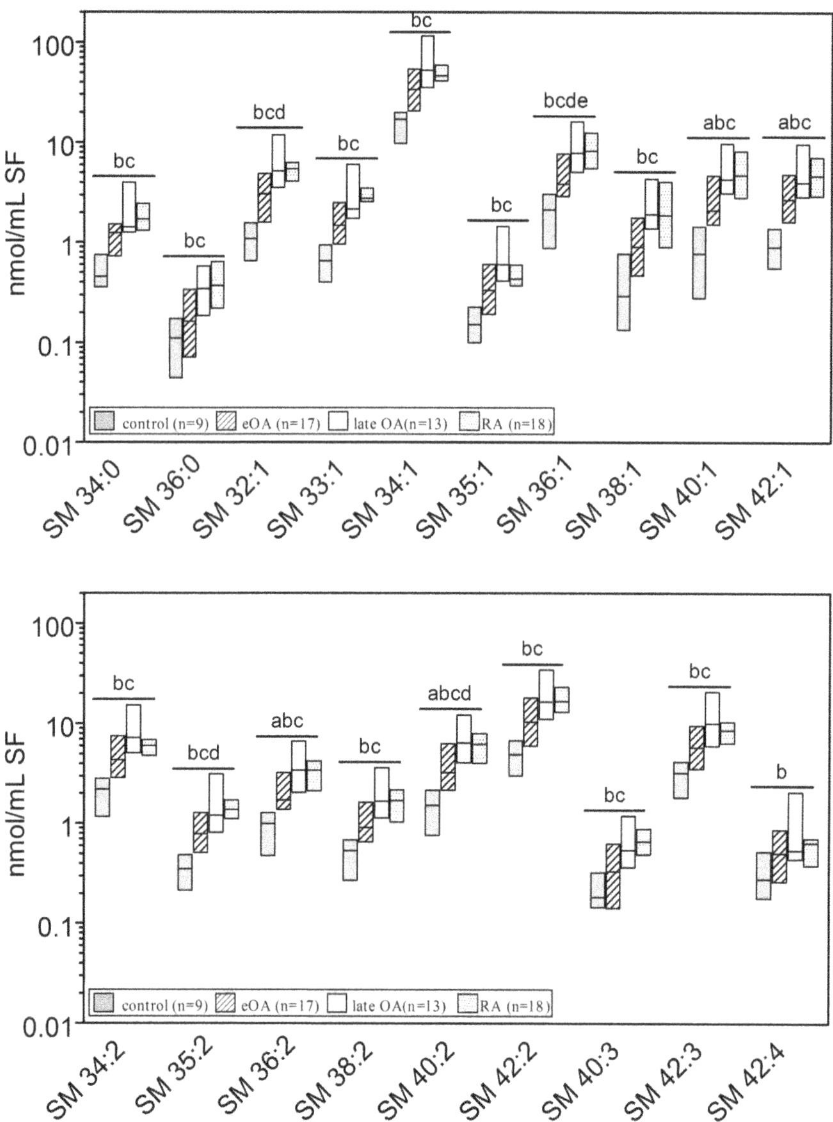

Figure 2. Concentrations of sphingomyelin species in human knee synovial fluid. Synovial fluid was obtained from donors serving as controls and from patients with early osteoarthritis (eOA), late OA (lOA), and rheumatoid arthritis (RA). SM species were determined by electrospray ionization tandem mass spectrometry as outlined in *Material and Methods*. Species annotation is based on the notion that 2 hydroxyl groups are linked to a sphingoid base. Values are presented as median and interquartile range. Significance was considered in the following way: a: p≤0.05: control vs eOA; b: p≤0.05: control vs lOA; c: p≤0.05: control vs RA; d: p≤0.05: eOA vs lOA; and e: p≤0.05: eOA vs RA. SM- sphingomyelin.

and in RA SF 5.8-fold (5.3–6.1-fold; p≤0.001) (Figure 3B), whereas Hex_2Cer species rose by 3.4-fold (3.2–5.5-fold; p≤0.001) in eOA, 4.5-fold (4.4–5.2-fold; p≤0.05) in lOA, and in RA SF 6.9-fold (6.9–7.3-fold; p≤0.001) (Figure 3B).

Lysosphingolipids and Their Phosphates

The values for S1P and sphinganine-1-phosphate in SF were below the limit of detection (6 pmol/ml for undiluted samples). We identified the following species in RA SF: SPH d18:0 [11.3 pmol/ml (0.0–21.2 pmol/ml)], SPH d18:1 [20.0 pmol/ml (15.2–24.8 pmol/ml)], SPC d18:0 [1.0 pmol/ml (0.0–1.8 pmol/ml)], and SPC d18:1 [16.1 pmol/ml (10.8–31.2 pmol/ml)]. Only 2 SL species in OA SF [SPH d18:1, 5.2 pmol/ml (0.0–16.9 pmol/ml) and SPC d18:1, 10.1 pmol/ml (4.6–19.5 pmol/ml)] were detected.

Molecular Species of Cardiolipins and BMPs

CLs possess a unique dimeric structure, bearing phosphatidyl moieties that are linked by a bridging glycerol, to which 4 FAs are attached. Our mass spectrometric analysis only enabled us to measure the sum of double bounds and carbon atoms in each of the 2 phosphatidyl moieties. The CL species concentrations were below the limit of detection, except for CL 36:4/36:4, which was elevated in RA SF.

Only 2 BMP species (BMP 18:1/18:1 and BMP 18:2/18:1) were above the limit of detection (Table 2). The highest levels of these species were observed in RA SF. In comparison with control SF, the levels of these BMP species rose by 1.6-fold (1.4–1.7-fold; ns) in all other cohorts.

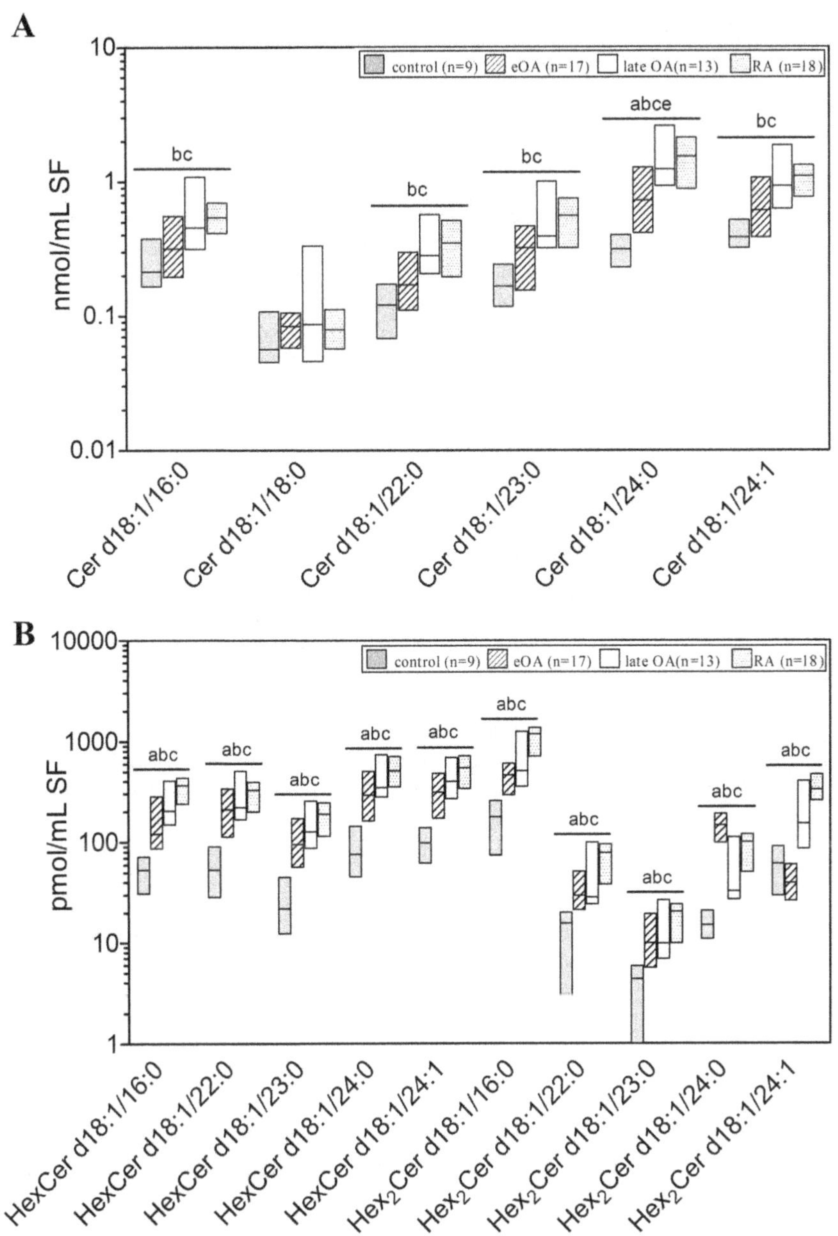

Figure 3. Concentrations of ceramide species in human knee synovial fluid. Synovial fluid was obtained from donors serving as controls and from patients with early osteoarthritis (eOA), late OA (lOA), and rheumatoid arthritis (RA). Cer species were determined by electrospray ionization tandem mass spectrometry as outlined in *Material and Methods*. Values are presented as median and interquartile range. Significance was considered in the following way: a: $p \leq 0.05$: control vs eOA; b: $p \leq 0.05$: control vs lOA; c: $p \leq 0.05$: control vs RA; d: $p \leq 0.05$: eOA vs lOA; and e: $p \leq 0.05$: eOA vs RA. (**A**): Cer species, (**B**): HexCer and Hex_2Cer species. Cer- ceramide, HexCer- hexosylceramide (most likely glucosylceramide), Hex_2Cer-dihexosylceramide (most likely lactosylceramide).

Molecular Species of PA, PG, and Lysophospholipids (LPA, LPG)

As a class, PAs and PGs contain 2 FA chains. Our mass spectrometric analysis allowed us only to determine the sum of double bonds as well as carbon atoms in the FAs, as shown in Figure 5A and 6.

Four PA and 5 LPA species, based on the number of double bounds and chain length, were detected in human SF (Figure 4B and 5). The relative distribution of these species was similar in all cohorts, except for high levels of LPA 18:0 in eOA and low levels of LPA 18:2 in eOA (Figure 4B). Notably, the concentrations of all PA and LPA species were similar in eOA, lOA, and RA SF. However, in comparison with control SF, the levels of all PA species increased 3.0-fold (2.3–3.8-fold; $p \leq 0.05$) in eOA, 4.5-fold (3.9–4.9; $p \leq 0.05$) in lOA, and in RA SF 6.7-fold (6.0–7.5; $p \leq 0.001$) (Figure 5A). Similarly, versus control SF, the levels of all LPA species rose by 2.7-fold (2.4–3.2-fold; $p \leq 0.01$) in eOA, 4.0-fold (3.6–4.4; $p \leq 0.01$) in lOA, and in RA SF 3.6-fold (3.2–4.1; $p \leq 0.001$) (Figure 5B).

The relative distribution of PG and LPG species did not differ between cohorts (Figure 5C). The major PG species in human SF were those with 34 and 36 C-atoms (PG 34:1, PG 36:1, and PG

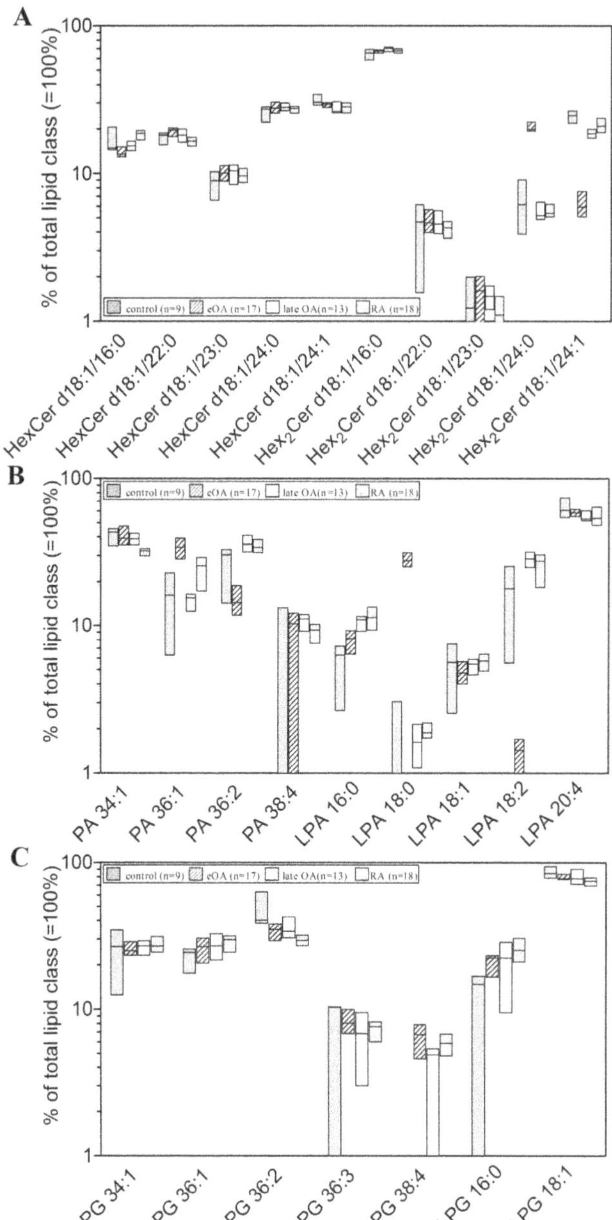

Figure 4. Relative distribution of HexCer and Hex_2Cer, PA, LPA, PG and LPG species in in human knee synovial fluid. Synovial fluid was obtained from donors serving as controls and from patients with early osteoarthritis (eOA), late OA (lOA), and rheumatoid arthritis (RA). The data show the percentage of the lipid species from the total corresponding lipid class (= 100%). Values are presented as median and interquartile range. (**A**): HexCer and Hex_2Cer species, (**B**): PA and LPA species, (**C**): PG and LPG species. HexCer- hexosylceramide (most likely glucosylceramide), Hex_2Cer- dihexosylceramide (most likely lactosylceramide), PA- phosphatidic acid, LPA- lysophosphatidic acid, PG- phosphatidylglycerol, LPG- lysophosphatidylglycerol.

36:2 with concentrations between 0.062 and 3.07 pmol/ml; Figure 6). Five PG and 2 LPG (LPG 16:0 and LPG 18:1) species were found in human SF at concentrations of 0.1–5.0 pmol/ml (Figure 6). Notably, in comparison with control SF, the levels of all PG and LPG species were elevated by 3.5-fold (2.5–5.6-fold; $p \leq 0.01$) in eOA, 3.6-fold (2.8–4.6; $p \leq 0.05$) in lOA, and in RA SF 2.9-fold (1.9–4.5; $p \leq 0.01$). However, the levels of PG and LPG species did not differ between eOA and lOA SF.

Post Mortem Stability of Sphingolipids in SF

The 9 postmortem donors died of intoxication (4×), multiple trauma (2×), cardiomyopathy (1×), pulmonary embolism (1×), and craniocerebral trauma (1×). The SF was obtained with a syringe during the autopsy of 9 adult donors without any known joint disease within a window of several hours to up to 5 days after the time-point of death. Since the stability of sphingolipids in SF as a function of the post-mortem time after time of death is unknown, the concentrations of several lipid species that exist at high levels in the SF (SM 34:1, SM 42:2, Cer d18: 1/24: 0) were plotted against the time between death and autopsy. Figure 6 show that no relevant changes occur in the level of sphingolipids within the time frame of sample collection. Furthermore, no discordant values is obvious in Figure 1 indicating that the cause of death appears to have no impact on the level of lipid species. However, the numbers of investigated SF per cause of death is too low to generalize this observation.

In order to confirm the stability of the lipid species mathematically, a linear regression of the data was obtained, and the slope of the line was calculated together with the 95% confidence interval. None of the slopes differed from 0 (values not shown).

Sphingolipids and Age of Donors

It is not known whether the level of sphingolipids in SF may be also dependent on the age of donors. Furthermore, the four cohorts of our study differ from each other with respect of their average age. Therefore the concentration of investigated lipid classes and species was plotted against the age of each donor within each cohort. Figure 7 as well as Figures S1, S2, S3 shows that the age of donors had no impact on the concentrations of lipids within the four investigated cohorts. Also, a linear regression of the data was calculated together with the slope and the 95% confidence interval revealing, that none of the slopes differed significantly from 0 (values not shown).

Adjustment of Data

The adjusted values were obtained from there corresponding nonadjusted concentrations by multiplying with a dilution factor [34] and resulting data are shown both for classes (Table 3) and individual species (Table S1). During OA water SF might be diluted by water due to inflammation-induced effusion. Therefore, the concentrations of lipid species were corrected for possible dilution. The concentrations of urea were determined within serum and SF in order to calculate a dilution factor for SF; this procedure was formerly developed to adjust for the dilution introduced by lavage during some biomarker studies. Compared with the level of lipids in SF of controls, eOA, lOA, and RA had elevated concentrations of most lipid species independent of whether they were adjusted or nonadjusted. However, the differences between most lipid species in eOA and lOA were more obvious using the adjusted values (Table S1)

Discussion

Lipids such as SLs, PAs, LPAs, LPGs, and BMPs and other groups of lipids are known to be bioactive molecules, but their location and function in SF of articular joints remain to be discovered. The lack of knowledge on the profile, quantity, and function of these lipids in human SF underscore the need for detailed studies in this area. Changes in the composition and

Table 2. Concentrations of bis(monoacylglycero)phosphate (BMP) species.

Concentration [pmol/ml]				
BMP-specie	**control (n = 9)**	**eOA (n = 17)**	**lOA (n = 13)**	**RA (n = 18)**
BMP 18:1/18:1	27.8 (17.5–46.8)	23.1 (15.4–37.9)	36.7 (22.9–74.7)	24.2 (19.8–30.9)
BMP 18:2/18:1	15.6 (9.27–20.0)	16.8 (11.5–25.5)	25.4 (15.9–46.3)	18.8 (13.9–23.6)

Concentrations of bis(monoacylglycero)phosphate (BMP) species in knee synovial fluid obtained from donors serving as controls and from patients with early osteoarthritis (eOA), late OA (lOA), and rheumatoid arthritis (RA). BMP species were determined by electrospray ionization tandem mass spectrometry as outlined in *Material and Methods*. Values are presented as median and interquartile range in the brackets. BMP-Bis(monoacylglycero)phosphate, eOA-early osteoarthritis, lOA-late osteoarthritis, RA-rheumatoid arthritis.

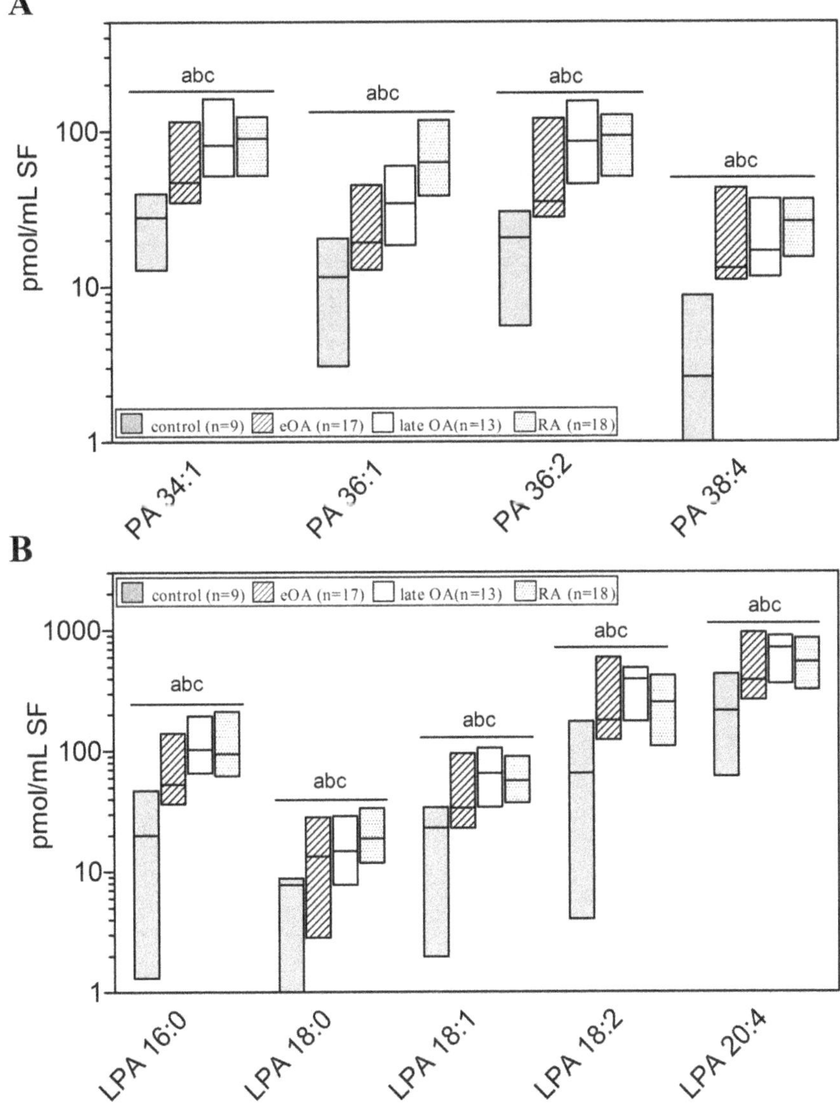

Figure 5. Concentrations of phosphatidic acid (PA) and lysophosphatidic acid (LPA) species in human knee synovial fluid. Synovial fluid was obtained from donors serving as controls and from patients with early osteoarthritis (eOA), late OA (lOA), and rheumatoid arthritis (RA). PA and LPA species were determined liquid chromatography coupled with tandem mass spectrometry as outlined in *Material and Methods*. Species annotation is based on the notion that only ester bonds are present. Values are presented as median and interquartile range. Significance was considered in the following way: a: $p \leq 0.05$: control vs eOA; b: $p \leq 0.05$: control vs lOA; and c: $p \leq 0.05$: control vs RA. (**A**): PA species, (**B**): LPA species. PA- phosphatidic acid, LPA- lysophosphatidic acid.

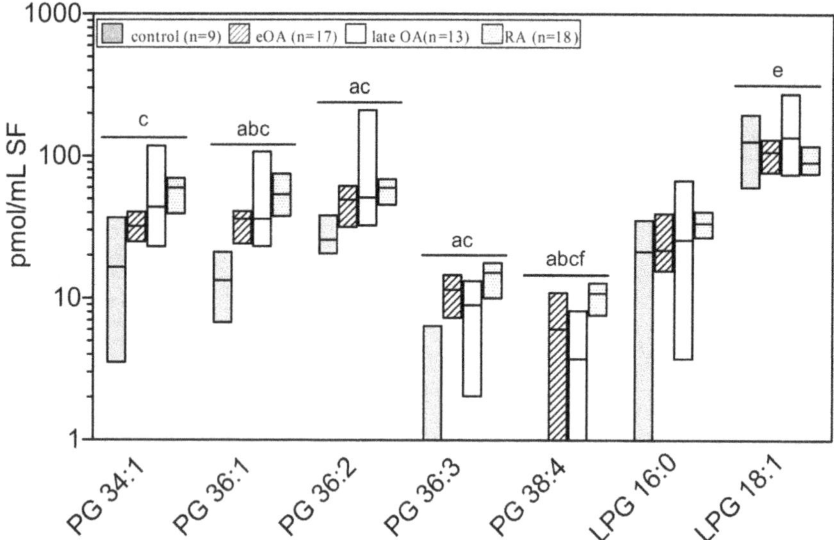

Figure 6. Concentrations of phosphatidylglycerol (PG) and lysophosphatidylglycerol (LPG) species in human knee synovial fluid. Synovial fluid was obtained from donors serving as controls and from patients with early osteoarthritis (eOA), late OA (lOA), and rheumatoid arthritis (RA). PG and LPG species were determined by liquid chromatography coupled with tandem mass spectrometry as outlined in *Material and Methods.* Species annotation is based on the notion that only ester bonds are present. Values are presented as median and interquartile range. Significance was considered in the following way: a: $p \leq 0.05$: control vs eOA; b: $p \leq 0.05$: control vs lOA; c: $p \leq 0.05$: control vs RA; d: $p \leq 0.05$: eOA vs lOA; e: $p \leq 0.05$: eOA vs RA; and f: $p \leq 0.05$: lOA vs RA. PG- phosphatidylglycerol, LPG- lysophosphatidylglycerol.

concentrations of various lipids have been already linked with several human disorders [19,26].

We have reported that concentrations of phospholipids species increase in SF of RA and OA compared with SF obtained from donors used as controls [26]. The principle finding of our current study is that a broad spectrum of SL species, their precursors, and intermediate metabolites was found in human SF. Moreover, the concentrations of 41 lipids in eOA SF, 48 species in lOA SF, and 50 species in RA SF increase significantly in comparison with control SF. Notably, the levels of 21 lipid species were altered between eOA and lOA SF, indicating that the lipid composition of SF reflects the severity of OA disease. Thus, our findings may be used to develop biomarkers to discriminate eOA from lOA, and eOA from healthy joints.

Until recently, there have been no sensitive methods to detect these species at low concentrations in biological materials. The lipidomic methods that we used in this study [28–32], allowed us to identify and quantify many lipid species that have not been reported in SF. This is why our lipidomic investigation reports for the first time about the composition of SL and minor glycerophospholipids species in human SF.

SMs and Cer species regulate many processes, including stress responses, proliferation and differentiation, apoptosis, and senescence [35–37]. Using chondrocytes and explants from rabbit articular cartilage, exogenous cell-permeable C2-Cer at concentrations over 25 μM were noted to induce apoptosis, up regulate MMP-1, -3, and -13, and ultimately induce articular cartilage matrix degradation by collagen type II cleavage and proteoglycan loss from cartilage [38–41]. Further, Cer species are reported to be mediators that induce proinflammatory cytokine production and possibly apoptosis in cultured human RA FLS [7,11] as well as cultured chondrocytes [38]. *In vitro* administration of synthetic exogenous C2- or C6-Cer at concentrations below 25 μM did not affect apoptosis but inhibited the proliferation of FLS in OA and RA [7]. However, intraarticular injection of 34.5 μg C2-Cer into the ankle joints of mice increased the population of apoptotic synovial cells [11].

We observed higher concentrations of several Cer species in SF from RA and lOA compared with control SF indicating that Cer species may be involved in the progression of OA and RA. However, the exact function of extracellular SM and Cer species, alone and in combination, in synovial joints is unknown. Further studies are needed to show whether Cer species are synthesized *de novo* or are the result of higher sphingomyelinase activity.

CLs are nearly exclusively a constituent of the mitochondrial inner membrane: extracellular CLs in body fluids have not been reported. We detected CLs only in RA SF. Thus, we speculate that the presence of CLs in SF is a hallmark of RA and that CLs can be used to develop a novel diagnostic tool for RA. However, it is unknown whether CLs in SF have functions. The source of CLs in RA SF is not known and further studies are needed to identify where the CLs come from. One possible source are the cells that are enriched in RA SF compared with OA and control SF and which can be damaged by normal joint movement so that mitochondrial lipids like CLs are released. Although we removed cells and cellular debris from SF by centrifugation and filtration, these techniques are unable to eliminate molecular micelles.

LPAs can promote the proliferation of many cell types. *In vitro* stimulation with 1 or 5 μM exogenous LPA stimulates the proliferation of rat primary chondrocytes [42,43]. Moreover, the expression of six G-protein-coupled LPA receptors increases in RA FLS. Thus, LPAs appear to function as lipid mediators between cells displaying growth factor-like activities [44]. We noted elevated levels of all PA and LPA species in SF of RA and OA compared with control SF, consistent with previous findings [45]. The higher concentration of LPAs is likely attributed to increased secretion and activity of enzymes for example phospholipase A_2 [46] and may point to a possible repair response. However, further studies need to evaluate the functions of LPA species as intercellular lipid mediators that induce cell proliferation and have growth factor-like activities in damaged articular cartilage.

A

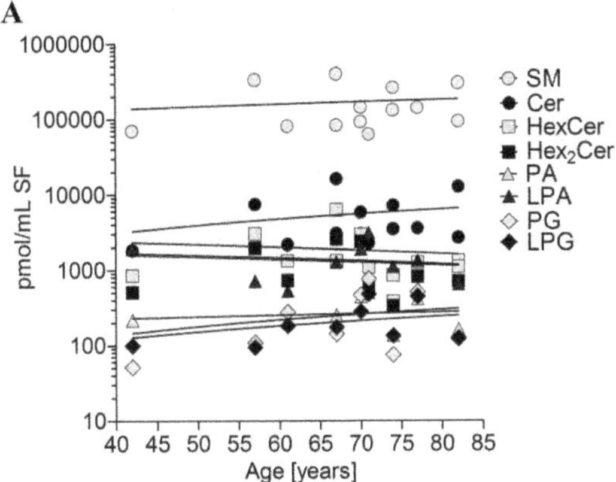

B

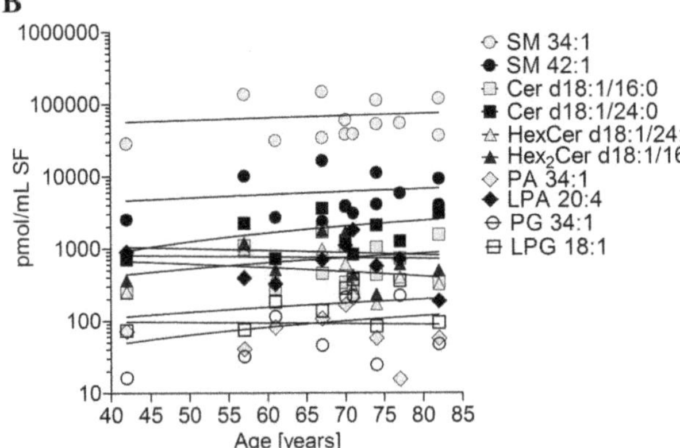

Figure 7. Concentrations of lipids in human synovial fluid as a function of the age of patients with late stage osteoarthritis. Lipids were determined by electrospray ionization tandem mass spectrometry (ESI-MS/MS) or liquid chromatography coupled with tandem mass spectrometry (LC-MS/MS) as outlined in *Material and Methods*. Values are displayed as a scatterplot of the concentration of each lipid class and species by age of donors. (**A**): Lipid classes, (**B**): Lipid species. SM-sphingomyelin, Cer-ceramide, HexCer-hexosylceramide (most likely glucosylceramide), Hex_2Cer-dihexosylceramide (most likely lactosylceramide), PA-phospatidic acid, LPA-lysophosphatidic acid, PG-phosphatidylglycerol, LPG-lysophosphatidylglycerol.

Recently, cPA was reported to stimulate the production of HA in human OA articular chondrocytes and to provide some anti-inflammatory and chondroprotective activities in a rabbit model of OA [23]. However, our methods applied did not allow us to quantify cPA in SF.

This study is the first to report about PG species in SF. PGs are important components of the pulmonary surfactant system [47]. Thus, we hypothesize that PG species have similar functions in synovial joints. However, our study demonstrates that PG species exist at low concentrations in human SF. Moreover, the PG species in human SF are also found in human plasma; albeit, human plasma appears to have more PG species than SF [20,48]. In, contrast to human plasma, in which only saturated LPG species (LPG16:0 and LPG 18:0) have been reported [49], human SF contains a high proportion of monounsaturated LPG 18:1. Notably, versus control SF, the concentrations of all PG species were significantly elevated in eOA, lOA, and RA SF. BMP, a structural isomer of PG, was also detected in SF at low levels, and 2 BMP species were identified. However, the function and source of extracellular PG, LPG, and BMP species are unknown.

Table 3. Impact of dilution factor on the concentrations of lipid classes.

Lipid class	eOA (n = 17) [%]	lOA (n = 13) [%]	RA (n = 18) [%]
SM	118.2 (110.5–123.8)	157.1 (146.5–173.5)	88.1 (83.4–89.2)
Cer	130.7 (122.6–132.9)	157.7 (154.9–164.1)	81.2 (78.4–87.3)
HexCer	110.1 (110.1–111.6)	153.1 (152.7–158.6)	86.0 (82.8–88.5)
Hex_2Cer	103.9 (99.8–105.4)	138.4 (135.5–139.8)	81.2 (77.5–81.9)
PA	103.3 (98.9–106.8)	180.0 (165.7–185.7)	82.8 (79.1–85.6)
LPA	109.9 (108.3–113.3)	176.3 (152.6–190.6)	84.2 (80.1–88.3)
PG	100.0 (98.9–108.5)	123.9 (121.1–126.4)	84.2 (80.8–86.4)
LPG	107.6 (101.9–113.3)	143.2 (133.0–153.4)	82.9 (81.9–83.9)
BMP	97.3 (95.4–99.3)	165.0 (165.0–165.0)	79.6 (77.9–81.2)

Impact of dilution factor on the concentrations of lipid classes as expressed as percentage of uncorrected values (= 100%). Lipids were determined by electrospray ionization tandem mass spectrometry or liquid chromatography coupled with tandem mass spectrometry, and corrected for possible dilution as outlined in *Material and Methods*. Values are median and interquartile range. eOA-early osteoarthritis, lOA-late osteoarthritis, RA-rheumatoid arthritis, SM-sphingomyelin, Cer-ceramide, HexCer-hexosylceramide (most likely glucosylceramide), Hex_2Cer-dihexosylceramide (most likely lactosylceramide), PA-phosphatidic acid, LPA-lysophosphatidic acid, PG-phosphatidylglycerol, LPG-lysophosphatidylglycerol, BMP-bis(monoglycero)phosphate.

In conclusion, this lipidomic investigation presents for the first time a comprehensive survey of SLs and minor glycerophospholipids in human SF. Our mass spectrometric analysis of lipids in SF from patients with eOA, lOA, and RA knee joints indicate disease and stage-dependent differences. Certain species of SM and Cer may, at least in part, be involved in the pathogenesis of OA and RA. The paucity of detailed data on the functions of lipid species in RA and OA underscore the necessity for further studies. Our study lays the foundation for addressing specific questions regarding the biosynthesis and function of lipid species in SF.

Supporting Information

Figure S1 Concentrations of lipids in human synovial fluid as a function of the age of donors used as controls. Synovial fluid was obtained post mortem from donors with healthy knee joints. Lipids were determined by electrospray ionization tandem mass spectrometry (ESI-MS/MS) or liquid chromatography coupled with tandem mass spectrometry (LC-MS/MS) as outlined in *Material and Methods.* Values are displayed as a scatterplot of the concentration of each lipid class and species by age of donors. (**A**): Lipid classes, (**B**): Lipid species. SM-sphingomyelin, Cer-ceramide, HexCer-hexosylceramide (most likely glucosylceramide), Hex_2Cer-dihexosylceramide (most likely lactosylceramide), PA-phospatidic acid, LPA-lysophosphatidic acid, PG-phosphatidylglycerol, LPG-lysophosphatidylglycerol.

Figure S2 Concentrations of lipids in human synovial fluid as a function of the age of patients with early stage osteoarthritis. Lipids were determined by electrospray ionization tandem mass spectrometry (ESI-MS/MS) or liquid chromatography coupled with tandem mass spectrometry (LC-MS/MS) as outlined in *Material and Methods.* Values are displayed as a scatterplot of the concentration of each lipid class and species by age of donors. (**A**): Lipid classes, (**B**): Lipid species. SM-sphingomyelin, Cer-ceramide, HexCer-hexosylceramide (most likely glucosylceramide), Hex_2Cer-dihexosylceramide (most likely lactosylceramide), PA-phospatidic acid, LPA-lysophosphatidic acid, PG-phosphatidylglycerol, LPG-lysophosphatidylglycerol.

Figure S3 Concentrations of lipids in human synovial fluid as a function of the age of patients with rheumatoid arthritis. Lipids were determined by electrospray ionization tandem mass spectrometry (ESI-MS/MS) or liquid chromatography coupled with tandem mass spectrometry (LC-MS/MS) as outlined in *Material and Methods*. Values are displayed as a scatterplot of the concentration of each lipid class and species by age of donors. (**A**): Lipid classes, (**B**): Lipid species. SM-sphingomyelin, Cer-ceramide, HexCer-hexosylceramide (most likely glucosylceramide), Hex_2Cer-dihexosylceramide (most likely lactosylceramide), PA-phospatidic acid, LPA-lysophosphatidic acid, PG-phosphatidylglycerol, LPG-lysophosphatidylglycerol.

Table S1 Concentrations of lipid species presented in Figure 1–7. Lipids were determined by electrospray ionization tandem mass spectrometry or liquid chromatography coupled with tandem mass spectrometry as outlined in *Material and Methods*. Data (nmol/ml or pmol/ml) obtained were either uncorrected (normal font) or corrected with the dilution factor per Kraus *et al.* (34, bold font). Values are median and interquartile range. The concentrations of urea were determined within serum and SF to calculate a dilution factor for SF; this procedure was formerly developed to adjust for the dilution introduced by lavage during some biomarker studies. eOA-early osteoarthritis, lOA-late osteoarthritis, RA-rheumatoid arthritis, SM-sphingomyelin, Cer-ceramide, HexCer-hexosylceramide (most likely glucosylceramide), Hex_2-Cer-dihexosylceramide (most likely lactosylceramide), PA-phospatidic acid, LPA-lysophosphatidic acid, PG-phosphatidylglycerol, LPG-lysophosphatidylglycerol, SPH-sphingosine, SPC-sphingosylphosphorylcholine, CL-cardiolipin, BMP-bis(monoglycero)phosphate.

Acknowledgments

The authors thank Magdalena Singer, Christiane Hild, and Simone Düchtel for excellent technical support and Manuela Döller for assistance with the study organization.

Author Contributions

Conceived and designed the experiments: MKK GS G. Lochnit JS. Performed the experiments: MKK G. Liebisch G. Lochnit JW HK UK G. Lasczkowski MR. Analyzed the data: MKK G. Liebisch GS JW JS. Contributed reagents/materials/analysis tools: G. Liebisch G. Lochnit JW HK UK G. Lasczkowski MR. Wrote the paper: MKK JS. Involved in drafting the article or revising it critically for important intellectual content, and approving the final version to be published: GLI GLO JW HK UK GL GS MR.

References

1. Bellamy N, Campbell J, Robinson V, Gee T, Bourne R, et al. (2006) Viscosupplementation for the treatment of osteoarthritis of the knee. Cochrane Database Syst Rev: CD005321.
2. Ludwig TE, McAllister JR, Lun V, Wiley JP, Schmidt TA (2012) Diminished cartilage-lubricating ability of human osteoarthritic synovial fluid deficient in proteoglycan 4: Restoration through proteoglycan 4 supplementation. Arthritis Rheum 64: 3963–3971.
3. Schmidt TA, Gastelum NS, Nguyen QT, Schumacher BL, Sah RL (2007) Boundary lubrication of articular cartilage: role of synovial fluid constituents. Arthritis Rheum 56: 882–891.
4. Lahiri S, Futerman AH (2007) The metabolism and function of sphingolipids and glycosphingolipids. Cell Mol Life Sci 64: 2270–2284.
5. Merrill AH Jr (2011) Sphingolipid and glycosphingolipid metabolic pathways in the era of sphingolipidomics. Chem Rev 111: 6387–6422.
6. Marchesini N, Hannun YA (2004) Acid and neutral sphingomyelinases: roles and mechanisms of regulation. Biochem Cell Biol 82: 27–44.
7. Gerritsen ME, Shen CP, Perry CA (1998) Synovial fibroblasts and the sphingomyelinase pathway: sphingomyelin turnover and ceramide generation are not signaling mechanisms for the actions of tumor necrosis factor-alpha. Am J Pathol 152: 505–512.
8. Cutler RG, Mattson MP (2001) Sphingomyelin and ceramide as regulators of development and lifespan. Mech Ageing Dev 122: 895–908.
9. Spiegel S, Milstien S (2003) Sphingosine-1-phosphate: an enigmatic signalling lipid. Nat Rev Mol Cell Biol 4: 397–407.
10. Luberto C, Kraveka JM, Hannun YA (2002) Ceramide regulation of apoptosis versus differentiation: a walk on a fine line. Lessons from neurobiology. Neurochem Res 27: 609–617.
11. Ichinose Y, Eguchi K, Migita K, Kawabe Y, Tsukada T, et al. (1998) Apoptosis induction in synovial fibroblasts by ceramide: in vitro and in vivo effects. J Lab Clin Med 131: 410–416.
12. Schlame M, Ren M (2009) The role of cardiolipin in the structural organization of mitochondrial membranes. Biochim Biophys Acta 1788: 2080–2083.
13. Houtkooper RH, Vaz FM (2008) Cardiolipin, the heart of mitochondrial metabolism. Cell Mol Life Sci 65: 2493–2506.
14. Schug ZT, Gottlieb E (2009) Cardiolipin acts as a mitochondrial signalling platform to launch apoptosis. Biochim Biophys Acta 1788: 2022–2031.
15. Yin H, Zhu M (2012) Free radical oxidation of cardiolipin: chemical mechanisms, detection and implication in apoptosis, mitochondrial dysfunction and human diseases. Free Radic Res 46: 959–974.
16. Ji J, Kline AE, Amoscato A, Samhan-Arias AK, Sparvero LJ, et al. (2012) Lipidomics identifies cardiolipin oxidation as a mitochondrial target for redox therapy of brain injury. Nat Neurosci 15: 1407–1413.
17. Ventura-Clapier R, Garnier A, Veksler V (2004) Energy metabolism in heart failure. J Physiol 555: 1–13.
18. Ellis CE, Murphy EJ, Mitchell DC, Golovko MY, Scaglia F, et al. (2005) Mitochondrial lipid abnormality and electron transport chain impairment in mice lacking alpha-synuclein. Mol Cell Biol 25: 10190–10201.
19. Schlame M, Ren M (2006) Barth syndrome, a human disorder of cardiolipin metabolism. FEBS Lett 580: 5450–5455.
20. Meikle PJ, Duplock S, Blacklock D, Whitfield PD, Macintosh G, et al. (2008) Effect of lysosomal storage on bis(monoacylglycero)phosphate. Biochem J 411: 71–78.
21. Hullin-Matsuda F, Luquain-Costaz C, Bouvier J, Delton-Vandenbroucke I (2009) Bis(monoacylglycero)phosphate, a peculiar phospholipid to control the fate of cholesterol: Implications in pathology. Prostaglandins Leukot Essent Fatty Acids 81: 313–324.
22. Tokumura A (2002) Physiological and pathophysiological roles of lysophosphatidic acids produced by secretory lysophospholipase D in body fluids. Biochim Biophys Acta 1582: 18–25.
23. Masuda I, Okada K, Momohara S (2013) Cyclic phosphatidic acid (CPA) stimulates the production of hyaluronic acid (HA) in human osteoarthritic articular chondrocytes, and intraarticular administration of CPA supresses pain, swelling, and cartilage destruction in rabbit experimental osteoarthritis. Osteoarthritis Cartilage 21: Abstracts:S296–S297.
24. Outerbridge RE (1961) The etiology of chondromalacia patellae. J Bone Joint Surg Br 43-B: 752–757.
25. Arnett FC, Edworthy SM, Bloch DA, McShane DJ, Fries JF, et al. (1988) The American Rheumatism Association 1987 revised criteria for the classification of rheumatoid arthritis. Arthritis Rheum 31: 315–324.
26. Kosinska MK, Liebisch G, Lochnit G, Wilhelm J, Klein H, et al. (2013) A lipidomic study of phospholipid classes and species in human synovial fluid. Arthritis Rheum 65: 2323–2333.
27. Berckmans RJ, Nieuwland R, Kraan MC, Schaap MC, Pots D, et al. (2005) Synovial microparticles from arthritic patients modulate chemokine and cytokine release by synoviocytes. Arthritis Res Ther 7: R536–544.
28. Liebisch G, Lieser B, Rathenberg J, Drobnik W, Schmitz G (2004) High-throughput quantification of phosphatidylcholine and sphingomyelin by electrospray ionization tandem mass spectrometry coupled with isotope correction algorithm. Biochim Biophys Acta 1686: 108–117.
29. Scherer M, Leuthauser-Jaschinski K, Ecker J, Schmitz G, Liebisch G (2010) A rapid and quantitative LC-MS/MS method to profile sphingolipids. J Lipid Res 51: 2001–2011.
30. Scherer M, Schmitz G, Liebisch G (2009) High-throughput analysis of sphingosine 1-phosphate, sphinganine 1-phosphate, and lysophosphatidic acid in plasma samples by liquid chromatography-tandem mass spectrometry. Clin Chem 55: 1218–1222.
31. Scherer M, Schmitz G, Liebisch G (2010) Simultaneous quantification of cardiolipin, bis(monoacylglycero)phosphate and their precursors by hydrophilic interaction LC-MS/MS including correction of isotopic overlap. Anal Chem 82: 8794–8799.
32. Liebisch G, Drobnik W, Reil M, Trumbach B, Arnecke R, et al. (1999) Quantitative measurement of different ceramide species from crude cellular extracts by electrospray ionization tandem mass spectrometry (ESI-MS/MS). J Lipid Res 40: 1539–1546.

33. Liebisch G, Vizcaino JA, Kofeler H, Trotzmuller M, Griffiths WJ, et al. (2013) Shorthand notation for lipid structures derived from mass spectrometry. J Lipid Res 54: 1523–1530.
34. Kraus VB, Huebner JL, Fink C, King JB, Brown S, et al. (2002) Urea as a passive transport marker for arthritis biomarker studies. Arthritis Rheum 46: 420–427.
35. Niemela PS, Hyvonen MT, Vattulainen I (2006) Influence of chain length and unsaturation on sphingomyelin bilayers. Biophys J 90: 851–863.
36. Drobnik W, Liebisch G, Audebert FX, Frohlich D, Gluck T, et al. (2003) Plasma ceramide and lysophosphatidylcholine inversely correlate with mortality in sepsis patients. J Lipid Res 44: 754–761.
37. Mizushima N, Kohsaka H, Miyasaka N (1998) Ceramide, a mediator of interleukin 1, tumour necrosis factor alpha, as well as Fas receptor signalling, induces apoptosis of rheumatoid arthritis synovial cells. Ann Rheum Dis 57: 495–499.
38. Sabatini M, Rolland G, Leonce S, Thomas M, Lesur C, et al. (2000) Effects of ceramide on apoptosis, proteoglycan degradation, and matrix metalloproteinase expression in rabbit articular cartilage. Biochem Biophys Res Commun 267: 438–444.
39. Sabatini M, Thomas M, Deschamps C, Lesur C, Rolland G, et al. (2001) Effects of ceramide on aggrecanase activity in rabbit articular cartilage. Biochem Biophys Res Commun 283: 1105–1110.
40. Tetlow LC, Adlam DJ, Woolley DE (2001) Matrix metalloproteinase and proinflammatory cytokine production by chondrocytes of human osteoarthritic cartilage: associations with degenerative changes. Arthritis Rheum 44: 585–594.
41. Colosimo M, McCarthy N, Jayasinghe R, Morton J, Taylor K, et al. (2000) Diagnosis and management of subdural haematoma complicating bone marrow transplantation. Bone Marrow Transplant 25: 549–552.
42. Kim MK, Lee HY, Park KS, Shin EH, Jo SH, et al. (2005) Lysophosphatidic acid stimulates cell proliferation in rat chondrocytes. Biochem Pharmacol 70: 1764–1771.
43. Hurst-Kennedy J, Boyan BD, Schwartz Z (2009) Lysophosphatidic acid signaling promotes proliferation, differentiation, and cell survival in rat growth plate chondrocytes. Biochim Biophys Acta 1793: 836–846.
44. Orosa B, Gonzalez A, Mera A, Gomez-Reino JJ, Conde C (2012) Lysophosphatidic acid receptor 1 suppression sensitizes rheumatoid fibroblast-like synoviocytes to tumor necrosis factor-induced apoptosis. Arthritis Rheum 64: 2460–2470.
45. Song HY, Lee MJ, Kim MY, Kim KH, Lee IH, et al. (2010) Lysophosphatidic acid mediates migration of human mesenchymal stem cells stimulated by synovial fluid of patients with rheumatoid arthritis. Biochim Biophys Acta 1801: 23–30.
46. Pruzanski W, Keystone EC, Sternby B, Bombardier C, Snow KM, et al. (1988) Serum phospholipase A2 correlates with disease activity in rheumatoid arthritis. J Rheumatol 15: 1351–1355.
47. Agassandian M, Mallampalli RK (2013) Surfactant phospholipid metabolism. Biochim Biophys Acta 1831: 612–625.
48. Quehenberger O, Armando AM, Brown AH, Milne SB, Myers DS, et al. (2010) Lipidomics reveals a remarkable diversity of lipids in human plasma. J Lipid Res 51: 3299–3305.
49. Lee JY, Min HK, Moon MH (2011) Simultaneous profiling of lysophospholipids and phospholipids from human plasma by nanoflow liquid chromatography-tandem mass spectrometry. Anal Bioanal Chem 400: 2953–2961.

21

A Randomized Clinical Trial to Evaluate Two Doses of an Intra-Articular Injection of LMWF-5A in Adults with Pain Due to Osteoarthritis of the Knee

David Bar-Or[1,2,3,4*], Kristin M. Salottolo[1,2,3], Holli Loose[3], Matthew J. Phillips[5], Brian McGrath[5], Nathan Wei[6], James L. Borders[7], John E. Ervin[8], Alan Kivitz[9], Mark Hermann[10], Tammi Shlotzhauer[11], Melvin Churchill[12], Donald Slappey[13], Vaughan Clift[3]

1 Trauma Research Department, Swedish Medical Center, Englewood, Colorado, United States of America, **2** Trauma Research Department, St Anthony Hospital, Lakewood, Colorado, United States of America, **3** Ampio Pharmaceuticals, Inc., Greenwood Village, Colorado, United States of America, **4** Rocky Vista University, Aurora Colorado, United States of America, **5** University Orthopaedic Center, Amherst, New York, United States of America, **6** Arthritis Treatment Center, Frederick Maryland, United States of America, **7** Central Kentucky Research Associates, Lexington, Kentucky, United States of America, **8** Center for Pharmaceutical Research, Kansas City, Missouri, United States of America, **9** Altoona Center for Clinical Research, Duncansville, Pennsylvania, United States of America, **10** Danville Orthopeadic Clinic, Danville Virginia, United States of America, **11** Rochester Medical Research, Rochester, New York, United States of America, **12** Physician Research Collaboration, Lincoln Nebraska, United States of America, **13** Alabama Clinical Therapeutics, LLC, Birmingham, Alabama, United States of America

Abstract

Objective: The Low Molecular Weight Fraction of 5% human serum Albumin (LMWF-5A) is being investigated as a treatment for knee pain from osteoarthritis.

Methods: This was a multicenter randomized, vehicle-controlled, double-blind, parallel study designed to evaluate the safety and efficacy of two doses of an intra-articular injection of LMWF-5A. Patients with symptomatic knee osteoarthritis were randomized 1:1:1:1 to receive a single 4 mL or 10 mL intra-articular knee injection of either LMWF-5A or vehicle control (saline). The primary efficacy endpoint was the difference between treatment groups in the Western Ontario and McMaster Universities (WOMAC) pain change from baseline over 12 weeks. Safety was examined as the incidence and severity of adverse events (AEs).

Results: A total of 329 patients were randomized and received treatment. LMWF-5A resulted in a significant decrease in pain at 12 weeks compared to vehicle control (−0.93 vs −0.72; estimated difference from control: −0.25, $p=0.004$); an injection volume effect was not observed ($p=0.64$). The effect of LMWF-5A on pain was even more pronounced in patients with severe knee OA (Kellgren Lawrence Grade IV): the estimated difference from control was −0.42 ($p=0.02$). Adverse events were generally mild and were similar in patients who received vehicle control (47%) and LMWF-5A (41%).

Conclusions: This clinical trial demonstrated that LMWF-5A is safe and effective at providing relief for the pain of moderate to severe OA of the knee over 12 weeks when administered by intra-articular injection into the knee.

Trial Registration: ClinicalTrials.gov NCT01839331

Editor: Arvind Chopra, Center for Rheumatic Diseases, India

Funding: Financial support provided by Ampio Pharmaceuticals, Inc. The following authors (employees of Ampio Pharmaceuticals, Inc). had a role in the design and conduct of the study (DBO, HL, VC); interpretation of the data (KMS, VC); preparation, review, and approval of the manuscript (DBO, KMS, HL, VC); and decision to submit the manuscript for publication (DBO).

Competing Interests: The authors have the following interests: Financial support for this study was provided by Ampio Pharmaceuticals, Inc., the employer of David Bar-Or, Kristin M. Salottolo, Vaughan Clift and Holli Loose who have stock/stock options in the company. David Bar-Or is also a board member, and inventor of patents (not paid) at Ampio Pharmaceuticals, Inc. Brian McGrath and Matthew Phillips have stock/stock options in the company. Ampion (LMWF-5A) is a product of Ampio Pharmaceuticals. There are no marketed products related to this work. There are several patents and products in development related to this work. Please see the supporting information file for more details. Donald Slappey is an employee of Alabama Clinical Therapeutics, LLC. This does not alter the authors' adherence to all the PLOS ONE policies on sharing data and materials, as detailed online in the guide for authors.

* E-mail: dbaror@ampiopharma.com

Introduction

Osteoarthritis (OA) is the most common form of arthritis affecting a conservatively estimated 27 million Americans in 2008 [1]. Symptomatic OA of the knee occurs in approximately 12% of individuals over the age of 60 [2]. OA is caused by inflammation of the soft tissue and bony structures of the joint which worsens over time and leads to progressive thinning of articular cartilage, narrowing of the joint space, synovial membrane thickening, osteophyte formation and increased density of subchondral bone. These changes eventually result in chronic pain and disability, and despite drug therapy may eventually require surgery for total joint replacement [3].

Current drug treatment for OA of the knee relies on pain control with analgesics, anti-inflammatory treatment with non-steroidal anti-inflammatory drugs (NSAIDs), intra-articular (IA) corticosteroids, and IA hyaluronan products. The only evidence based treatment recommendations by the American Academy of Orthopaedic Surgeons (AAOS) for pain due to OA are self-management/physical activity, weight loss, and NSAIDs or Tramadol; patients with pain that is not controlled by these recommended treatments rely on non-recommended alternatives, or eventually knee replacement [4]. Therefore, there is a need for additional anti-inflammatory and analgesic treatments for OA, particularly as the population ages and the prevalence of obesity, a contributing factor to the development of OA, continues to rise [2,5,6,7].

Human Serum Albumin (HSA) has been commercially approved and in use for over 30 years. It has been safely administered intravenously to humans worldwide and has an excellent safety profile. In common clinical use, HSA is administered as a 5% solution in volumes of 100–500 mL per day in treatment for shock, burns, and plasma volume expansion [8,9,10].

The Low Molecular Weight Fraction of 5% HSA (LMWF-5A) has not previously been used for the indication of OA. The low molecular weight fraction (< 5,000 Da) of pharmaceutical HSA contains aspartyl-alanyl diketopiperazine (DA-DKP), which is formed after the dipeptide aspartate-alanine is cleaved from the N-terminus of albumin and cyclizes into a diketopiperazine [8,11,12,13,14]. DA-DKP has been shown to have multiple anti-inflammatory and immune modulating effects [12,13,15], and is believed to be one of the active ingredients in the pharmacological effects of commercial HAS.

LMWF-5A is being developed to provide relief for the pain of moderate to severe OA of the knee. A previous randomized, placebo-controlled, double-blind study conducted in 43 adults in Australia demonstrated that a single 4 mL IA injection of LMWF-5A is considered safe and well tolerated, and is efficacious at reducing pain in adults with OA of the knee (unpublished).

The purpose of this study was to investigate the safety and efficacy of two doses of a single IA knee injection of LMWF-5A on joint pain in OA of the knee. The primary trial objective was to evaluate the greater efficacy of 10 mL LMWF-5A versus 10 mL vehicle control than 4 mL LMWF-5A versus 4 mL vehicle control IA injection in improving knee pain, when applied to patients suffering from OA of the knee. The secondary trial objectives included: the safety of an IA injection of LMWF-5A, and the efficacy of an IA of LMWF-5A on stiffness, function, and overall disease severity.

Methods

Ethics statement

The study was performed in accordance with the principles of good clinical practice guidelines and received institutional review board (IRB) approval from the SUNY-Buffalo Health Sciences IRB and Liberty IRB; written informed consent was obtained from all participants involved in the study. Registration on ClinicalTrials.gov was initiated on March 25, 2013 and preceded patient recruitment (Identifier: NCT01839331).

Study design

We conducted a randomized, vehicle-controlled, double-blind, parallel study designed to evaluate the effect of two doses of a single IA knee injection of LMWF-5A in patients with symptomatic knee OA. The study was conducted at nine clinics across the United States, and consisted of a 28 day screening period and a 12 week participation period. Patients were enrolled and received treatment between March 29, 2013 and May 1, 2013, with follow-up through July 17, 2013.

Patient selection

Patients were recruited from the population being seen by Investigators at the clinics participating in the study. In addition, we recruited patients through notifications sent to referring physicians as well as radio and web-based campaigns.

Eligible patients were between the ages of 40 to 85 years old, fully ambulatory, with symptomatic index knee OA of at least 6 months preceding screening and a clinical diagnosis of OA supported by recent radiologic evidence within 6 months of screening, with moderate-to-severe OA pain in the index knee (baseline pain rating of ≥ 1.5 on the Western Ontario and McMaster Universities Arthritis Index (WOMAC®) osteoarthritis Index 3.1 5-point Likert pain subscale [16] without evidence of analgesia use 12 hours preceding screening/baseline efficacy measures, and no clinically significant liver abnormality.

Exclusion criteria included: A history of allergic reactions to albumin and its excipients; any human albumin treatment in the 3 months before randomization; concurrent arthritic conditions such as inflammatory or crystal arthropathies, previous major injury, and any other disease or condition interfering with the free use and evaluation of the index knee for the duration of the trial; any pharmacological or non-pharmacological treatment targeting OA started or changed during the 4 weeks prior to randomization; use of the following medications during the study: IA-injected pain medication or topical treatment in the index knee, analgesics containing opioids, significant anticoagulant therapy, immunosuppressants, systemic treatments, or corticosteroids > 10 mg prednisolone equivalent per day.

Randomization and blinding

If both knees were osteoarthritic, then at screening the investigator selected the knee that best satisfied the requirements for the study. In cases where both knees satisfied all inclusion and exclusion criteria, the study knee was selected based on greater baseline WOMAC A pain score. Patients were assigned to treatment by a sequential (by clinical site) randomization schedule in blocks of 4 following confirmation of eligibility before study medication was administered as a single intra-articular injection into the knee joint space (inferior lateral to the patella). Randomization was developed and maintained by an independent statistician. Treatments were provided in kits containing blinded study vials, syringes, needles and acetaminophen (rescue medication). The Sponsor, the investigator, and all study staff having a role in the day-to-day conduct of the study remained blinded to treatment.

Interventions

A total of 329 patients with OA knee pain were randomized 1:1:1:1 across 4 study arms: 4 mL LMWF-5A, 4 mL saline vehicle control, 10 mL LMWF-5A or 10 mL saline vehicle control.

The starting material of LMWF-5A, HSA purchased from OctaPharma (Lachen, Switzerland), was subjected to centrifugation/ultrafiltration under sterile conditions and the ultrafiltrate, containing species with a MW less than 5000 Da, was separated. The ultrafiltrate contained DA-DKP (approximately 50 – 200 μM) and the excipients (i.e. sodium caprylate and sodium acetyltryptophanate). The ultrafiltrate was transferred for aseptic filling, to afford sterile drug product. The control arm in this study was saline vehicle control, rather than a true 'placebo', as saline has been shown to induce significant pain relief, especially in trials involving intra-articular injections [17].

The clinical effects of treatment on OA were evaluated during clinic visits at 6 and 12 weeks and telephone contacts at 2, 4, 8 and 10 weeks, using the WOMAC® osteoarthritis Index 3.1 5-point Likert score, the Patient's Global Assessment of disease severity (PGA) using a 5-point Likert Score, and the amount of acetaminophen after intra-articular injection. Acetaminophen was supplied in 500 mg tablets at baseline as a rescue medication, and allowed as 1 tablet every 4 hours as needed.

Safety was evaluated by recording adverse events (through 24 hours post-dose and at all follow-up contacts), vital signs and physical examination results (baseline, weeks 6 and 12).

Outcomes

The primary endpoint was the change in the WOMAC average pain subscore by 5-point Likert scale between baseline and week 12. Both the Likert and VAS scales are validated[18]; the Likert scale may be more favorable over the VAS version[16,19].

Secondary endpoints included: the incidence and severity of AEs; change in the WOMAC average subscore by 5-point Likert scale for stiffness (WOMAC B subscore), physical function (WOMAC C subscore), and pain with movement and pain at rest (WOMAC A subscore questions 1–2 and 3–5, respectively); change in PGA; use of rescue analgesia (acetaminophen).

Power and sample size

We estimated the sample size based on the mean difference in the WOMAC A pain change from baseline at week 12 using a 2-way ANOVA. The estimate was based on detecting a treatment difference of 1.0 and 0.5 for 10 ml and 4 ml volumes, respectively (with a common SD of 0.9) using a 2 tailed alpha of 0.05. We estimated a sample size of 80 patients into each study arm for a total of 320 patients in a 1:1:1:1 ratio across all 4 study arms (4 mL vehicle control, 4 mL LMWF-5A, 10 mL vehicle control, 10 mL LMWF-5A) in order to achieve power of at least 80% to demonstrate both main effects (treatment effect, volume effect) or an interaction between the two main effects.

Statistical analysis

The primary endpoint, change in WOMAC A Pain subscore between baseline and week 12, was analysed using analysis of covariance (ANCOVA) to test the main effects of LMWF-5A vs vehicle control and 4 mL vs 10 mL, and their interaction. The WOMAC A baseline measure was used as the covariate; clinical site effect was non-significant, and therefore was not included (p = 0.42). Residuals of the model were assessed for normalcy and heteroscedasticity to ensure that the model was appropriate.

The following secondary endpoints were evaluated between treatment groups using a mixed-effects repeated measures ANCOVA, adjusted for the respective baseline value: change in WOMAC B stiffness, WOMAC C physical function, WOMAC A pain at rest, WOMAC A pain with movement, and PGA. The mixed-effects repeated measures ANCOVA covariance structure was modelled as first-order autoregressive with subject as a repeated effect, and treatment arm and time included in the model; the interaction between treatment arm and time was removed if not significant. Amount of rescue medication (overall pill count use of acetaminophen) followed a non-normal distribution and was analysed using a Wilcoxon rank-sum test; the study-wide mean pill count was used for imputation of missing data in 29 patients.

Adverse events were examined in all patients who were randomized and received study medication; no safety data was imputed. All efficacy analyses were performed in the intent-to-treat (ITT) population, defined as all patients who were randomized, received study medication and had at least one post-baseline observation. The ITT population was analyzed as randomized; data were imputed using a last observation carried forward approach (4.9% of missing data were imputed). The primary endpoint was also examined in subgroups according to Kellgren Lawrence Grade, and prior IA knee injection for pain due to OA.

Statistical analyses were performed using SAS® software, version 9.1.3 or later (SAS Institute, Cary, NC). All analyses were defined *a priori* and performed in accordance with the study Protocol and the Statistical Analysis Plan. The protocol and Statistical Analysis Plan for this trial and supporting CONSORT checklist are available as supporting information; see Checklist S1, Protocol S1 and SAP S1.There was no adjustment for multiple comparison testing; the change from baseline to week 12 was considered the primary endpoint, and all other time points were supportive. Statistical significance was set at p value < 0.05 for all analyses.

Results

Subject disposition, baseline data

Patient disposition can be seen in Figure 1, reported according to the CONSORT guidelines [20,21]. A total of 329 patients were enrolled and received treatment, as follows: LMWF-5A 4 mL (n = 83), LMWF-5A 10 mL (n = 82) vehicle control 4 mL (n = 83) and vehicle control 10 mL (n = 81).

Baseline data is shown in Table 1. Enrolled patients ranged in age from 41 to 84 years, of whom 63.5% were female and 90.9% were white. The Kellgren Lawrence Grade was Grade II for 35%, III for 42%, and IV for 22%. There were no differences between treatment groups in demographic characteristics, baseline WOMAC scores or PGA.

Treatment efficacy

LMWF-5A resulted in a statistically significant improvement in pain as compared to vehicle control (−0.93 vs −0.72, respectively), Table 2. An injection volume effect was not observed (p = 0.64). The estimated difference from control was −0.25 (95% CI: −0.08 – −0.41), p = 0.004. The reduction in pain with LMWF-5A compared to vehicle control was observed as early as week 4 (p = 0.03), and persisted to week 12 (p = 0.004). The percent reduction in pain over time was significantly greater for LMWF-5A as compared to vehicle control (week 12: 42.3% and 31.7%, respectively), Figure 2.

Patients treated with LMWF-5A demonstrated significant improvements in the following secondary endpoints, as compared to vehicle control: PGA (−0.87 vs −0.65, p = 0.01), physical function, (−0.78 vs −0.64, p = 0.04); pain at rest (−0.91 vs −0.70, p = 0.004); pain with movement (−0.96 vs −0.75, p = 0.01), Table 3. There were no differences in reduced stiffness between treatment groups. There was a trend towards a reduced number of acetaminophen pills used over the study period for LMWF-5A as compared to vehicle control (median (IQR)): 24.0 (0, 62) vs 34.0 (5, 85.5), p = 0.09.

Subgroup analyses

The effect of LMWF-5A was most pronounced in patients with severe knee OA (Table 3). In particular, LMWF-5A resulted in a significant improvement in pain in patients with severe OA

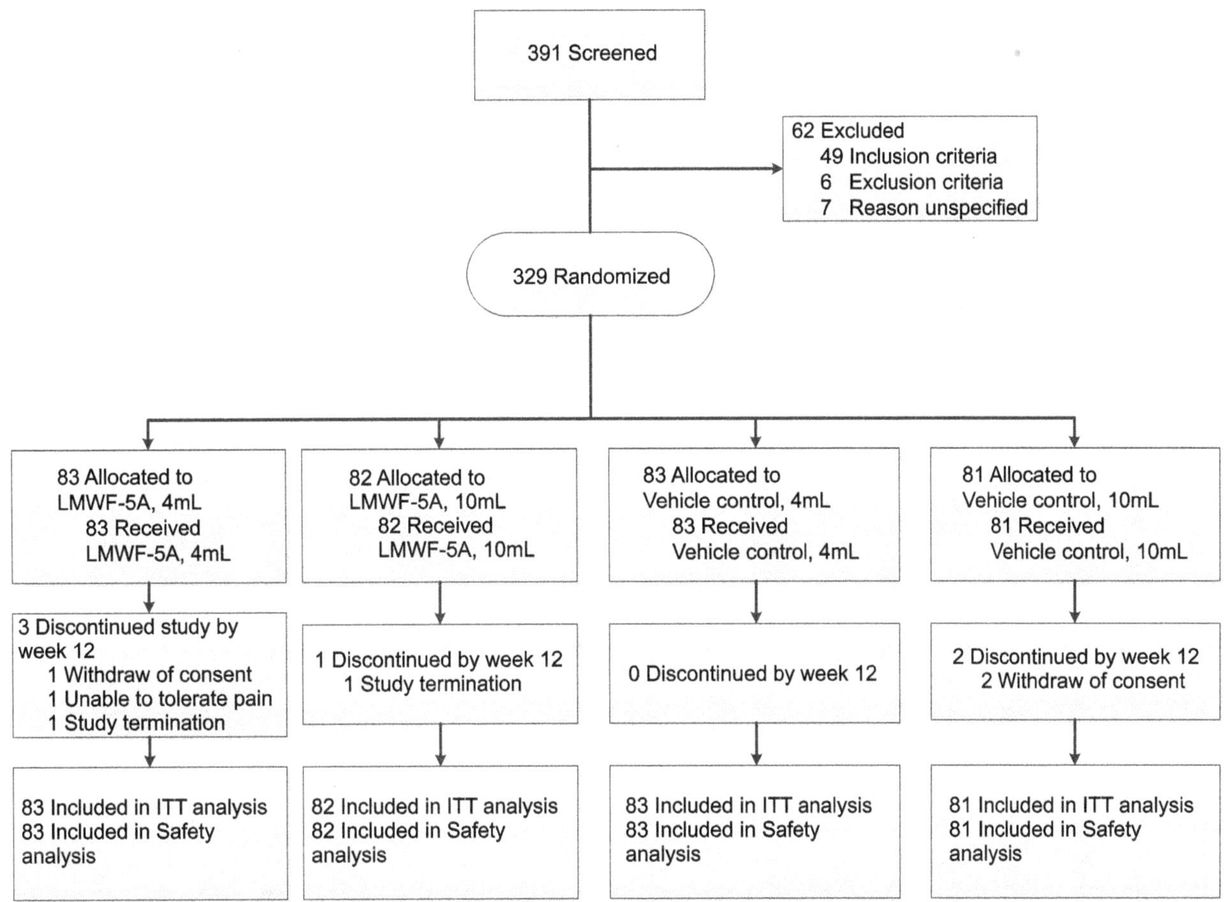

Figure 1. CONSORT Flow diagram.

(Kellgren Lawrence Grade IV), with an estimated difference from vehicle control of −0.42 (95% CI: −0.08 – −0.77), p = 0.02.

Patients with prior knee injection observed a significant improvement in mean pain with LMWF-5A as compared to vehicle control at week 12, while patients without prior knee injection saw a borderline significant improvement in pain with LMWF-5A as compared to vehicle control at week 12 (table 3).

Safety

Adverse events were reported for 144 patients (44%), and were similar in patients who received LMWF-5A (41%) and vehicle control (47%), Table 4. Only arthralgia was reported in at least 5% of patients (7% LMWF-5A, 15% vehicle control). AEs were generally mild; severe AEs were observed in 5% and 6% of patients treated with LMWF-5A and vehicle control, respectively. There were no deaths and no AEs resulting in treatment change or study discontinuation. There were 7 reported SAEs (2% incidence in both treatment groups); no SAE was considered related to study drug.

The percent of patients reporting treatment-related AEs was 10% with LMWF-5A and 13% with vehicle control; the most commonly occurring treatment-related AE was arthralgia (n = 17) and injection site pain (n = 7).

Discussion

This randomized clinical trial demonstrated that a single intra-articular injection of LMWF-5A is safe and effective at both 4 mL and 10 mL volumes. Our study represents a potential major breakthrough in identifying a treatment for pain due to moderate to severe OA. Our trial's primary and secondary efficacy endpoints of improvements in pain, function, and overall assessment of disease severity support significant efficacy of LMWF-5A. The clinically and statistically significant reduction in study outcomes with LMWF-5A was observed after only a single IA injection into the knee. Both treatments were well tolerated, with a low incidence of treatment-related adverse events.

This is the first published study to evaluate an intra-articular injection of the low molecular weight fraction of HSA (LMWF-5A) to patients with OA. This low molecular weight fraction of HSA has been extensively evaluated *in vitro* and *in vivo* for its contents and its anti-inflammatory properties. One of the active ingredients, DA-DKP, has been shown to have multiple anti-inflammatory and immune modulating effects [12,13,15]. In a previous unpublished randomized controlled trial of 43 patients, LMWF-5A was efficacious at reducing pain in adults with OA of the knee, and was well tolerated with only minor treatment-related AEs reported. LMWF-5A resulted in a trend towards a significant decrease in overall pain NRS at 12 weeks compared to placebo (−1.6 vs. −0.36, p = 0.07), which became statistically significant when patients who received betamethasone rescue injection after week 1 were excluded (−2.22 vs. −0.46, p = 0.04).

Intra-articular corticosteroids have been used historically for the treatment of OA, but they are believed to be associated with significant safety [22] and efficacy limitations [4,23]. Intra-articular hyaluronan products have been licensed in the USA for

Table 1. Demographics and baseline characteristics: ITT population.

	Randomized arms				Combined arms	
N (%)	**Control, 4 mL (N=83)**	**Control, 10 mL (N=81)**	**LMWF-5A, 4 mL (N=83)**	**LMWF-5A, 10 mL (N=81)**	**Control (N=164)**	**LMWF-5A (N=165)**
Female sex	57 (69%)	50 (62%)	56 (67%)	46 (56%)	107 (65%)	102 (62%)
White race	74 (89%)	77 (95%)	74 (89%)	74 (90%)	151 (92%)	148 (90%)
Hispanic	0 (0%)	2 (2%)	0 (0%)	2 (2%)	2 (1%)	2 (1%)
Age - Mean (SD)	60.7 (8.3)	63.8 (10.0)	62.7 (9.3)	62.8 (8.4)	62.2 (9.3)	62.7 (8.8)
BMI - Mean (SD)	34.5 (8.0)	32.1 (6.5)	33.2 (7.8)	32.8 (6.6)	33.3 (7.4)	33.0 (7.2)
Left study knee	42 (51%)	40 (49%)	35 (42%)	41 (50%)	82 (50%)	76 (46%)
Previous injection	58 (70%)	54 (67%)	49 (59%)	58 (71%)	112 (68%)	107 (65%)
Injection Type						
Steroid	32 (55%)	24 (44%)	25 (51%)	26 (45%)	56 (50%)	51 (48%)
Hyaluronic acid	20 (34%)	19 (35%)	17 (35%)	20 (34%)	39 (35%)	37 (35%)
Other	6 (10%)	11 (20%)	7 (14%)	12 (21%)	17 (15%)	19 (18%)
K-L Grade						
II	29 (35%)	26 (32%)	28 (34%)	32 (39%)	55 (34%)	60 (36%)
III	32 (39%)	34 (42%)	38 (46%)	35 (43%)	66 (40%)	73 (44%)
IV	22 (27%)	21 (26%)	17 (20%)	15 (18%)	42 (26%)	32 (19%)
PGA - Mean (SD)	3.4 (0.8)	3.4 (0.8)	3.4 (0.65)	3.4 (0.8)	3.4 (0.8)	3.4 (0.7)
WOMAC- Mean (SD)						
Pain	2.3 (0.5)	2.2 (0.6)	2.2 (0.5)	2.2 (0.5)	2.3 (0.5)	2.2 (0.5)
Stiffness	2.4 (0.8)	2.4 (0.8)	2.3 (0.7)	2.4 (0.8)	2.4 (0.8)	2.3 (0.8)
Function	2.3 (0.6)	2.2 (0.6)	2.1 (0.6)	2.2 (0.6)	2.2 (0.6)	2.2 (0.6)

Control, saline vehicle control; BMI, Body Mass Index; K-L Grade, Kellgren Lawrence Grade; PGA, Patient Global Assessment; WOMAC, Western Ontario and McMaster Universities Osteoarthritis Index.
The BMI is the weight in kilograms divided by the square of the height in meters. The PGA scores can range from 0 to 5. Scores for the WOMAC can range from 0 to 5.

the treatment of knee OA since 1997. However, the magnitude of the therapeutic effects of IA hyaluronan products on OA of the knee is controversial due to low trial quality, publication bias and questionable efficacy [7,24,25,26,27], with inconclusive recommendations from the AHRQ [28] and a strong recommendation against their use by the AAOS [4].

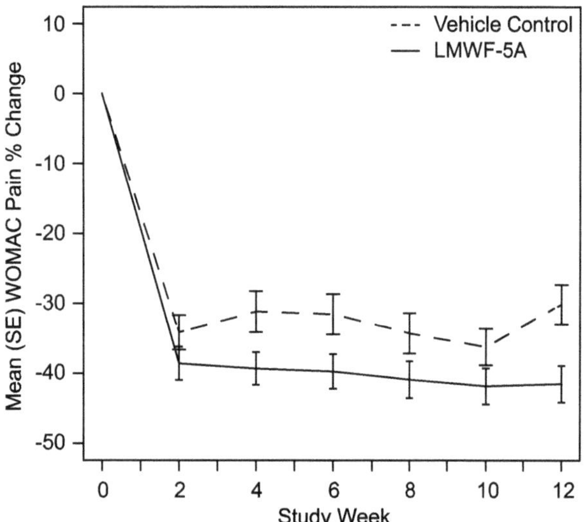

Figure 2. Summary of the percent improvement in the Western Ontario and McMaster Universities Osteoarthritis (WOMAC) pain subscore.

Despite recommendations against their use, Hylan G-F 20 is the current treatment of choice in patients who cannot be managed with analgesics. In the pivotal trial of a single IA injection of 6 ml Hylan G-F 20, a borderline statistically significant reduction in pain was demonstrated, with an estimated difference from control of −0.15 (95% CI: −0.30 to −0.002), p = 0.047), corresponding to a 31.3% improvement in pain over 26 weeks in patients treated with Hylan G-F20. In comparison, our study demonstrated that a single IA injection of LMWF-5A resulted in a clinically and statistically significant reduction in pain, with an estimated difference from control at the study endpoint of −0.25 (95% CI: −0.41 to −0.08), p = 0.004, corresponding to a 42.3% improvement in pain at 12 weeks in patients treated with LMWF-5A. The accepted threshold for a minimum clinically important improvement (MCII), defined as the smallest change in a measurement that signifies important improvement in a patient's symptom, is −40.8% in WOMAC A pain change from baseline with knee OA, which only LMWF-5A exceeded [29].

Our results were even more robust in patients with severe OA (Kellgren-Lawrence Grade IV), with a non-significant treatment effect in patients with minimal OA (Kellgren-Lawrence Grade II), a finding worth discussing. The severity of disease (i.e. pathology at presentation) appeared to result in differing treatment effects in our study. We believe our results are partially due to a pronounced saline effect in patients with minimal OA (Grade II), resulting in a

Table 2. Summary of the Western Ontario and McMaster Universities Osteoarthritis Index (WOMAC) Mean Change in Pain (SE) over Time.

	Randomized arms				Combined arms		
Week	**Control, 4 mL (n = 83)**	**Control, 10 mL (n = 81)**	**LMWF-5A, 4 mL (n = 83)**	**LMWF-5A, 10 mL (n = 82)**	**Control (n = 164)**	**LMWF-5A (n = 165)**	**p value†**
Week 2	−0.75 (0.08)	−0.88 (0.10)	−0.86 (0.08)	−0.90 (0.08)	−0.81 (0.06)	−0.88 (0.06)	.14
Week 4	−0.68 (0.10)	−0.83 (0.10)	−0.84 (0.08)	−0.93 (0.07)	−0.76 (0.07)	−0.88 (0.05)	**.03**
Week 6*	−0.71 (0.09)	−0.82 (0.11)	−0.88 (0.08)	−0.91 (0.08)	−0.77 (0.07)	−0.89 (0.06)	**.04**
Week 8	−0.74 (0.09)	−0.89 (0.11)	−0.92 (0.09)	−0.94 (0.09)	−0.81 (0.07)	−0.93 (0.06)	.06
Week 10	−0.79 (0.08)	−0.91 (0.10)	−0.97 (0.08)	−0.90 (0.09)	−0.85 (0.06)	−0.94 (0.06)	.11
Week 12*	−0.71 (0.08)	−0.73 (0.11)	−0.93 (0.08)	−0.92 (0.09)	−0.72 (0.07)	−0.93 (0.06)	**.004**

Control: Saline vehicle control.
*Data were collected at in-person clinic visits; data at all other Weeks were collected via telephone.
†P values were calculated using ANCOVA, with adjustment for baseline WOMAC A pain score.

non-significant reduction in pain for patients treated with LMWF-5A over saline placebo in this subgroup. The effect of saline was less pronounced in patients with moderate-to-severe OA, resulting in a clinically and statistically significant reduction in pain with LMWF-5A over saline. We believe LMWF-5A represents an alternative IA treatment, providing relief for the pain of moderate to severe OA of the knee, particularly in patients with severe OA in whom there are currently no pharmacologic treatments.

The primary limitation is that our study was designed to follow patients to 12 weeks following IA injection, which may not capture the maximum difference between groups. Systematic reviews of intra-articular injections suggest that the primary endpoint of change in pain is generally measured at 13–26 weeks for IA hyaluronan products [25] and at 4 weeks for IA corticosteroids [23], in which the maximum treatment effect was demonstrated at 5–13 weeks for IA hyaluronan products [25,30] and 2–3 weeks for IA corticosteroids [23]. In our study, patients treated with vehicle control observed an initial decrease in pain of −0.81 (36%) at week 2, which gradually worsened to −0.72 (32%) by week 12; on the contrary, patients treated with LMWF-5A observed an initial decrease in pain of −0.88 (40%) at week 2, with further decreases in pain of −0.93 (42%) by week 12. We are conducting an additional pivotal trial of LMWF-5A with a longer observation period of at least 20 weeks to identify maximum treatment effect. Secondarily, patients routinely present with bilateral OA, and it is likely that efficacy measures may be affected by pain due to OA of the contra lateral (non-treated) knee. We did not record the presence of bilateral OA in this study, and thus cannot determine whether the treatment effect differed between patients with unilateral vs. bilateral OA. Lastly, we included all patients with radiologic OA, defined by Kellgren Lawrence Grades II, III and IV [31]. Patients with varying stages of disease severity present with differing pathologies; the pathology at presentation may result in a different treatment effect at each severity grade. While this heterogeneity of our population may be considered a potential limitation, we believe this to also be a strength of our study, making it more generalizable than previously published studies of intra-articular injection for treatment of OA of the knee.

Table 3. Summary of Additional Efficacy endpoints, reported as Mean Change (SE) at Week 12, ITT.

Mean (SE) change	**Control, 4 mL (n = 83)**	**Control, 10 mL (n = 81)**	**LMWF-5A, 4 mL (n = 83)**	**LMWF-5A, 10 mL (n = 82)**	**Control (n = 164)**	**LMWF-5A (n = 165)**	**p value†**
			Secondary efficacy endpoint				
Stiffness*	−0.55 (0.10)	−0.80 (0.11)	−0.66 (0.10)	−0.79 (0.10)	−0.67 (0.08)	−0.72 (0.07)	.41
Physical function*	−0.58 (0.08)	−0.69 (0.11)	−0.72 (0.09)	−0.83 (0.09)	−0.64 (0.07)	−0.78 (0.06)	**.04**
Resting pain*	−0.71 (0.09)	−0.68 (0.11)	−0.90 (0.09)	−0.91 (0.09)	−0.70 (0.07)	−0.91 (0.06)	**.004**
Moving Pain*	−0.69 (0.09)	−0.81 (0.11)	−0.98 (0.09)	−0.94 (0.10)	−0.75 (0.07)	−0.96 (0.07)	**.01**
PGA subscale	−0.55 (0.12)	−0.74 (0.13)	−0.96 (0.11)	−0.77 (0.13)	−0.65 (0.09)	−0.87 (0.08)	**.01**
			Subgroup population, WOMAC A Pain				
Prior injection	−0.66 (0.10)	−0.71 (0.12)	−0.81 (0.12)	−0.87 (0.11)	−0.68 (0.08)	−0.84 (0.08)	**.04**
No prior injection	−0.82 (0.15)	−0.77 (0.22)	−1.11 (0.11)	−1.05 (0.13)	−0.80 (0.13)	−1.09 (0.08)	.051
K-L Grade II	−0.83 (0.15)	−1.01 (0.22)	−0.94 (0.12)	−1.07 (0.14)	−0.92 (0.13)	−1.01 (0.09)	.70
K-L Grade III	−0.62 (0.11)	−0.76 (0.14)	−0.95 (0.13)	−0.82 (0.15)	−0.69 (0.09)	−0.89 (0.10)	**.04**
K-L Grade IV	−0.67 (0.19)	−0.34 (0.21)	−0.88 (0.22)	−0.83 (0.16)	−0.51 (0.14)	−0.86 (0.14)	**.02**

*WOMAC, Western Ontario and McMaster Universities Osteoarthritis.
Control: Saline vehicle control; Index. PGA, Patient Global Assessment of disease severity; K-L, Kellgren-Lawrence.
†P values were calculated using mixed-effects repeated measures ANCOVA, with adjustment for baseline score.

Table 4. Summary of Adverse Events (AEs).

n (%)	Randomized arms				Combined arms	
	Control, 4 mL (n = 83)	**Control, 10 mL (n = 81)**	**LMWF-5A, 4 mL (n = 83)**	**LMWF-5A, 10 mL (n = 82)**	**Control (n = 164)**	**LMWF-5A (n = 165)**
Overall summary of AEs						
Any AE	41 (49%)	36 (44%)	35 (42%)	32 (39%)	77 (47%)	67 (41%)
Any Related AE	13 (16%)	8 (10%)	9 (11%)	8 (10%)	21 (13%)	17 (10%)
Any severe AE	5 (6%)	5 (6%)	5 (6%)	3 (4%)	10 (6%)	8 (5%)
Any SAE	2 (2%)	2 (2%)	0 (0%)	3 (4%)	4 (2%)	3 (2%)
Any Related SAE	0 (0%)	0 (0%)	0 (0%)	0 (0%)	0 (0%)	0 (0%)
Related AEs, by preferred term, descending order						
Arthralgia	7 (8%)	3 (4%)	3 (4%)	4 (5%)	10 (6%)	7 (4%)
Injection site pain	2 (2%)	2 (2%)	2 (2%)	1 (1%)	4 (2%)	3 (2%)
Headache	3 (4%)	1 (1%)	1 (1%)		4 (2%)	1 (< 1%)
Joint stiffness	2 (2%)		1 (1%)	2 (2%)	2 (1%)	3 (2%)
Joint swelling		1 (1%)		1 (1%)	2 (1%)	1 (< 1%)
Flushing	1 (1%)			1 (1%)	1 (< 1%)	1 (< 1%)
Nausea		1 (1%)	1 (1%)		1 (< 1%)	1 (< 1%)
Anxiety	1 (1%)				1 (< 1%)	
Injection site joint pain	1 (1%)				1 (< 1%)	
Muscle spasms	1 (1%)				1 (< 1%)	
Musculoskeletal discomfort	1 (1%)				1 (< 1%)	
Myalgia				1 (1%)		1 (< 1%)
Osteoarthritis			1 (1%)			1 (< 1%)
Urticaria				1 (1%)		1 (< 1%)

In conclusion, this randomized, controlled clinical trial demonstrated that a single intra-articular injection of LMWF-5A is a safe and effective treatment for osteoarthritis. Our results demonstrate improvements in pain and function, as well as overall disease severity with LMWF-5A as compared to vehicle control. These findings represent a potential major breakthrough in identifying a treatment for pain due to osteoarthritis, particularly in patients with severe osteoarthritis where no other safe and effective therapies exists prior to joint replacement.

Supporting Information

Protocol S1 Protocol AP-003A (Version 2.0, 15 May 2013).

SAP S1 Statistical Analysis Plan AP-003-A (Version 2.0, 8 August 2013).

Checklist S1 CONSORT 2010 checklist of information to include when reporting a randomised trial.

Issued Patents S1 Issued Patents for "AMPION", as of December 5, 2013.

Acknowledgments

We would like to acknowledge the following for their role in the clinical trial: Promedica International and Gerard Smits, PhD for the conduct and management of the study, acquisition of data, and data analysis.

Author Contributions

Conceived and designed the experiments: DBO VC HL. Performed the experiments: BM MJP NW JLB JEE AK MH TS MC DS. Analyzed the data: KMS VC. Wrote the paper: KMS DBO.

References

1. Lawrence RC, Felson DT, Helmick CG, Arnold LM, Choi H, et al. (2008) Estimates of the prevalence of arthritis and other rheumatic conditions in the United States. Part II. Arthritis and rheumatism 58: 26–35.
2. Dillon CF, Rasch EK, Gu Q, Hirsch R (2006) Prevalence of knee osteoarthritis in the United States: arthritis data from the Third National Health and Nutrition Examination Survey 1991-94. The Journal of rheumatology 33: 2271–2279.
3. Quintana JM, Arostegui I, Escobar A, Azkarate J, Goenaga JI, et al. (2008) Prevalence of knee and hip osteoarthritis and the appropriateness of joint replacement in an older population. Archives of internal medicine 168: 1576–1584.
4. American Academy of Orthopaedic Surgeons (2013) Treatment of osteoarthritis of the knee: Evidence-based guideline. 2nd ed. Rosemont, IL: American Academy of Orthopaedic Surgeons.
5. Dunlop DD, Manheim LM, Song J, Chang RW (2001) Arthritis prevalence and activity limitations in older adults. Arthritis and rheumatism 44: 212–221.
6. Guccione AA, Felson DT, Anderson JJ, Anthony JM, Zhang Y, et al. (1994) The effects of specific medical conditions on the functional limitations of elders in the Framingham Study. American journal of public health 84: 351–358.
7. Zhang W, Nuki G, Moskowitz RW, Abramson S, Altman RD, et al. (2010) OARSI recommendations for the management of hip and knee osteoarthritis: part III: Changes in evidence following systematic cumulative update of research

published through January 2009. Osteoarthritis and cartilage/OARS, Osteoarthritis Research Society 18: 476–499.

8. Bar-Or D, Bar-Or R, Rael LT, Gardner DK, Slone DS, et al. (2005) Heterogeneity and oxidation status of commercial human albumin preparations in clinical use. Critical care medicine 33: 1638–1641.
9. Evans TW (2002) Review article: albumin as a drug–biological effects of albumin unrelated to oncotic pressure. Alimentary pharmacology & therapeutics 16 Suppl 5: 6–11.
10. Quinlan GJ, Martin GS, Evans TW (2005) Albumin: biochemical properties and therapeutic potential. Hepatology 41: 1211–1219.
11. Bar-Or D, Rael LT, Lau EP, Rao NK, Thomas GW, et al. (2001) An analog of the human albumin N-terminus (Asp-Ala-His-Lys) prevents formation of copper-induced reactive oxygen species. Biochemical and biophysical research communications 284: 856–862.
12. Bar-Or D, Thomas GW, Bar-Or R, Rael LT, Scarborough K, et al. (2006) Commercial human albumin preparations for clinical use are immunosuppressive in vitro. Critical care medicine 34: 1707–1712.
13. Shimonkevitz R, Thomas G, Slone DS, Craun M, Mains C, et al. (2008) A diketopiperazine fragment of human serum albumin modulates T-lymphocyte cytokine production through rap1. The Journal of trauma 64: 35–41.
14. Bar-Or D, Slone DS, Mains CW, Rael LT (2013) Dipeptidyl peptidase IV activity in commercial solutions of human serum albumin. Analytical biochemistry 441: 13–17.
15. Rael LT, Bar-Or R, Shimonkevitz R, Mains CW, Slone DS, et al. (2010) Anti-inflammatory effect of a diketopiperazine by-product of commercial albumin in TBI patients [abstract]. J Neurotrauma 27: A1–A97.
16. Bellamy N, Buchanan WW, Goldsmith CH, Campbell J, Stitt LW (1988) Validation study of WOMAC: a health status instrument for measuring clinically important patient relevant outcomes to antirheumatic drug therapy in patients with osteoarthritis of the hip or knee. The Journal of rheumatology 15: 1833–1840.
17. Zhang W, Robertson J, Jones AC, Dieppe PA, Doherty M (2008) The placebo effect and its determinants in osteoarthritis: meta-analysis of randomised controlled trials. Annals of the rheumatic diseases 67: 1716–1723.
18. Bellamy N (2002) WOMAC Osteoarthritis Index User Guide. Version V. Brisbane, Australia.
19. Kersten P, White PJ, Tennant A (2010) The visual analogue WOMAC 3.0 scale–internal validity and responsiveness of the VAS version. BMC musculoskeletal disorders 11: 80.
20. Moher D, Hopewell S, Schulz KF, Montori V, Gotzsche PC, et al. (2010) CONSORT 2010 explanation and elaboration: updated guidelines for reporting parallel group randomised trials. BMJ 340: c869.
21. Schulz KF, Altman DG, Moher D (2010) CONSORT 2010 statement: updated guidelines for reporting parallel group randomised trials. BMJ 340: c332.
22. Cole BJ, Schumacher Jr HR (2005) Injectable corticosteroids in modern practice. The Journal of the American Academy of Orthopaedic Surgeons 13: 37–46.
23. Bellamy N, Campbell J, Robinson V, Gee T, Bourne R, et al. (2006) Intraarticular corticosteroid for treatment of osteoarthritis of the knee. Cochrane database of systematic reviews: CD005328.
24. Arrich J, Piribauer F, Mad P, Schmid D, Klaushofer K, et al. (2005) Intra-articular hyaluronic acid for the treatment of osteoarthritis of the knee: systematic review and meta-analysis. CMAJ: Canadian Medical Association journal = journal de l'Association medicale canadienne 172: 1039–1043.
25. Bellamy N, Campbell J, Robinson V, Gee T, Bourne R, et al. (2006) Viscosupplementation for the treatment of osteoarthritis of the knee. Cochrane database of systematic reviews: CD005321.
26. Lo GH, LaValley M, McAlindon T, Felson DT (2003) Intra-articular hyaluronic acid in treatment of knee osteoarthritis: a meta-analysis. JAMA: the journal of the American Medical Association 290: 3115–3121.
27. Printz JO, Lee JJ, Knesek M, Urquhart AG (2013) Conflict of Interest in the Assessment of Hyaluronic Acid Injections for Osteoarthritis of the Knee: An Updated Systematic Review. The Journal of arthroplasty.
28. (2007) Three Treatments for Osteoarthritis of the Knee: Evidence Shows Lack of Benefit. Comparative Effectiveness Review Summary Guides for Clinicians. Rockville (MD).
29. Tubach F, Ravaud P, Baron G, Falissard B, Logeart I, et al. (2005) Evaluation of clinically relevant changes in patient reported outcomes in knee and hip osteoarthritis: the minimal clinically important improvement. Annals of the rheumatic diseases 64: 29–33.
30. Bannuru RR, Natov NS, Dasi UR, Schmid CH, McAlindon TE (2011) Therapeutic trajectory following intra-articular hyaluronic acid injection in knee osteoarthritis–meta-analysis. Osteoarthritis and cartilage/OARS, Osteoarthritis Research Society 19: 611–619.
31. Kellgren JH, Lawrence JS (1957) Radiological assessment of osteo-arthrosis. Annals of the rheumatic diseases 16: 494–502.

Melanocortin 1 Receptor-Signaling Deficiency Results in an Articular Cartilage Phenotype and Accelerates Pathogenesis of Surgically Induced Murine Osteoarthritis

Julia Lorenz[1,7], **Elisabeth Seebach[2]**, **Gerit Hackmayer[1,6]**, **Carina Greth[2]**, **Richard J. Bauer[3]**, **Kerstin Kleinschmidt[4]**, **Dominik Bettenworth[5]**, **Markus Böhm[6]**, **Joachim Grifka[7]**, **Susanne Grässel[1,7]***

1 Experimental Orthopedics, University Hospital of Regensburg, Regensburg, Bavaria, Germany, **2** Research Centre for Experimental Orthopedics, Orthopedic University Hospital Heidelberg, Heidelberg, Baden-Württemberg, Germany, **3** Oral and Maxillofacial Surgery, University Hospital of Regensburg, Regensburg, Bavaria, Germany, **4** TIP Immunology, Merck Serono Global Research & Development, Darmstadt, Hessen, Germany, **5** Medical Hospital B, University Hospital of Münster, Münster, North Rhine-Westphalia, Germany, **6** Dermatology, University Hospital of Münster, Münster, North Rhine-Westphalia, Germany, **7** Orthopedic Surgery, University Hospital of Regensburg, Bad Abbach, Bavaria, Germany

Abstract

Proopiomelanocortin-derived peptides exert pleiotropic effects via binding to melanocortin receptors (MCR). MCR-subtypes have been detected in cartilage and bone and mediate an increasing number of effects in diathrodial joints. This study aims to determine the role of MC1-receptors (MC1) in joint physiology and pathogenesis of osteoarthritis (OA) using MC1-signaling deficient mice (Mc1re/e). OA was surgically induced in Mc1re/e and wild-type (WT) mice by transection of the medial meniscotibial ligament. Histomorphometry of Safranin O stained articular cartilage was performed with non-operated controls (11 weeks and 6 months) and 4/8 weeks past surgery. μCT–analysis for assessing epiphyseal bone architecture was performed as a longitudinal study at 4/8 weeks after OA-induction. Collagen II, ICAM-1 and MC1 expression was analysed by immunohistochemistry. Mc1re/e mice display less Safranin O and collagen II stained articular cartilage area compared to WT prior to OA-induction without signs of spontaneous cartilage surface erosion. This MC1-signaling deficiency related cartilage phenotype persisted in 6 month animals. At 4/8 weeks after OA-induction cartilage erosions were increased in Mc1re/e knees paralleled by weaker collagen II staining. Prior to OA-induction, Mc1re/e mice do not differ from WT with respect to bone parameters. During OA, Mc1re/e mice developed more osteophytes and had higher epiphyseal bone density and mass. Trabecular thickness was increased while concomitantly trabecular separation was decreased in Mc1re/e mice. Numbers of ICAM-positive chondrocytes were equal in non-operated 11 weeks Mc1re/e and WT whereas number of positive chondrocytes decreased during OA-progression. Unchallenged Mc1re/e mice display smaller articular cartilage covered area without OA-related surface erosions indicating that MC1-signaling is critical for proper cartilage matrix integrity and formation. When challenged with OA, Mc1re/e mice develop a more severe OA-pathology. Our data suggest that MC1-signaling protects against cartilage degradation and subchondral bone sclerosis in OA indicating a beneficial role of the POMC system in joint pathophysiology.

Editor: Luc Malaval, Université Jean Monnet, France

Funding: This work was funded by the DFG, and the grant No. GR1301/9-1 was assigned to SG and MB. The funders had no role in study design, data collection and analysis, decision to publish, or preparation of the manuscript.

Competing Interests: Neither Merck nor KK have any conflict of interest with the data published in the manuscript. KK was involved in the work done independently from Merck, only because of KK's expertise in microCT imaging. The work that KK contributed was done while employed at Merck, but at KK's former employer (Research Centre for Experimental Orthopaedics, Heidelberg University Hospital, Germany) during free time. Neither Merck nor KK have any financial interest in the work or outcomes described nor has Merck funded any of the work done. Merck has as to KK's knowledge no patents that are related to the content of the manuscript. Please note that even though KK is employed by Merck SG can assure that this does not alter adherence to PLOS ONE policies on sharing data and materials.

* Email: susanne.graessel@klinik.uni-regensburg.de

These authors contributed equally to this work.

Introduction

Osteoarthritis is an age-related and/or trauma-induced multifactorial, slowly progressing degenerative disorder of the synovial joints culminating in the irreversible destruction of the articular cartilage. Clinical symptoms of OA appear in more than 10% of the world population affecting almost everyone over the age of 65. As a consequence of the increasing longevity and obesity in the European Community, the burden caused by OA rapidly grows substantially influencing life quality of the affected individuals with enormous costs to the health care system. Current therapeutic strategies seek to ameliorate pain and increase mobility, however, to date none of them halts disease progression or regenerates damaged cartilage. Thus, there is an ultimate need for the development of non-invasive treatments that could substitute joint replacement. OA exact aetiology is still unclear. Genetic disorders, limb mal-alignment and overuse as well as metabolic problems (obesity, immune responses, inflammation) play an important role in the onset of OA. [1–4]. Besides chondrocytes and cartilage as mediators of OA also other cells and tissues of the joint like synovium or subchondral bone modulate OA-pathogenesis. Subchondral bone and articular cartilage are separated through the tide mark region and have a close relationship during progression of OA. Abnormal calcification of this tide mark region during OA leads to a decrease in cartilage thickness and increased subchondral plate thickness [5] preceded by increased turnover of subchondral bone, thinning trabecular structures, sclerosis of the subchondral plate, bone marrow lesions and subchondral bone cysts [6,7]. Alterations in subchondral bone remodeling add to biomechanical changes and enhance OA progression [8,9].

Proopiomelanocortin (POMC) is a multifunctional precursor protein for several biologically active hormones which include the melanocyte-stimulating hormones (α-, β- and γ-MSH) and adrenocorticotropic hormone (ACTH). These peptides play an important role in a diversity of physiological processes including energy homeostasis, adrenal function, sexual activity, thermoregulation, nociception, exocrine gland activity, immune function, and pigmentation. Although originally characterized as neurohormones induced by stressful signals in context of the classical hypothalamic-pituitary-adrenal (HPA) stress axis, it is now established that POMC and its derived peptides can also be autonomously generated in a number of peripheral tissues, e. g. the skin and diathrodial joints. Here, receptors for POMC peptides, the melanocortin receptors (MCR) have been identified in various resident cell types where they elicit biological effects far beyond the initially identified action of their ligands. A very fascinating aspect of POMC-derived peptides is their immunomodulatory potential, especially that of melanocortin-derived peptides [10–12].

The melanocortin peptides ACTH as well as α-, β- and γ-MSH bind with high affinity to melanocortin receptors [13]. Five MCR subtypes, MC1 to MC5, have been cloned and which bind melanocortins with different affinities. With respect to diathrodial joints, initially the MC3 was detected in rat bone marrow stroma-like cells and in chondrocytes isolated from ribcages of young rats [14]. Our group recently demonstrated the presence of MC1, MC2 and MC5 transcripts in human articular chondrocytes derived from patients with OA [15]. Protein expression of the MC1 in these cells was confirmed on OA cartilage explants. Here, chondrocytes located in the middle and deep cartilage layers were immuno-reactive for MC1 while chondrocytes in the superficial zone were mostly negative. Treatment of these chondrocytes with α-MSH was associated with functional coupling as shown by cAMP assays but not with a Ca^{2+} response. The detection of MC1 in human articular chondrocytes is in accordance with the observation that also a human chondrosarcoma cell line, likewise expresses functional MC1 [16]. In addition, transcripts of all five MCR were found in normal human osteoblasts as well as in MG63 and SAOS-2 osteosarcoma cells, albeit not all receptors were present in each cell type [17].

For analyzing the role of the MC1 in pathogenesis of OA, we have induced OA surgically in mice using the model of destabilization of the medial meniscus (DMM) as it induces OA with great ease and reproducibility. It is less invasive than the anterior cruciate ligament transaction (ACLT) procedure and resembles more closely slowly progressive human OA. It has been shown to be sufficiently sensitive to detect significant protection against OA progression in ADAMTS-5 and IL-1β knockout joints at 4–8 weeks following DMM [18,19]. We assume that the DMM-OA model will thus be sensitive enough to allow evaluation of the hypothesized chondroprotective role of endogenously expressed Mc1r in murine articular cartilage.

As a tool for analysis of the melanocortin system in OA, we have used yellow colored MC1 signaling-deficient (Mc1*re/e*) mice. The Mc1*re/e*- recessive yellow allele (e) results from a frameshift between the IV. and V. transmembrane domain that produces a prematurely terminated, non-functioning MC1 which does not functionally couple to adenylate cyclase [20] but is still expressed and transported to the cell membrane.

Materials and Methods

Mouse model

To evaluate the role of MC1 signaling during osteoarthritis pathogenesis, Mc1re/e mice on a C57BL/6 background were used [20]. C57BL/6 mice (Charles River) served as wild type (WT) control group.

Study design

Right knees of Mc1re/e mice and WT received DMM while left knee served as sham control with just the surgical access set. Cartilage matrix was evaluated after histological assessment with scoring [21] and histomorphometry whereas changes in subchondral bone were evaluated with X-ray scoring and µCT. The experimental protocol was approved by the local animal experimental ethics committee (Az.: 54-2532.1-36/11) and all procedures were performed according to the European Laboratory Animal Science Guidelines.

For histological assessment, 22 male WT and 21 male Mc1re/e mice were included in study. 11 weeks (5 WT, 4 Mc1re/e) and 6 months (5 WT, 5 Mc1re/e) old, male mice received no DMM and represent non-operated control group whereas 12 WT and 12 Mc1re/e received DMM (6 WT and 6 Mc1re/e mice for 4 and 8 weeks each). To analyze OA progression, Safranin O/Fast green stained knee joint sections were scored and evaluated morphometrically.

For X-ray scoring and µCT analysis, 7 WT (2 female, 5 male) and 7 Mc1re/e (2 female, 5 male) mice received DMM. Changes in epiphyseal bone micro-architecture and osteophyte number were assessed directly before surgery (day 0) and 4 and 8 weeks after OA-induction.

Surgically induced osteoarthritis

10–11 week old mice were anaesthetized by intraperitoneal injection of ketamine-hydrochloride (90–120 mg/kg body weight, Bela-pharma, Vechta) and Xylazin (6–8 mg/kg body weight, Serumwerk Bernburg). DMM was performed as described previously [19] from Dr. med. vet. Gerit Hackmayer (doctor of veterinary medicine). In both knees, a 3 mm longitudinal incision between the distal patella and proximal tibia plateau was set and the joint capsule was opened medial to the patellar tendon. In the right knee, the medial meniscotibial ligament (MMTL) was carefully transected, while in left knee MMTL was visualized but not transected (sham surgery). Joint capsule, subcutaneous layer and skin were closed and mice were allowed full activity. Mice were administered subcutaneous sodium chloride infusion (10 ml/kg body weight) and Buprenorphin (0.09 mg/kg body weight, Bayer vital) 12 and 24 h after operation in a longitudinal study.

Histological preparation, OA-scoring and histomorphometry

For histological preparation and morphometry, we correspond mainly to the recommendation of OARSI [21]. Knee joints were fixed for 18–24 h in 4% paraformaldehyde and decalcified with 25% EDTA for 2 weeks at room temperature and embedded in paraffin. 5 µm frontal sections through the weight bearing area of each knee joint were taken. 5–6 sections in 60–80 µm intervals from 6 mice per time point were stained with Safranin O, Weigerts iron haematoxylin and fast green and scored by two independent observers.

Additionally, histomorphometry was performed with the same sections used for OA-scoring using graphic tablet Bamboo (Wacom) and image J software (NIH, Bethesda). On sections of knee joints from non-operated mice, total cartilage area was determined in pixel. On sections of knee joints from non-operated mice, 4 and 8 weeks after OA-induction, total articular cartilage area and cartilage area without cells/Safranin O staining (destroyed cartilage) was determined in pixel. Destroyed cartilage area was related to total cartilage area which was set as 100%.

For both methods medial regions of the knee joints were analyzed and mean values of femur and tibia scores were included in statistical analysis.

Localization of MC1, collagen II, matrix metalloproteinase 13 (MMP-13), aggrecan neoepitope DIPEN(341)/(342)FFGVG (DIPEN) and intracellular adhesion molecule 1(ICAM-1)

For each antigen, 1–3 representative sections in the weight bearing area of 4–6 different mice per time point were chosen and included in staining. For immunostaining of MC1, collagen II, MMP-13, DIPEN and ICAM-1, following antibodies were used: rabbit anti-mouse mc1r [22], mouse anti-mouse collagen II (DSHB), rabbit-anti MMP-13 (Abcam), rabbit anti-DIPEN (a generous gift from Amanda Fosang (University of Melbourne)) and rabbit-anti-ICAM (BioVision).

Sections were deparaffinized, rehydrated and endogenous peroxidase activity was blocked with 3% H_2O_2 for 5 min at RT. For MC1, collagen II, MMP-13 and DIPEN staining, sections were pre-incubated with protease XXIV (0.05% in PBS for 10 min at 37°C, Sigma-Aldrich) and with testicular hyaluronidase (0.1% in acetate buffer pH 6.0 for 90 min at 37°C, Sigma-Aldrich). For staining of specimen with antibodies against ICAM, heat induced epitope retrieval was performed for 20 min at 98 °C in 10 mM sodium citrate buffer, pH 6.0. This was followed by a cooling period at room temperature for 20 min.

Sections were incubated over night at 4°C with MC1, MMP-13, DIPEN or ICAM-1 antibodies (1:75 dilution in blocking solution for MC1-ab, 1:600 for MMP-13-ab, 1:5000 for DIPEN-ab and 1:100 for ICAM-1-ab), after blocking with 1% bovine serum albumin (Biomol) and 5% swine serum (Dako). 1 h incubation with a biotinylated swine anti-rabbit (1:500 diluted in PBS, Dako) was followed by an incubation with streptavidin-peroxidase and buffered substrate solution containing H_20_2 and 3,3-diaminobenzidine chromogen solution (Dako). The secondary antibody for the ICAM-1-staining was provided with the Envision kit (Dako) according to manufacturer's instruction (incubation time was 30 min). Sections were counterstained with hematoxylin modified after Gil (Merck), dehydrated and mounted.

For staining of sections with antibodies against collagen II, a commercial biotinylation kit was used according to manufactor's instructions (Dako) with a 1:125 dilution of primary antibody. Sections were counterstained with Weigert's hematoxylin, dehydrated and mounted.

For MC1, collagen II, MMP-13, DIPEN and ICAM-1 staining, images from both groups of each condition were compared and evaluated microscopically. To quantify collagen II, MMP-13, DIPEN and ICAM-1 stained sections, a scoring system was applied. For collagen II stained sections, percentage of stained cartilage area (see Tab. 1), for MMP-13 staining, percentage of positive non-hypertrophic articular chondrocytes (see Tab. 2) and for ICAM-1 and DIPEN, percentage of stained articular chondrocytes was estimated (see Tab. 3). To evaluate scoring systems for collagen II, MMP-13, DIPEN and ICAM-1 staining, intra- and inter-observer agreement was determined with cohens kappa coefficients. Therefore 7 independent observers scored 10 frontal sections of each staining and 4 of them scored the same images after 1 week again. To score the images, observers got no further information except for scoring tables (Tab. 1–3) and 4 exemplary images with scores according to [21] (Fig. S4).

Sections incubated with appropriate isotype control antibody served as negative control and showed no staining (Fig. S1).

X-ray Scoring

Mice were scanned under anesthesia by intraperitoneal injection of ketamine hydrochloride (Ketavet: 120 mg/kg body weight, Pfizer, Berlin, Germany) und medetomidine hydrochloride (Domitor: 0.5 mg/kg body weight, Orion Pharma, Hamburg, Germany) in the Sky-Scan 1076 in vivo x-ray microtomograph (Skyscan, Antwerpen). Anesthesia was antagonized after µCT-scan by subcutaneous administration of atipamezole hydrochloride (Antisedan: 2.5 mg/kg body weight, Orion Pharma, Hamburg, Germany). 2 Mc1re/e mice died due to anesthesia reducing the group size to 5 mice (1 female, 4 male). Legs were hold in a stretched position by a small styrofoam cylinder taped between hind legs. Following settings were used for µCT analysis: 1 mm aluminium filter, voxel size 8.85 µm, voltage 40 kV, current 250 µA, exposure time 2550 ms, frame averaging 2 [23]. Data were recorded every 1.5 degree rotation step through 180 degrees. Both legs were scanned in the same scan session and a shutter was set to reduce X-ray exposure time ($<$20 min).

Micro-CT analysis

Reconstruction of X-ray scans was performed using NRecon software (version 1.6.3.2, Skyscan). Datasets were separated using DataViewer (Skyscan). Knees were manually analyzed for osteophytes based on the reconstructed images in transaxial, sagittal and coronal plane. Osteophytes were defined as abnormal bony projections along the bony margin of the knee joints appearing after 4 and 8 weeks of OA progression. Presence of osteophytes was assessed by two independent investigators. For further 3D analysis, tibia plateau was oriented along the growth plate and tibial diaphysis according to transaxial, sagittal and cortical plane. A volume of interest (VOI) of 400×400×100 slices per knee was set. Bone parameters were analyzed with CTAn analysis software (Skyscan) with a threshold set at 55 to define mineralized callous tissue. An interpolated VOI was set along the outer bone boundaries of the tibia plateau excluding the growth plate. For evaluating bone density the mean grayscale within the VOI was determined. Changes in bone nature were calculated regarding following 3D parameters: bone volume/tissue volume (BV/TV), trabecular number (Tb.N), trabecular thickness (Tb.Th) and trabecular separation (Tb.Sp). Parameters are shown following ASBMR nomenclature [24].

Statistical analysis

For statistical evaluation of histological and morphometric scoring non-parametric Mann-Whitney-U test was used. A two-tailed significance value of $p<0.05$ was considered statistically significant. Data analysis was performed with GraphPad Prism 5 (San Diego).

After consultation of a statistician, the intra- and inter-observer agreement of histological scoring systems was calculated using

Table 1. Scoring system for collagen type II immunohistochemistry.

Grade	collagen type II staining in articular cartilage
0	articular cartilage is not stained
1	<25% of articular cartilage area is stained
2	25–50% of articular cartilage area is stained
3	50–75% of articular cartilage area is stained
4	>75% of articular cartilage area is stained

Cohens kappa coefficient. Hereby, a kappa value of 0 corresponds to no agreement and a kappa value of 1.0 to complete agreement. Kappa values between 0–0.20 indicate slight agreement, 0.21–0.40 indicate fair agreement, 0.41–0.60 indicate moderate agreement, 0.61–0.80 indicate substantial agreement and 0.81–1.00 indicate excellent agreement. [25]. Data analysis was performed with SPSS for Windows 22.0 (SPSS Inc., Chicago).

For µCT analysis all parameters were referred to the respective value at day 0. For statistical comparison of Mc1re/e mice (n = 5) with WT mice (n = 7), Mann-Whitney-U Signed-Rank tests was conducted. For comparison of time points (day 0, 4 weeks and 8 weeks) Friedman-overall-test with post-hoc Wilcoxon-tests was conducted. Only if Friedman-overall-test indicated significance, data were analyzed post-hoc. Comparison of the right and the left knee was done by a paired Wilcoxon-test. A two-tailed significance value of $p<0.05$ was considered statistically significant. Data analysis was performed with SPSS for Windows 16.0 (SPSS Inc., Chicago).

Results

Morphometric analysis of knee joint articular cartilage from non-operated Mc1re/e and WT mice

Fig. 1A depicts representative Safranin O/fast green stained image from a frontal section through a mouse knee joint. For OA – induction always the meniscotibial ligament of the medial meniscus (MM) was transected. For further evaluation always the medial femoral condyle (MFC) and the medial tibial plateau (MTP) were used. Articular cartilage morphology was assessed by morphometric evaluation of Safranin O stained area of knee joints of non-operated 11 weeks (Fig. 1B, C) and 6 months old animals (Fig. 1D, E). In both age groups, cartilage area was smaller in Mc1re/e mice compared to WT which was statistically significant. Notably, we were unable to detect any signs of spontaneous OA-related cartilage surface erosions.

Table 2. Scoring system for MMP-13 immunohistochemistry.

Grade	MMP-13 stained non-hypertrophic chondrocytes in articular cartilage
0	no chondrocytes are stained
1	<25% of chondrocytes are stained
2	25–50% of chondrocytes are stained
3	50–75% of chondrocytes are stained
4	>75% of chondrocytes are stained

Analysis of cartilage degradation during OA-pathogenesis

Scoring and histomorphometric analysis of Safranin O stained articular cartilage revealed that OA was successfully induced in right knee joints of both Mc1re/e and WT mice (Fig. 2A). Both evaluation methods indicated significant increase in severity of cartilage degradation during OA progression in both groups. OA scoring of non-operated Mc1re/e and WT mice reveal that there is no spontaneous osteoarthritis induction in 11 weeks old (non-op; Fig. 2B–E) and 6 months old (data not shown) animals. Osteoarthritic related cartilage alterations as increasing loss of ECM macromolecules and cartilage surface erosions were more severe in Mc1re/e knee joints 4 and 8 weeks after OA induction (p.o.) for both evaluation methods (Fig. 2B, C) while sham-operated knees were unaffected (Fig. 2D, E).

Distribution of MC1 in DMM- and non-operated knee joints of Mc1re/e and WT mice

Immunoreactivity for MC1 was tested on sections of knee joints from non-operated 11 week old and 6 month old Mc1re/e and WT animals and from mice 4 and 8 weeks after OA-induction with DMM. Representative images are shown in Figure 3.

Immunostaining demonstrates the presence of MC1 in knee joints of mice. Chondrocytes in menisci and the upper and the adjunct part of the middle zone of articular cartilage are immunopositive for MC1. In addition, chondrocytes of the growth plate stain positive for MC1, here mainly cells in the proliferating zone which are organized into columns are stained (Fig. S2). Mostly, hypertrophic chondrocytes and also subpopulations of bone cells in the subchondral bone area remain negative. There is no difference in staining intensity or profile between WT and Mc1re/e mice detectable after OA-induction. Also, in 11 weeks and 6 months old non-operated mice MC1 distribution appears not to be altered between mutant and WT group and during aging (Fig. 3).

Collagen II, MMP-13, ICAM-1 and DIPEN in DMM- and non-operated knee joints of WT and Mc1re/e mice

Immunoreactivity for collagen II, MMP-13, ICAM-1 and DIPEN was tested on sections of knee joints from non-operated 11 week old and 6 month old Mc1re/e and WT animals and from mice 4 and 8 weeks after OA-induction with DMM. Representative images of MC1, collagen II, MMP-13 and ICAM-1 were shown in figure 3. Additionally a 0–4 point scoring system was applied for all groups and antigens (Tab. 1, 2 and 3) and data are presented for collagen II (Fig. 4A,), MMP-13 (Fig. 4B) and ICAM-1 (Fig. 4C) staining. Images of DIPEN staining and quantitative scoring is shown in Fig. S3. Immunohistology with appropriate isotype control antibodies served as negative control and remained unstained (Fig. S1).

In sections of 6 month old non-operated WT animals and of WT mice 4 and 8 weeks after OA-induction, collagen II stained articular cartilage is significantly decreased compared to non-operated 11 week old control. In contrast, articular cartilage of Mc1re/e showed no loss of collagen II staining in sections of 6 month old non-operated WT animals and of WT mice 4 and 8 weeks after OA-induction compared to non-operated 11 week old controls. Between non-operated 11 weeks old Mc1re/e and WT mice, collagen II stained knee joints revealed differences in stained cartilage area with significantly less collagen II staining in Mc1re/e joints. Also, 4 weeks after OA-induction there are significantly more cartilage regions without collagen II staining in Mc1re/e mice compared to WT. At 8 weeks after DMM this is reflected by

Table 3. Scoring system for ICAM-1 and DIPEN immunohistochemistry.

Grade	ICAM-1/DIPEN stained chondrocytes in articular cartilage
0	no chondrocytes are stained
1	<25% of chondrocytes are stained
2	25–50% of chondrocytes are stained
3	50–75% of chondrocytes are stained
4	>75% of chondrocytes are stained

trend only. At 6 month of age, collagen II staining pattern did not differ between WT and Mc1re/e mice (Fig. 3 and Fig. 4A). Cohens kappa coefficients showed a substantial (MFC: 0.64) and moderate (MTP: 0.55) intra-observer agreement and a moderate (MFC: 0.40, MTP: 0.46) inter-observer agreement (Fig. S4).

Immunoreactivity for MMP-13 was significantly increased in MMP-13 positive non-hypertrophic articular chondrocytes 8 weeks after OA-induction and in sections of non-operated 6 months old animals compared to non-operated 11 weeks old mice. In contrast, articular chondrocytes of Mc1re/e did not show an increase of MMP-13 positive cells during OA-progression or ageing compared to 11 weeks old non-operated mice. We observed a significant higher number of MMP-13 positive non-hypertrophic chondrocytes in Mc1re/e mice compared to WT in

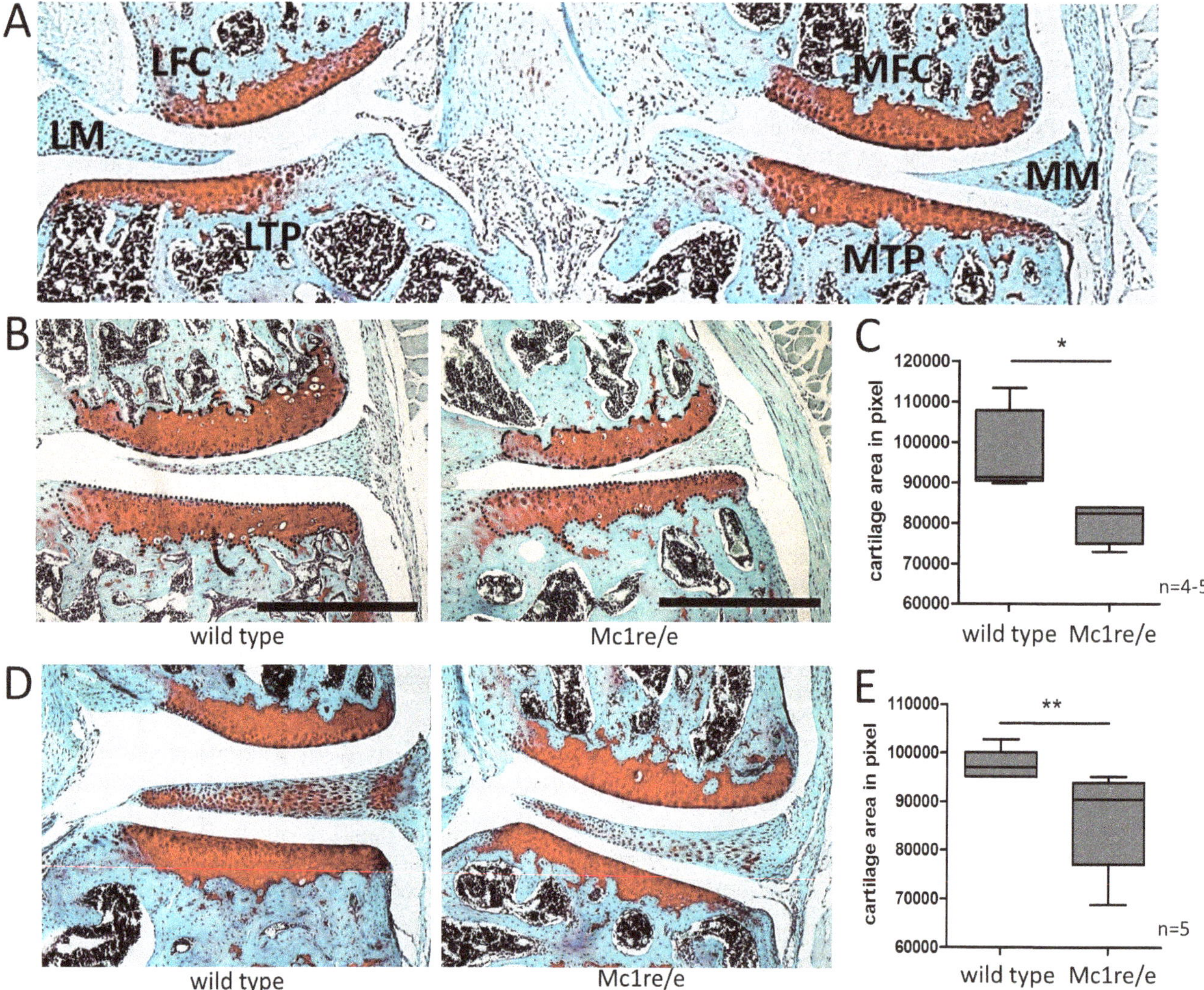

Figure 1. Histomorphometric comparison of knee joint morphology between non-operated Mc1re/e and WT mice. A) Overview of Safranin O/Fast green stained frontal section of a right mouse knee joint from a non-operated 11 week old Mc1re/e mouse (40× magnification). Lateral femoral condyle (LFC), lateral tibial plateau (LTP) and lateral meniscus (LM) as well as medial femoral condyle (MFC), medial tibial plateau (MTP) and medial meniscus (MM) are labeled. For osteoarthritis induction with DMM, the medial meniscotibial ligament is transected. B–E) Histological evaluation of cartilage area was performed with Safranin O/Fast green stained frontal sections of right knee joints from non-operated 11 weeks old and 6 months old WT and Mc1re/e mice. B+D) Medial, tibial (dotted line) and femoral (broken line) Safranin O stained cartilage was circuited with Bamboo tablet. C+E) Cartilage area of Mc1re/e mice was significantly smaller in 11 weeks ($p = 0.0159$) and 6 months old ($p = 0.0079$) animals compared to cartilage area of WT mice. For statistical analyses mean values of tibial and femoral cartilage areas of 5–6 section per knee joint was determined. Data are presented as boxplots reflecting the 25th and 75th percentile as boxes, the median as horizontal line and minimum and maximum values as whiskers. Bars = 500 µm, * $p<0.05$ and ** $p<0.01$ wild type vs. Mc1re/e.

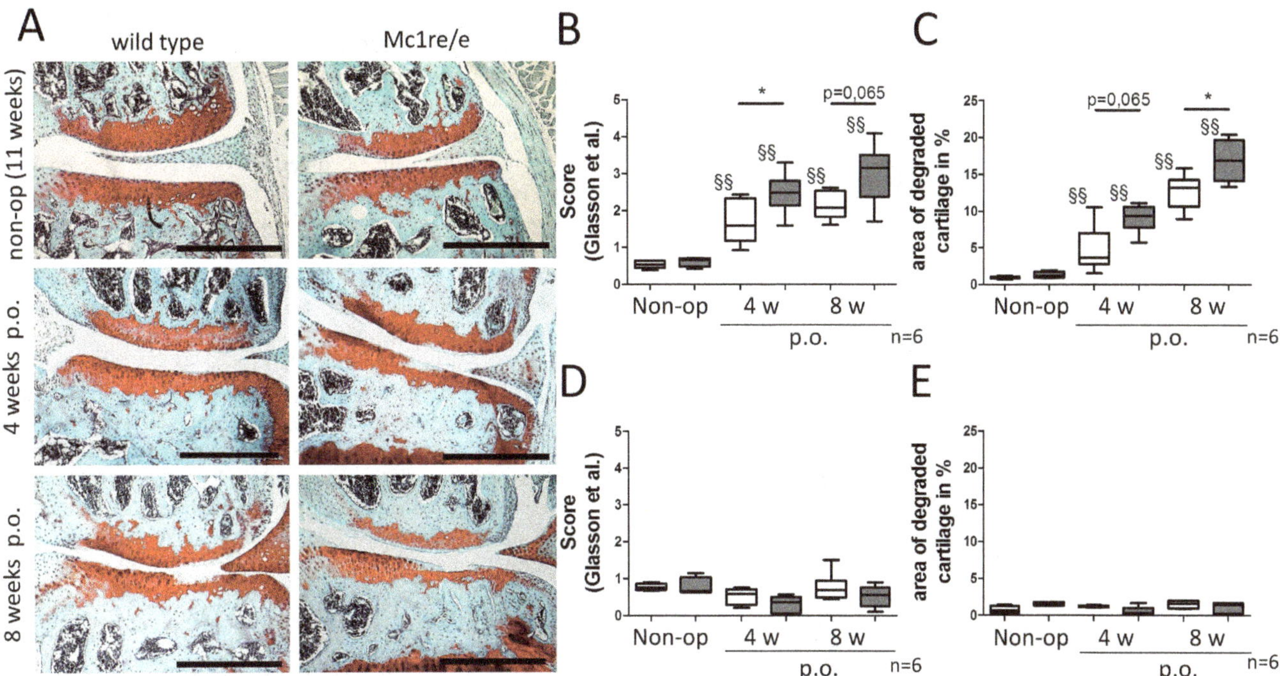

Figure 2. Assessment of cartilage degradation 4 and 8 weeks after osteoarthritis induction. A-E) Frontal sections of knee joints from WT and Mc1re/e mice of non-operated (non-op) 11 week old animals, and of animals 4 and 8 weeks post operation (p.o.) by DMM were stained with Safranin O/Fast green. A) Representative images of the medial area from sections of right knee joints from non-operated 11 weeks old animals and from mice 4 and 8 weeks after osteoarthritis induction (p.o.) show disease progression over the time. B–E) 5–6 sections in 60–80 μm intervals of right knees (DMM, B, C) and left knees (Sham, D, E) were scored histological according to Glasson et al. [21] (B, D) and morphometrically (C, E). B) We observed OA-progression over time in WT ($p = 0.0043$) and Mc1re/e ($p = 0.0095$) mice compared to non-operated controls. Mc1re/e mice had higher scores 4 weeks ($p = 0.0411$) and 8 weeks ($p = 0.0649$) after OA-induction. C) Percentages of degraded cartilage area also indicated an OA-progression over time in WT ($p = 0.0043$) and Mc1re/e ($p = 0.0095$) compared to non-operated controls. Mc1re/e mice had more degraded cartilage 4 weeks ($p = 0.0649$) and 8 weeks ($p = 0.0411$) after OA-induction compared to WT animals. D+E) Sham operated knee joints showed similar scores (D) and area of degraded cartilage (E) compared to non-operated controls. Mean scores of medial tibia and femur were included in statistical analysis. Data are presented as box plots reflecting the 25th and 75th percentile as boxes, the median as horizontal line and minimum and maximum values as whiskers. White bars indicate wild type and grey bars indicate mutant group. Bars = 500 μm, §§ $p < 0.01$ 4/8 weeks post-surgery vs. non-operated, * $p < 0.05$ wild type vs. Mc1re/e.

non-operated 11 weeks old animals. This difference persisted 4 weeks after OA-inductions and was not observed 8 weeks after OA-induction and in non-operated 6 month old animals (Fig. 3 and Fig 4B). Cohens kappa coefficients showed a fair (MFC: 0.25) and moderate (MTP: 0.50) intra-observer agreement and a moderate (MFC: 0.40, MTP: 0.46) inter-observer agreement (Fig. S4).

Notably, staining for ICAM-1 revealed strong signals in chondrocytes of the articular cartilage and in chondrocytes mainly of the hypertrophic zone of the growth plate (Fig. S2). In WT and Mc1re/e animals, 6 month old non-operated animals and mice 4 and 8 weeks after OA-induction contain fewer ICAM-1 positive articular chondrocytes compared to non-operated 11 week old control. We detected no differences in ICAM-1 staining between Mc1re/e and WT mice in non-operated 11 weeks old and 6 month old animals. 4 and 8 weeks after OA-induction, Mc1re/e mice showed significantly less ICAM-1 positive articular chondrocytes in the medial part of the joints compared to WT (Fig. 3 and Fig. 4C). Cohens kappa coefficients showed a substantial (MFC/MTP: 0.74) intra-observer agreement and a fair (MFC: 0.37, MTP: 0.32) inter-observer agreement (Fig. S4).

Staining for MMP-generated aggrecan neoepitope DIPEN revealed highest immunoreactivity in articular cartilage chondrocytes of 11 weeks old WT and Mc1re/e mice. 4 weeks after OA-induction, number of DIPEN positive chondrocytes was lower compared to 11 weeks old mice of both groups. Numbers of DIPEN positive chondrocytes did not differ between WT and Mc1re/e in age-matched mice and 4 and 8 weeks after OA-induction (Fig. S3). Cohens kappa coefficients showed a substantial (MFC: 0.61, MTP: 0.71) intra-observer agreement and a fair (MFC: 0.26, MTP: 0.36) inter-observer agreement (Fig. S4).

Analysis of bone architecture at the day of surgery (day 0)

Bone morphology of the epiphysis of the right tibia was recorded at the day of surgery (day 0) by μCT analysis within a VOI excluding the growth plate (Fig. 5A). The mean grayscale was calculated as an indicator for bone density (Fig. 5). Bone volume (BV) was calculated relative to total volume (TV) to normalize on knee size and was used as an indicator for bone mass (Fig. 5C). Bone density and BV/TV were similar between WT and Mc1re/e mice at the day of surgery indicating no differences in epiphyseal bone density and mass prior to OA induction. Trabecular number (Tb.N, Fig. 5D) and trabecular thickness (Tb.Th, Fig. 5E) did not differ between the groups at day 0

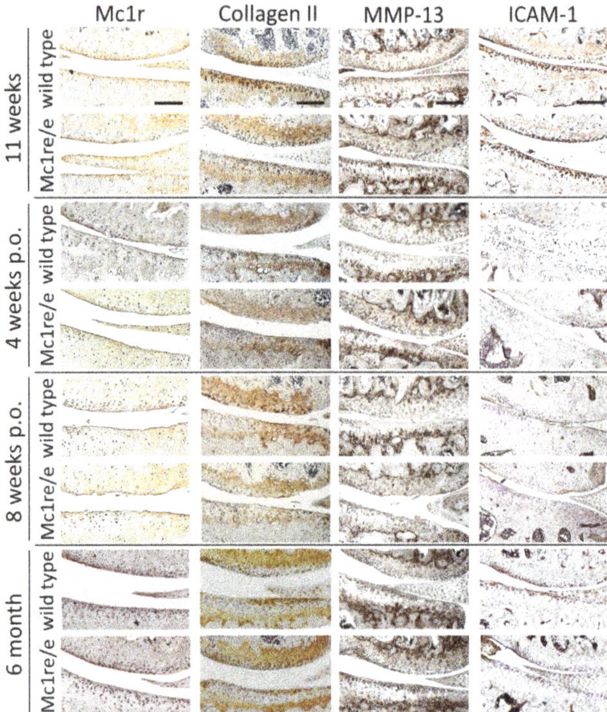

Figure 3. Localization of MC1, collagen II, MMP-13 and ICAM-1 in knee joints of Mc1re/e and wild type mice. A+C) Frontal sections of right knee joints from WT and Mc1re/e mice of non-operated (non-op) 11 weeks old and 6 months old animals, and of mice 4 and 8 weeks after osteoarthritis induction (post operation (p.o.)) were stained with antibodies against MC1, collagen II, MMP-13 and ICAM-1 as described in material and methods. Representative pictures of medial parts of the knee joints from each time point are shown. Bars = 200 μm.

whereas mutants showed an increased trabecular separation (Tb.Sp, Fig. 5F).

Development of osteophytes in the joints of Mc1re/e mice after OA-induction

Osteophytes were evident 4 weeks after OA-induction in 2 of 7 animals of the WT- and in 4 of 5 animals of the Mc1re/e group (Fig. 6A–C). Only the right knee (DMM) was affected, sham-operated knees did not develop osteophytes. Osteophytes were increased in size at 8 weeks, but no additional novel osteophytes became apparent 8 weeks after OA-induction (Fig. 6D).

Increased bone density and bone volume in knees of Mc1re/e mice after OA-induction

DMM-knees developed areas of increased mineral deposition during OA progression according to reconstructed images (Fig. 7A, B). At 4 weeks the mean grayscale as an indicator for bone density was significantly increased in the Mc1re/e group compared to day 0. Eight weeks after OA-induction WT animals revealed a significantly elevated bone density. At both time points, Mc1re/e mice had higher bone density in the epiphysis (Fig. 7C). BV/TV as an indicator of bone mass increased in the knee joints of the Mc1re/e group only compared to day 0 and was higher compared to the WT group 4 weeks and 8 weeks after OA-induction (Fig. 7D).

Alterations in bone architecture are significant more pronounced in Mc1re/e mice affecting also the contra-lateral knee joints

In destabilized DMM knee joints, trabecular number (Tb.N) declined significantly in WT and Mc1re/e at 4 and 8 weeks compared to day 0 with no differences observed between both groups (Fig. 8A).

Trabecular thickness (Tb.Th) was significantly increased in DMM-knees of the Mc1re/e group at 4 and 8 weeks compared to day 0. In the WT group an increase in Tb.Th was evident only at 8 weeks with trabeculae being significantly thinner compared to the Mc1re/e group at both time points (Fig. 8B).

In line with an increase of Tb.Th was a decrease in Tb.Sp in DMM knee joints of the Mc1re/e group reaching significance at 8 weeks compared to day 0. This decrease was not observed in the WT group at these time points. At both time points, Mc1re/e animals showed less Tb.Sp versus the WT group (Fig. 8C).

Interestingly, mild alterations in trabecular structure also occurred in sham operated contra-lateral knees in both groups within the set time span (Fig. 8D–E) but to a significantly lesser extend compared to destabilized knees. However, no significant changes in BV/TV were detected in contra-lateral knees of animals of both groups (data not shown).

Discussion

Hallmark features of OA are structural changes including cartilage destruction as well as alterations in synovial membrane and subchondral bone. Synovial tissue and subchondral bone are considered to play decisive roles in OA-pathology, but up to now cartilage is the main target for therapeutic approaches because of its paramount importance in joint articulation. However, current therapies are palliative and there are no disease-modifying drugs available for effective clinical use. One major reason for the lack of curative therapies is that OA is mostly diagnosed in late or end stage of the disease where joint replacement by endoprotheses remains the only treatment option [26]. Thus, it is of great importance to understand basic mechanisms of OA-pathology in an early stage of the disease in order to develop effective regenerative therapies. For that approach we have chosen surgical OA induction with DMM in mice which allows to detect alteration in cartilage and subchondral bone already early after induction of OA and resembles quite closely slowly progressive human OA [19].

There is compelling evidence that the osteoarticular system is a direct target organ and source of POMC peptides [12]. Our study provides novel evidence for a role of the POMC system in the osteoarticular system and in OA-pathology. Mice which lack a functional MC1 develop a cartilage phenotype which is reflected in a smaller cartilage area, lower immunoreactivity for collagen II and a higher number of MMP-13 positive chondrocytes. After OA-induction, they develop more severe cartilage erosions and tissue loss compared to WT. Of note, immunoreactivity for ICAM-1 decreases during OA progression which is significantly more pronounced in articular chondrocytes of Mc1re/e mice as in WT. This effect supports our observation that MC1 signaling helps to stabilize cartilage matrix integrity. Immunostaining for MC1 revealed no difference between WT and MC1re/e mice. Reduced collagen II and increased MMP-13 immunostaining in non-operated Mc1re/e knees indicates a cartilage phenotype in the mutant mice independent of OA pathology suggesting a premature appearance of age – related structural ECM alterations in the absence of a functional MC1.

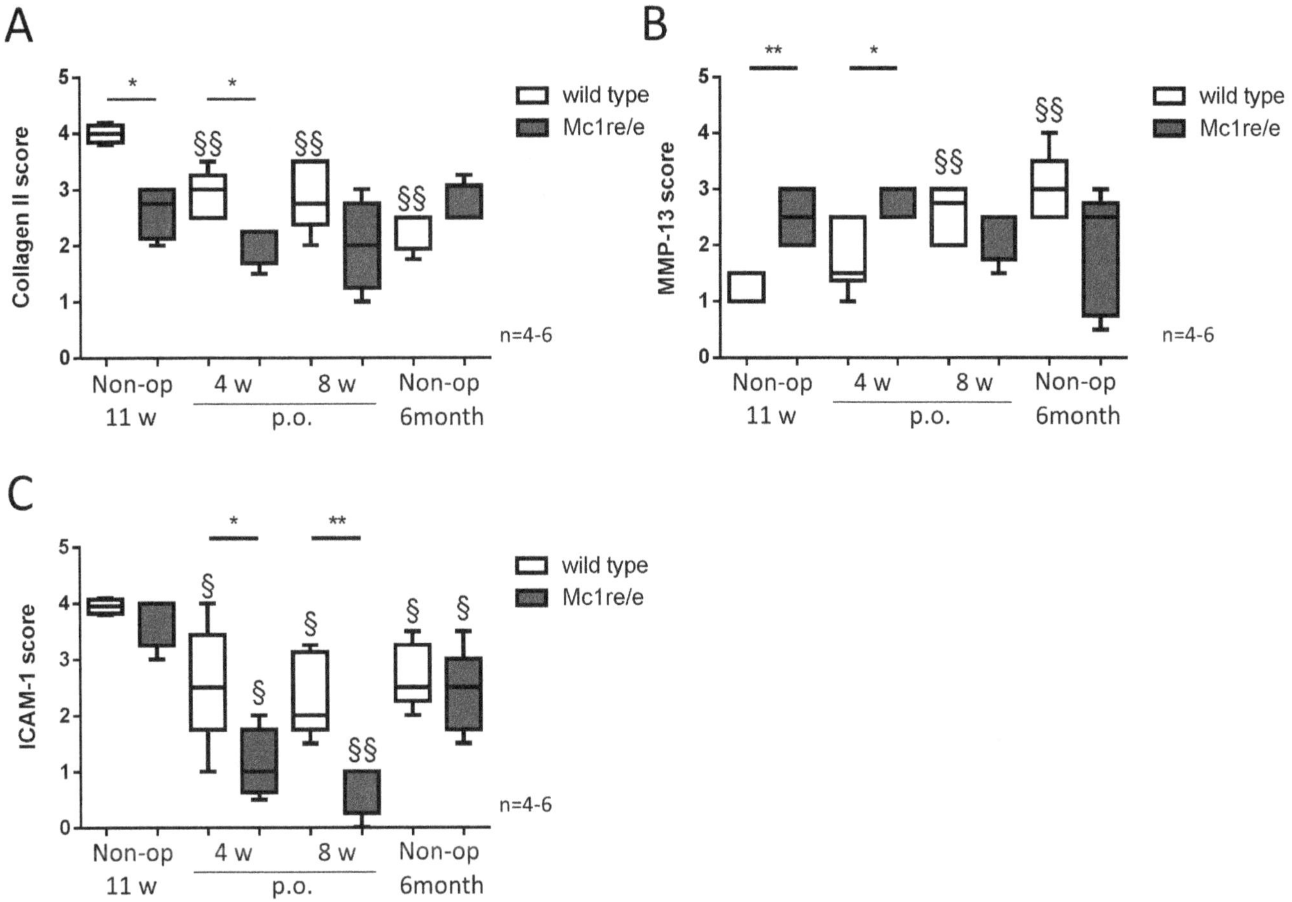

Figure 4. Quantitative scoring of collagen II, MMP-13 and ICAM-1 immunohistochemistry. Medial parts of frontal sections of right knee joints from WT and Mc1re/e mice of non-operated (non-op) 11 weeks old and 6 months old animals, and of mice 4 and 8 weeks after osteoarthritis induction (post operation (p.o.)) were scored after staining. 1-3 sections of right knees (DMM) were scored histological according to the scoring system illustrated in Tab. 1 for collagen II, in Tab. 2 for MMP-13 and in Tab. 3 for ICAM-1 staining. A) Compared to non-operated controls collagen II stained cartilage area of WT knee joints is decreased 4 weeks ($p = 0.0079$) and 8 weeks ($p = 0.0043$) after OA-induction as well as in non-operated 6 month old animals ($p = 0.0159$). Sections of Mc1re/e knee joints showed no difference over time. Collagen II stained cartilage area of non-operated 11 weeks old Mc1re/e mice ($p = 0.0159$) and Mc1re/e mice 4 weeks ($p = 0.0159$) after OA induction is decreased compared to WT mice. B) Compared to non-operated controls number of MMP-13 positive non-hypertrophic articular chondrocytes of WT knee joints is increased 8 weeks ($p = 0.0022$) after OA-induction as well as in non-operated 6 month old animals ($p = 0.0076$). Sections of Mc1re/e knee joints showed no difference over time. MMP-13 positive chondrocytes of non-operated 11 weeks old Mc1re/e mice ($p = 0.0079$) and Mc1re/e mice 4 weeks ($p = 0.035$) after OA induction are increased compared to WT mice. C) Compared to non-operated controls number of ICAM-1 positive articular chondrocytes of Mc1re/e and WT knee joints are decreased 4 weeks (Mc1re/e: $p = 0.0159$; WT: $p = 0.0381$) and 8 weeks (Mc1re/e: $p = 0.0159$; WT: $p = 0.0159$) after OA-induction as well as in non-operated 6 month old animals (Mc1re/e: $p = 0.0317$; WT: $p = 0.0159$). There is no difference between WT and Mc1re/e regarding the number of ICAM-1 positive chondrocytes in non-operated controls whereas Mc1re/e mice 4 ($p = 0.0303$) and 8 weeks ($p = 0.0079$) after OA-induction showed lower numbers of ICAM-1 positive cells. Mean scores of medial tibia and femur were included in statistical analysis. Data are presented as box plots reflecting the 25th and 75th percentile as boxes, the median as horizontal line and minimum and maximum values as whiskers. §§ $p<0.01$ 4/8 weeks post-surgery vs. non-operated, § $p<0.05$ 4/8 weeks post-surgery vs. non-operated, ** $p<0.01$ wild type vs. Mc1re/e, * $p<0.05$ wild type vs. Mc1re/e.

With respect to epiphyseal bone architecture, we did not detect obvious differences between Mc1re/e and WT mice regarding bone density and mass at the day of DMM surgery. However, trabecular separation was increased in Mc1re/e mice indicating a slight, but distinct effect on bone marrow thickness. We cannot exclude compensatory effects of other MCR subtypes in bone tissue, i.e. MC2 and MC4, for which at least mRNA transcripts are found in osteoblasts [17,27]. In addition to matrix producing osteoblasts, bone contains also matrix degrading cells, the osteoclasts which express MC2, MC3, MC4 and MC5 transcripts [17]. Presumably, it needs challenging by inflicting traumata in order to reveal physiological relevance of an individual MCR subtype. With respect to cartilage morphology, histomorphometry demonstrates that the area in knee joints covered by articular cartilage surface was smaller in non-operated Mc1re/e mice compared to WT. This observation indicates, together with less collagen II stained area and a higher number of MMP-13 positive chondrocytes in sections of knee joints of 11 weeks old mutant mice, an OA – independent cartilage phenotype, however without signs of OA typical surface erosions. Notably, immunoreactivity for cellular MMP-generated aggrecan neoepitope DIPEN does not differ between WT and Mc1re/e in articular chondrocytes at any time point. Besides DIPEN, various other aggrecan neoepitopes generated by MMPs and aggrecanases are known which indicate aggrecan degradation. Our data suggest that presumably MMP-13 might not be the major proteinase causative for reduction of area of safranin O stained cartilage in Mc1re/e mice. Again, there might be some compensation as mRNA transcripts of other MCR

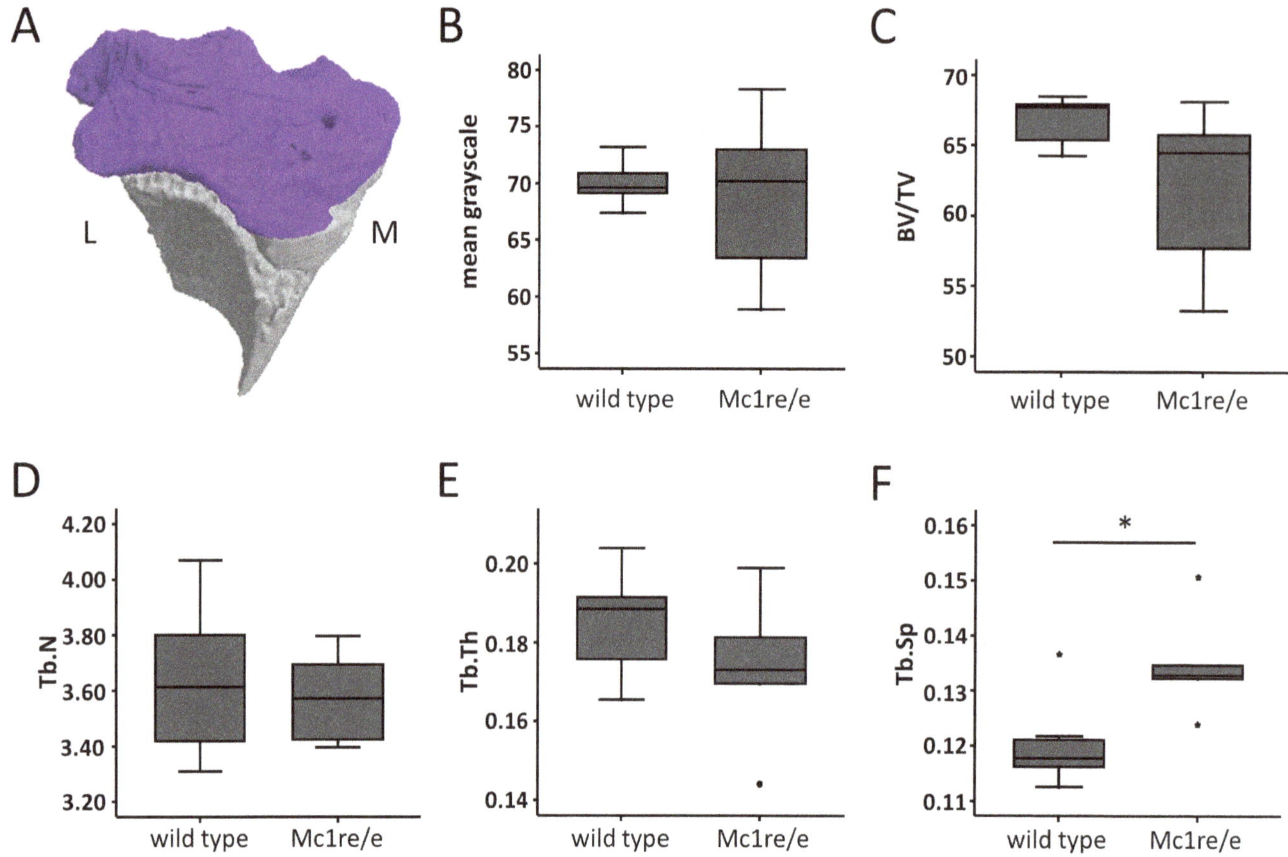

Figure 5. Comparison of bone architecture between Mc1re/e and WT mice at the day of DMM surgery (day 0) using μCT. A–F) μCT 3D analysis of bone parameters was performed within a defined VOI including the tibia epiphysis of both knees respectively. A) Frontal view on 3D model of the proximal tibia of the right leg showing the VOI marked in purple (L: lateral, M: medial). B) μCT analysis of mean grayscale within the VOI as an indicator for bone density indicated no difference between WT and Mc1re/e mice. C) 3D calculation of BV/TV within the VOI as an indicator of bone mass also revealed no difference between both groups. In Trabecular number (Tb.N, D) and trabecular thickness (Tb.Th, E) no difference was observed whereas trabecular separation (Tb.Sp, F) was increased in Mc1re/e compared to controls ($p = 0.028$). Values of left and right knees were combined. Data are presented as boxplots reflecting the 25th and 75th percentile as boxes, the median as horizontal line and minimum and maximum values as whiskers, stars indicating extreme outliers. * $p<0.05$ wild type vs. Mc1re/e.

subtypes, i.e. MC2 and MC5 were detected in articular cartilage from newborn mice (data not shown). In contrast to bone, chondrocytes are the only cell type in cartilage and for them MC1 signaling might be more important than signaling through other MCR subtypes. Recently, we demonstrated that α-MSH, the high affinity ligand of MC1, modulated metabolism of articular chondrocytes by altering gene expression and protein secretion of several collagens, MMPs and cytokines [15].

In this study we provide evidence that the POMC system can be chondro-osseo protective and ameliorates OA pathogenesis. In vivo effects of melanocortin peptides which affect the osteoarticular system are mainly anti-inflammatory and affect bone turnover and -volume. α-MSH, the high-affinity ligand of MC1 besides ACTH [12], is reported to reduce collagen-induced arthritis in mice [28] and to lead to reduced arthritis scores as well as reduced articular erosions in rat adjuvant arthritis [29]. Interestingly, α-MSH also reduces tibial perimeter and length. In primary cultures of osteoblasts and chondrocytes, α-MSH dose dependently stimulated cell proliferation while in bone marrow cultures, α-MSH stimulated osteoclastogenesis. Systemic administration of α-MSH to mice decreased trabecular bone volume in the proximal tibiae and reduced trabecular number. From this it can be concluded that α-MSH acts directly on bone, increasing bone turnover, and, when administered systemically, decreasing bone volume [30]. These observations are nicely in line with our data showing increased bone density and bone mass in MC1-signaling deficient mice after OA-induction. With respect to cartilage matrix formation, α-MSH and ACTH stimulate matrix production by increasing collagen II and aggrecan expression in committed murine and rat chondrocytes [14,15]. This anabolic effect of melanocortins would help to explain our observation of a articular cartilage phenotype in native Mc1re/e mice and of more severe cartilage matrix degradation and loss in OA.

Together with our observation that functional MC1 signaling delays cartilage degradation and loss during experimental OA pathogenesis, we also observed alterations in subchondral bone micro-architecture and osteophyte number in MC1 signaling-deficient mice after induction of OA. Mutant mice develop clearly more and larger osteophytes as WT. Osteophyte formation is besides joint space narrowing, subchondral sclerosis and subchondral cyst formation one of the main radiographic features of OA and an important criterion for this disease. Osteophytes have a significant clinical impact and can be a source of pain and loss of function [31]. In addition to increased osteophyte formation, lack of MC1 signaling leads to increased subchondral bone mass and bone density after OA-induction. In early OA, a marked thinning,

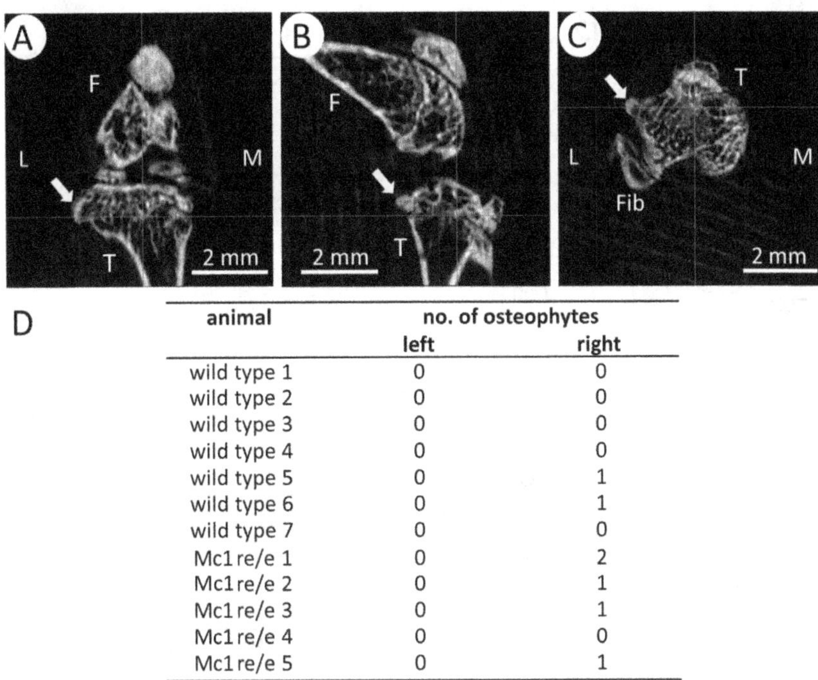

animal	no. of osteophytes	
	left	right
wild type 1	0	0
wild type 2	0	0
wild type 3	0	0
wild type 4	0	0
wild type 5	0	1
wild type 6	0	1
wild type 7	0	0
Mc1re/e 1	0	2
Mc1re/e 2	0	1
Mc1re/e 3	0	1
Mc1re/e 4	0	0
Mc1re/e 5	0	1

Figure 6. Radiographic evaluation of osteophytes at 4 and 8 weeks past OA induction. A–C) Knees were oriented as described in material and methods section and were analyzed for osteophytes (white arrow) in transaxial (A), sagittal (B) and coronal (C) plane. F: femur, T: tibia, Fib: fibula, L: lateral and M: medial. D) At 4 and 8 weeks the number and size of osteophytes was calculated for the right and the left knee of each animal, respectively. 4 of 5 Mc1re/e mice developed osteophytes whereas only 2 from 7 WT mice developed one osteophyte after OA-induction.

increase in porosity [23] and hypomineralization of subchondral bone is observed due to an abnormal high turnover [32] while in late OA-stages subchondral bone thickening occurs followed by sclerosis [33]. In line with a significant increase in trabecular thickness and decrease of trabecular separation, our observations indicate a more severe and clearly faster progression of subchondral OA-related sclerosis in Mc1re/e mice. Notably, we observed similar effects, however less pronounced in sham-operated knees at

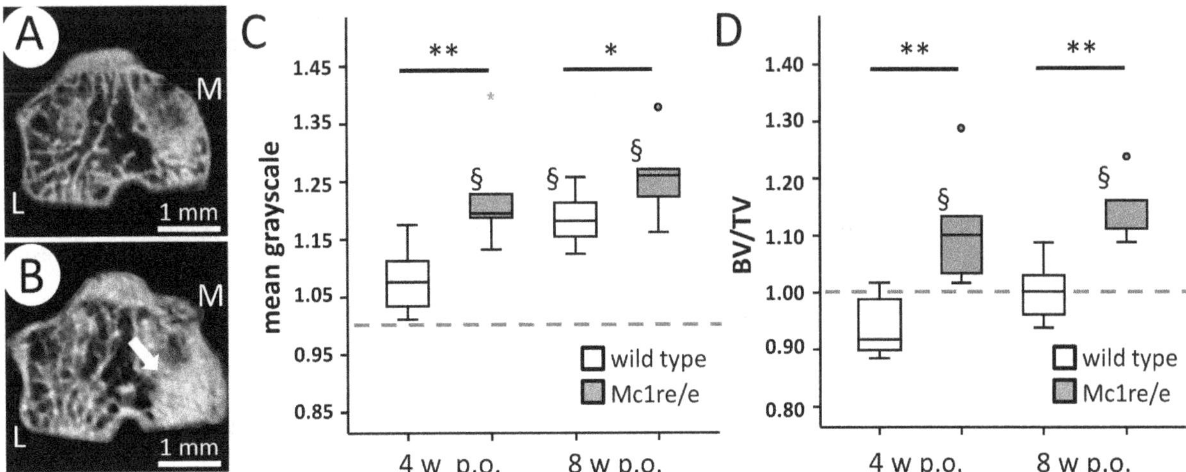

Figure 7. Alteration of bone density and bone volume at 4 and 8 weeks past OA induction. A–B) Reconstructed coronal image of Mc1re/e knee joints at the day of OA-surgery (day 0) (A) and 8 weeks after OA-surgery (B). White arrow marks an area of increased mineral deposition (L: lateral, M: medial). C) µCT analysis of mean grayscale within the VOI of the right knees as an indicator for bone density revealed an increase in bone densitiy 4 ($p = 0.043$) and 8 weeks ($p = 0.043$) after OA-indution in Mc1re/e mice and 8 weeks ($p = 0.018$) after OA-induction in WT animals. Mc1re/e mice showed a higher bone density 4 ($p = 0.007$) and 8 weeks ($p = 0.042$) after OA-induction compared to WT mice. D) In Mc1re/e mice but not in WT animals, BV/TV within the VOI of the right knee as an indicator of bone mass was increased at both time points after OA-induction compared to day 0 ($p = 0.043$). There was a higher bone mass in the epiphysis of Mc1re/e mice 4 ($p = 0.007$) and 8 weeks ($p = 0.004$) after OA-induction compared to WT animals. Data were normalized to the values at day 0 (day of surgery, (set as 1, grey dotted line). Data are presented as boxplots reflecting the 25th and 75th percentile as boxes, the median as horizontal line and minimum and maximum values as whiskers with dots indicating outliers and stars indicating extreme outliers. § $p<0.05$ 4/8 weeks post-surgery vs. day 0, * $p<0.05$ and ** $p<0.01$ wild type vs. mutant.

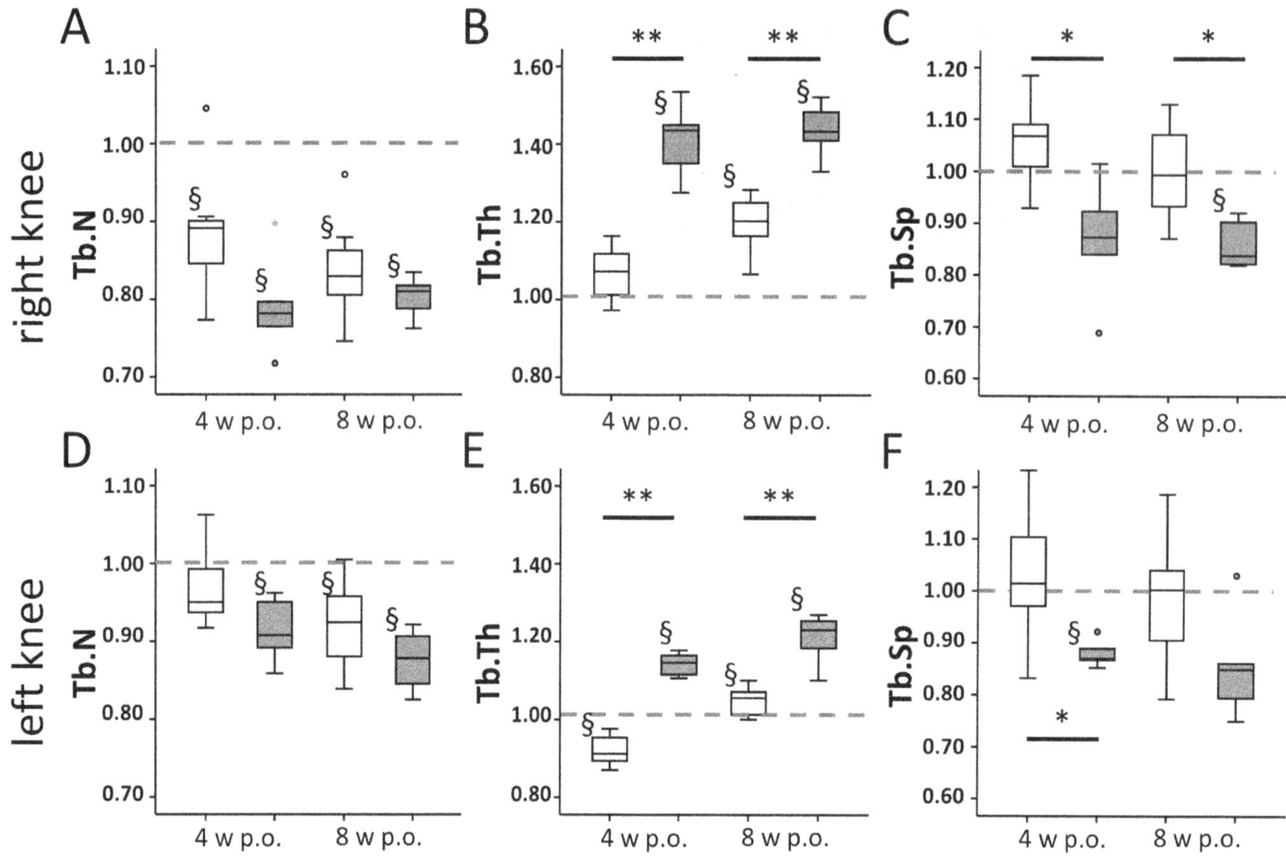

Figure 8. Alteration of bone architecture after OA induction. µCT 3D-analysis of trabecular parameters in the right knee joint (DMM, A–C) and the left knee joint (Sham, D–F) depicted as trabecular number (Tb.N, A,D), trabecular thickness (Tb.Th, B,E) and trabecular separation (Tb.Sp, C,F). A) Tb.N declined in WT (p = 0.018) and Mc1re/e (p = 0.043) at both time points after OA-induction compared to day 0 with no differences observed between both groups. B) Compared to day 0 animals Tb.Th was increased in Mc1re/e mice at both time points (p = 0.043) after OA-induction whereas WT mice showed an increase only 8 weeks after operation (p = 0.018). Mc1re/e mice had thicker trabeculae at both time points compared to WT animals (p = 0.004) C) Th.Sp was decreased in Mc1re/e animals reaching significance 8 weeks after OA-induction compared to day 0 mice (p = 0.043). At both time points, Mc1re/e animals developed less Th.Sp compared to WT group (p = 0.019). Mild alterations in trabecular structure also occurred in sham operated contra-lateral knees in both groups but to a significantly lesser extend compared to destabilized knees. Data were normalized to the values at day 0 (day of surgery, set as 1, grey dotted line). Data are presented as box plots reflecting the 25th and 75th percentile as boxes, the median as horizontal line and minimum and maximum values as whiskers with dots indicating outliers and stars indicating extreme outliers. White bars indicate wild type and grey bars indicate Mc1re/e group. § $p<0.05$ 4/8 weeks post-surgery vs. day 0, * $p<0.05$ and ** $p<0.01$ wild type vs. mutant.

4 and 8 weeks after DMM with increased severity in Mc1re/e mice. We were unable to detect OA related cartilage matrix alterations in sham-knees in both groups during that time points indicating that during early OA alterations in subchondral bone morphology precede OA related phenotypical changes in cartilage matrix.

We did not detect obvious differences in MC1 immunostaining between WT and Mc1re/e mice or during OA progression indicating that MC1 synthesis per se is not affected by the disease. Contrary to human OA-cartilage [15], mostly chondrocytes of the upper and partly the middle layer were MC1 positive while chondrocytes close to the tide mark remained unstained. These differences in MC1 distribution might be due to the profound thinner articular cartilage in mice which consists of only a few cell layers. Notably, in line with Zhong et al., we also found that chondrocytes mainly in the proliferative zone of the growth plate stained positive for the MC1 whereas chondrocytes of the hypertrophic zone lack not only MC1 expression but mRNA for all other MCR subtypes [17]. Our unpublished observations indicated an induction of ICAM-1 gene and protein expression in human articular OA-chondrocytes in vitro when stimulated with α-MSH which prompted us to analyze ICAM-1 protein expression in mouse joints with immunohistochemistry. Notably, we found strong ICAM-1 immunoreactivity in articular chondrocytes of non-operated 11 week old Mc1re/e and WT mice which was decreased in 6 month old animals. Moreover, during pathogenesis of OA, in cartilage of Mc1re/e mice even less ICAM-1 positive chondrocytes were detected compared to WT. ICAM-1 is constitutively expressed on articular chondrocytes [34] and is a cell surface receptor for hyaluronan (HA) [35,36]. Hyaluronan and collagen II are two major components of cartilage ECM which, among other roles, serve as structural components for cell adhesion. One can speculate that imbalance of these ECM molecules feeds back on the expression of associated adhesion molecules like ICAM-1. Loss of ICAM-1 expression after OA-induction could add to the aggravated degradation of cartilage in Mc1re/e mice when challenged with DMM. The study of Yasuda et al. indicate that the interaction of ICAM-1 and HA suppresses cartilage destruction induced via collagen II peptides and MMP-13 production [37] suggesting that increased loss of ICAM-1 in this context might facilitate OA pathology. Moreover, Lisignoli et al., demonstrated an anti-apoptotic effect of HA bound to its receptors CD44 and ICAM-1 [38] not only after OA induction but already in unchallenged mice.

Conclusions

Inflammatory-like processes originated from OA increase bone and cartilage turnover and eventually lead to degradation of these tissues. The osteoarticular system presumably responds to this with an evolutionary conserved stress response in analogy to the classical HPA axis, that is increased synthesis of POMC-derived peptides. The release of such POMC peptides will subsequently not only modulate the activity of immune cells but also of resident cells as osteoclasts, osteoblasts, chondrocytes, synoviocytes and their progenitor cells which carry the appropriate MC-receptors. Inactivation of the MC1, which is present on chondrocytes and cells of epiphyseal bone will thus consequently have an effect on physiology and pathophysiology of diathrodial joint tissues. Our study demonstrates that signal-deficient Mc1re/e mice have a cartilage phenotype prior to OA induction which increases in severity during OA-pathogenesis already in an early stage. In addition, we suggest that absence of MC1-signaling accelerates age-related structural cartilage ECM alterations as demonstrated by loss of collagen II and increased number of MMP-13 positive chondrocytes. Notably, our data from sham – operated joints suggest that OA-pathogenesis related alterations in epiphyseal bone architecture precede alterations in articular cartilage which is more pronounced in Mc1re/e joints. Understanding the underlying molecular mechanisms of the functional role of the POMC system in joints will eventually help to tailor efficient future therapies against degenerative joint diseases as OA.

Supporting Information

Figure S1 Isotype control staining for MC1, collagen II, MMP-13, DIPEN and ICAM-1 immunohistochemistry. Frontal sections of right knee joints from WT and Mc1re/e mice of non-operated 11 weeks old (Collagen II and DIPEN) and 6 months old (MC1, MMP-13 and ICAM-1) animals were stained with antibodies against MC1, collagen II, MMP-13, DIPEN and ICAM-1and appreciate isotype control antibodies. Representative pictures of medial parts of the knee joints from WT and Mc1re/e stained with specific antibodies and isotype control antibodies are shown. Staining with isotype control antibodies revealed no staining. Black bars = 200 μm.

Figure S2 Localization of MC1, collagen II, MMP-13 and ICAM-1 in articular cartilage and tibial growth plate of Mc1re/e and WT mice. Frontal sections of right knee joints from WT and Mc1re/e mice of non-operated 11 weeks old and 6 months old animals and of mice 4 and 8 weeks after OA-induction were stained with antibodies against MC1, collagen II, MMP-13 and ICAM-1 as described in material and methods. Representative pictures of a 520× magnification of medial, tibial articular cartilage and tibial growth plate of the knee joints from 11 weeks old (Collagen II, Col II and MMP-13) and 6 months old (MC1 and ICAM-1) mice are shown. Black bars = 200 μm, white bars = 25 μm.

Figure S3 Localization of aggrecan neoepitope DIPEN in knee joints of Mc1re/e and wild type mice. Frontal sections of right knee joints from WT and Mc1re/e mice of non-operated (non-op) 11 weeks old and 6 months old animals, and of mice 4 and 8 weeks after osteoarthritis induction (post operation (p.o.)) were stained with antibodies against DIPEN as described in material and methods. A) Representative pictures of medial parts of the knee joints from each time point are shown. B) Number of DIPEN positive chondrocytes was scored according to Tab. 3. Compared to 11 weeks old non-op mice number of DIPEN positive decreased 4 weeks after OA-induction in both groups (WT: $p = 0{,}0186$ and Mc1re/e: $p = 0{,}0647$). Mean scores of medial tibia and femur were included in statistical analysis. Data are presented as box plots reflecting the 25th and 75th percentile as boxes, the median as horizontal line and minimum and maximum values as whiskers. Bars = 200 μm; § $p<0.05$ 4/8 weeks post-surgery vs. non-operated; (§) $p<0.0647$ 4/8 weeks post-surgery vs. non-operated.

Figure S4 Intra- and inter-observer agreement of histological scoring systems. Histological scoring systems for collagen II (A–B), MMP-13 (C-D), ICAM-1 (E–F) and DIPEN (G–H) staining were evaluated. Therefore 7 independent observer scored 10 frontal sections of each staining to obtain inter-observer agreement and 4 observer scored twice within one week to get intra-observer variability. Summed scores of medial femoral condyle (MFC) and medial tibial plateau (MTP) were shown for collagen II (A), MMP-13 (C), ICAM-1 (E) and DIPEN (G) scoring. To determine intra-observer agreement, cohens kappa coefficient between scores of measurement 1 and scores of measurement 2 of each observer (MV, RB, SG and TN) was calculated. For inter-observer agreement, cohens kappa coefficient between each observer of measurement 1 was determined. Mean of cohens kappa coefficients of collagen II (B), MMP-13 (B), ICAM-1 (F) and DIPEN (H) scorings were shown.

Acknowledgments

We thank Anja Pasoldt for her superior technical assistance.

Author Contributions

Conceived and designed the experiments: JL ES MB SG. Performed the experiments: JL ES RJB CG KK DB GH. Analyzed the data: JL ES RJB CG MB SG GH. Contributed reagents/materials/analysis tools: KK MB JG. Wrote the paper: JL ES SG.

References

1. Pitsillides AA, Beier F (2011) Cartilage biology in osteoarthritis-lessons from developmental biology. Nat Rev Rheumatol 7: 654–663.
2. van den Berg WB (2011) Osteoarthritis year 2010 in review: pathomechanisms. Osteoarthritis Cartilage 19: 338–341.
3. Dreier R (2010) Hypertrophic differentiation of chondrocytes in osteoarthritis: the developmental aspect of degenerative joint disorders. Arthritis Res Ther 12: 216.
4. Goldring MB, Marcu KB (2009) Cartilage homeostasis in health and rheumatic diseases. Arthritis Res Ther 11: 224.
5. Burr DB (2004) The importance of subchondral bone in the progression of osteoarthritis. J Rheumatol Suppl 70: 77–80.
6. Karsdal MA, Leeming DJ, Dam EB, Henriksen K, Alexandersen P, et al. (2008) Should subchondral bone turnover be targeted when treating osteoarthritis? Osteoarthritis Cartilage 16: 638–646. S1063-4584(08)00022-8 [pii];10.1016/j.joca.2008.01.014 [doi].
7. Felson DT, Neogi T (2004) Osteoarthritis: is it a disease of cartilage or of bone? Arthritis Rheum 50: 341–344. 10.1002/art.20051 [doi].
8. Goldring MB, Goldring SR (2007) Osteoarthritis. J Cell Physiol 213: 626–634.
9. Goldring MB, Goldring SR (2010) Articular cartilage and subchondral bone in the pathogenesis of osteoarthritis. Ann N Y Acad Sci 1192: 230–237.

10. Slominski A, Wortsman J, Luger T, Paus R, Solomon S (2000) Corticotropin releasing hormone and proopiomelanocortin involvement in the cutaneous response to stress. Physiol Rev 80: 979–1020.
11. Brzoska T, Luger TA, Maaser C, Abels C, Bohm M (2008) Alpha-melanocyte-stimulating hormone and related tripeptides: biochemistry, antiinflammatory and protective effects in vitro and in vivo, and future perspectives for the treatment of immune-mediated inflammatory diseases. Endocr Rev 29: 581–602.
12. Bohm M, Grassel S (2012) Role of Proopiomelanocortin-Derived Peptides and Their Receptors in the Osteoarticular System: From Basic to Translational Research. Endocr Rev. er.2011–1016 [pii];10.1210/er.2011-1016 [doi].
13. Schioth HB (2001) The physiological role of melanocortin receptors. Vitam Horm 63: 195–232.
14. Evans JF, Niu QT, Canas JA, Shen CL, Aloia JF, et al. (2004) ACTH enhances chondrogenesis in multipotential progenitor cells and matrix production in chondrocytes. Bone 35: 96–107.
15. Grassel S, Opolka A, Anders S, Straub RH, Grifka J, et al. (2009) The melanocortin system in articular chondrocytes: melanocortin receptors, pro-opiomelanocortin, precursor proteases, and a regulatory effect of alpha-melanocyte-stimulating hormone on proinflammatory cytokines and extracellular matrix components. Arthritis Rheum 60: 3017–3027.
16. Yoon SW, Chun JS, Sung MH, Kim JY, Poo H (2008) alpha-MSH inhibits TNF-alpha-induced matrix metalloproteinase-13 expression by modulating p38 kinase and nuclear factor kappaB signaling in human chondrosarcoma HTB-94 cells. Osteoarthritis Cartilage 16: 115–124.
17. Zhong Q, Sridhar S, Ruan L, Ding KH, Xie D, et al. (2005) Multiple melanocortin receptors are expressed in bone cells. Bone 36: 820–831.
18. Glasson SS, Askew R, Sheppard B, Carito B, Blanchet T, et al. (2005) Deletion of active ADAMTS5 prevents cartilage degradation in a murine model of osteoarthritis. Nature 434: 644–648.
19. Glasson SS, Blanchet TJ, Morris EA (2007) The surgical destabilization of the medial meniscus (DMM) model of osteoarthritis in the 129/SvEv mouse. Osteoarthritis Cartilage 15: 1061–1069.
20. Robbins LS, Nadeau JH, Johnson KR, Kelly MA, Roselli-Rehfuss L, et al. (1993) Pigmentation phenotypes of variant extension locus alleles result from point mutations that alter MSH receptor function. Cell 72: 827–834.
21. Glasson SS, Chambers MG, van den Berg WB, Little CB (2010) The OARSI histopathology initiative - recommendations for histological assessments of osteoarthritis in the mouse. Osteoarthritis Cartilage 18 Suppl 3: S17–S23. S1063-4584(10)00238-4 [pii];10.1016/j.joca.2010.05.025 [doi].
22. Bohm M, Brzoska T, Schulte U, Schiller M, Kubitscheck U, et al. (1999) Characterization of a polyclonal antibody raised against the human melanocortin-1 receptor. Ann N Y Acad Sci 885: 372–382.
23. Botter SM, van Osch GJ, Clockaerts S, Waarsing JH, Weinans H, et al. (2011) Osteoarthritis induction leads to early and temporal subchondral plate porosity in the tibial plateau of mice: an in vivo microfocal computed tomography study. Arthritis Rheum 63: 2690–2699.
24. Parfitt AM, Drezner MK, Glorieux FH, Kanis JA, Malluche H, et al. (1987) Bone histomorphometry: standardization of nomenclature, symbols, and units. Report of the ASBMR Histomorphometry Nomenclature Committee. J Bone Miner Res 2: 595–610. 10.1002/jbmr.5650020617 [doi].
25. Friedrich-Rust M, Meyer G, Dauth N, Berner C, Bogdanou D, et al. (2013) Interobserver agreement of Thyroid Imaging Reporting and Data System (TIRADS) and strain elastography for the assessment of thyroid nodules. PLoS One. 8(10): e77927
26. Sinusas K (2012) Osteoarthritis: diagnosis and treatment. Am Fam Physician 85: 49–56. d10073 [pii]s.
27. Dumont LM, Wu CS, Tatnell MA, Cornish J, Mountjoy KG (2005) Evidence for direct actions of melanocortin peptides on bone metabolism. Peptides 26: 1929–1935. S0196-9781(05)00239-1 [pii];10.1016/j.peptides.2004.12.034 [doi].
28. Vessillier S, Adams G, Montero-Melendez T, Jones R, Seed M, et al. (2012) Molecular engineering of short half-life small peptides (VIP, alphaMSH and gamma(3)MSH) fused to latency-associated peptide results in improved anti-inflammatory therapeutics. Ann Rheum Dis 71: 143–149. annrheumdis-2011-200100 [pii];10.1136/annrheumdis-2011-200100 [doi].
29. Ceriani G, Diaz J, Murphree S, Catania A, Lipton JM (1994) The neuropeptide alpha-melanocyte-stimulating hormone inhibits experimental arthritis in rats. Neuroimmunomodulation 1: 28–32.
30. Cornish J, Callon KE, Mountjoy KG, Bava U, Lin JM, et al. (2003) alpha - melanocyte-stimulating hormone is a novel regulator of bone. Am J Physiol Endocrinol Metab 284: E1181–E1190.
31. van der Kraan PM, van den Berg WB (2007) Osteophytes: relevance and biology. Osteoarthritis Cartilage 15: 237–244. S1063-4584(06)00327-X [pii];10.1016/j.joca.2006.11.006 [doi].
32. Bettica P, Cline G, Hart DJ, Meyer J, Spector TD (2002) Evidence for increased bone resorption in patients with progressive knee osteoarthritis: longitudinal results from the Chingford study. Arthritis Rheum 46: 3178–3184.
33. Botter SM, van Osch GJ, Waarsing JH, van der Linden JC, Verhaar JA, et al. (2008) Cartilage damage pattern in relation to subchondral plate thickness in a collagenase-induced model of osteoarthritis. Osteoarthritis Cartilage 16: 506–514.
34. Davies ME, Dingle JT, Pigott R, Power C, Sharma H (1991) Expression of intercellular adhesion molecule 1 (ICAM-1) on human articular cartilage chondrocytes. Connect Tissue Res 26: 207–216. 10.3109/03008209109152439 [doi].
35. McCourt PA, Ek B, Forsberg N, Gustafson S (1994) Intercellular adhesion molecule-1 is a cell surface receptor for hyaluronan. J Biol Chem 269: 30081–30084.
36. Yasuda T (2010) Hyaluronan inhibits p38 mitogen-activated protein kinase via the receptors in rheumatoid arthritis chondrocytes stimulated with fibronectin fragment. Clin Rheumatol 29: 1259–1267. 10.1007/s10067-010-1512-5 [doi].
37. Yasuda T (2012) Activation of p38 mitogen-activated protein kinase is inhibited by hyaluronan via intercellular adhesion molecule-1 in articular chondrocytes stimulated with type II collagen peptide. J Pharmacol Sci 118: 25–32. JST.JSTAGE/jphs/11044FP [pii].
38. Lisignoli G, Grassi F, Zini N, Toneguzzi S, Piacentini A, et al. (2001) Anti-Fas-induced apoptosis in chondrocytes reduced by hyaluronan: evidence for CD44 and CD54 (intercellular adhesion molecule 1) invovement. Arthritis Rheum 44: 1800–1807. 10.1002/1529-0131(200108)44:8<1800::AID-ART317> 3.0.CO;2-1 [doi].

Adiponectin Enhances Intercellular Adhesion Molecule-1 Expression and Promotes Monocyte Adhesion in Human Synovial Fibroblasts

Hsien-Te Chen[1,2], Hsi-Kai Tsou[3,4], Jui-Chieh Chen[7,9], James Meng-Kun Shih[5], Yen-Jen Chen[2,6], Chih-Hsin Tang[6,7,8]*

1 School of Chinese Medicine, College of Chinese Medicine, China Medical University, Taichung, Taiwan, **2** Department of Orthopaedic Surgery, China Medical University Hospital, Taichung, Taiwan, **3** Department of Neurosurgery, Taichung Veterans General Hospital, Taichung, Taiwan, **4** Department of Early Childhood Care and Education, Jen-Teh Junior College of Medicine, Nursing and Management, Miaoli County, Taiwan, **5** Department of Orthopaedic Surgery, Lin Sen Hospital, Taichung, Taiwan, **6** School of Medicine, China Medical University, Taichung, Taiwan, **7** Graduate Institute of Basic Medical Science, China Medical University, Taichung, Taiwan, **8** Department of Biotechnology, College of Health Science, Asia University, Taichung, Taiwan, **9** National Institute of Cancer Research, National Health Research Institutes, Miaoli County, Zhunan, Taiwan

Abstract

Adiponectin is a protein hormone secreted predominantly by differentiated adipocytes and is involved in energy homeostasis. Adiponectin expression is significantly high in the synovial fluid of patients with osteoarthritis (OA). Intercellular adhesion molecule-1 (ICAM-1) is an important adhesion molecule that mediates monocyte adhesion and infiltration during OA pathogenesis. Adiponectin-induced expression of ICAM-1 in human OA synovial fibroblasts (OASFs) was examined by using qPCR, flow cytometry and western blotting. The intracellular signaling pathways were investigated by pretreated with inhibitors or transfection with siRNA. The monocyte THP-1 cell line was used for an adhesion assay with OASFs. Stimulation of OASFs with adiponectin induced ICAM-1 expression. Pretreatment with AMP-activated protein kinase (AMPK) inhibitors (AraA and compound C) or transfection with siRNA against AMPKα1 and two AMPK upstream activator-liver kinase B1 (LKB1) and calmodulin-dependent protein kinase II (CaMKII) diminished the adiponectin-induced ICAM-1 expression. Stimulation of OASFs with adiponectin increased phosphorylation of LKB1, CaMKII, AMPK, and c-Jun, resulting in c-Jun binding to AP-1 element of ICAM-1 promoter. In addition, adiponectin-induced activation of the LKB1/CaMKII, AMPK, and AP-1 pathway increased the adhesion of monocytes to the OASF monolayer. Our results suggest that adiponectin increases ICAM-1 expression in human OASFs via the LKB1/CaMKII, AMPK, c-Jun, and AP-1 signaling pathway. Adiponectin-induced ICAM-1 expression promoted the adhesion of monocytes to human OASFs. These findings may provide a better understanding of the pathogenesis of OA and can utilize this knowledge to design a new therapeutic strategy.

Editor: Chuen-Mao Yang, Chang Gung University, Taiwan

Funding: This work was supported by grants from the National Science Council of Taiwan (NSC100-2320-B-039-028-MY3) and China Medical University Hospital (DMR-102-055). The funders had no role in study design, data collection and analysis, decision to publish, or preparation of the manuscript.

Competing Interests: The authors have declared that no competing interests exist.

* E-mail: chtang@mail.cmu.edu.tw

Introduction

Osteoarthritis (OA) is the most common chronic degenerative joint disorder in elderly individuals, which is often characterized by infiltration of inflammatory cells and production of multiple potent inflammatory mediators and matrix-degrading proteinases in synovium, leading to disabling pain, stiffness, cartilage breakdown, and a loss of joint function [1]. To date, the etiology of OA is still not fully understood. Nevertheless, emerging evidence has revealed that adipose tissue is capable of secreting a number of adipokines, which have a critical role in the development and progression of OA [2–6].

Adiponectin (also known as Acrp30, AdipoQ, and GBP28), one of the most abundant adipokines, is highly expressed in the synovial fluid of patients with OA and closely associated with the severity [7–10]. Previous studies showed that adiponectin could be expressed not only by articular adipocytes but also by synovial fibroblasts [11]. In addition, adiponectin receptors have also been identified on the surface of synovial fibroblasts, which are necessary to exert the adiponectin-dependent signals to increase the production of cartilage-degrading matrix metalloproteinase (MMP) enzymes, cytokines and prostaglandin E2 [11–13]. Besides release of inflammatory mediators, infiltration of inflammatory cells has also been detected in the inflamed synovium of OA patients, which plays a critical role in persistent inflammation and joint destruction [14]. The movement of mononuclear cells into the inflammatory sites is regulated by adhesion molecules, such as intercellular adhesion molecule-1 (ICAM-1).

ICAM-1 is an inducible surface glycoprotein that belongs to the immunoglobulin superfamily and mediates adhesion-dependent cell-to-cell interactions [15,16]. The extracellular domain of ICAM-1 plays a crucial role in migration of leukocytes out of blood vessels into sites of inflammation [17]. More recently, a study further demonstrated that tumor-associated fibroblasts isolated from tumor tissues exhibit increased ICAM-1 expression and affinity for monocytes [18]. Up-regulation of ICAM-1 has been shown in synovium of OA patients, which may be an important regulator of leukocyte recruitment into the synovial tissue [19,20]. Furthermore, reducing the levels of ICAM-1 in synovial fluid also proposed effective method to suppress the inflammatory response and to ameliorate symptoms of physiological distress in OA [21,22].

Although the roles of adiponectin have emerged as key a regulator of immune responses and inflammatory arthritis, little is known about the mechanisms underlying the interaction between monocytes and human OASFs by which adiponectin induce ICAM-1 expression. In the present study, we explored the possible intracellular signaling pathways involved in adiponectin-induced ICAM-1 expression in human OASFs.

Materials and Methods

Material

Rabbit polyclonal antibodies specific for ICAM-1, p-AMPK, AMPK, p-LKB1, LKB1, p-CaMKII, CaMKII, p-c-Jun, c-Jun, and β-actin, anti-mouse and anti-rabbit IgG-conjugated horseradish peroxidase, and Protein A/G beads were purchased from Santa Cruz Biotechnology (Santa Cruz, CA, USA). Compound C and adenosine-9-β-D-arabino-furanoside (AraA) were purchased from Calbiochem (San Diego, CA). Human full-length adiponectin was purchased from R&D Systems (Minneapolis, MN). The AP-1 luciferase plasmid was purchased from Stratagene (La Jolla, CA). The pSV-β-galactosidase vector and luciferase assay kit were purchased from Promega (Madison, MA). All other chemicals were purchased from Sigma-Aldrich (St. Louis, MO).

Cell cultures

Human synovial fibroblasts were isolated using collagenase treatment of synovial tissues obtained from knee replacement surgeries of 18 patients with OA. OASFs were isolated, cultured, and characterized as previously described [23,24]. Experiments were performed using cells grown in vitro for 3–6 passages. The study protocol was approved by the Institutional Review Board of China Medical University Hospital, and all subjects gave informed written consent before enrollment. THP-1, a human leukemia cell line of the monocyte/macrophage lineage, was obtained from the American Type Culture Collection (Manassas, VA, USA) and grown in RPMI-1640 medium with 10% fetal bovine serum.

Quantitative real-time PCR

Total RNA was extracted from OASFs using a TRIzol kit (MDBio Inc., Taipei, Taiwan). The reverse transcription reaction was performed from 2 μg of total RNA using M-MLV reverse transcriptase (Invitrogen) according to the manufacturer's instructions. The quantitative real-time PCR (qPCR) analysis was carried out using Taqman one-step PCR Master Mix (Applied Biosystems, Foster City, CA). The cDNA templates (2 μl) were added per 25-μl reaction with sequence-specific primers and Taqman probes. All target gene primers and probes were purchased commercially (β-actin was used as internal control) (Applied Biosystems). The qPCR assays were carried out in triplicate using a StepOnePlus sequence detection system. Amplification curves were generated with an initial denaturing step at 95°C for10 min, followed by 40 cycles at 95°C for 15 s and 60°C for 60 s. The threshold was set above the non-template control background and within the linear phase of the target gene amplification to calculate the cycle number at which the transcript was detected (denoted CT). Reactions were normalized to copies of β-actin mRNA within the same sample using the $-\Delta\Delta CT$ method. The levels of mRNA are expressed as the fold change in expression compared with that of controls.

Western blot analysis

Cells were lysed in RIPA buffer containing protease inhibitor cocktail. Protein concentration was determined by the BCA assay (Pierce). Proteins (30 μg) were resolved on SDS-PAGE and transferred to immobilon polyvinyldifluoride (PVDF) membranes. The blots were blocked with 5% BSA for 1 h at room temperature and then probed with rabbit anti-human antibodies against ICAM-1, p-AMPK, AMPK, p-CaMKII, CaMKII, p-LKB1, or LKB1 (1:1000) for 1 h at room temperature. β-actin was used as an internal control of protein loading. After three washes, the blots were subsequently incubated with the appropriate secondary antibodies conjugated to horseradish peroxidase. Membranes were then washed and bound antibodies were visualized using ECL reagents (PerkinElmer, MA, USA) and autoradiography.

Flow cytometry analysis

Human synovial fibroblasts were seeded in six-well plates. The cells were then washed with PBS and detached with trypsin at 37°C. After fixation with 1% paraformaldehyde for 10 min at room temperature, cells were resuspended in PBS with mouse anti-human antibody against ICAM-1 (1:100) for 1 h at 4°C. Cells were then washed again and incubated with FITC-conjugated goat anti-mouse secondary IgG (1:100; Leinco Technologies Inc., St. Louis, MO, USA) for 45 min and analyzed by flow cytometry using FACS Calibur (10,000 cells were collected for each experiment) and CellQuest software (BD Biosciences).

Transfection of siRNAs

ON-TARGETplus siRNA of AMPKα1, CaMKII, LKB1, c-Jun, c-fos, and control were purchased from Dharmacon Research (Lafayette, CO). Transient transfection of siRNAs (100 nM) was carried out using DharmaFECT1 transfection reagent, according to the manufacturer's instructions.

Chromatin immunoprecipitation assay

Chromatin immunoprecipitation (ChIP) analysis was performed as described previously [25]. Briefly, the DNA/protein complex was immunoprecipitated by protein G-agarose beads with anti-c-Jun monoclonal antibody (mAb). After incubation, the beads were washed with the low-salt wash buffer, the high-salt wash buffer, the LiCl wash buffer and finally two times with Tris-EDTA buffer. The bound protein was eluted with elution buffer containing 1% SDS and 100 mM NaHCO3. The crosslinks were reversed by overnight incubation at 65°C. The DNA was then extracted with phenol-chloroform. The purified DNA pellet was subjected to PCR. PCR products were then resolved by 1.5% agarose gel electrophoresis and visualized by UV transillumination. The primers 5′-AGACCTTAGCGCGGTGTAGA-3′ and 5′-AGTAGCAGAGGAGCTCAGCG-3′ were utilized to amplify across the ICAM-1 promoter region (−346 to −24).

Reporter assay

Human OASF cells were transfected with a reporter plasmid (ICAM-1 luciferase plasmid or AP-1 luciferase) using Lipofectamine 2000 (Invitrogen) according to the manufacturer's recommendations. At 24 h after transfection, the cells were exposed to various doses (0.3–3 μM/ml) of adiponectin for 24 h or pretreated with inhibitors for 30 min, and then, adiponectin or vehicle was

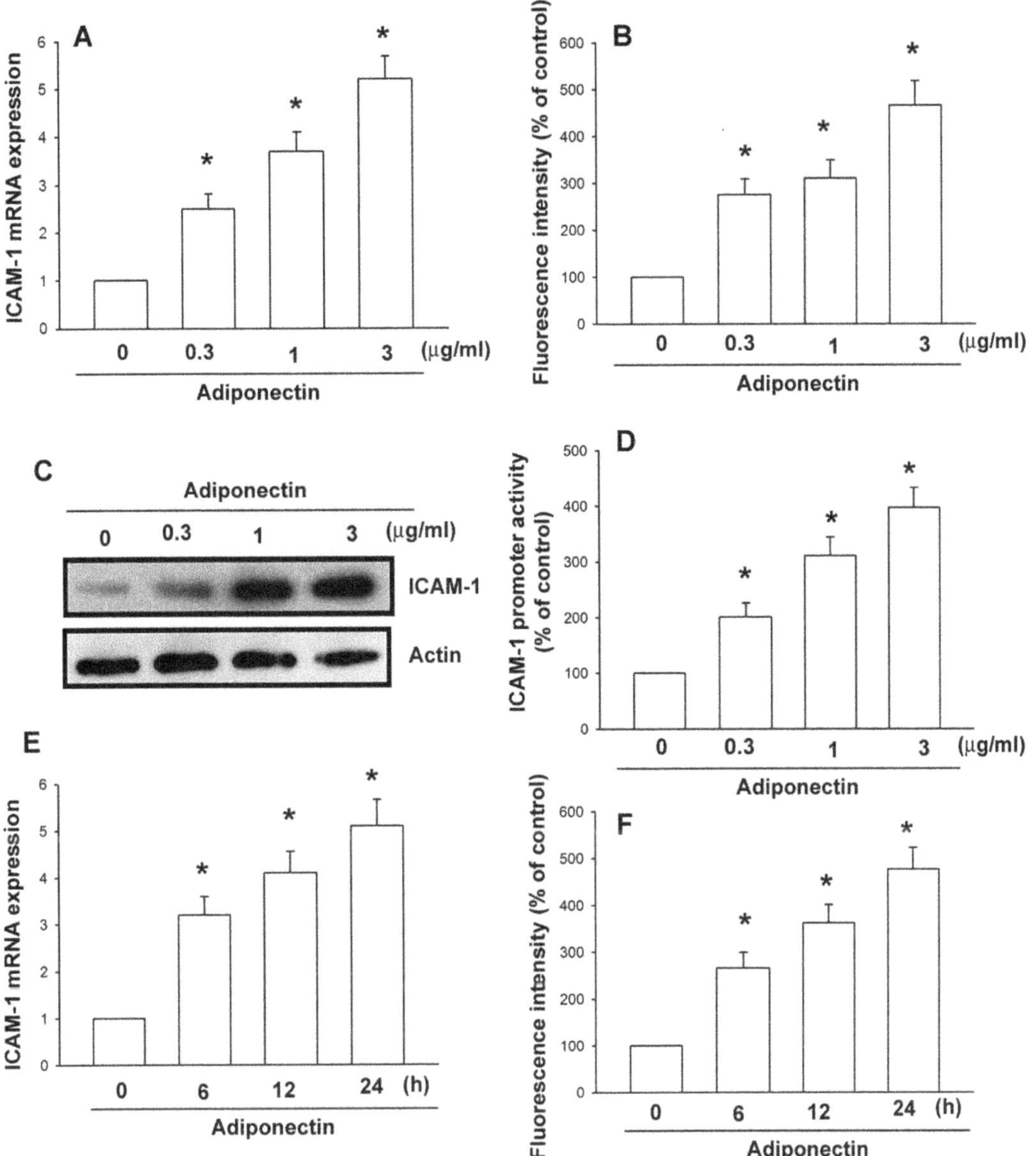

Figure 1. Adiponectin increases ICAM-1 expression. OASFs were incubated with various concentrations of adiponectin for 24 h. The levels of ICAM-1 mRNA (A), cell surface (B), and protein expression (C) were examined by qPCR, flow cytometry, and western blotting. (D) OASFs were transfected with ICAM-1 promoter-luciferase construct to examine the adiponectin-induced promoter activity in a dose-dependent manner. (E, F) OASFs were incubated with adiponectin (3 μg/ml) for the indicated time intervals. The levels of ICAM-1 mRNA (E) and cell surface (F) expression were examined by qPCR and flow cytometry. Results are expressed as the mean ± S.E. *$p<0.05$, compared to basal expression levels. #$p<0.05$, compared to expression levels in the adiponectin-treated group.

added for 24 h. Cell extracts were then prepared, and luciferase and β-galactosidase activities were measured.

Cell adhesion assay

THP-1 cells were labeled with BCECF-AM (10 μM) at 37°C for 1 h in RPMI-1640 medium and subsequently washed by centrifugation. OASFs grown on glass coverslips were incubated with adiponectin for 6 h. Confluent adiponectin-treated OASFs were incubated with THP-1 cells (2×10^6 cells/ml) at 37°C for 1 h. Non-adherent THP-1 cells were then removed and gently washed with PBS. The number of adherent THP-1 cells was counted in four randomly chosen fields per well at a high magnification of 200× using a fluorescence microscope (Zeiss, Axiovert 200 M).

Statistics

The values reported are means ± S.E. Statistical comparisons between two samples were performed using the Student's *t*-test. Statistical comparisons of more than two groups were performed using one-way analysis of variance (ANOVA) with a Bonferroni's *post-hoc* test. In all cases, a p-value of <0.05 was considered significant.

Results

Adiponectin induces ICAM-1 expression in human synovial fibroblasts

We initially assessed the effects of adiponectin on the expression of ICAM-1 in human OASFs. The treatment of OASFs with

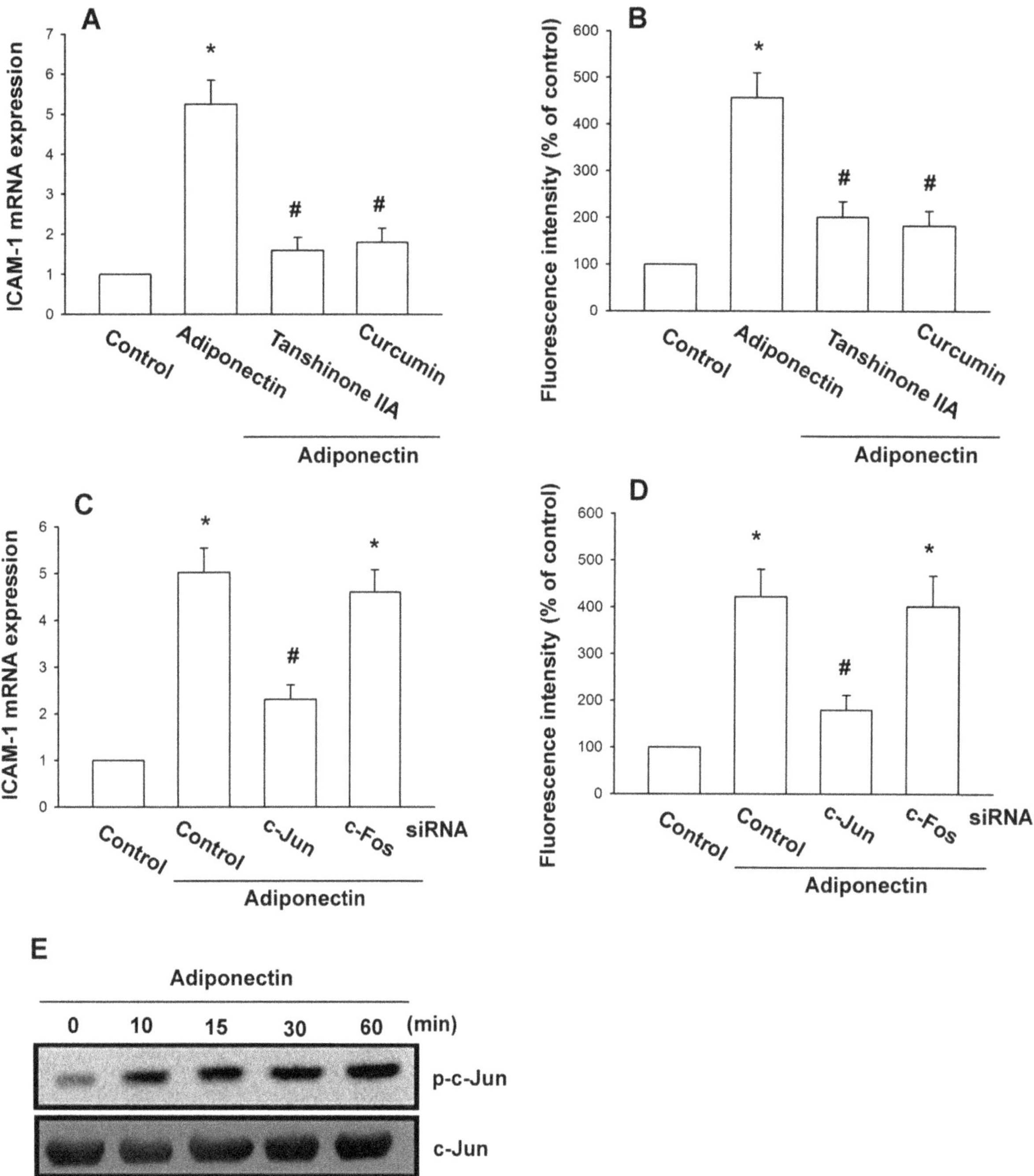

Figure 2. AP-1 is involved in the potentiation of ICAM-1 expression by adiponectin. OASFs were pretreated for 30 min with curcumin (3 μM) or tanshinone IIA (5 μM) followed by stimulation with adiponectin (3 μg/ml) for 24 h, and ICAM-1 expression was examined by qPCR (A) and flow cytometry (B). OASFs were transfected with c-Jun siRNA or c-fos siRNA for 24 h followed by stimulation with adiponectin (3 μg/ml) for 24 h, and ICAM-1 expression was examined by qPCR (C) and flow cytometry (D). (E) OASFs were incubated with adiponectin (3 μg/ml) for the indicated time intervals and c-Jun phosphorylation was determined by western blot. Results are expressed as the mean ± S.E. $*p<0.05$, compared to basal expression levels. $\#p<0.05$, compared to expression levels in the adiponectin-treated group.

adiponectin resulted in a dose-dependent increase in mRNA and cell surface ICAM-1 expression, as assessed by qPCR (Fig. 1A) and flow cytometry (Fig. 1B). The expression of ICAM-1 was further validated by western blot analysis (Fig. 1C). To clarify whether adiponectin is able to stimulate activation of ICAM-1 promoter in human synovial fibroblasts cells, the human ICAM-1 promoter-luciferase construct was transfected into cells to examine the adiponectin-induced promoter activity. As shown in Fig. 1D, adiponectin increased ICAM-1 promoter activity in a dose-dependent manner. Furthermore, the expression levels of ICAM-1 were also increased in OASFs after treatment with adiponectin in a time dependent (Fig. 1E, F). These data indicate that adiponectin increases ICAM-1 expression in human OASFs.

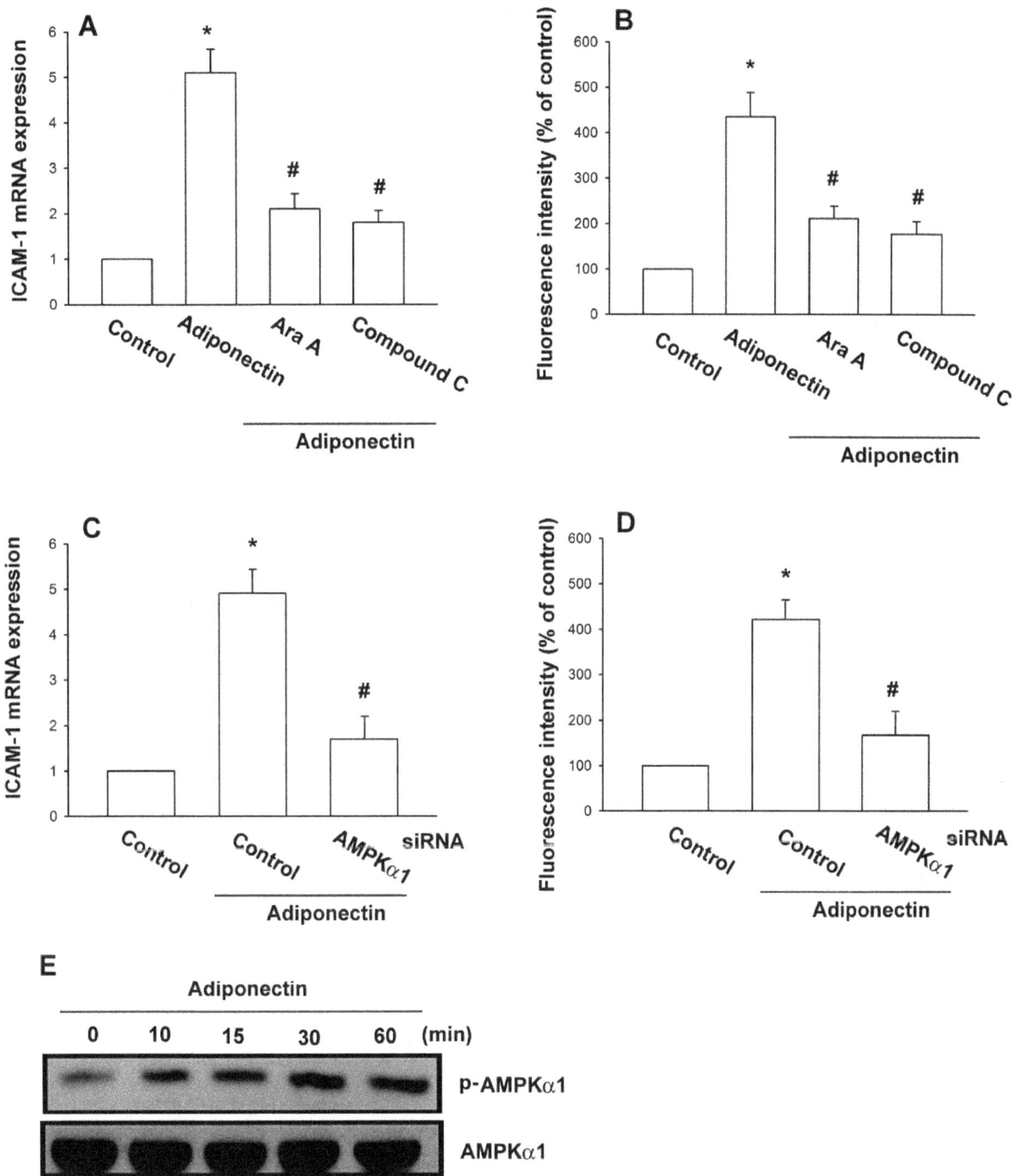

Figure 3. AMPK is involved in adiponectin-induced ICAM-1 expression in synovial fibroblasts. OASFs were pretreated for 30 min with Ara A (0.5 mM) or compound C (10 μM) followed by stimulation with adiponectin (3 μg/ml) for 24 h, and ICAM-1 expression was examined by qPCR (A) and flow cytometry (B). OASFs were transfected with AMPKα1 siRNA for 24 h followed by stimulation with adiponectin (3 μg/ml) for 24 h, and ICAM-1 expression was examined by qPCR (C) and flow cytometry (D). (E) OASFs were incubated with adiponectin (3 μg/ml) for the indicated time intervals and AMPKα1 phosphorylation was determined by western blot. Results are expressed as the mean ± S.E. *$p<0.05$, compared to basal expression levels. #$p<0.05$, compared to expression levels in the adiponectin-treated group.

AP-1 is involved in the adiponectin-mediated increase of ICAM-1 expression

Because it has been reported that the ICAM-1 promoter includes binding sites for AP-1 [26], we sought to investigate whether the transcription factor is responsible for adiponectin-mediated ICAM-1 expression on OASFs observed above. Pretreatment of cells for 30 min with AP-1 inhibitors (curcumin and tanshinone IIA) antagonized adiponectin-induced ICAM-1 expression (Fig. 2A, B). We then investigated whether the presence of c-Jun and/or c-Fos is critical for adiponectin-mediated increase of ICAM-1 expression. As shown in Fig. 2C, D, the adiponectin-mediated increase of ICAM-1 expression was inhibited by

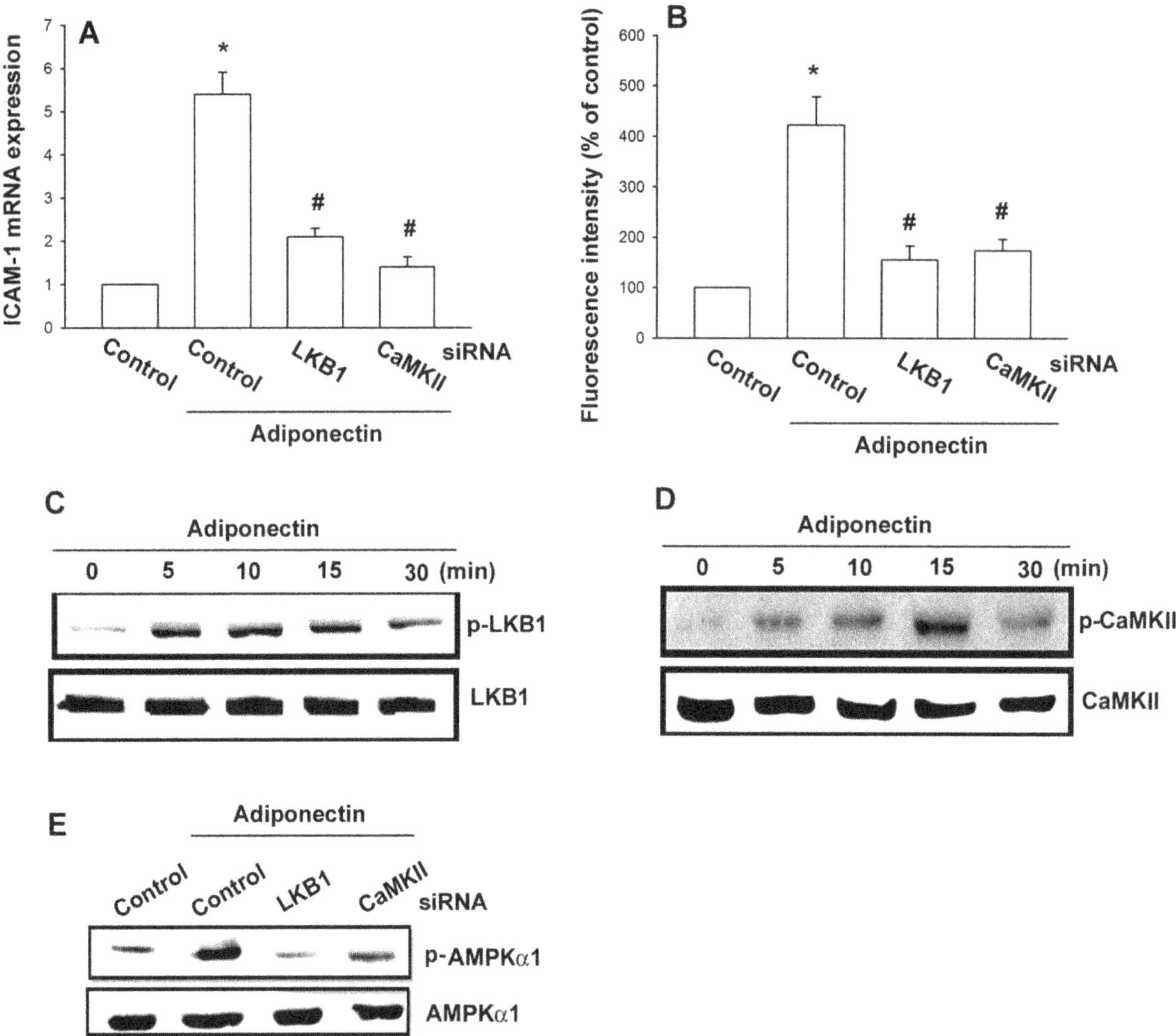

Figure 4. LKB1 and CaMKII are involved in adiponectin-induced ICAM-1 expression in synovial fibroblasts. OASFs were transfected with LKB1 or CaMKII siRNA for 24 h followed by stimulation with adiponectin (3 μg/ml) for 24 h, and ICAM-1 expression was examined by qPCR (A) and flow cytometry (B). (C, D) OASFs were incubated with adiponectin (3 μg/ml) for indicated time intervals and LKB1 and CaMKII phosphorylation was determined by western blot. (E) OASFs were transfected with LKB1 siRNA or CaMKII siRNA for 24 h followed by stimulation with adiponectin (3 μg/ml) for 30 min. AMPK phosphorylation was determined by western blot. Results are expressed as the mean ± S.E. *$p<0.05$, compared to basal expression levels. #$p<0.05$, compared to expression levels in the adiponectin-treated group.

knocking down c-Jun with siRNA, but not by knocking down c-fos. Next, we further examined c-Jun phosphorylation after adiponectin treatment. Stimulation of OASFs with adiponectin promoted c-Jun phosphorylation (Fig. 2E). These data indicated that AP-1 transactivation by the c-Jun homodimer is involved in adiponectin-induced ICAM-1 expression.

The AMPK signaling pathway is involved in the adiponectin-mediated increase of ICAM-1 expression

Previously studies have reported that adiponectin is able to increase fatty acid oxidation via activation of AMP-activated protein kinase (AMPK) in adipocytes [27,28]. To determine whether AMPK is involved in adiponectin triggered ICAM-1 expression, the AMPK inhibitors Ara A and compound C were used. As seen in Fig. 3A, B, pretreatment with Ara A and compound C reduced adiponectin-induced ICAM-1 expression. Further, we knocked down the expression of AMPKα1 by its specific siRNAs in OASFs and investigated the effects of adiponectin on the ICAM-1 production. Indeed, transfection of cells with AMPKα1 siRNA diminished adiponectin-induced ICAM-1 expression (Fig. 3C, D). We then directly measured AMPK phosphorylation in response to adiponectin and found that stimulation of OASFs led to a significant increase in phosphorylation of AMPK (Fig. 3E). These data suggest that AMPK activation is involved in adiponectin-induced ICAM-1 expression in human OASFs.

LKB1 and CaMKII signaling pathways are involved in adiponectin-induced ICAM-1 expression

AMPK is regulated by upstream kinases which have been identified as LKB1 or CaMKII [29,30]. In addition, a study indicates that adiponectin also activates AMPK upstream kinase LKB1 and CaMKII, which plays a critical role in AMPK activation [31]. To examine the role of LKB1 and CaMKII in adiponectin-mediated ICAM-1, we generated LKB1- and CaMKII- suppressed OASFs by siRNA knockdown. Both siRNA

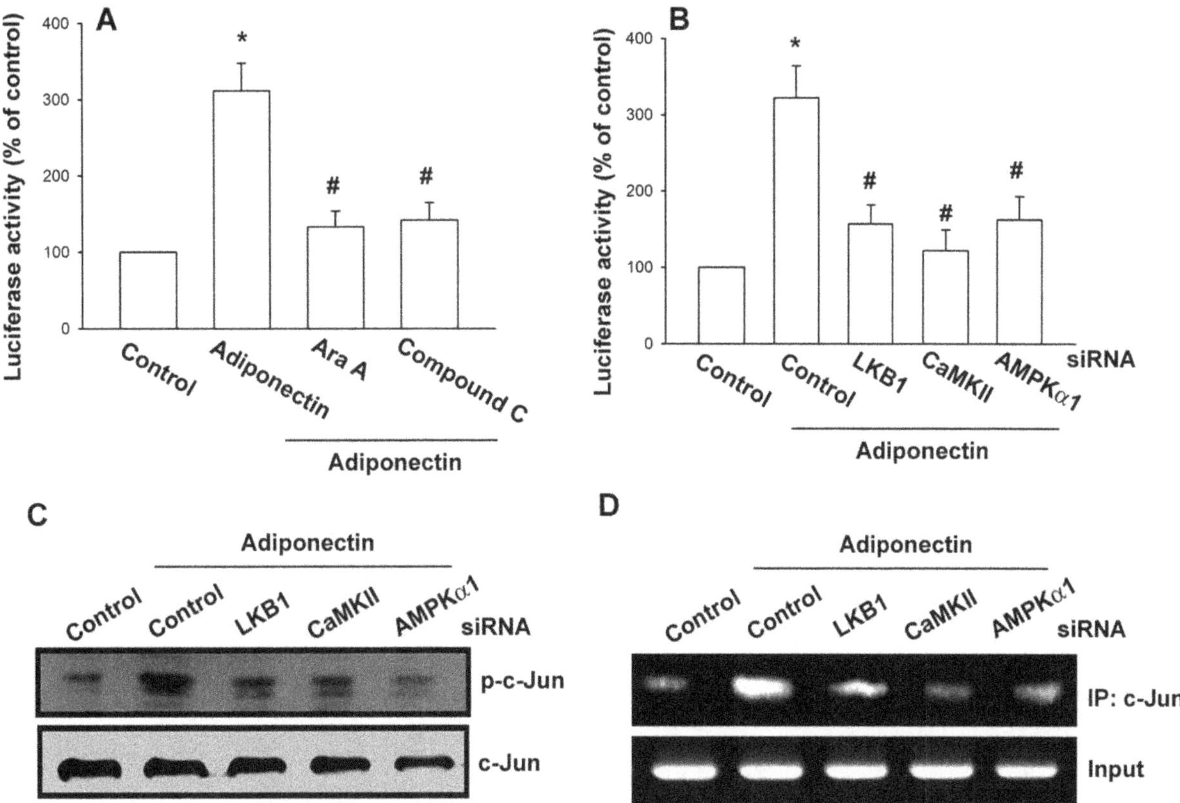

Figure 5. The LKB1, CaMKII, and AMPK signaling pathway is involved in adiponectin-induced AP-1 activation. OASFs transiently transfected with AP-1-luciferase plasmid for 24 h and then pretreated with Ara A and compound C (A) for 30 min or cotransfected with LKB1, CaMKII, and AMPKα1 siRNA (B) for 24 h before incubation with adiponectin for 24 h. Luciferase activity was measured, and the results were normalized to the β-galactosidase activity. OASFs were transfected with LKB1, CaMKII, or AMPKα1 siRNA for 24 h followed by stimulation with adiponectin (3 μg/ml), and c-Jun phosphorylation and c-Jun binding to the ICAM-1 promoter were examined by western blot (C) and chromatin immunoprecipitation assay (D). Results are expressed as the mean ± S.E. **p*<0.05, compared to basal expression levels. #*p*<0.05, compared to expression levels in the adiponectin-treated group.

constructs significantly restricted increases in adiponectin-induced expression of ICAM-1, as determined by qPCR (Fig. 4A) and flow cytometry (Fig. 4B). Direct incubation of cells with adiponectin caused a time-dependent increase in phosphorylation of LKB1 and CaMKII (Fig. 4C, D). In addition, knockdown of LKB1 or CaMKII led to a decrease in adiponectin-induced AMPK1 phosphorylation (Fig. 4E). Taken together, these results indicate that the LKB1/CaMKII-dependent AMPK activation is involved in the regulation of ICAM-1 expression.

LKB1/CaMKII/AMPK signaling pathway is involved in adiponectin-induced AP-1 activation

To further evaluate the LKB1/CaMKII/AMPK signaling pathway involved in adiponectin-induced AP-1 activation, OASFs were transiently transfected with AP-1 promoter-luciferase construct as an indicator of AP-1 activation. As shown in Fig. 5A, treatment of OASFs with adiponectin caused an increase in AP-1-luciferase activity, whereas pretreatment of cells with Ara A or compound C reduced adiponectin-mediated AP-1 activity. Moreover, co-transfection of cells with LKB1, CaMKII, or AMPK1 siRNA also reduced adiponectin-induced AP-1 activity (Fig. 5B)

Finally, AP-1 activation was further validated using western blot analysis and ChIP. As shown in Fig. 5C, transfection of cells with LKB1, CaMKII, and AMPK1 siRNA inhibited adiponectin-mediated c-Jun phosphorylation. ChIP analysis reveals that adiponectin significantly increased c-Jun binding to AP-1 element of ICAM-1 promoter, but this phenomenon was attenuated by transfection of cells with LKB1, CaMKII, and AMPK1 siRNA (Fig. 5D).

Adiponectin induces monocyte adhesion through the LKB1/CaMKII/AMPK pathway

In order to identify whether adiponectin is involved in the interaction between OASFs and monocytes, we carried out adhesion assays using the THP-1 cell line as a monocyte model. Treatment of OASFs with adiponectin enhanced the adhesion between OASFs and THP-1 cells in a dose-dependent fashion (Fig. 6A). To further evaluate the LKB1/CaMKII/AMPK pathway is able to induce monocytes to adhere to the monolayer of OASFs, we pretreated OASFs with Ara A and compound C, and also transfected them with LKB1, CaMKII, and AMPK1 siRNA. Both the pretreatment and transfection significantly inhibited monocyte adhesion to OASFs (Fig. 6B). These results indicate that adiponectin promoted the adhesion of monocytes to OASFs via the LKB1/CaMKII/AMPK pathway.

Discussion

OA is a chronic inflammatory disease with cytokine production that may play a key role in the recruitment and infiltration of leucocyte to the joint, resulting in degradation and loss of articular

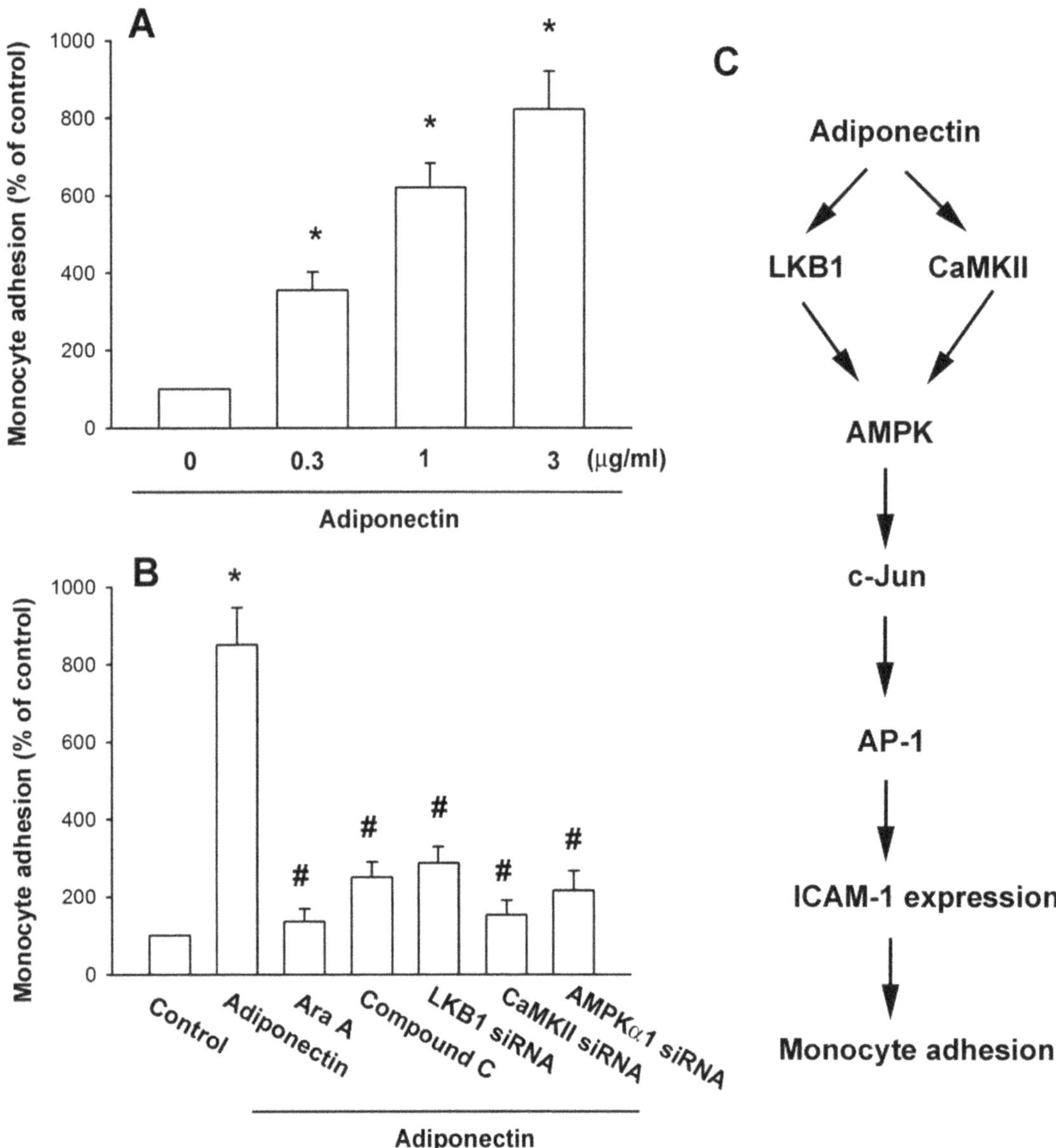

Figure 6. Adiponectin induces monocyte adhesion through the LKB1, CaMKII, AMPK, and AP-1 pathway. OASFs were incubated with various concentrations of adiponectin for 24 h (A), pretreated with Ara A and compound C for 30 min, or transfected with LKB1, CaMKII, and AMPKα1 siRNA followed by stimulation with adiponectin for 24 h (B). THP-1 cells labeled with BCECF-AM were added to OASFs for 6 h, and then the adherence of THP-1 cells was measured by fluorescence microscopy. Results are expressed as the mean ± S.E. *$p<0.05$, compared to basal expression levels. #$p<0.05$, compared to expression levels in the adiponectin-treated group. (C) Schematic presentation of the signaling pathways involved in adiponectin-induced ICAM-1 expression and monocyte adhesion to human synovial fibroblasts.

tissues. However, detailed mechanisms responsible for attracting immune cells to the site of inflamed synovium are still unclear. In this study, we characterized the effect of adiponectin on the expression of ICAM-1 in synovial fibroblasts, which may mediate the interaction of fibroblasts with immune cells. Furthermore, we also showed that potentiation of ICAM-1 by adiponectin requires the activation of the LKB1/CaMKII, AMPK, and AP-1 signaling pathway and promotes the adhesion of monocytes to OASFs (Fig. 6C).

Adiponectin is an adipocytokine originally found to be secreted exclusively by adipose tissue, but meanwhile, adiponectin was found to be expressed by bone-forming cells as well [32]. In synovial fibroblasts and articular adipocytes of rheumatoid arthritis (RA) and OA patients, high levels of adiponectin expression were also detected, which may contribute to inflammation in the fluid of the joint [11]. A previous study showed that plasma adiponectin levels were significantly higher in OA patients than in healthy controls [33]. Another study also found that increased plasma adiponectin levels were positively correlated with synovial fluid adiponectin concentrations in OA patients [9]. Adiponectin exists both as full-length and globular forms. Globular adiponectin is proteolytically cleaved from the full-length protein, which consists of the C-terminal domain of the full-length adiponectin [34]. Contrary to full-length adiponectin, globular form constitutes about 25% of adiponectin in synovial fluid from patients with arthritis [35]. Moreover, other research has shown cleavage of adiponectin by leukocyte elastase secreted from activated monocytes is able to generate the globular adiponectin

[36], which may be involved in the generation of the globular fragment of adiponectin in inflamed joints. Adiponectin interacts with at least two known cellular receptors (AdipoR1 and AdipoR2). AdipoR1 is abundantly expressed in skeletal muscle, whereas AdipoR2 is predominantly expressed in the liver [37]. However, our previous studies have demonstrated that RASF and OASF cells express both AdipoR1 and AdipoR2 receptor isoforms. Furthermore, adiponectin increased IL-6 production in human synovial fibroblasts via the AdipoR1 receptor but not AdipoR2 [12]. In the present study, we found similar results. Our data indicate that adiponectin can induce ICAM-1 expression in human OASFs via AdipoR1 (Fig. S1).

Interestingly, the ability to respond to adiponectin is not exclusive to synovial fibroblasts. AdipoRs have also been identified on the surface of human chondrocytes. In chondrocytes, the binding of adiponectin to its receptor causes the increased production of IL-6, IL-8, monocyte chemoattractant protein-1 (MCP-1), prostaglandin E2, matrix metalloproteinase (MMP), and nitric oxide, which contribute to inflammation and joint destruction in OA [38–42]. In addition, adiponectin could elicit persistent cartilage-degrading processes by inducing expression of vascular cell adhesion molecules-1 (VCAM-1) in chondrocytes, which is responsible for infiltration of leukocyte and monocyte into inflamed joints [43]. We therefore investigated whether adiponectin can also stimulate expression of VCAM-1 on OASFs. As shown in Fig. S2A, adiponectin was also able to induce VCAM-1 expression in a dose-dependent manner. To further determine which of adhesion molecules is primarily responsible for recruitment of leukocytes on adiponectin-stimulated OASFs, we performed siRNA experiments to knock down VCAM-1 or ICAM-1 in OASFs. Our results revealed ICAM-1 kncokdown exerted more potent effect on inhibiting the adhesion of monocytes when compared with VCAM-1 kncokdown (Fig. S2B).

On the contrary, some studies have shown contradictory results. In an animal model, adiponectin has been shown to ameliorate the severity of collagen-induced arthritis [44]. Moreover, adiponectin may play a protective role against OA by inducing tissue inhibitor of metalloproteinase-2 (TIMP-2) expression and suppressing IL-1β-induced MMP-13 production in chondrocytes [45]. A clinical report has also indicated that decreased adiponectin levels in both plasma and synovial fluid is associated with severity of OA [9]. The explanation for the above discrepancies may be attributable to differences in methodologies, disease progression, populations, and inappropriate controls for normalization.

AMPK, a heterotrimeric serine/threonine kinase, consists of a catalytic α subunit, and regulatory β and γ subunits [46]. Previous studies have demonstrated that AMPK is involved in the adiponectin signaling pathway [47–49]. We observed that AMPK inhibitors, namely, Ara A and compound C, antagonize adiponectin-mediated ICAM-1 expression, suggesting that AMPK activation is required for adiponectin-induced ICAM-1 expression in synovial fibroblasts. In addition, it has been shown that AMPK1 is more important than AMPK2 in adiponectin-mediated gene expression in human synovial fibroblasts [12]. Thus, we attempted to investigate whether the catalytic subunit of AMPKα1 mediates adiponectin signaling in human OASFs cells. The results revealed that siRNA against AMPKα1 reduced adiponectin-mediated ICAM-1 production, implying that AMPKα1 is involved in adiponectin-induced expression of ICAM-1.

Histologically, OA synovium shows an increased number of mixed immune cells infiltrate, particularly macrophages in early OA [50]. Additionally, numerous studies have shown that activated synovial macrophages play a pivotal role in ongoing inflammation in OA through an increase in production of cytokines and destructive enzymes [51–53]. Another study also found that synovial fluid macrophages are capable of differentiating into mature osteoclasts to promote OA pathology [54]. The results from these reports imply that prevention of macrophage infiltration into inflamed synovium could be an attractive strategy for OA therapy.

Conclusion

We have explored the signaling mechanisms of adiponectin in the regulation of ICAM-1 expression in human synovial fibroblasts. Our results demonstrated that adiponectin increases ICAM-1 production by activating LKB1/CaMKII and AMPK, which in turn enhances the binding of AP-1 transcription factor to the ICAM-1 promoter, leading to the transactivation of ICAM-1 expression. In addition, we also showed that the adiponectin-mediated LKB1/CaMKII, AMPK, and AP-1 pathway promotes the adhesion of monocytes to human OASFs. These findings may provide a better understanding of the mechanisms underlying OA pathogenesis and can utilize this knowledge translationally for novel treatment strategies for OA.

Supporting Information

Figure S1 AdipoR1, but not AdipoR2 is involved in adiponectin-induced ICAM-1 expression in synovial fibroblasts. OASFs were transfected with AdipoR1 or AdipoR2 siRNA for 24 h followed by stimulation with adiponectin (3 μg/ml) for 24 h, and ICAM-1 expression was examined by qPCR.

Figure S2 Adiponectin can also increase VCAM-1 expression to induce monocyte adhesion. (A) OASFs were incubated with various concentrations of adiponectin for 24 h. The level of VCAM-1 mRNA was examined by qPCR. (B) OASFs were transfected with ICAM-1 or VCAM-1 siRNA for 24 h followed by stimulation with adiponectin (3 μg/ml) for 24 h. THP-1 cells labeled with BCECF-AM were added to OASFs for 6 h, and then the adherence of THP-1 cells was measured by fluorescence microscopy. Results are expressed as the mean ± S.E. *$p<0.05$, compared to basal expression levels. #$p<0.05$, compared to expression levels in the adiponectin-treated group.

Author Contributions

Conceived and designed the experiments: HTC HKT CHT. Performed the experiments: HTC HKT JCC JMKS YJC. Analyzed the data: HTC HKT JCC JMKS YJC. Contributed reagents/materials/analysis tools: HTC HKT JCC JMKS YJC. Wrote the paper: HTC JCC CHT.

References

1. Scanzello CR, Goldring SR (2012) The role of synovitis in osteoarthritis pathogenesis. Bone 51: 249–257.
2. Pottie P, Presle N, Terlain B, Netter P, Mainard D, et al. (2006) Obesity and osteoarthritis: more complex than predicted! Ann Rheum Dis 65: 1403–1405.
3. Toussirot E, Streit G, Wendling D (2007) The contribution of adipose tissue and adipokines to inflammation in joint diseases. Curr Med Chem 14: 1095–1100.
4. Dozio E, Corsi MM, Ruscica M, Passafaro L, Steffani L, et al. (2011) Adipokine actions on cartilage homeostasis. Adv Clin Chem 55: 61–79.
5. Hu PF, Bao JP, Wu LD (2011) The emerging role of adipokines in osteoarthritis: a narrative review. Mol Biol Rep 38: 873–878.
6. Huang C-Y (2012) Cardiovascular disease and cancer progression—A brief insight. BioMedicine 2: 129.

7. Schaffler A, Ehling A, Neumann E, Herfarth H, Tarner I, et al. (2003) Adipocytokines in synovial fluid. JAMA 290: 1709–1710.
8. Filkova M, Liskova M, Hulejova H, Haluzik M, Gatterova J, et al. (2009) Increased serum adiponectin levels in female patients with erosive compared with non-erosive osteoarthritis. Ann Rheum Dis 68: 295–296.
9. Honsawek S, Chayanupatkul M (2010) Correlation of plasma and synovial fluid adiponectin with knee osteoarthritis severity. Arch Med Res 41: 593–598.
10. Koskinen A, Juslin S, Nieminen R, Moilanen T, Vuolteenaho K, et al. (2011) Adiponectin associates with markers of cartilage degradation in osteoarthritis and induces production of proinflammatory and catabolic factors through mitogen-activated protein kinase pathways. Arthritis Res Ther 13: R184.
11. Ehling A, Schaffler A, Herfarth H, Tarner IH, Anders S, et al. (2006) The potential of adiponectin in driving arthritis. J Immunol 176: 4468–4478.
12. Tang CH, Chiu YC, Tan TW, Yang RS, Fu WM (2007) Adiponectin enhances IL-6 production in human synovial fibroblast via an AdipoR1 receptor, AMPK, p38, and NF-kappa B pathway. J Immunol 179: 5483–5492.
13. Kusunoki N, Kitahara K, Kojima F, Tanaka N, Kaneko K, et al. (2010) Adiponectin stimulates prostaglandin E(2) production in rheumatoid arthritis synovial fibroblasts. Arthritis Rheum 62: 1641–1649.
14. de Lange-Brokaar BJ, Ioan-Facsinay A, van Osch GJ, Zuurmond AM, Schoones J, et al. (2012) Synovial inflammation, immune cells and their cytokines in osteoarthritis: a review. Osteoarthritis Cartilage 20: 1484–1499.
15. van de Stolpe A, van der Saag PT (1996) Intercellular adhesion molecule-1. J Mol Med (Berl) 74: 13–33.
16. Zimmerman T, Blanco FJ (2008) Inhibitors targeting the LFA-1/ICAM-1 cell-adhesion interaction: design and mechanism of action. Curr Pharm Des 14: 2128–2139.
17. Long EO (2011) ICAM-1: getting a grip on leukocyte adhesion. J Immunol 186: 5021–5023.
18. Schellerer VS, Langheinrich M, Hohenberger W, Croner RS, Merkel S, et al. (2014) Tumor-associated fibroblasts isolated from colorectal cancer tissues exhibit increased ICAM-1 expression and affinity for monocytes. Oncol Rep 31: 255–261.
19. Koller M, Aringer M, Kiener H, Erlacher L, Machold K, et al. (1999) Expression of adhesion molecules on synovial fluid and peripheral blood monocytes in patients with inflammatory joint disease and osteoarthritis. Ann Rheum Dis 58: 709–712.
20. Lavigne P, Benderdour M, Lajeunesse D, Shi Q, Fernandes JC (2004) Expression of ICAM-1 by osteoblasts in healthy individuals and in patients suffering from osteoarthritis and osteoporosis. Bone 35: 463–470.
21. Karatay S, Kiziltunc A, Yildirim K, Karanfil RC, Senel K (2004) Effects of different hyaluronic acid products on synovial fluid levels of intercellular adhesion molecule-1 and vascular cell adhesion molecule-1 in knee osteoarthritis. Ann Clin Lab Sci 34: 330–335.
22. Lavigne P, Benderdour M, Shi Q, Lajeunesse D, Fernandes JC (2005) Involvement of ICAM-1 in bone metabolism: a potential target in the treatment of bone diseases? Expert Opin Biol Ther 5: 313–320.
23. Tang CH, Chiu YC, Tan TW, Yang RS, Fu WM (2007) Adiponectin enhances IL-6 production in human synovial fibroblast via an AdipoR1 receptor, AMPK, p38, and NF-kappa B pathway. Journal of immunology 179: 5483–5492.
24. Tang CH, Hsu CJ, Fong YC (2010) The CCL5/CCR5 axis promotes interleukin-6 production in human synovial fibroblasts. Arthritis and rheumatism 62: 3615–3624.
25. Yu HS, Lin TH, Tang CH (2013) Involvement of intercellular adhesion molecule-1 up-regulation in bradykinin promotes cell motility in human prostate cancers. International journal of molecular sciences 14: 13329–13345.
26. Roebuck KA, Finnegan A (1999) Regulation of intercellular adhesion molecule-1 (CD54) gene expression. J Leukoc Biol 66: 876–888.
27. Tomas E, Tsao TS, Saha AK, Murrey HE, Zhang Cc C, et al. (2002) Enhanced muscle fat oxidation and glucose transport by ACRP30 globular domain: acetyl-CoA carboxylase inhibition and AMP-activated protein kinase activation. Proc Natl Acad Sci U S A 99: 16309–16313.
28. Liu Q, Gauthier MS, Sun L, Ruderman N, Lodish H (2010) Activation of AMP-activated protein kinase signaling pathway by adiponectin and insulin in mouse adipocytes: requirement of acyl-CoA synthetases FATP1 and Acsl1 and association with an elevation in AMP/ATP ratio. FASEB J 24: 4229–4239.
29. Woods A, Johnstone SR, Dickerson K, Leiper FC, Fryer LG, et al. (2003) LKB1 is the upstream kinase in the AMP-activated protein kinase cascade. Curr Biol 13: 2004–2008.
30. Hurley RL, Anderson KA, Franzone JM, Kemp BE, Means AR, et al. (2005) The Ca2+/calmodulin-dependent protein kinase kinases are AMP-activated protein kinase kinases. J Biol Chem 280: 29060–29066.
31. Zhou L, Deepa SS, Etzler JC, Ryu J, Mao X, et al. (2009) Adiponectin activates AMP-activated protein kinase in muscle cells via APPL1/LKB1-dependent and phospholipase C/Ca2+/Ca2+/calmodulin-dependent protein kinase kinase-dependent pathways. J Biol Chem 284: 22426–22435.
32. Berner HS, Lyngstadaas SP, Spahr A, Monjo M, Thommesen L, et al. (2004) Adiponectin and its receptors are expressed in bone-forming cells. Bone 35: 842–849.
33. Laurberg TB, Frystyk J, Ellingsen T, Hansen IT, Jorgensen A, et al. (2009) Plasma adiponectin in patients with active, early, and chronic rheumatoid arthritis who are steroid- and disease-modifying antirheumatic drug-naive compared with patients with osteoarthritis and controls. J Rheumatol 36: 1885–1891.
34. Kadowaki T, Yamauchi T (2005) Adiponectin and adiponectin receptors. Endocr Rev 26: 439–451.
35. Chedid P, Hurtado-Nedelec M, Marion-Gaber B, Bournier O, Hayem G, et al. (2012) Adiponectin and its globular fragment differentially modulate the oxidative burst of primary human phagocytes. Am J Pathol 180: 682–692.
36. Waki H, Yamauchi T, Kamon J, Kita S, Ito Y, et al. (2005) Generation of globular fragment of adiponectin by leukocyte elastase secreted by monocytic cell line THP-1. Endocrinology 146: 790–796.
37. Yamauchi T, Kamon J, Ito Y, Tsuchida A, Yokomizo T, et al. (2003) Cloning of adiponectin receptors that mediate antidiabetic metabolic effects. Nature 423: 762–769.
38. Lago R, Gomez R, Otero M, Lago F, Gallego R, et al. (2008) A new player in cartilage homeostasis: adiponectin induces nitric oxide synthase type II and pro-inflammatory cytokines in chondrocytes. Osteoarthritis Cartilage 16: 1101–1109.
39. Kang EH, Lee YJ, Kim TK, Chang CB, Chung JH, et al. (2010) Adiponectin is a potential catabolic mediator in osteoarthritis cartilage. Arthritis Res Ther 12: R231.
40. Tong KM, Chen CP, Huang KC, Shieh DC, Cheng HC, et al. (2011) Adiponectin increases MMP-3 expression in human chondrocytes through AdipoR1 signaling pathway. J Cell Biochem 112: 1431–1440.
41. Gomez R, Scotece M, Conde J, Gomez-Reino JJ, Lago F, et al. (2011) Adiponectin and leptin increase IL-8 production in human chondrocytes. Ann Rheum Dis 70: 2052–2054.
42. Priya T, Chowdhury MG, Vasanth K, Vijayakumar TM, Ilango K, et al. (2013) Correlation of serum leptin and resistin levels with the metabolic risk factors of pre- and postmenopausal women in South India. BioMedicine 3: 167–173.
43. Conde J, Scotece M, Lopez V, Gomez R, Lago F, et al. (2012) Adiponectin and leptin induce VCAM-1 expression in human and murine chondrocytes. PLoS One 7: e52533.
44. Lee SW, Kim JH, Park MC, Park YB, Lee SK (2008) Adiponectin mitigates the severity of arthritis in mice with collagen-induced arthritis. Scand J Rheumatol 37: 260–268.
45. Chen TH, Chen L, Hsieh MS, Chang CP, Chou DT, et al. (2006) Evidence for a protective role for adiponectin in osteoarthritis. Biochim Biophys Acta 1762: 711–718.
46. Hardie DG, Ross FA, Hawley SA (2012) AMP-activated protein kinase: a target for drugs both ancient and modern. Chem Biol 19: 1222–1236.
47. Tang CH, Lu ME (2009) Adiponectin increases motility of human prostate cancer cells via adipoR, p38, AMPK, and NF-kappaB pathways. Prostate 69: 1781–1789.
48. Huang CY, Lee CY, Chen MY, Tsai HC, Hsu HC, et al. (2010) Adiponectin increases BMP-2 expression in osteoblasts via AdipoR receptor signaling pathway. J Cell Physiol 224: 475–483.
49. Ding C, Li L, Su YC, Xiang RL, Cong X, et al. (2013) Adiponectin increases secretion of rat submandibular gland via adiponectin receptors-mediated AMPK signaling. PLoS One 8: e63878.
50. Benito MJ, Veale DJ, FitzGerald O, van den Berg WB, Bresnihan B (2005) Synovial tissue inflammation in early and late osteoarthritis. Ann Rheum Dis 64: 1263–1267.
51. Bondeson J, Wainwright SD, Lauder S, Amos N, Hughes CE (2006) The role of synovial macrophages and macrophage-produced cytokines in driving aggrecanases, matrix metalloproteinases, and other destructive and inflammatory responses in osteoarthritis. Arthritis Res Ther 8: R187.
52. Shen PC, Lu CS, Shiau AL, Lee CH, Jou IM, et al. (2013) Lentiviral small hairpin RNA knockdown of macrophage inflammatory protein-1gamma ameliorates experimentally induced osteoarthritis in mice. Hum Gene Ther 24: 871–882.
53. Blasioli DJ, Matthews GL, Kaplan DL (2014) The degradation of chondrogenic pellets using cocultures of synovial fibroblasts and U937 cells. Biomaterials 35: 1185–1191.
54. Adamopoulos IE, Sabokbar A, Wordsworth BP, Carr A, Ferguson DJ, et al. (2006) Synovial fluid macrophages are capable of osteoclast formation and resorption. J Pathol 208: 35–43.

Angelica Sinensis Polysaccharides Stimulated UDP-Sugar Synthase Genes through Promoting Gene Expression of *IGF-1* and *IGF1R* in Chondrocytes: Promoting Anti-Osteoarthritic Activity

Yinxian Wen[1], Jing Li[2], Yang Tan[1], Jun Qin[1], Xianfei Xie[2], Linlong Wang[1], Qibing Mei[3], Hui Wang[2,4], Jacques Magdalou[5], Liaobin Chen[1,4]*

1 Department of Orthopedic Surgery, Zhongnan Hospital of Wuhan University, Wuhan, China, **2** Department of pharmacology, Basic Medical School of Wuhan University, Wuhan, China, **3** Department of Pharmacology, School of Pharmacy, The Fourth Military Medical University, Xi'an, China, **4** Hubei Provincial Key Laboratory of Developmentally Originated Disease, Wuhan, China, **5** UMR 7365 CNRS-Université de Lorraine, Faculté de Médecine, Vandœuvre-lès-Nancy, France

Abstract

Background: Osteoarthritis (OA) is a chronic joints disease characterized by progressive degeneration of articular cartilage due to the loss of cartilage matrix. Previously, we found, for the first time, that an acidic glycan from *Angelica Sinensis* Polysaccharides (APSs), namely the APS-3c, could protect rat cartilage from OA due to promoting glycosaminoglycan (GAG) synthesis in chondrocytes. In the present work, we tried to further the understanding of ASP-3c's anti-OA activity.

Methodology/Principal Findings: Human primary chondrocytes were treated with APS-3c or/and recombinant human interleukin 1β (IL-1β). It turned out that APS-3c promoted synthesis of UDP-xylose and GAG, as well as the gene expression of UDP-sugar synthases (USSs), insulin like growth factor 1 (*IGF1*) and IGF1 receptor (*IGF1R*), and attenuated the degenerative phenotypes, suppressed biosynthesis of UDP-sugars and GAG, and inhibited the gene expression of *USSs*, *IGF1* and *IGF1R* induced by IL-1β. Then, we induced a rat OA model with papain, and found that APS-3c also stimulated GAG synthesis and gene expression of *USSs*, *IGF1* and *IGF1R in vivo*. Additionally, recombinant human IGF1 and IGF1R inhibitor NP-AEW541 were applied to figure out the correlation between stimulated gene expression of USSs, *IGF1* and *IGF1R* induced by APS-3c. It tuned out that the promoted GAG synthesis and USSs gene expression induced by APS-3c was mediated by the stimulated *IGF1* and *IGF1R* gene expression, but not through directly activation of IGF1R signaling pathway.

Conclusions/Significances: We demonstrated for the first time that APS-3c presented anti-OA activity through stimulating *IGF-1* and *IGF1R* gene expression, but not directly activating the IGF1R signaling pathway, which consequently promoted UDP-sugars and GAG synthesis due to up-regulating gene expression of USSs. Our findings presented a better understanding of APS-3c's anti-OA activity and suggested that APS-3c could potentially be a novel therapeutic agent for OA.

Editor: Joy Marilyn Burchell, King's College London, United Kingdom

Funding: This work was supported by Grants from the National Natural Science Foundation of China (No. 81220108026, 81430089, 81371940, 81001617, 81401832), International science and technology cooperation projects of Hubei province (2012IHA01202).

Competing Interests: The authors have declared that no competing interests exist.

* Email: lbchen@whu.edu.cn

Introduction

Osteoarthritis (OA) is a chronic joint disease with a high prevalence in elderly people, which is characterized by progressive degradation of articular cartilage [1,2]. An imbalance between anabolism and catabolism of chondrocytes leads to loss of matrix components including collagens and glycosaminoglycan (GAG) chains, which consequently triggers the continuous degradation of articular cartilage [3]. Current pharmacological therapies for OA are mainly analgesics, nonsteroidal anti-inflammatory drugs and other symptomatic slow-acting drugs (SYSADOA), which mainly act on pain relief and mobility improvement but with dissatisfactory effects on alleviating cartilage degeneration [4,5,6].

Angelica sinensis is a traditional herbal medicine that has long been applied to relieve the pain and slow the progress of OA. But what the therapeutic ingredient is and how it works still remains unclear. *Angelica sinensis* polysaccharides (APSs) are natural polysaccharides extracted from the root of *Angelica sinensis*, which have been proved beneficial in multiple disease models including cancer, ischemia-reperfusion, inflammation, leukopenia, ulcerative colitis and hepatic injury [7,8,9,10,11,12,13]. APS-3c is an acidic glycan from APSs [14]. In the previous work, we found,

Table 1. Primer sequences and the optimal PCR conditions.

Genes	Accession number	Sequence	Product size (bp)	Tm (°C)
GALE	NM_000403	F: 5′-GGCAGACAAGACTTGGAACGC-3′	131	58
		R: 5′-TCGCCACCTGGGAGACATAA-3′		
GALT	NM_000155.3	F: 5′-AGCGTGATGATCTAGCCTCCA-3′	217	60
		R: 5′-GCAAGCATTTCGTAGCCAACC-3′		
UGDH	NM_003359.3	F: 5′-CAGGCTATGTTGGAGGACCC-3′	162	60
		R: 5′-TCGACAGGATTCTACCACTTCTT-3′		
UXS1	NM_001253875.1	F: 5′-TCCCGCTGGAGGAAGGTTTA-3′	101	60
		R: 5′-TCTGGCAGGCTTTGGTTTGG-3′		
IGF-1	NM_001111285.1	F: 5′-GATGTATTGCGCACCCCTCA-3′	168	60
		R: 5′-TTCTGTTCCCCTCCTGGATGT-3′		
IGF1R	NM_000875.3	F: 5′-GAGAACATGGAGAGCGTCCC-3′	220	60
		R: 5′-CCAAGGATCAGCAGGTCGAA-3′		
GAPDH	NM_002046.4	F: 5′-GAAATCCCATCACCATCTTCCAG-3′	313	60
		R: 5′-GAGTCCTTCCACGATACCAAAG-3′		

RT-PCR, real time quantitative polymerase chain reaction; *GALE*, UDP-galactose-4-epimerase; *GALT*, galactose-1-phosphate uridylyltransferase; *UGDH*, UDP-glucose 6-dehydrogenase; *UXS1*, UDP-xyl synthase 1; *IGF-1*, insulin like growth factor 1; *IGF1R*, IGF-1 receptor; *GAPD*, glyceraldehyde-3-phosphate dehydrogenase.

for the first time, that ASP-3c could protect rat cartilage from OA due to promoting GAG synthesis [15]. However, more detailed study on the anti-OA activity of APS-3c is still needed.

In mammals, GAG synthesis starts with the step-wise addition of carbohydrate moieties from the corresponding high energy donors, uridine diphosphate sugars (UDP-sugar) onto the serine residues of the core protein by certain glycosyltransferases (GTs) [16]. These compounds are the products of a series of UDP-sugar synthases (USSs). The UDP-xylose synthase 1 (UXS1) catalyzes the formation of UDP-xylose (UDP-xyl) through decarboxylation of UDP-glucuronic acid (UDP-GlcA) [17], the product of UDP-glucose 6-dehydrogenase (UGDH) from UDP-glucose [18]. In the Leloir pathway of galactose metabolism, galactose-1-phosphate uridylyltransferase (GALT) catalyzes the conversion of UDP-glucose and UDP-galactose [19], while UDP-galactose-4-epimerase (GALE) catalyzes the reversible conversion of UDP-galactose to UDP-glucose and from Uridine diphospho-N-acetylglucosamine (UDP-GlcNAc) to UDP-N-acetylgalactosamine (UDP-GalNAc) [19]. All these UDP-sugars are essential for GAG chain elongation and/or sorting [20].

The process of GAG synthesis in articular cartilage is regulated by multiple cytokines and growth factors, among which are interleukin β (IL-1β) and insulin like growth factor 1 (IGF-1) [21,22]. As a typical pro-inflammatory factor in OA pathophysiology, IL-1β could inhibit synthesis of GAG due to decrease gene expression and enzyme activity of GTs [23,24]. On the contrary, IGF-1 is one of the key protective factors of cartilage. It reported that IGF-1 could attenuate the catabolic and degenerative changes induced by IL-1β in chondrocytes [25]. The binding of IGF1 to IGF1 receptor (IGF1R) leads to the autophosphorylation of the receptor, and subsequently induces insulin receptor substrates (IRS) and Src homology/collagen domain protein, which consequently activate the PI3K/Akt and MEK/ERK signaling pathways [26,27,28]. However, IGF-1 enhances GAG synthesis in human primary chondrocyte mainly through the PI3K/Akt pathway but not the MEK/ERK pathway [29].

To further investigate the possible mechanism involved in the anti-OA activities of APS-3c, we tested the effects of APS-3c on UDP-sugar synthesis *in vitro*, as well as the gene expression of USSs, *IGF-1* and *IGF1R* both *in vivo* and *in vitro*. Then, exogenous IGF-1, IL-1β and IGF1R inhibitor NVP-AEW541 were used to figure out whether IGF-1 and IGF1R mediated the promotion of APS-3c on the USSs gene expression and the consequent GAG synthesis in human primary chondrocytes. As such, this study would contribute to a better understanding of the anti-OA activities of APS-3c.

Materials and Methods

Materials

DMEM/F12 (1:1) and fetal bovine serum (FBS) were supplied by Thermo Scientific (Beijing, China). Recombinant human IL-1β and IGF-1 were bought from PeproTech (NJ, USA). Cell Counting Kit-8 (CCK-8) was acquired from Dojindo (Kumamoto, Japan). Collagenase type II, Chondroitin sulfate sodium salt from shark cartilage, 1,9-dimethylmethylene Blue (DMB), Alcian blue dye and Uridine 5′-diphospho-N-acetylglucosamine sodium salt (UDP-GlcNAc) were obtained from Sigma-Aldrich (MO, USA). UDP-xyl was obtained from CarboSource Services (GA, USA). Ultrafiltration membranes were obtained from Millipore (MA, USA). CarboPac PA20 Carbohydrate Column was supplied by Dionex (CA, USA). TRIzol reagent was obtained from Life Technologies (NY, USA). First Strand cDNA Synthesis Kit and real time quantitative polymerase chain reaction (RT-PCR) kits were purchased from Takara Biotechnology (Dalian, China). Oligonucleotide primers were synthesized by Sangon Biotech (Shanghai, China). Anti-GALE, anti-GALT, anti-UGDH, anti-UXS1, anti-IGF1 and anti-GAPDH polyclonal antibodies were obtained from Proteintech (CHI, USA). Anti-IGF1R and anti-IRS1 polyclonal antibodies were obtained from Santa Cruz Biotechnology (CA, USA). Anti-phosphorylated-IRS1 (Y612) antibody was supplied by Abcam (Cambridge, UK). Western Bright ECL HRP substrate was purchased from Advansta (CA, USA). RIPA lysis buffer and BCA Protein Assay Kit were purchased from Beyotime Institute of Biotechnology (Haimen, China). NVP-AEW541 was obtained from Novartis Pharma AG (Basel, Switzerland). APS-3c was a gift from Professor Mei Qibing

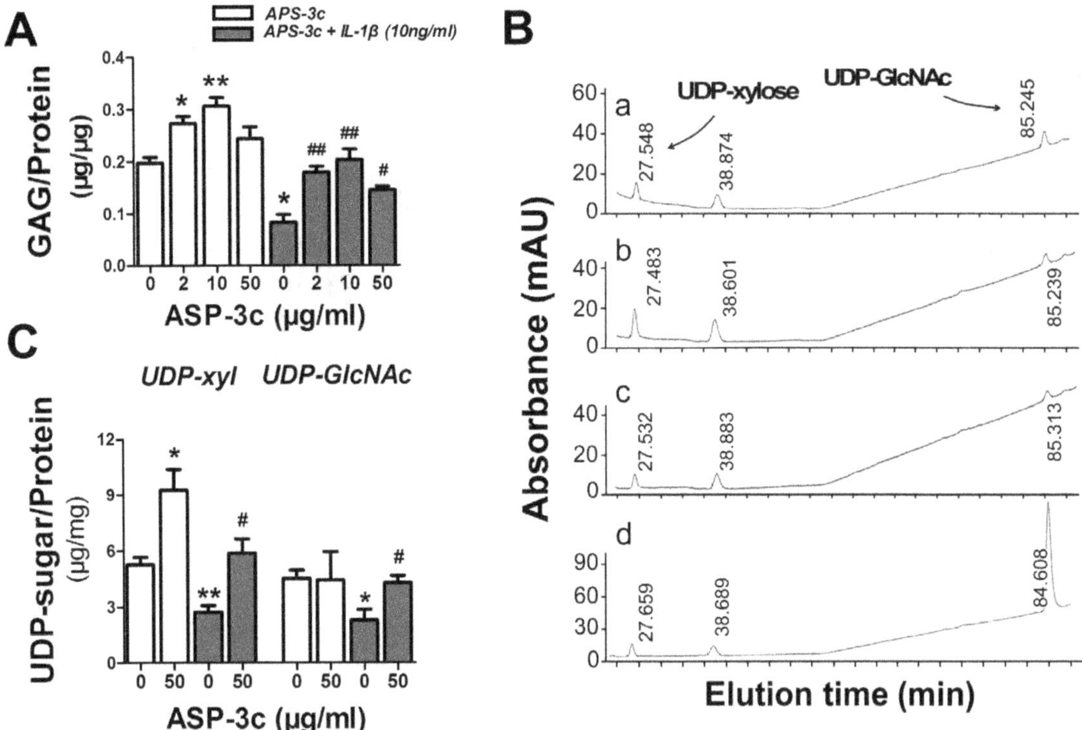

Figure 1. APS-3c stimulated glycosaminoglycan (GAG) and UDP-sugar synthesis *in vitro*. A, Total GAG were detected in chondrocytes treated with 2,10 and 50 µg/ml ASP-3c, or pre-treated with 10 ng/ml interleukin 1 beta (IL-1β) for 30 min and consequently co-treated with IL-1β and ASP-3c for another 48 h using DMB assay. B, UDP-sugar content in chondrocytes was also detected with high-performance anion-exchange chromatography using a CarboPac PA20 carbohydrate column. a, control; b, chondrocytes treated with 50 µg/ml ASP-3c for 48 h; c, chondrocytes treated with 10 ng/ml IL-1β for 48 h; d, chondrocytes pre-treated with 10 ng/ml IL-1β for 30 min, and subsequently co-treated with the IL-1β and 50 µg/ml ASP-3c for another 48 h. C, UDP-sugar contents were presented as peak areas compared with standards and normalized to the total protein. Values were presented as mean ± S.E.M. from three independent experiments. mAU, milli absorbance unit. *$P<0.05$ *versus* control group; #$P<0.05$, ##$P<0.01$ *versus* IL-1β group.

from the Fourth Military Medical University of China [14]. Other chemicals and reagents were of analytical grade.

Cartilage specimen

Human articular cartilage was obtained in total knee replacement surgery from patients (11 knees of 8 female patients, aged 66±10 years), who were diagnosed with OA using the criteria of the American College of Rheumatology for OA [30]. The protocol was in accordance to the ethical guidelines of the Declaration of Helsinki and approved by Medical Ethics Committee of the Zhongnan Hospital of Wuhan University (Approval Number, 2012030). Informed consent was obtained from each donor as written form.

Pathogen-free male adult Wistar rats (weighed 220–280 g) were supplied by Experimental Centre of Medical Scientific Academy of Hubei province, which also approved animal study protocol applied in the study (No. 2008–0005). The protocol was in accordance with the Guide for the Care and Use of Laboratory Animals (eighth edition) by the National Research Council of the United States National Academies. The animal study was performed in the Animal Biosafety Level 3 Laboratory of Wuhan University (Wuhan, China) accredited by the AAALAC International. The OA model was induced as described previously [15]. Then, all the rats were anaesthetized using isoflurane through inhalation, and subsequently sacrificed by cervical dislocation for the knee joints.

Histopathology assay

Cartilage samples from the weight-bearing area of the knee joint were applied in pathological test, which were fixed in 4% paraformaldehyde overnight and embedded in paraffin wax, successively. Then, cartilage sections of 5 µm were obtained perpendicularly to the surface of articular cartilage. Safranin O staining was performed according to the standard protocol. Moreover, protein level of UGDH, GALE, IGF-1 and IGF1R of the cartilage was also detected using immunohistochemistry (IHC) assay as previously described [31,32]. And relative protein level was presented as mean optical density (MOD) of each chondrocytes using NIS-elements software (Nikon, Tokyo, Japan).

Isolation and treatment of human primary chondrocytes

Chondrocytes were obtained from macroscopically normal areas of cartilage and cultured as a monolayer using DMEM/F12 (1:1) with 10% (v/v) fetal bovine serum, 100 IU/ml penicillin, 100 µg/ml streptomycin, and 2 mM glutamine at 37°C with 5% CO_2. Then, chondrocytes were treated with 2, 10 and 50 µg/ml APS-3c (or 2, 10 and 50 ng/ml IGF-1) alone for 48 h, or pre-treated with 10 ng/ml IL-1β for 30 min and subsequently co-treated with the IL-1β and 2, 10 and 50 µg/ml APS-3c (or 50 ng/ml IGF1) for another 48 h, to detect the GAG synthesis and USSs gene expression. Chondrocytes were also treated with 50 ng/ml IGF1 or 10 µg/ml APS-3c for 30 min, or pre-treated with 1 µM NVP-AEW541 for 30 min and then co-treated with the NVP-AEW541 and 10 µg/ml APS-3c or NVP-AEW541 and 50 ng/ml

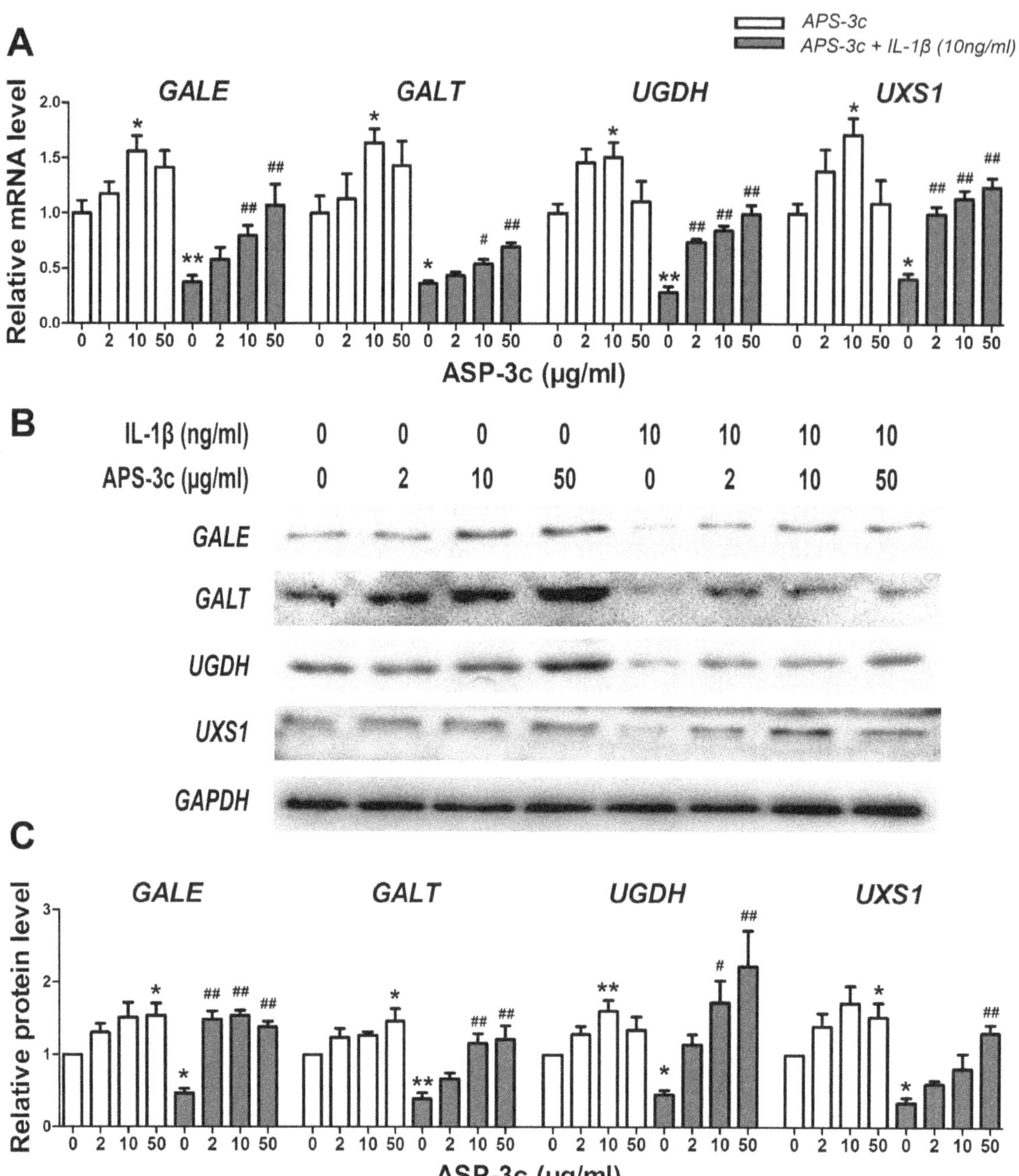

Figure 2. APS-3c modulated gene expression of UDP-sugar synthases *in vitro*. A, The mRNA levels of UDP-galactose-4-epimerase (*GALE*), galactose-1-phosphate uridylyltransferase (*GALT*), UDP-glucose 6-dehydrogenase (*UGDH*), and UDP-xyl synthase 1 (*UXS1*) were detected in chondrocytes treated with 2,10 and 50 μg/ml ASP-3c, or pre-treated with 10 ng/ml interleukin 1 beta (IL-1β) for 30 min and consequently co-treated with IL-1β and ASP-3c for another 48 h using real time quantitative PCR assay. B and C, The protein level of GALE, GALT, UGDH and UXS1 was also detected using Western blotting assay. Then, the mean optical density of each lane was analyzed. Values were presented as mean ± SEM from three independent experiments. **P*<0.05, ***P*<0.01 *versus* control group; #*P*<0.05, ##*P*<0.01*versus* IL-1β group.

IGF1 for another 30 min, to detect the phosphorylated IRS-1. Moreover, for the assay of GAG synthesis and USSs gene expression, chondrocytes were also pre-treated with 1 μM NVP-AEW541 for 30 min and then co-treated with the NVP-AEW541 and 10 μg/ml APS-3c for another 48 h.

Cell viability assay

Chondrocytes were cultured in 96-well plates at 2×10^4 cells/ml and treated as described above. Then, the medium was replaced with 100 μl serum-free DMEM/F12 containing 10 μl CCK-8 reagent. Absorbance of each well was determined at 450 nm using a UV-1601 spectrophotometer (Shimadzu, Kyoto, Japan).

Transmission electron microscopy

Transmission electron microscopy observation was performed as previously described [33]. The chondrocytes were fixed in Karnovsky's fixative for 30 min and post-fixed in a 1% OsO4 solution. Then, samples were dehydrated in increasing ethyl

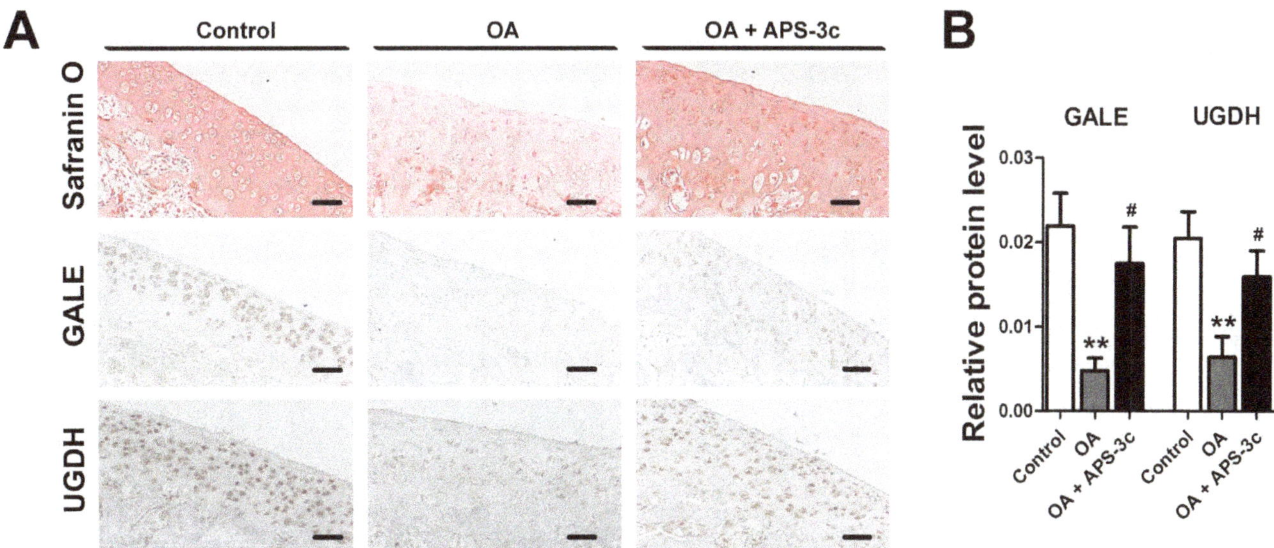

Figure 3. ***Angelica sinensis*** **polysaccharides (APS-3c) increased protein expression of UDP-sugar synthases** ***in vivo.*** A, Glycosaminoglycan content of rat cartilage from knee joints was detected using Safranin O staining. The protein expression of UDP-galactose-4-epimerase (*GALE*) and UDP-glucose 6-dehydrogenase (*UGDH*) was detected in the cartilage using immunohistochemistry. All the sections were photographed using NIS-Elements software (Nikon, Tokyo, Japan). Scale bars, 100 µm. B, Relative protein level of GALE and UGDH was presented as mean optical density of each chondrocyte. $^{**}P<0.01$ *versus* control; $^{\#}P<0.05$, $^{\#\#}P<0.01$ *versus* osteoarthritis (OA) group.

alcohol concentrations, embedded in Epon, and cut on a LKB-V ultramicrotome (Bromma, Kista, Sweden). 2% (w/v) uranyl acetate/lead citrate was used for contrasting these ultrathin sections. Then, the ultrastructures of chondrocytes were observed and photographed using a H-600 TEM (Hitachi, Tokyo, Japan) at a magnification of 15,000.

GAG assay

Both supernatant and chondrocyte-associated GAG were collected using papain extraction reagent and dyed using DMB color reagent as reported [34,35]. Absorbance was detected using a UV-1601 spectrophotometer. A standard curve constructed using chondroitin sulfate sodium salt was applied to quantify the total GAG of the chondrocyte cultures. Total protein of the cultures was also quantified to calibrate the total GAG of each chondrocyte culture. Then, Chondrocytes cultured on coverslips were fixed in 10% (w/v) neutral formalin for 15 min at room temperature, stained overnight at 4°C with 0.5% (w/v) Alcian blue dye and photographed using an AZ100 Microscopes (Nikon, Tokyo, Japan). MOD of each chondrocyte was obtained using NIS-Elements software.

Real time quantitative PCR assay

Total RNA was isolated by TRIzol reagent following the manufacturer's protocol. Single-strand cDNA was obtained from purified total RNA using the reverse transcription kit. Primers used in this study were designed using Primer Premier 5.0 (Premier Biosoft, CA, USA) and the NCBI BLAST database. Primer sequences and the optimal PCR conditions were shown in Table 1. RT-PCR assay was performed on a StepOne thermal cycler (Applied Biosystems, NY, USA) following the procedure: pre-denaturation at 95°C for 30 sec, denaturation at 95°C for 5 sec, annealing at Tm for 30 sec, and extension at 72°C for 30 sec. The last 3 steps ran for 40 cycles. Relative standard curves were applied to quantify the mRNA level of each sample, while GAPDH mRNA level was detected and used as internal reference.

Western blotting analysis

Total proteins were obtained using RIPA lysis buffer and quantified using a BCA kit following the protocol. Then, total proteins were loaded as 40 µg per lane, separated by SDS-PAGE (5 and 10% gels) and blotted onto nitrocellulose membranes. Membranes were blocked in 5% skimmed milk, probed with anti-human GALE (1:1000), GALT (1:500), UGDH (1:1000), UXS1 (1:800), IGF-1 (1:800), IGF1R (1:1000), IRS1(1:1000), phosphorylated IRS1 (Y612, 1:500) and GAPDH (1:1000) primary antibodies, incubated with horseradish peroxidase-conjugated secondary antibody (goat anti-rabbit IgG, 1:5000) and visualized using ECL HRP substrate. Then, relative protein level was standardized with normal control and the GAPDH protein level obtained using Quantity One software (Version 4.6, Bio-Rad Laboratories Inc., CA, USA).

UDP-sugars detection

High-performance anion-exchange chromatography (HPEAC) assay was performed to detect the UDP-sugars content in chondrocytes. UDP-sugar samples were obtained as previously described [36,37]. Protein concentration of each sample was detected and adjusted to 100 µg/µl. UDP-xyl and UDP-GlcNAc were used as standards. Then, contents of UDP-xyl and UDP-GlcNAc in each chondrocyte culture were detected using a CarboPac PA20 carbohydrate column with a loading quantity of 20 µl. The gradient elution assay was performed as reported [36]. The UDP-sugar contents of each sample were presented as peak areas.

Statistical analysis

Data analysis was performed using SPSS 17.0 (SPSS Science Inc., CHI, USA) and Prism 5.0 (GraphPad Software, CA, USA). Results were presented as mean ± S.E.M. Analysis of variance (ANOVA) and Student *t* test were applied in the study. Statistical significance was defined as $P<0.05$.

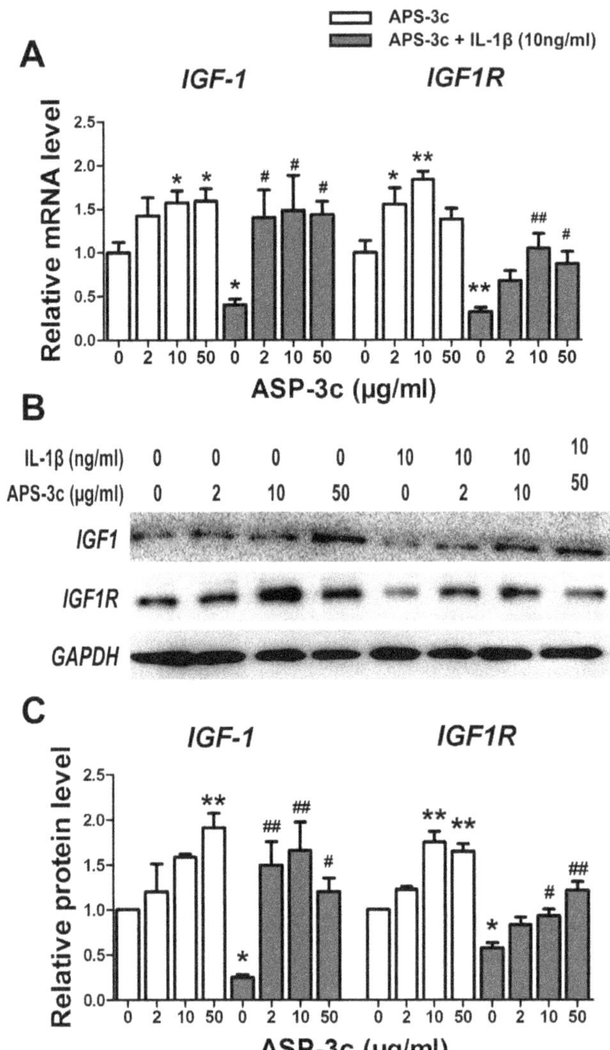

Figure 4. APS-3c stimulated expression of insulin like growth factor (IGF1) and its receptor (IGF1R) ***in vitro.*** The mRNA and protein level of IGF1 and IGF1R were detected in human primary chondrocytes treated with ASP-3c (2,10 and 50 μg/ml) or/and interleukin 1 beta (IL-1β) for 48 h. Values were presented as mean ± SEM from three independent experiments. *$P<0.05$, **$P<0.01$ *versus* control group; #$P<0.05$, ##$P<0.01$*versus* IL-1β group.

Results

Promoted GAG and UDP-sugars synthesis of human primary chondrocyte by APS-3c

Total GAG contents in human primary chondrocytes cultures treated with APS-3c were 38.4% (2 μg/ml) and 55.3% (10 μg/ml) higher than the control (Figure 1A, $P<0.05$), while the chondrocyte-associated GAG contents were also elevated up to 165.4% (50 μg/ml) of the control in APS-3c groups (Figure S1, $P<0.05$). Although IL-1β significantly suppressed GAG synthesis of the chondrocytes, APS-3c significantly inhibited the suppression of IL-1β on the total GAG contents by 116.7% (2 μg/ml), 145.9% (10 μg/ml) and 75.5% (50 μg/ml) after 48 h (Figure 1A, $P<0.05$), and the chondrocyte-associated GAG contents by 78.4% (2 μg/ml), 134.3% (10 μg/ml) and 196.5% (50 μg/ml) as well (Figure S1, $P<0.05$), compared with the IL-1β groups. Meanwhile, intracellular content of UDP-xyl and UDP-GlcNAc, the substrates for GAG synthesis, was detected using HPEAC assay, with the elution time around 27 min and 85 min, respectively (Figure 1B). The content of UDP-xyl but not UDP-GlcNAc inside the chondrocytes was 76.3% higher in APS-3c group than the control group. Both UDP-xyl and UDP-GlcNAc content were decreased in IL-1β group, to 51.8% and 50.6% of the corresponding control, respectively. However, subsequent APS-3c treatment significantly inhibited the IL-1β-induced decrease of UDP-xyl content by 115.4% and UDP-GlcNAc content by 87.1%, compared with the IL-1β group (Figure 1C, $P<0.05$).

Sitimulated USSs gene expression *in vitro* and *in vivo* by APS-3c

Gene expression and protein levels of *GALE*, *GALT*, *UGDH* and *UXS1* were seen to increase respectively by 56.2%, 63.5%, 50.9%, 71.6% and 54.0%, 46.0%, 60.2%, 51.2% in human primary chondrocytes after 48 h treatment with APS-3c at a concentration of 10 μg/ml or 50 μg/ml (Figure 2 $P<0.05$). While IL-1β induced a markedly suppression of those genes by more than 50%, the subsequent APS-3c treatment led to a multiplied increased of the USSs expression in a concentration-dependent manner (Figures 2, $P<0.05$). Moreover, GALE and UGDH protein expression in rat OA cartilage was markedly lower than that of normal cartilage by 78.1% and 68.6%, respectively (Figure 3, $P<0.05$), which was accompanied by the decrease of GAG content. However, obviously improvements in the degenerative features and a markedly increase in the GAG contents of the rat OA cartilage were observed. Meanwhile, protein level of GALE and UGDH were increased in APS-c group to 364.6% and 247.8% of the control group, respectively (Figure 3, $P<0.05$).

Up-regulated IGF-1 and IGF1R gene expression *in vitro* and *in vivo* by APS-3c

As one of the most important cartilage-protective growth factor in OA, gene expression of *IGF-1* and its receptor drew our attention. It turned out that the mRNA level of *IGF-1* and *IGF1R* was increased in APS-3c-treated chondrocytes up to 159.3% (50 μg/ml) and 183.7% (10 μg/ml), and the protein level to 192.4% (50 μg/ml) and 180.7% (10 μg/ml) of the control (Figure 4, $P<0.05$). However, both the mRNA and protein level of *IGF1* and *IGF1R* were significantly inhibited by IL-1β (Figure 4, $P<0.05$). Then, remarkable increases up to 366.7% and 328.7% in the mRNA levels, and 687.6% and 199.3% in the protein levels, of *IGF-1* and *IGF1R* were detected in chondrocytes pre-treated with IL-1β and then co-treated with IL-1β and APS-3c, when compared with the IL-1β-treated chondrocytes (Figure 4, $P<0.05$). Meanwhile, both *IGF1* and *IGF1R* protein level in rat OA cartilage was decreased to 23.8% and 42.1% of the control, which was accompanied by the decrease of GAG content and USSs protein level in the cartilage (Figure 5, $P<0.05$). However, the cartilage protein level of *IGF1* and *IGF1R* in rats from the APS-3c group was 178.4% and 105.4% higher than the OA group, respectively (Figure 5, $P<0.05$).

Gene expression of USSs induced by exogenous recombinant human IGF-1

To uncover whether the promotion of USSs gene expression by APS-3c was related to the up-regulated IGF-1 gene expression, we also detected USSs gene expression in chondrocytes treated with exogenous IGF-1 and/or IL-1β. It turned out that mRNA expression level of *GALE*, *GALT*, *UGDH* and *UXS1* was up to 139.4%, 79.7%, 87.3% and 196.7% higher in the IGF-1 groups

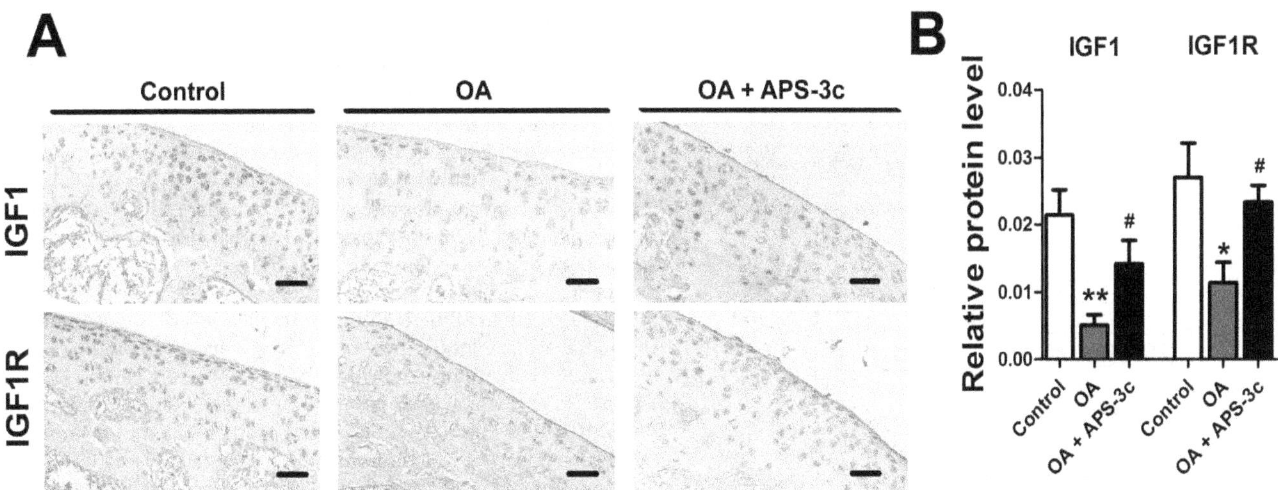

Figure 5. APS-3c stimulated expression of insulin like growth factor (IGF1) and its receptor (IGF1R) *in vivo.* Protein expression of IGF1 and IGF1R were detected in rat cartilage and relative protein level of IGF1 and IGF1R was presented as mean optical density of each chondrocyte. Scale bars, 100 μm. $^{**}P<0.01$ *versus* control; $^{\#}P<0.05$, $^{\#\#}P<0.01$*versus* osteoarthritis (OA) group.

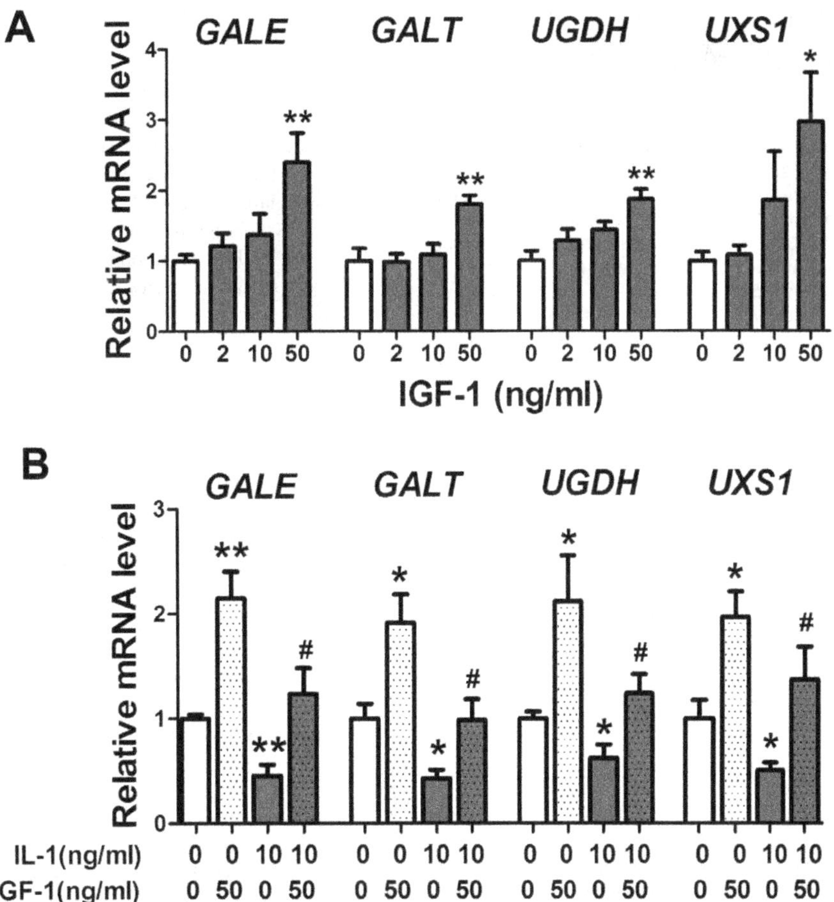

Figure 6. Insulin like growth factor (IGF1) modulated UDP-sugar synthases (USSs) gene expression *in vitro.* A, The mRNA expression of the USSs was detected in human primary chondrocytes treated with recombinant human IGF1 (2, 10 and 50 ng/ml) for 48 h. B, Chondrocytes were pre-treated with 10 ng/ml interleukin 1beta (IL-1β) for 30 min, then co-treated with the IL-1β and 50 ng/ml IGF1 for 48 h. Then, mRNA level of the USSs was detected. Values were presented as mean ± SEM from at least two independent experiments. $^{*}P<0.05$ *versus* control group; $^{\#}P<0.05$ *versus* IL-1β group.

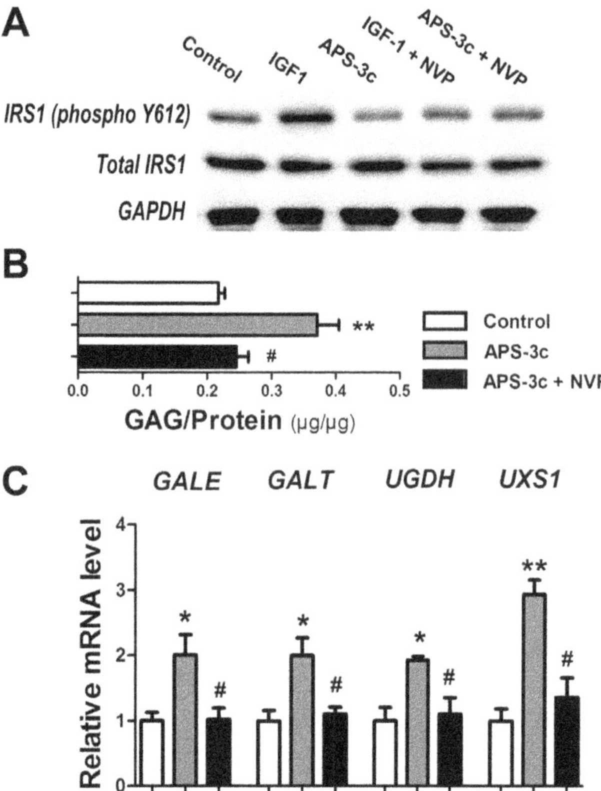

Figure 7. NVP-AEW541 attenuated GAG synthesis and UDP-sugar synthases (USSs) gene expression induced by APS-3c. A, Phosphorylated and total insulin receptor substrate 1 (IRS-1) was detected in the chondrocytes treated with 50 ng/ml recombinant human insulin like growth factor 1 (IGF-1) or 10 μg/ml *Angelica sinensis* polysaccharides (APS-3c) for 30 min, or pretreated with IGF1 receptor (IGF1R) inhibitor 1 μM NVP-AEW541 for 30 min and subsequently co-treated with IGF1 and NVP-AEW541 or APS-3c and NVP-AEW541 for another 30 min. B and C, Total GAG and mRNA level of the USSs was assayed in the chondrocytes treated with 10 μg/ml APS-3c for 48 h, or pretreated with 1 μM NVP-AEW541 for 30 min and subsequently co-treated with APS-3c and NVP-AEW541 for another 48 h. Values were presented as mean ± SEM from at least two independent experiments. *$P<0.05$ and **$P<0.01$ *versus* control group; #$P<0.05$ *versus* IL-1β group.

compared with the control, while IGF-1 also significantly up-regulated the IL-1β-inhibited USSs mRNA level to 271.8%, 230.0%, 200.4% and 271.8% of the IL-1β group (Figure 6, $P<0.05$), which was synchronous with the GAG synthesis and secretion modulated by exogenous IGF1 (Figure S2).

NVP-AEW541 attenuated the stimulation of USSs gene expression by APS-3c

Exogenous recombinant human IGF-1 markedly increased the phosphorylated IRS1 level in the chondrocytes after 30 min, while APS-3c did not (Figure 7 A). However, the pre-treated NVP-AEW541 significantly suppressed the phosphorylation of IRS-1 induced by IGF1 (Figure 7 A). Although GAG content and USSs mRNA expression was stimulated in chondrocytes treated with 10 μg/ml APS-3c, NVP-AEW541 significantly reduced the GAG synthesis to 66.1%, and *GALE*, *GALT*, *UGDH*, *UXS1* mRNA expression to 50.9%, 55.1%, 57.3% and 46.4% of the APS-3c group (Figure 7 B and C, $P<0.05$).

Discussion

APS-3c stimulated GAG synthesis in chondrocytes due to the up-regulated USSs gene expression

As GAG synthesis depends on the biosynthesis of UDP-sugar by USSs, modulating USSs gene expression or enzyme activity modulates GAG synthesis in chondrocytes. Over-expression of *UGDH* gene with retrovirus led to a remarkable increase of GAG synthesis and hyaluronic acid release in articular surface cells from chicken embryonic joints [38]. UXS1 activity is also essential for the production and organization of cartilage extracellular matrix [17]. Mutation of the *UXS1* gene resulted in a dramatic reduction and defective localization of proteoglycans in zebrafish, which consequently disturbed cartilage and bone morphogenesis [17]. In the present work, both *in vivo* and *in vitro* studies showed that ASP-3c obviously promoted GAG synthesis in the chondrocyte (Figure 1 and 3), which was mediated by the stimulated USSs gene expression (Figure 2 and 3). These findings are consistent with our previous work that APS-3c promoted expression of GTs genes and consequently enhanced GAG synthesis in rat primary chondrocytes [15]. However, how APS-3c stimulated gene expression of these USSs was still unknown.

The up-regulation of USSs gene expression by ASP-3c was mediated by the enhanced gene expression of *IGF-1* and *IGF1R*

IGF-1 has long been proved essential in chondrogenesis, chondrocyte-phenotype maintenance and cartilage repair [39,40]. IGF1 inhibited IL-1β-induced activation of NF-kB and apoptosis of chondrocytes partly through inhibiting phosphorylation, degradation and kinase activity of IkBα, which consequently inhibited NF-kB-mediated expression of some inflammation- and apoptosis-related genes [33,41]. Meanwhile, IGF-1 also helped to retain the typical features in chondrocytes and enhances synthesis and release of PGs and collagen II mainly through activation of PI3K/Akt signaling pathway [29,41,42]. In the present study, exogenous IGF-1 promoted GAG synthesis and secretion in chondrocytes (Figure S2), increased mRNA level of USSs and abolished the inhibition of IL-1β on USSs mRNA expression (Figure 6), which agreed with the report by Maneix *et al* that IGF-1 up-stimulated *UGDH* gene expression and consequently promoted GAG synthesis in chondrocytes [43]. Interestingly, we also found that APS-3c stimulated both *IGF1* and *IGF1R* gene expression *in vivo* and *in vitro* (Figure 4 and 5), which indicated that the up-regulation of USSs gene expression by APS-3c was possibly mediated by IGF1/IGF1R pathway.

IRSs are signaling adaptor proteins which act as intermediates of the activated cell surface receptors, mostly the insulin receptor and IGF1R [44]. Binding of IGF1 to IGF1R leads to phosphorylation of IRS-1, and consequently the activation of the downstream signal cascades [26]. Here, we found that it was IGF1, not APS-3c, that induced an obvious increase of phosphorylated IRS-1 protein level within 30 min (Figure 7A), which indicated that APS-3c functioned mainly though up-regulating *IGF-1* and *IGF1R* gene expression but not through directly activating the IGF1R signaling pathway. Moreover, IGF1R inhibitor NVP-AEW541 markedly attenuated the USSs gene expression stimulated by APS-3c (Figure 7C). Altogether, these data indicated that promoted USSs gene expression and consequent GAG synthesis induced by APS-3c was due to the stimulated gene expression of *IGF-1* and *IGF1R* in the chondrocytes. This was further supported by our findings that APS-3c attenuated the IL-1β-induced degenerative ultrastructure of monolayer-cultured chondrocytes (Figure S3), as IGF-1 alone or co-treated with platelet-derived growth factor could attenuate the degenerative features and apoptosis induced by IL-1β in chondrocytes of monolayer culture [33]. Moreover, as APS-3c also helped to restore cartilage matrix, retain the integrality of cartilage surface and decrease the Mankin score of rat OA cartilage in our present and previous work [15], we guess that the cartilage-repair activities of ASP-3c were possibly mediated by the stimulation of *IGF1* and *IGF1R* gene expression.

Take APS-3c as a novel SYSADOA?

APS-3c is a natural glycan with about 1.4×10^4 Da molecular weight and containing 61.0% of sugars and 35.7% of uronic acids [14]. Sugar component of APS-3c was determined to be glucose, galactose, arabinose, rhamnose, mannose and xylose in a molar ratio of 6.3:4.7:6.7:6.5:1.6:1.0 [14]. It's reported that APS was a (1→4)-α-D-glucan with side chains at the glucosyl residues of the main chain [45,46], indicating a similarity of the composition and molecular structure of APS-3c with chondroitin sulfate (CS), which is a natural sulfated GAG composed of the repeated disaccharide units of D-GlcA and D-GalNAc [47]. CS is a widely used SYSADOA, which partly modify, stabilize and postpone the pathology of OA [48,49,50], through promoting cartilage matrix synthesis and presenting anti-catabolic, anti-inflammatory, anti-apoptotic and anti-oxidant effects [47,51]. In the present work, we found that APS-3c promoted GAG synthesis of articular chondrocytes and presented anti-inflammation and anti-degeneration effects against IL-1β through stimulating IGF1/IGF1R gene expression. Additionally, we also found that intra-gastric administration of APS-3c could increase the GAG content of OA rat cartilage and attenuate the inflammation of the OA synovium, but not affect the body weight of the rats (unpublished data). Moreover, APS-3c affected neither the cell viability of the primary chondrocytes (Figure S4), nor the integrality of normal rat cartilage [15]. Altogether, these data suggest that APS-3c might potentially be a novel SYSADOA.

Conclusion

In conclusion, APS-3c promoted GAG synthesis and cartilage repair through stimulating USSs gene expression, which was mediated by the enhanced IGF1/IGF1R gene expression but not the direct activation of the IGF1R signaling pathway. Our findings presented a better understanding of the pharmacological effects of APS-3c on OA and suggested that APS-3c might potentially be a novel SYSADOA.

Supporting Information

Figure S1 ***Angelica sinensis*** **polysaccharides (APS-3c) stimulated glycosaminoglycan (GAG) synthesis and secretion of human primary chondrocyte.** A, Chondrocytes-associated GAG was stained with Alcian blue dye (original magnification of 200); B, The optical density analysis of Alcian blue positive spots was performed using NIS-Elements software (Nikon, Tokyo, Japan). Values are presented as mean ± SEM from at least three independent experiments. *$P<0.05$, **$P<0.01$ *versus* control group; #$P<0.05$, ##$P<0.01$*versus* IL-1β group.

Figure S2 Insulin like growth factor 1 (IGF1) stimulated glycosaminoglycan (GAG) synthesis of human primary chondrocytes. Chondrocytes were treated with IGF-1 (2, 10 and 50 ng/ml) or IL-1β (10 ng/ml) alone for 48 h, respectively. Meanwhile, chondrocytes were pre-treated with IL-1β (10 ng/ml) for 30 min and then co-treated with IL-1β and IGF-1 (2, 10 and 50 ng/ml) for another 48 h. Then, 1,9-dimethylmethylene Blue was applied to detect the GAG of chondrocyte cultures. Values are presented as mean ± SEM from at least two independent experiments. *$P<0.05$, **$P<0.01$ *versus* control group; #$P<0.05$, ##$P<0.01$*versus* IL-1β group.

Figure S3 Effects of *Angelica sinensis* polysaccharides (APS-3c) on the ultrastructure of human primary chondrocytes. A, Control group; B–D, Chondrocytes treated with 2, 10 and 50 μg/ml APS-3c for 48 h; E, Chondrocytes induced by 10 ng/ml IL-1β for 48 h;F–H, Chondrocytes pre-treated with 10 ng/ml IL-1β for 30 min and then co-treated with IL-1β and 2, 10 and 50 μg/ml APS-3c for 48 h. All photographs were taken at an original magnification of 15,000. N, nucleus;M, mitochondrion; rER, rough surfaced endoplasmic reticulum; G, Golgi apparatus; V, vacuole; AV, autophagic vacuole; SV, secretory vesicle.

Figure S4 Effects of *Angelica sinensis* polysaccharides (APS-3c) on cell viability of human primary chondrocytes. Chondrocytes were treated with 2, 10 and 50 μg/ml APS-3c for 48 h or pre-treated with IL-1β (10 ng/ml) for 30 min, and then co-treated with IL-1β and APS-3c (2, 10 and 50 μg/ml) for 48 h. Values are presented as mean ± SEM from at least three independent experiments. *$P<0.05$*versus* control group.

Author Contributions

Conceived and designed the experiments: YXW JL YT JQ XFX LLW QBM HW JM LBC. Performed the experiments: YXW JL YT JQ XFX LLW. Analyzed the data: YXW HW JM LBC. Contributed reagents/materials/analysis tools: QBM HW LBC. Contributed to the writing of the manuscript: YXW JL YT JQ XFX LLW QBM HW JM LBC.

References

1. Goldring MB, Goldring SR (2007) Osteoarthritis. J Cell Physiol 213: 626–634.
2. Loeser RF, Goldring SR, Scanzello CR, Goldring MB (2012) Osteoarthritis: a disease of the joint as an organ. Arthritis Rheum 64: 1697–1707.
3. Heinegard D, Saxne T (2011) The role of the cartilage matrix in osteoarthritis. Nat Rev Rheumatol 7: 50–56.
4. Adatia A, Rainsford KD, Kean WF (2012) Osteoarthritis of the knee and hip. Part I: aetiology and pathogenesis as a basis for pharmacotherapy. J Pharm Pharmacol 64: 617–625.
5. Berenbaum F (2011) Osteoarthritis year 2010 in review: pharmacological therapies. Osteoarthritis Cartilage 19: 361–365.
6. Jerosch J (2011) Effects of Glucosamine and Chondroitin Sulfate on Cartilage Metabolism in OA: Outlook on Other Nutrient Partners Especially Omega-3 Fatty Acids. Int J Rheumatol 2011: 969012.
7. Chao WW, Hong YH, Chen ML, Lin BF (2010) Inhibitory effects of *Angelica sinensis* ethyl acetate extract and major compounds on NF-kappaB trans-activation activity and LPS-induced inflammation. J Ethnopharmacol 129: 244–249.
8. Chao WW, Lin BF (2011) Bioactivities of major constituents isolated from *Angelica sinensis* (Danggui). Chin Med 6: 29.
9. Hui MK, Wu WK, Shin VY, So WH, Cho CH (2006) Polysaccharides from the root of *Angelica sinensis* protect bone marrow and gastrointestinal tissues against the cytotoxicity of cyclophosphamide in mice. Int J Med Sci 3: 1–6.
10. Lee JG, Hsieh WT, Chen SU, Chiang BH (2012) Hematopoietic and myeloprotective activities of an acidic *Angelica sinensis* polysaccharide on human CD34+ stem cells. J Ethnopharmacol 139: 739–745.
11. Wong VK, Yu L, Cho CH (2008) Protective effect of polysaccharides from *Angelica sinensis* on ulcerative colitis in rats. Inflammopharmacology 16: 162–167.
12. Yang T, Jia M, Meng J, Wu H, Mei Q (2006) Immunomodulatory activity of polysaccharide isolated from *Angelica sinensis*. Int J Biol Macromol 39: 179–184.

13. Ye YN, Liu ES, Li Y, So HL, Cho CC, et al. (2001) Protective effect of polysaccharides-enriched fraction from *Angelica sinensis* on hepatic injury. Life Sci 69: 637–646.
14. Cao W, Li XQ, Wang X, Li T, Chen X, et al. (2010) Characterizations and anti-tumor activities of three acidic polysaccharides from *Angelica sinensis* (Oliv.) Diels. Int J Biol Macromol 46: 115–122.
15. Qin J, Liu YS, Liu J, Li J, Tan Y, et al. (2013) Effect of *Angelica sinensis* Polysaccharides on osteoarthritis *in vivo* and *in vitro*: A possible mechanism to promote proteoglycans synthesis. Evid Based Complement Alternat Med 2013: 794761.
16. Schwartz N (2000) Biosynthesis and regulation of expression of proteoglycans. Front Biosci 5: D649–D655.
17. Eames BF, Singer A, Smith GA, Wood ZA, Yan YL, et al. (2010) UDP xylose synthase 1 is required for morphogenesis and histogenesis of the craniofacial skeleton. Dev Biol 341: 400–415.
18. Egger S, Chaikuad A, Kavanagh KL, Oppermann U, Nidetzky B (2010) UDP-glucose dehydrogenase: structure and function of a potential drug target. Biochem Soc Trans 38: 1378–1385.
19. Frey PA (1996) The Leloir pathway: a mechanistic imperative for three enzymes to change the stereochemical configuration of a single carbon in galactose. FASEB J 10: 461–470.
20. Prydz K, Dalen KT (2000) Synthesis and sorting of proteoglycans. J Cell Sci 113 Pt 2: 193–205.
21. Caterson B, Flannery CR, Hughes CE, Little CB (2000) Mechanisms involved in cartilage proteoglycan catabolism. Matrix Biol 19: 333–344.
22. Porter RM, Akers RM, Howard RD, Forsten-Williams K (2006) Transcriptional and proteolytic regulation of the insulin-like growth factor-I system of equine articular chondrocytes by recombinant equine interleukin-1beta. J Cell Physiol 209: 542–550.
23. Khair M, Bourhim M, Barre L, Li D, Netter P, et al. (2013) Regulation of xylosyltransferase I gene expression by interleukin 1beta in human primary chondrocyte cells: mechanism and impact on proteoglycan synthesis. J Biol Chem 288: 1774–1784.
24. Gouze JN, Bordji K, Gulberti S, Terlain B, Netter P, et al. (2001) Interleukin-1beta down-regulates the expression of glucuronosyltransferase I, a key enzyme priming glycosaminoglycan biosynthesis: influence of glucosamine on interleukin-1beta-mediated effects in rat chondrocytes. Arthritis Rheum 44: 351–360.
25. Goldring SR, Goldring MB (2004) The role of cytokines in cartilage matrix degeneration in osteoarthritis. Clin Orthop Relat Res: S27–S36.
26. Li R, Pourpak A, Morris SW (2009) Inhibition of the insulin-like growth factor-1 receptor (IGF1R) tyrosine kinase as a novel cancer therapy approach. J Med Chem 52: 4981–5004.
27. Shelton JG, Steelman LS, White ER, McCubrey JA (2004) Synergy between PI3K/Akt and Raf/MEK/ERK pathways in IGF-1R mediated cell cycle progression and prevention of apoptosis in hematopoietic cells. Cell Cycle 3: 372–379.
28. Haisa M (2013) The type 1 insulin-like growth factor receptor signalling system and targeted tyrosine kinase inhibition in cancer. J Int Med Res 41: 253–264.
29. Starkman BG, Cravero JD, Delcarlo M, Loeser RF (2005) IGF-I stimulation of proteoglycan synthesis by chondrocytes requires activation of the PI 3-kinase pathway but not ERK MAPK. Biochem J 389: 723–729.
30. Altman R, Asch E, Bloch D, Bole G, Borenstein D, et al. (1986) Development of criteria for the classification and reporting of osteoarthritis. Classification of osteoarthritis of the knee. Diagnostic and Therapeutic Criteria Committee of the American Rheumatism Association. Arthritis Rheum 29: 1039–1049.
31. Naumann A, Dennis JE, Awadallah A, Carrino DA, Mansour JM, et al. (2002) Immunochemical and mechanical characterization of cartilage subtypes in rabbit. J Histochem Cytochem 50: 1049–1058.
32. Tan Y, Liu J, Deng Y, Cao H, Xu D, et al. (2012) Caffeine-induced fetal rat over-exposure to maternal glucocorticoid and histone methylation of liver IGF-1 might cause skeletal growth retardation. Toxicol Lett 214: 279–287.
33. Montaseri A, Busch F, Mobasheri A, Buhrmann C, Aldinger C, et al. (2011) IGF-1 and PDGF-bb suppress IL-1beta-induced cartilage degradation through down-regulation of NF-kappaB signaling: involvement of Src/PI-3K/AKT pathway. PLOS ONE 6: e28663.
34. Farndale RW, Buttle DJ, Barrett AJ (1986) Improved quantitation and discrimination of sulphated glycosaminoglycans by use of dimethylmethylene blue. Biochim Biophys Acta 883: 173–177.
35. Enobakhare BO, Bader DL, Lee DA (1996) Quantification of sulfated glycosaminoglycans in chondrocyte/alginate cultures, by use of 1,9-dimethylmethylene blue. Anal Biochem 243: 189–191.
36. Tomiya N, Ailor E, Lawrence SM, Betenbaugh MJ, Lee YC (2001) Determination of nucleotides and sugar nucleotides involved in protein glycosylation by high-performance anion-exchange chromatography: sugar nucleotide contents in cultured insect cells and mammalian cells. Anal Biochem 293: 129–137.
37. Hull SR, Montgomery R (1994) Separation and analysis of 4′-epimeric UDP-sugars, nucleotides, and sugar phosphates by anion-exchange high-performance liquid chromatography with conductimetric detection. Anal Biochem 222: 49–54.
38. Clarkin CE, Allen S, Kuiper NJ, Wheeler BT, Wheeler-Jones CP, et al. (2011) Regulation of UDP-glucose dehydrogenase is sufficient to modulate hyaluronan production and release, control sulfated GAG synthesis, and promote chondrogenesis. J Cell Physiol 226: 749–761.
39. Fortier LA, Barker JU, Strauss EJ, McCarrel TM, Cole BJ (2011) The role of growth factors in cartilage repair. Clin Orthop Relat Res 469: 2706–2715.
40. Gaissmaier C, Koh JL, Weise K (2008) Growth and differentiation factors for cartilage healing and repair. Injury 39 Suppl 1: S88–S96.
41. Zhang M, Zhou Q, Liang QQ, Li CG, Holz JD, et al. (2009) IGF-1 regulation of type II collagen and MMP-13 expression in rat endplate chondrocytes via distinct signaling pathways. Osteoarthritis Cartilage 17: 100–106.
42. Shakibaei M, Seifarth C, John T, Rahmanzadeh M, Mobasheri A (2006) Igf-I extends the chondrogenic potential of human articular chondrocytes in vitro: molecular association between Sox9 and Erk1/2. Biochem Pharmacol 72: 1382–1395.
43. Maneix L, Beauchef G, Servent A, Wegrowski Y, Maquart FX, et al. (2008) 17Beta-oestradiol up-regulates the expression of a functional UDP-glucose dehydrogenase in articular chondrocytes: comparison with effects of cytokines and growth factors. Rheumatology (Oxford) 47: 281–288.
44. Metz HE, Houghton AM (2011) Insulin receptor substrate regulation of phosphoinositide 3-kinase. Clin Cancer Res 17: 206–211.
45. Yamada H, Kiyohara H, Cyong JC, Kojima Y, Kumazawa Y, et al. (1984) Studies on polysaccharides from Angelica acutiloba. Part 1. Fractionation and biological properties of polysaccharides. Planta Med 50: 163–167.
46. Cao W, Li XQ, Liu L, Wang M, Fan HT, et al. (2006) Structural analysis of water-soluble glucans from the root of Angelica sinensis (Oliv.) Diels. Carbohydr Res 341: 1870–1877.
47. David-Raoudi M, Deschrevel B, Leclercq S, Galera P, Boumediene K, et al. (2009) Chondroitin sulfate increases hyaluronan production by human synoviocytes through differential regulation of hyaluronan synthases: Role of p38 and Akt. Arthritis Rheum 60: 760–770.
48. Clegg DO, Reda DJ, Harris CL, Klein MA, O'Dell JR, et al. (2006) Glucosamine, chondroitin sulfate, and the two in combination for painful knee osteoarthritis. N Engl J Med 354: 795–808.
49. Hochberg MC (2010) Structure-modifying effects of chondroitin sulfate in knee osteoarthritis: an updated meta-analysis of randomized placebo-controlled trials of 2-year duration. Osteoarthritis Cartilage 18 Suppl 1: S28–S31.
50. Hochberg M, Chevalier X, Henrotin Y, Hunter DJ, Uebelhart D (2013) Symptom and structure modification in osteoarthritis with pharmaceutical-grade chondroitin sulfate: what's the evidence? Curr Med Res Opin 29: 259–267.
51. Henrotin Y, Lambert C (2013) Chondroitin and glucosamine in the management of osteoarthritis: an update. Curr Rheumatol Rep 15: 361.

Permissions

All chapters in this book were first published in PLOS ONE, by The Public Library of Science; hereby published with permission under the Creative Commons Attribution License or equivalent. Every chapter published in this book has been scrutinized by our experts. Their significance has been extensively debated. The topics covered herein carry significant findings which will fuel the growth of the discipline. They may even be implemented as practical applications or may be referred to as a beginning point for another development.

The contributors of this book come from diverse backgrounds, making this book a truly international effort. This book will bring forth new frontiers with its revolutionizing research information and detailed analysis of the nascent developments around the world.

We would like to thank all the contributing authors for lending their expertise to make the book truly unique. They have played a crucial role in the development of this book. Without their invaluable contributions this book wouldn't have been possible. They have made vital efforts to compile up to date information on the varied aspects of this subject to make this book a valuable addition to the collection of many professionals and students.

This book was conceptualized with the vision of imparting up-to-date information and advanced data in this field. To ensure the same, a matchless editorial board was set up. Every individual on the board went through rigorous rounds of assessment to prove their worth. After which they invested a large part of their time researching and compiling the most relevant data for our readers.

The editorial board has been involved in producing this book since its inception. They have spent rigorous hours researching and exploring the diverse topics which have resulted in the successful publishing of this book. They have passed on their knowledge of decades through this book. To expedite this challenging task, the publisher supported the team at every step. A small team of assistant editors was also appointed to further simplify the editing procedure and attain best results for the readers.

Apart from the editorial board, the designing team has also invested a significant amount of their time in understanding the subject and creating the most relevant covers. They scrutinized every image to scout for the most suitable representation of the subject and create an appropriate cover for the book.

The publishing team has been an ardent support to the editorial, designing and production team. Their endless efforts to recruit the best for this project, has resulted in the accomplishment of this book. They are a veteran in the field of academics and their pool of knowledge is as vast as their experience in printing. Their expertise and guidance has proved useful at every step. Their uncompromising quality standards have made this book an exceptional effort. Their encouragement from time to time has been an inspiration for everyone.

The publisher and the editorial board hope that this book will prove to be a valuable piece of knowledge for researchers, students, practitioners and scholars across the globe.

List of Contributors

Martin Guillot, Pascale Rialland, Mary P. Klinck and Eric Troncy
Groupe de Recherche en Pharmacologie Animale du Québec (GREPAQ), Department of Biomedical Sciences, Faculty of Veterinary Medicine - Universite´ de Montréal, Saint-Hyacinthe, Quebec, Canada

Johanne Martel-Pelletier and Jean-Pierre Pelletier
Osteoarthritis Research Unit, Université de Montréal Hospital Centre, Notre-Dame Hospital, Montreal, Quebec, Canada

Polly M. Taylor
Topcat Metrology, Gravel Head Farm, Downham Common, Little Downham, Nr Ely, Cambridgeshire, United Kingdom

Christelle Nguyen
INSERM, UMR-S 606, Hospital Lariboisière, Paris, France

Hang-Korng Ea and Frédéric Lioté
INSERM, UMR-S 606, Hospital Lariboisière, Paris, France
University Paris Diderot (UFR de Me´decine), Sorbonne Paris Cité, Paris, France

Véronique Chobaz, Sonia Nasi, Annette Ives, Daniel Van Linthoudt, Alexander So and Nathalie Busso
Department of Musculoskeletal Medicine, Service of Rheumatology, CHUV and University of Lausanne, Lausanne, Switzerland

Peter van Lent
Department of Rheumatology, Rheumatology Research and Advanced Therapeutics, Radboud University Nijmegen Medical Centre, Nijmegen, The Netherlands

Michel Daudon
Service des Explorations Fonctionnelles, Hô pital Tenon, AP-HP, Paris, France

Arnaud Dessombz and Dominique Bazin
Laboratoire de Physique des Solides, Université Paris Sud, Orsay, France

Geraldine McCarthy
Mater Misericordiae University Hospital, Dublin, Ireland

Brigitte Jolles-Haeberli
Service de chirurgie orthope´dique et traumatologique de l'appareil moteur, Department of Musculoskeletal Medicine, CHUV and University of Lausanne, Lausanne, Switzerland

Yiru Elizabeth Wu and David A. Hart
Department of Surgery, University of Calgary, Calgary, Alberta, Canada

Roman J. Krawetz
Department of Surgery, University of Calgary, Calgary, Alberta, Canada
Department of Cell Biology and Anatomy, University of Calgary, Calgary, Alberta, Canada

Jerome B. Rattner
Department of Cell Biology and Anatomy, University of Calgary, Calgary, Alberta, Canada

Liam Martin
Department of Medicine, University of Calgary, Calgary, Alberta, Canada

John R. Matyas
Department of Comparative Biology and Experimental Medicine, Faculty of Veterinary Medicine, University of Calgary, Calgary, Alberta, Canada

Javier Conde, Morena Scotece, Verónica López, Juan Jesús Gómez-Reino and Oreste Gualillo
NEIRID Lab (NeuroEndocrine Interaction in Rheumatology and Inflammatory Diseases), SERGAS, Santiago University Clinical Hospital, Institute of Medical Research (IDIS), Santiago de Compostela, Spain

Rodolfo Gómez
Division of Rheumatology, Fundación Jiménez Diaz, Madrid, Spain

Francisca Lago
Research Laboratory 7 (Molecular and Cellular Cardiology), SERGAS Santiago University Clinical Hospital, Institute of Medical Research (IDIS), Santiago de Compostela, Spain

Jesús Pino
Division of Orthopaedics Surgery and Traumatology, SERGAS, Santiago University Clinical Hospital, Santiago de Compostela, Spain

Mathilde Benhamou
Service de Rééducation et Réadaptation de l'Appareil Locomoteur et des Pathologies du Rachis, Assistance Publique-Hôpitaux de Paris; Université Paris Descartes; INSERM IFR 25 Handicap, Paris, France

François Rannou and Serge Poiraudeau
Service de Rééducation et Réadaptation de l'Appareil Locomoteur et des Pathologies du Rachis, Assistance Publique-Hôpitaux de Paris; Université Paris Descartes; INSERM IFR 25 Handicap, Paris, France
Section Arthrose de la Société Française de Rhumatologie, Paris, France

Gabriel Baron, Marie Dalichampt, Isabelle Boutron and Philippe Ravaud
Centre d'Epidémiologie Clinique, Assistance Publique-Hôpitaux de Paris; Universite´ Paris Descartes, Paris, France

Sophie Alami
Department of Sociology, Université Paris Descartes, Interlis, Paris, France

Erfan Aref-Eshghi, Yuhua Zhang, Andrew Furey, Glynn Martin, Guang Sun and Proton Rahman
Faculty of Medicine, Memorial University of Newfoundland, St. John's, Newfoundland, Canada

Guangju Zhai
Faculty of Medicine, Memorial University of Newfoundland, St. John's, Newfoundland, Canada
Department of Twin Research and Genetic Epidemiology, King's College London, London, United Kingdom

Deborah Hart, Ana M. Valdes and Tim D. Spector
Department of Twin Research and Genetic Epidemiology, King's College London, London, United Kingdom

Nigel Arden
Musculoskeletal Epidemiology and Biobank, University of Oxford, Oxford, United Kingdom

J. Christiaan Keurentjes, Thea P. M. Vliet Vlieland and Rob G. Nelissen
Department of Orthopaedic Surgery, Leiden University Medical Center, Leiden, The Netherlands

Marta Fiocco
Department of Medical Statistics and BioInformatics, Leiden University Medical Center, Leiden, The Netherlands

Cynthia So-Osman
Department of Research and Development, Sanquin Blood Supply South West Region, Leiden, The Netherlands

Ron Onstenk
Department of Orthopaedic Surgery, Groene Hart Hospital, Gouda, The Netherlands

Ankie W. M. M. Koopman- Van Gemert
Department of Anaesthesiology, Albert Schweitzer Hospital, Dordrecht, The Netherlands

Ruud G. Pöll
Department of Orthopaedic Surgery, Slotervaart Hospital, Amsterdam, The Netherlands

Herman M. Kroon
Department of Radiology, Leiden University Medical Center, Leiden, The Netherlands

Kai Jiao, Jing Zhang, Mian Zhang, Zhong Ying Qiu, Jianjun He and Mei-Qing Wang
Department of Oral Anatomy and Physiology and TMD, School of Stomatology, Fourth Military Medical University, Xi'an, China

Yuying Wei, Yunxin Cao, Jintao Hu and Kun Yang
Department of Immunology, Fourth Military Medical University, Xi'an, China

Yaoping Wu and Han Zhu
Department of Orthopedics, Xijing Hospital, Fourth Military Medical University, Xi'an, China

Li-Na Niu
Department of of Prosthodontics, School of Stomatology, Fourth Military Medical University, Xi'an, China

Xu Cao
Department of Orthopaedic Surgery, The Johns Hopkins University, School of Medicine, Baltimore, Maryland, United States of America

Jun-Hong Yan, Jian Sun, Wen-Xiao Zhang and Bao-Wei Li
Department of Clinical Medical Technology, Affiliated Hospital of Binzhou Medical College, Binzhou, PR China

Wan-Jie Gu
Department of Anaesthesiology, The First Affiliated Hospital, Guangxi Medical University, Nanning, Guangxi, PR China

Lei Pan
Department of Internal Medicine, The First Affiliated Hospital, Guangzhou Medical College, Guangzhou, PR China

Xue-Dong Wang, Xiao-Xing Kou, Dan-Qing He, Min-Min Zeng, Yan Liu, Jie-Ni Zhang and Yan-Heng Zhou
Department of Orthodontics, Peking University School and Hospital of Stomatology, Beijing, China

Zhen Meng, Rui-Yun Bi and Ye-Hua Gan
Center for Temporomandibular Disorders and Orofacial Pain, Peking University School and Hospital of Stomatology, Beijing, China

Feliks Kogan, Hari Hariharan and Ravinder Reddy
CMROI, Department of Radiology, University of Pennsylvania, Philadelphia, Pennsylvania, United States of America

Anup Singh
CMROI, Department of Radiology, University of Pennsylvania, Philadelphia, Pennsylvania, United States of America
Center for Biomedical Engineering, Indian Institute of Technology Delhi, Delhi, India

Mohammad Haris
CMROI, Department of Radiology, University of Pennsylvania, Philadelphia, Pennsylvania, United States of America
Research Branch, Sidra Medical and Research Center, Doha, Qatar

Kejia Cai
CMROI, Department of Radiology, University of Pennsylvania, Philadelphia, Pennsylvania, United States of America
Radiology, University of Illinois at Chicago, Chicago, Illinois, United States of America

Erika Terzuoli, Antonio Giachetti, Marina Ziche and Sandra Donnini
Department of Life Sciences, University of Siena, Siena, Italy

Stefania Meini, Paola Cucchi, Claudio Catalani, Cecilia Cialdai and Carlo Alberto Maggi
Pharmacology Department, Menarini Ricerche S.p.A, Florence, Italy

Ming-Chih Chou
Institute of Medicine, Chung Shan Medical University, Taichung, Taiwan

Yu-Min Lin
Institute of Medicine, Chung Shan Medical University, Taichung, Taiwan
Department of Orthopedic Surgery, Taichung Veterans General Hospital, Taichung, Taiwan

Chin-Jung Hsu
School of Chinese Medicine, China Medical University, Taichung, Taiwan
Department of Orthopaedics, China Medical University Hospital, Taichung, Taiwan

Yuan-Ya Liao
Department of Surgery, Chung Shan Medical University Hospital, Taichung, Taiwan

Chih-Hsin Tang
Department of Pharmacology, School of Medicine, China Medical University, Taichung, Taiwan
Graduate Institute of Basic Medical Science, China Medical University, Taichung, Taiwan

Shamsul B. Sulaiman and Ng Min-Hwei
Tissue Engineering Centre, Universiti Kebangsaan Malaysia Medical Centre, Cheras, Selangor, Malaysia

Aminuddin B. Saim
Tissue Engineering Centre, Universiti Kebangsaan Malaysia Medical Centre, Cheras, Selangor, Malaysia
ENT Consultant Clinic, Ampang Putri Specialist Hospital, Ampang, Selangor, Malaysia

Chinedu C. Ude and Ruszymah B. H. Idrus
Tissue Engineering Centre, Universiti Kebangsaan Malaysia Medical Centre, Cheras, Selangor, Malaysia
Department of Physiology, Faculty of Medicine, Universiti Kebangsaan Malaysia, Kuala Lumpur, Selangor, Malaysia

Chen Hui-Cheng
Department of Clinical Veterinary, Faculty of Veterinary Medicine Universiti Putra Malaysia, Serdang, Selangor, Malaysia

Johan Ahmad and Norhamdan M. Yahaya
Department of Orthopedic and Traumatology, Universiti Kebangsaan Malaysia Medical Center, Cheras, Selangor, Malaysia

Richard F. Loeser
Department of Internal Medicine, Section of Molecular Medicine, Wake Forest University School of Medicine, Winston-Salem, North Carolina, United States of America

Amy L. Olex
Department of Computer Science, Wake Forest University, Winston-Salem, North Carolina, United States of America

Jacquelyn S. Fetrow
Department of Computer Science, Wake Forest University, Winston-Salem, North Carolina, United States of America
Department of Physics, Wake Forest University, Winston-Salem, North Carolina, United States of America

Margaret A. McNulty and Cathy S. Carlson
Department of Veterinary Population Medicine, College of Veterinary Medicine, University of Minnesota, St. Paul, Minneapolis, United States of America

Michael Callahan and Cristin Ferguson
Department of Orthopedic Surgery, Wake Forest University School of Medicine, Winston-Salem, North Carolina, United States of America

Dong-Dong Wu and Yan Li
State Key Laboratory of Genetic Resources and Evolution, Kunming Institute of Zoology, Chinese Academy of Sciences, Kunming, China

Ya-Ping Zhang
State Key Laboratory of Genetic Resources and Evolution, Kunming Institute of Zoology, Chinese Academy of Sciences, Kunming, China
Laboratory for Conservation and Utilization of Bio-resource, Yunnan University, Kunming, China

Gui-Mei Li and Wei Jin
Laboratory for Conservation and Utilization of Bio-resource, Yunnan University, Kunming, China

Zhan-Chun Li, Jian-Wei Chen, Tao Ma, Guang-Qi Cheng, Yu-Qi Dong, Wei-li Wang and Zu-De Liu
Department of Orthopaedic Surgery, Ren Ji Hospital, School of Medicine, Shanghai Jiao Tong University, Shanghai, P. R. China

Jie Xiao
Department of Anesthesiology, Ren Ji Hospital, School of Medicine, Shanghai Jiao Tong University, Shanghai, P. R. China

Jin-Liang Peng
School of Biomedical Engineering/MED-X Research Institute, Shanghai Jiao Tong University, Shanghai, P. R. China

MinHee Lee, Kyung-Won Kang, Jung Eun Kim, Joo-Hee Kim, Seunghoon Lee, Mi-Suk Shin, So-Young Jung, Ae-Ran Kim, Hyo-Ju Park, Hee- Jung Jung and Sun-Mi Choi
Korea Institute of Oriental Medicine, Dae-Jeon, South Korea

Tae-Hun Kim
Korea Institute of Oriental Medicine, Dae-Jeon, South Korea
College of Korean medicine, Gachon University, Seongnam, South Korea

Kun Hyung Kim
Korea Institute of Oriental Medicine, Dae-Jeon, South Korea
Department of Acupuncture and Moxibustion, Korean medicine hospital, Pusan National University, Yangsan, South Korea

Jung Won Kang
Department of Acupuncture and Moxibustion, College of Korean Medicine, Kyung-Hee University, Seoul, South Korea

Ho Sueb Song
Kyungwon University Incheon Gill Oriental Medical Hospital, Incheon, South Korea

Hyeong Jun Kim
Semyung University Jecheon Oriental Medical Hospital, Jecheon, South Korea

Jin-Bong Choi
Dongshin University Gwangju Oriental Hospital, Gwangju, South Korea

Kwon Eui Hong
Department of Acupuncture and Moxibustion, Daejeon University, Daejeon, South Korea

Kohei Nishitani, Masahiko Kobayashi, Takaaki Shirai, Tsuyoshi Satake, Shinnichiro Nakamura, Ryuzo Arai and Shuichi Matsuda
Department of Orthopaedic Surgery, Graduate School of Medicine, Kyoto University, Kyoto, Japan

Yasuaki Nakagawa and Takashi Nakamura
Department of Orthopaedic Surgery, Graduate School of Medicine, Kyoto University, Kyoto, Japan
Department of Orthopaedic surgery, National Hospital Organization Kyoto Medical Center, Kyoto, Japan

Hiroshi Kuroki
Department of Physical Therapy, Human Health Sciences, Graduate School of Medicine, Kyoto University, Kyoto, Japan

Koji Mori
Department of Applied Medical Engineering Science, Graduate School of Medicine, Yamaguchi University, Ube, Japan

Marta Krystyna Kosinska, Heiko Klein, Markus Rickert and Juergen Steinmeyer
Department of Orthopedics, Justus-Liebig-University Giessen, Giessen, Germany

Gerhard Liebisch and Gerd Schmitz
Department of Clinical Chemistry and Laboratory Medicine, University Hospital Regensburg, Regensburg, Germany

Guenter Lochnit
Department of Biochemistry, Justus-Liebig-University Giessen, Giessen, Germany

Jochen Wilhelm
Medical Clinic II/IV, Justus-Liebig-University Giessen, Giessen, Germany

Ulrich Kaesser
Internistisches Praxiszentrum am Krankenhaus Balserische Stiftung, Giessen, Germany

Gabriele Lasczkowski
Institute of Forensic Medicine, Justus-Liebig- University Giessen, Giessen, Germany

Hugh MacPherson
Department of Health Sciences, University of York, York, United Kingdom

Emily Vertosick and Andrew J. Vickers
Memorial Sloan-Kettering Cancer Center, New York, New York, United States of America

George Lewith
Faculty of Medicine, Primary Care and Population Sciences, University of Southampton, Southampton, United Kingdom

Klaus Linde
Institute of General Practice, Technische Universität München, Munich, Germany

Karen J. Sherman
Group Health Research Institute, Seattle, Washington, United States of America

Claudia M. Witt
Center for Complementary and Integrative Medicine, University Hospital Zurich, Zurich, Switzerland
Institute for Social Medicine, Epidemiology and Health Economics, Charite´ - Universitätsmedizin, Berlin, Germany

Kristin M. Salottolo
Trauma Research Department, Swedish Medical Center, Englewood, Colorado, United States of America
Trauma Research Department, St Anthony Hospital, Lakewood, Colorado, United States of America
Ampio Pharmaceuticals, Inc., Greenwood Village, Colorado, United States of America

David Bar-Or
Trauma Research Department, Swedish Medical Center, Englewood, Colorado, United States of America
Trauma Research Department, St Anthony Hospital, Lakewood, Colorado, United States of America
Ampio Pharmaceuticals, Inc., Greenwood Village, Colorado, United States of America
Rocky Vista University, Aurora Colorado, United States of America

Holli Loose and Vaughan Clift
Ampio Pharmaceuticals, Inc., Greenwood Village, Colorado, United States of America

Matthew J. Phillips and Brian McGrath
University Orthopaedic Center, Amherst, New York, United States of America

Nathan Wei
Arthritis Treatment Center, Frederick Maryland, United States of America

James L. Borders
Central Kentucky Research Associates, Lexington, Kentucky, United States of America

John E. Ervin
Center for Pharmaceutical Research, Kansas City, Missouri, United States of America

Alan Kivitz
Altoona Center for Clinical Research, Duncansville, Pennsylvania, United States of America

Mark Hermann
Danville Orthopeadic Clinic, Danville Virginia, United States of America

Tammi Shlotzhauer
Rochester Medical Research, Rochester, New York, United States of America

Melvin Churchill
Physician Research Collaboration, Lincoln Nebraska, United States of America

Donald Slappey
Alabama Clinical Therapeutics, LLC, Birmingham, Alabama, United States of America

Gerit Hackmayer
Experimental Orthopedics, University Hospital of Regensburg, Regensburg, Bavaria, Germany
Dermatology, University Hospital of Münster, Münster, North Rhine-Westphalia, Germany

Julia Lorenz and Susanne Grässel
Experimental Orthopedics, University Hospital of Regensburg, Regensburg, Bavaria, Germany
Orthopedic Surgery, University Hospital of Regensburg, Bad Abbach, Bavaria, Germany

Elisabeth Seebach and Carina Greth
Research Centre for Experimental Orthopedics, Orthopedic University Hospital Heidelberg, Heidelberg, Baden-Württemberg, Germany

Richard J. Bauer
Oral and Maxillofacial Surgery, University Hospital of Regensburg, Regensburg, Bavaria, Germany

Kerstin Kleinschmidt
TIP Immunology, Merck Serono Global Research and Development, Darmstadt, Hessen, Germany

Dominik Bettenworth
Medical Hospital B, University Hospital of Münster, Münster, North Rhine- Westphalia, Germany

Markus Böhm
Dermatology, University Hospital of Mu¨ nster, Münster, North Rhine-Westphalia, Germany

Joachim Grifka
Orthopedic Surgery, University Hospital of Regensburg, Bad Abbach, Bavaria, Germany

Hsien-Te Chen
School of Chinese Medicine, College of Chinese Medicine, China Medical University, Taichung, Taiwan
Department of Orthopaedic Surgery, China Medical University Hospital, Taichung, Taiwan

Yen-Jen Chen
Department of Orthopaedic Surgery, China Medical University Hospital, Taichung, Taiwan
School of Medicine, China Medical University, Taichung, Taiwan

Hsi-Kai Tsou
Department of Neurosurgery, Taichung Veterans General Hospital, Taichung, Taiwan
Department of Early Childhood Care and Education, Jen-Teh Junior College of Medicine, Nursing and Management, Miaoli County, Taiwan

James Meng-Kun Shih
Department of Orthopaedic Surgery, Lin Sen Hospital, Taichung, Taiwan

Chih-Hsin Tang
School of Medicine, China Medical University, Taichung, Taiwan
Graduate Institute of Basic Medical Science, China Medical University, Taichung, Taiwan
Department of Biotechnology, College of Health Science, Asia University, Taichung, Taiwan

Jui-Chieh Chen
Graduate Institute of Basic Medical Science, China Medical University, Taichung, Taiwan
National Institute of Cancer Research, National Health Research Institutes, Miaoli County, Zhunan, Taiwa

Jing Li and Xianfei Xie
Department of pharmacology, Basic Medical School of Wuhan University, Wuhan, China

Hui Wang
Department of pharmacology, Basic Medical School of Wuhan University, Wuhan, China
Hubei Provincial Key Laboratory of Developmentally Originated Disease, Wuhan, China

Qibing Mei
Department of Pharmacology, School of Pharmacy, The Fourth Military Medical University, Xi'an, China

Jacques Magdalou
UMR 7365 CNRS-Universite´ de Lorraine, Faculte´ de Me´decine, Vandoeuvre-le`s-Nancy, France

Philippe Ravaud
U1153, Institut National de la Santé et de la Recherche Médicale, Paris, France
Centre d'E´pide´miologie Clinique, Hôpital Hôtel Dieu AP-HP, Paris, France
Universite´Paris Descartes, PRES Sorbonne Paris Cité, Paris, France

Clémence Palazzo
U1153, Institut National de la Santé et de la Recherche Médicale, Paris, France
Centre d'E´pide´miologie Clinique, Hôpital Hôtel Dieu AP-HP, Paris, France
Universite´Paris Descartes, PRES Sorbonne Paris Cité, Paris, France
Service de rée´ducation et réadaptation de l'appareil locomoteur et des pathologies du rachis, Hôpital Cochin AP-HP, Paris, France

Serge Poiraudeau
U1153, Institut National de la Santé et de la Recherche Médicale, Paris, France
Universite´Paris Descartes, PRES Sorbonne Paris Cité, Paris, France
Service de rée´ducation et réadaptation de l'appareil locomoteur et des pathologies du rachis, Hôpital Cochin AP-HP, Paris, France
Institut fédé ratif de recherche sur le handicap, Institut National de la Sante´ et de la Recherche Me´ dicale, Paris, France

Agathe Papelard
Service de rée´ducation et réadaptation de l'appareil locomoteur et des pathologies du rachis, Hôpital Cochin AP-HP, Paris, France
Institut fédé ratif de recherche sur le handicap, Institut National de la Sante´ et de la Recherche Me´ dicale, Paris, France

Jean-François Ravaud
Institut fédé ratif de recherche sur le handicap, Institut National de la Sante´ et de la Recherche Me´ dicale, Paris, France
U988, Institut National de la Sante´ et de la Recherche Me´dicale, Villejuif, France
UMR 8211, Centre national de la recherche scientifique, Villejuif, France

Yi-Ming Chen
Faculty of Medicine, National Yang-Ming University, Taipei, Taiwan, R.O.C
Division of Allergy, Immunology and Rheumatology, Taichung Veterans General Hospital, Taichung, Taiwan, R.O.C

Yinxian Wen, Yang Tan, Jun Qin and Linlong Wang
Department of Orthopedic Surgery, Zhongnan Hospital of Wuhan University, Wuhan, China

Liaobin Chen
Department of Orthopedic Surgery, Zhongnan Hospital of Wuhan University, Wuhan, China
Hubei Provincial Key Laboratory of Developmentally Originated Disease, Wuhan, China

Index

P

R

S

T

www.ingramcontent.com/pod-product-compliance
Lightning Source LLC
Chambersburg PA
CBHW080513200326
41458CB00012B/4189
* 9 7 8 1 6 3 2 4 1 7 2 1 3 *